Problem Solving in Clinical Medicine

From Data to Diagnosis

Third Edition

Problem Solving in Clinical Medicine

From Data to Diagnosis

Third Edition

Paul Cutler, MD, FACP
Honorary Clinical Professor of Medicine
The Jefferson Medical College
of The Thomas Jefferson University
Philadelphia, Pennsylvania

Dean Emeritus
St. George's University
School of Medicine
Grenada, West Indies

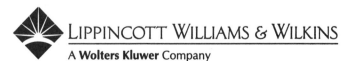

LIPPINCOTT WILLIAMS & WILKINS
A **Wolters Kluwer** Company
Philadelphia • Baltimore • New York • London
Buenos Aires • Hong Kong • Sydney • Tokyo

Editor: Paul Kelly
Managing Editor: Crystal Taylor
Marketing Manager: Rebecca Himmelheber
Development Editor: Susan E. Kimner
Production Coordinator: Felecia R. Weber
Project Editor: Karen M. Ruppert
Designer: Circa 86
Illustration Planner: Wayne Hubbel
Cover Designer: Mario Fernandez
Typesetter: Peirce Graphic Services, Inc.
Digitized Illustrations: Chansky, Inc.

351 West Camden Street
Baltimore, Maryland 21201-2436 USA

Accurate indications, adverse reactions and dosage schedules for drugs are provided in this book, but it is possible that they may change. The reader is urged to review the package information data of the manufacturers of the medications mentioned.

Printed in the United States of America

Second Edition, 1985

Library of Congress Cataloging-in-Publication Data
Cutler, Paul, 1920–
    Problem solving in clinical medicine : from data to diagnosis /
Paul Cutler. — 3rd ed.
        p.   cm.
    Includes bibliographical references and index.
    ISBN 13: 978-0-683-30167-0
    ISBN 10: 0-683-30167-5
    1. Diagnosis—Problems, exercises, etc.   2. Medical logic—
Problems, exercises, etc.   3. Clinical medicine—Problems,
exercises, etc.   I. Title.
    [DNLM: 1. Diagnosis.   2. Clinical medicine—methods.   3. Problem
Solving.   WB 141 C989p 1998]
RC71.3.C88   1998
616.07′5—dc21
DNLM/DLC
for Library of Congress   97-5523
                                                        CIP

The publishers have made every effort to trace the copyright holders for borrowed material. If they have inadvertently overlooked any, they will be pleased to make the necessary arrangements at the first opportunity.

8 9 10

Dedication

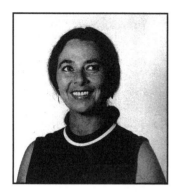

To Helene, who will always be with me.

Preface to the Third Edition

In spite of the recent profusion of high-technology diagnostic procedures and tests, the majority of patient problems can still be solved during the first two minutes of the patient interview.

While guided biopsies, microminiaturized assays, and sophisticated imagery may be the trump cards in selected cases, most diagnoses are still made simply on the basis of the patient's symptoms plus one or two physical findings.

Like an embryo, the diagnosis is conceived, germinates, develops, and is most often delivered during the dynamics of taking the history, and the entire drama of medical problem-solving may unfold without leaving the stage set of two chairs and a desk.

Rookie problem solvers must know not only how to elicit information about the patient's history and physical examination but also how to evaluate this data in light of the underlying pathophysiology.

The idea that experienced clinicians use complex, indefinable tactics to unravel diagnostic mysteries is a myth. The clinical reasoning process can be fragmented into clearly described, recognizable, and duplicable heuristic strategies that include the formation of an initial concept, the generation of single or multiple hypotheses, the further expansion of inquiry tactics, and the application of appropriate clinical skills.

It is with these concepts in mind that the editor plans to teach students how to solve medical problems and how to find out what is wrong with the patient.

The book is divided into two sections. *Section 1* consists of sample cases wherein the reader learns why certain questions are asked and which specific areas must be examined. Attention is given to the respective roles and relative values of the history, the physical examination, and tests and procedures in the construction of an adequate database in each case. This section goes on further to describe and give examples of the numerous problem-solving techniques used by clinicians as they unravel puzzles in an almost subconscious manner.

Additional chapters delve more deeply into the convolutions of the problem solver's mind through the medium of a series of more complex cases that are solved in a think-along-with-me style. The reader learns how the clinician uses Kipling's six honest serving men (What, Why, When, How, Where, and Who) to elicit the details of the chief complaint; to decide which areas to examine; to evaluate this information; and to decide what else needs to be done. All this is described synchronously with the patient-doctor encounter, thereby allowing the reader to enter the diagnostician's mind during the gathering of data.

Section 2 is composed of many carefully selected cases in which chunks of data are interspersed with corresponding chunks of logic, generally in the order in which the information is garnered. These cases are designed to cover the most common clinical presentations seen in medical practice, as well as to present the reader with a respectable and extensive body of medical knowledge. By the iterative process of following the data-logic-data-logic sequence portrayed in each case and by identifying the strategies used, the student can begin to solve problems in much the same way. This format, used in both previous editions, was designed not only to demonstrate the clinician's thought processes and logic but also to encourage the reader to cultivate his or her problem-solving skills by providing his or her own logic after each parcel of data, and then comparing them to those of the clinician-author.

It was never intended that yet another edition of *Problem Solving in Clinical Medicine* would be necessary. But during the past 10 years, while medical education has spawned the concepts of problem-based learning, objective-structured clinical evaluations, standardized patients, and decision analysis, the costs of medical diagnosis and medical care have risen dramatically, at least in some part because of the seemingly indiscriminate use of costly and often unnecessary diagnostic interventions. And therein lies the justification for the third edition of a book that preaches simple, inexpensive, and effective methods for reaching medical solutions.

The third edition has many new authors, and the number of clinical case discussions in Section 2 has been increased from 65 to 86. All cases were newly written and brought up-to-date. The chapters in Section 1 were also rewritten and additional educational tools were introduced to enhance the reader's clinical skills. The abridgement of many chapters has permitted the introduction of more than 150 case-related graphics, as well as additional tables, outlines, and icons, thus providing more attractive spacing, less density, and easier reading, without increasing the size of the book.

The objectives of this edition, as before, are to teach the reader how to:

- elicit and process patient data
- use problem-solving techniques
- establish diagnostic game plans
- deal with common patient presentations
- achieve diagnostic closure with reasonable certainty

The author hereby enters into a covenant with his readers that they will be better informed and better solvers of medical problems if the process and content of the materials contained herein are carefully read and learned.

Paul Cutler, MD, FACP
Philadelphia, Pennsylvania

Preface to the Second Edition

An author usually writes a second edition because 4 years have elapsed since the first, because small changes have occurred which render the book's contents obsolete in a few areas, and because competition with publishers of similar books makes a new edition economically advisable.

Such is not the case here. Except for books written primarily for educators, I know of no comparable text that teaches and exemplifies medical problem solving at the elementary level compatible with student comprehension.

Since 1979, problem solving, problem-based learning, probability theory, and decision analysis have become key concept in educational circles, and they have started to flood the medical literature, to creep slightly into standard textbooks, and even to enter into formalized undergraduate courses in a few schools.

The blind men from beyond Ghor have begun to confer with each other, and a more holistic and accurate concept of both the elephant and the profession of medicine is under construction.

Much ongoing research aims to determine how the mind works, how patient information is processed, and how the clinician solves problems and makes decisions. The transactions of the young Society for Medical Decision Making are testimony to the progress being made in these areas.

Patients and their families, hospital and public policy, and administrators, politicians, attorneys, and clergy—all demand that students practice medicine with ever increasing new concerns in mind. Simply providing the best possible care is not enough. Consideration must be given to accountability, cost containment, health care rationing, and the various legal, moral, and ethical issues that are implicated by these new slants.

And at long last the concrete curricula of ivied and ivory towers are being eroded by the realization that students learn better by teaching themselves than by rote memorization and regurgitation of didactic lectures. Not since the days of Flexner have curricula been under such scrutiny, criticism, reevaluation, and revision. Students must be inspired to think, to read, to learn, to solve, to decide—not to memorize. Demonstrating the intellectual beauty of problem solving should do much to restore the enthusiasm and scholarly attitude of medical students who are being drowned by thousands of facts which they will mostly never use again.

Greater stress is being laid on protocols, flow charts, algorithms, and decision trees. Nevertheless, the fact remains that problem solving begins with and depends primarily on the taking of the history and on the processing of patient data—two skills in which students are notoriously weak.

Any book that attempts to teach students of the 80's to deal with patient problems must include: the concept of imperfect information; the consideration of informed consent and cost of medical care; the intelligent selection of tests and treatment; the availability of new but expensive procedures that may short-cut, although sometimes complicate, the diagnostic process; attempts to make computer programs that simulate natural intelligence; and efforts to construct mathematical models that add precision to intuitive and judgmental decisions.

To accomplish these objectives, the section on the problem-solving process was rewritten, revised, and expanded. Chapters on data processing, data relevance, decision making, the impact of new diagnostic tools, and the ordering and interpretation of tests were added. All case studies and their associated "Suggested Readings" lists were updated. An introductory chapter instructs the student or teacher how, where, and when to best use this book. Numerous exercises and self-evaluation procedures have been interspersed throughout the text; the answers follow.

It is hoped that this book will increasingly serve as a model for teaching students how to think—to learn—then think again.

May I express even greater gratitude than before to my wife and friend, Helene, not only for her encouragement and forbearance (perfunctory functions of most spouses), but for her exceptional typing, proofreading, and editing—and for the remarkable ways in which her Betz cells have filled the void created by those which may have disappeared from my own cortex.

Paul Cutler, M.D.
Philadelphia, Pennsylvania

Preface to the First Edition

Just as King Savatthi's blind men described the elephant—students, teacher, practitioner, and patient each sees medicine in his own way. The student asks, "How much must I learn? What's important, and how do I put it all together to solve the patient's problems?" The teacher answers, "Learn it all! $a+b+c = x$. Proceed in an orderly complete fashion." The practitioner is concerned with shortcuts, speed, experience, and clinical judgment. The patient wants to know, "What's wrong, can you cure me, and how much will it cost?"

And each is right.

And each is wrong.

Having observed medicine for 38 years from all four viewpoints—as student, teacher, practitioner, and patient—not like the blind men, but in a holistic and overlapping manner—I have noted that the effectiveness of many students and physicians is impaired because they have never really learned or acquired certain vital skills and categories of information. These include:

1. Collection and interpretation of data
2. Pathophysiology of disease
3. Processing of data into what is relevant
4. Many presentations of a disease
5. Many diseases causing a presentation
6. Appreciation of what is common and likely
7. Solution of problems.

In addition to being covered in many good books, the first two items are now taught intensively at most medical schools. Physical Diagnosis and Introduction to Clinical Medicine take care of data collection (1); the pathophysiology of disease (2) is taught in an integrated modular fashion or in traditional separate subjects, depending on the curricular structure of each school. Yet few schools, and almost no books, teach the student how to process or synthesize acquired data into diagnoses or problem lists—a skill requiring knowledge of items 3 to 7. This book is concerned mainly with these last five items; principal emphasis, however, is on problem solving, since mastery of its intricacies differentiates the outstanding from the mediocre student or physician.

Sometimes data synthesis and problem solving are half-heartedly included in Physical Diagnosis or Introduction to Clinical Medicine. More often they are left for the third-year medicine clerkship, where it is hoped the student will somehow acquire those skills by himself, from the busy intern or resident, at the foot of the attending physician, by observation or by osmosis—but rarely is time allotted for the formal teaching of this material.

Modern curricula are accelerated. The student usually sees patients in his first year, and on completion of this third year he has seen, felt, heard, and learned more than the previous generation had experienced after 5 to 10 years in practice. Everything is taught earlier. Why not problem solving?

Sometime between the second and fifth years of medical education, the student must learn to think, to solve, to relate, and to manage. Some do. Many do not. A few never do!

To illustrate: I used to know a physician who had quick indiscriminate recall of thousands of facts.

He attended all conferences, read numerous journals, and took assiduous notes. Yet he did not know how to handle facts and could not solve patient problems. He had no judgment, no common sense, and was a failure so far as patient care was concerned. If he saw someone who was sick, he could list 10 possible diseases, but he could not tell what was *most likely* to be wrong. Patients were usually frightened away by his imposing differential diagnoses. Once at 2 AM he saw a 65-year-old woman who had epigastric discomfort and vomiting due to a dietary indiscretion. As possible causes of her illness he listed everything from acute gastritis, perforated ulcer, and cancer of the stomach to coronary thrombosis and dissections aneurysm—all unlikely except for the first. By 8 AM she had placed herself under the çare of another physician who recognized that she needed only a tranquilizer and reassurance. The first physician had never learned problem solving—either in school or 20 years after.

Should the medical student be expected to know disease probabilities, odds, and likelihoods? How does he deal with the absence of a crucial clue or the presence of one that does not fit? Can he learn to categorize symptoms or groups of symptoms which overlap into many diseases? Should he be able to cope with the varied presentations of a single disease? Which clues form a plausible cluster? Can he deal with the specificity and sensitivity of clues in the history, physical examination, and laboratory profile? What about the orderly selection of appropriate diagnostic studies? Are we dealing with one disease or are there several? Indeed, is it possible to teach the student to think in these terms and can we give him guidelines for solving problems?

I believe so.

This book purports to teach the student to reason in a logical, rational manner. After a general discussion of preliminary key issues, it goes on to describe and give examples of more than 25 methods of problem solving called upon daily by the clinician. As a rule these techniques are used almost subconsciously in a manner which the capable physician does not conceptualize and may not even be aware of.

After a second section on data synthesis, 65 common patient presentations in Section Three demonstrate the use of previously discussed techniques. Different methods are used in each case, depending upon the nature of the problem and the approach of each contributing author. Section Four contains specialized aspects of problem solving.

Some of this material is derived from scattered references. Much is the distillate of 30 years' experience in private practice, primitive medicine in central Asia, and academia. I regret not being able to give due credit for the numerous "pearls, nuggets, and aphorisms" incorporated into my own knowledge base from long-forgotten sources, but who can remember where he learned or read all that he knows?

Sincere thanks to my more identifiable sources of assistance: the contributors; the students who taught me what they needed to know; those of the Williams & Wilkins Co. who gave guidance and planning; Leon Cander, M.D., the chairman of medicine who gave me his friendship and the freedom, advice, and support needed to develop new ways to teach students to think and learn; Terry Mikiten, Ph.D., for his early suggestions regarding clarity and content; Lee B. Lusted, M.D., Edmond A. Murphy, M.D., and Alvan R. Feinstein, M.D., whose writings were inspirational; my wife, Helene, for her encouragement, critiques, manuscript typing, proofreading, and editing; and last, my father, Meyer Melechovitch Kotlyarenko, but for whose emigration 75 years ago this book might have been written in Russian or not at all.

Paul Cutler, M.D.
San Antonio, Texas

Acknowledgment

My sincere thanks to Crystal Taylor, Susan Kimner, Felecia R. Weber, and Karen M. Ruppert of Williams and Wilkins, whose labors and support throughout the entire editing process were outstanding.

My very special thanks to Helene Cutler, my wife, for word processing the entire original manuscript and for her exceptional proofreading skills, but mostly for the inspiration, advice, encouragement, love, and caring throughout the 50 years of our lives together.

P.C.

Contributors

Juan Albino, MD
Assistant Professor of Medicine
University of Medicine and Dentistry
  of New Jersey
Newark, New Jersey

Frank Beardell, MD
Instructor in Medicine
Jefferson Medical College
Philadelphia, Pennsylvania

H. Leonard Bentch, MD
Clinical Professor of Medicine
University of Texas
Health Sciences Center at San Antonio
San Antonio, Texas

Richard P. Borge, Jr, MD
Fellow in Cardiology
Jefferson Medical College
Philadelphia, Pennsylvania

Timothy N. Caris, MD
Clinical Professor of Medicine
University of Texas
Health Sciences Center at San Antonio
San Antonio, Texas

Chul Joon Choi, MD
Fellow in Cardiology
Jefferson Medical College
Philadelphia, Pennsylvania

Edward K. Chung, MD
Professor of Medicine
Jefferson Medical College
Philadelphia, Pennsylvania

Michael H. Crawford, MD
Professor of Medicine
University of New Mexico
School of Medicine
Albuquerque, New Mexico

Paul Cutler, MD
Honorary Clinical Professor of Medicine
Jefferson Medical College
Philadelphia, Pennsylvania

Lisa L. Dever, MD
Assistant Professor of Medicine
University of Medicine and Dentistry
  of New Jersey
Newark, New Jersey

Herschel L. Douglas, MD
Professor of Family Medicine
University of Florida
College of Medicine
Health Science Center at Jacksonville
Jacksonville, Florida

Sherry S. Durica, MD
Assistant Professor of Medicine
University of Oklahoma
School of Medicine
Oklahoma City, Oklahoma

Kenneth R. Epstein, MD
Clinical Assistant Professor of Medicine
Jefferson Medical College
Philadelphia, Pennsylvania

Allan J. Erslev, MD
Distinguished Professor of Medicine
Jefferson Medical College
Philadelphia, Pennsylvania

Marvin Forland, MD
Professor of Medicine
University of Texas
Health Sciences Center at San Antonio
San Antonio, Texas

James N. George, MD
Professor of Medicine
University of Oklahoma
School of Medicine
Oklahoma City, Oklahoma

Barry Goldstein, MD
Associate Professor of Medicine
Jefferson Medical College
Philadelphia, Pennsylvania

Glenn W.W. Gross, MD
Assistant Professor of Medicine
University of Texas
Health Sciences Center at San Antonio
San Antonio, Texas

Gary D. Harris, MD
Professor of Medicine
University of Texas
Health Sciences Center at San Antonio
San Antonio, Texas

James D. Heckman, MD
Professor of Orthopaedics
University of Texas
Health Sciences Center at San Antonio
San Antonio, Texas

Waldemar G. Johanson, Jr, MD
Professor of Medicine
University of Medicine and Dentistry
   of New Jersey
Newark, New Jersey

Karen Kelley, MD
Clinical Assistant Professor of Medicine
Jefferson Medical College
Philadelphia, Pennsylvania

Barbara A. Konkle, MD
Associate Professor of Medicine
Jefferson Medical College
Philadelphia, Pennsylvania

David J. Kudzma, MD
Assistant Professor of Medicine
University of Miami
School of Medicine
Miami, Florida

M. James Lenhard, MD
Clinical Assistant Professor of Medicine
Jefferson Medical College
Philadelphia, Pennsylvania

Shirley Parker Levine, MD
Professor of Medicine
Albert Einstein College of Medicine
New York, New York

Meyer D. Lifschitz, MD
Professor of Medicine
University of Texas
Health Sciences Center at San Antonio
San Antonio, Texas

Roger M. Lyons, MD
Associate Professor of Medicine
University of Texas
Health Sciences Center at San Antonio
San Antonio, Texas

Arthur S. McFee, MD, PhD
Professor of Surgery
University of Texas
Health Sciences Center at San Antonio
San Antonio, Texas

Carlos A. Moreno, MD
Professor of Family Practice
University of Texas
Health Sciences Center at Houston
Houston, Texas

Carlos Pestana, MD, PhD
Professor of Surgery
University of Texas
Health Sciences Center at San Antonio
San Antonio, Texas

Suzanne Rose, MD
Assistant Professor of Medicine
University of Pittsburgh Medical School
Pittsburgh, Pennsylvania

Raymond A. Rubin, MD
Atlanta Gastroenterology Associates
Atlanta, Georgia

David A. Sears, MD
Professor of Medicine
Baylor College of Medicine
Houston, Texas

Jamie A. Selingo, MD
Fellow in Medicine
Jefferson Medical College
Philadelphia, Pennsylvania

Sandor S. Shapiro, MD
Professor of Medicine
Jefferson Medical College
Philadelphia, Pennsylvania

Ernest Urban, MBBS
Professor of Medicine
University of Pittsburgh
School of Medicine
Pittsburgh, Pennsylvania

Elliot Weser, MD
Professor of Medicine
University of Texas
Health Sciences Center at San Antonio
San Antonio, Texas

Michael A. Wirth, MD
Assistant Professor of Orthopaedics
University of Texas
Health Sciences Center at San Antonio
San Antonio, Texas

Hiroshi Yamasaki, MD
Fellow in Cardiology
Jefferson Medical College
Philadelphia, Pennsylvania

Contents

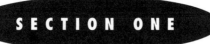

SECTION ONE

The Problem-Solving Process

Dissection of a Symptom

Paul Cutler

A BREATHLESS DAY IN THE EMERGENCY DEPARTMENT

During a recent 24-hour period of time, six patients came to the University Hospital emergency department complaining of shortness of breath. Each case was different.

To find out what was wrong, the house officer asked about the precise nature of the complaint, how it began, how it progressed, the accompanying symptoms, the patient's identifying data, and the past medical history.

Only 2 minutes into each patient encounter, and on the basis of limited information, the house officer was able to decide what was the most likely diagnosis out of a group of contending hypotheses. She then proceeded to gather additional information that would uphold or reject her initial impression, rule out contenders, and rerank the order of likelihoods. This was done by asking carefully selected questions and performing a subset of the physical examination that focused on areas of concern. Once reasonably certain of what was wrong, she ordered tests to sustain her primary impression and rule out others.

Because of the urgency of the situation in some cases, treatment was begun before the diagnosis was confirmed, but in most cases appropriate treatment followed the establishment of a diagnosis.

CASE 1

Patient 1 arrived at the emergency department at 12:10 AM. He was a 65-year-old man who could not get to sleep because he "could not breathe right" when he laid down. Recently he had noted some mild shortness of breath on walking up a flight of stairs and on walking to the mailbox, activities that had never before given him problems. There were no other symptoms. Three years earlier, he had suffered a heart attack for which he was hospitalized for 10 days and made a "complete recovery."

Physical examination revealed normal color, normal vital signs, neck veins distended at a 45-degree reclining position, a few fine rales at each lung base, an apex beat that was 11 cm tangentially from the midsternal line and in the sixth left intercostal space, and an audible fourth heart sound at the apex.

The chest radiograph showed moderately severe cardiac enlargement and clear lungs (Fig. 1.1). The electrocardiogram (ECG) showed an old anterior wall myocardial infarction (Fig. 1.2).

The intern concluded that the patient had mild left and beginning right ventricular failure

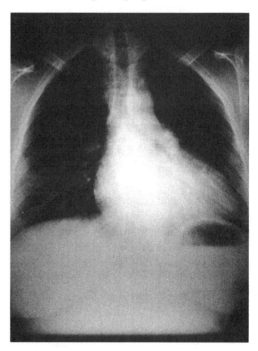

▶ **Figure 1.1.** Enlarged heart and clear lungs.

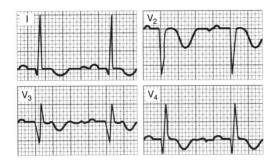

► **Figure 1.2.** Old anterior wall myocardial infarction. Q waves and inverted T waves in leads I, V_2, V_3, V_4. ST segments are isoelectric.

as a result of coronary artery disease and an old myocardial infarction. She prescribed a low-salt diet, a mild diuretic, the use of two or more pillows, and referred the patient to the medicine outpatient clinic for further care.

CASE 2

Approximately 2 hours later, at 2:37 AM, a young mother rushed into the emergency department. She carried a 2-year-old child who was in obvious respiratory distress. The child was breathing rapidly; cyanotic; and emitted a high-pitched, crowing noise each time he breathed. The mother said that her child had had a cough and fever for the past 2 or 3 days and had not been playing with any of his toys.

Examination showed blue nails and lips; respirations, 32 per minute; temperature 100°F; and retraction of the supraclavicular and intercostal spaces and a stridulous sound on inspiration. The chest was difficult to examine because of noisy breathing.

Chest radiographic findings were normal. There were 12000 white blood cells (WBC) per mm³ with 75% polymorphonuclear neutrophils.

The intern opted for the diagnosis of acute infectious laryngotracheobronchitis, but was somewhat concerned about possible aspiration of a non-radiopaque foreign body. Having read a recent journal article about acute epiglottitis, she was even more concerned. She admitted the patient to the pediatric intensive care unit and suggested antibiotics, a humidifier, and a tracheostomy set at the bedside.

A 72-year-old man arrived with his wife at the emergency department at 7:00 AM. Shortly after awakening, he had suddenly become extremely dyspneic. There were no other symptoms. Carcinoma of the prostate had been diagnosed 1 year previously, and he had been taking "some kind of female hormones" for the past few months. Otherwise his past health had been good.

Examination revealed respirations, 26 per minute; pulse, 138 beats per minute; blood pressure (BP), 80/60; dyspnea; cyanosis; a loud and palpable pulmonic second sound; and clear lungs. The apex beat was in the normal position and was barely perceptible. The legs were not swollen; the calves were not tender; and Homans' sign was not present.

The intern recognized the seriousness of the situation and requested help from the resident. She considered acute myocardial infarction and pulmonary embolus equally probable, although the resident leaned more toward pulmonary embolus because of estrogen intake, the history of cancer, and clinical evidence of pulmonary hypertension.

Sedation was given; oxygen was administered; and thrombolysis was begun.

The ECG showed right bundle branch block, sinus tachycardia, and occasional atrial premature contractions (Fig. 1.3). Chest radiographic findings were normal. A ventilation-perfusion scan showed an extensive perfusion defect in the upper half of the right lung, as well as a small defect on the left, which confirmed the diagnosis of pulmonary emboli (Fig. 1.4).

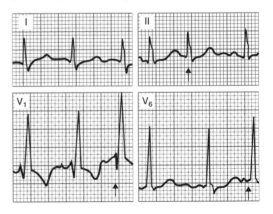

► **Figure 1.3.** Pulmonary embolus. Sinus tachycardia, right bundle branch block, premature atrial contractions (*arrows*).

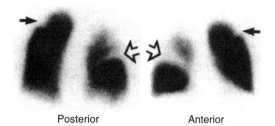

Posterior   Anterior

▶ **Figure 1.4.** Pulmonary embolus. Technetium perfusion scan shows large defect on the right (*open arrow*) and segment defect on the left (*closed arrow*). The xenon ventilation scan showed normal findings.

C A S E   4

While the intern was waiting for the results of the scan for the patient in Case 3, a 38-year-old woman walked into the emergency department. She was visibly short of breath. She reported that she had had similar episodes of dyspnea associated with wheezing for the past 15 years. Usually the episodes were relieved by a few whiffs from an inhaler, but this time the shortness of breath started quite suddenly, and it had never been this bad before. In addition, she reported having had a cough and fever with pains in the arms and legs for the past few days.

Examination revealed a temperature of 101° F; pulse, 120 beats per minute; respirations, 28 per minute; BP, 106/86; dyspnea; cyanosis; a few faint expiratory wheezes on the left side; absent breath sounds, absent fremitus and tympany on the right; and the trachea shifted slightly to the left. These findings were not confirmed by the resident.

The intern and resident discussed the diagnostic possibilities before ordering tests to strengthen their impressions. The patient had bronchial asthma that was clearly episodic, but how did this incident differ? Although the possibilities included pneumonia, the sudden onset of dyspnea and the intern's physical findings suggested acute pneumothorax resulting from hyperinflated lung tissue or a ruptured bleb. The severe distress and tracheal shift, if confirmed, implied a tension pneumothorax. The absence of chest pain was disturbing.

The chest radiograph showed that the right chest was filled with air, the lung was collapsed around the hilum, and the trachea and mediastinum were indeed shifted to the left. WBCs were 8,500/mm³.

The patient had an acute respiratory infection, chronic recurrent bronchial asthma, and an acute tension pneumothorax. A needle was inserted under the right second rib anteriorly; there was marked relief of symptoms as air was collected into a water bottle, and an antibiotic was administered. The patient was then admitted to the hospital.

C A S E   5

A 56-year-old woman was seen at 1:00 PM. She had been sitting in the waiting room for an hour and was visibly disturbed. She complained of not having been able to catch her breath off and on all morning. She did not notice it while cleaning up after breakfast, but it again began to disturb her while watching a morning TV show. She had had a heart murmur since childhood, and she had adult-onset diabetes mellitus for which she adhered to a diet and took an oral hypoglycemic drug.

Physical examination revealed normal vital signs, and chest findings that were normal except for a grade 2/6 systolic aortic ejection murmur that did not radiate. During the examination she was noted to take occasional deep breaths and to yawn.

The intern concluded that the patient had the hyperventilation syndrome, and that the heart murmur and diabetes were unrelated to the chief complaint. She asked a few more questions about numbness and tingling in the fingers and around the mouth. These signs were absent. She asked whether physical exertion seemed to worsen the dyspnea, and the patient replied that it did not. She tapped the facial nerve in front of the tragus; the face and mouth did not twitch. There was no evidence of alkalosis. In the course of further conversation, the patient reported that an older sister also had a heart murmur and died suddenly at the age of 60.

The patient went home with a prescription for sedatives and reassurance that there was no serious organic problem, and was advised to try as much as possible to divert her thoughts from the conscious act of breathing.

C A S E   6

Next, the intern was introduced to a 64-year-old man who was thin, nervous, and smelled from cigarette smoking. He complained that he could no longer walk to the convenience store without getting very short of breath. In fact, more recently, he felt short of breath even while at rest. He came to the emergency department because he had just coughed up some blood-tinged sputum and feared he might have cancer.

Additional questions revealed chronic cough and expectoration for 15 years, a 100-pack-year history, and gradually worsening shortness of breath for the past 2 years. The sputum had always been greenish gray. He claimed to have had a heart attack 5 years previously, at which time he had been told to stop smoking.

Physical examination showed normal vital signs, minimal clubbing of tobacco-stained fingers, fine and medium moist crackles and faint expiratory wheezes at both lung bases, and no cardiac abnormalities. The liver was not enlarged, cervical veins were not distended, and no abnormal lymph nodes could be found.

The patient was referred to the general medical clinic for definitive diagnosis and care. The intern signed the chart as follows: chronic obstructive pulmonary disease (COPD), rule out carcinoma of the lung. She knew that COPD acts this way: that after years of obstructive bronchial and bronchiolar disease with destruction of alveoli, dyspnea may occur, first on exertion, but later even at rest. She did not feel that the old myocardial infarction was related because there was no evidence of cardiac enlargement and congestive failure. But she did express concern about carcinoma because of the continuation of cigarette smoking, hemoptysis, and early clubbing.

Comment

In order for the emergency department house officer to find out what was wrong in each case, he or she not only had to elicit meaningful information, but also had to have knowledge and understanding of the basic pathophysiologic processes that might be operative in patients complaining of shortness of breath.

The initial part of the doctor-patient encounter is where the problem solver's wheels begin to turn, where provisional hypotheses are formed, and where the interviewer first starts to organize his or her thoughts and decides what additional information is needed. Indeed, this is the point at which the "star trek" through the universe of pathophysiology begins, and the patient's clinical features are matched to a template of disease patterns.

Because each of the patients in the preceding six cases had dyspnea as a chief complaint, this symptom will be analyzed as to its meaning, its causes, and its underlying mechanisms. Such an analysis should serve as a prototype for the understanding of all other clinical presentations.

THE PATHOPHYSIOLOGY OF DYSPNEA

An Analysis of the Chief Complaint

Never was a symptom so common and so important, yet so poorly understood, as is dyspnea. It is not clearly definable; patients have difficulty describing it; there are many diseases and mechanisms that cause it; and the nerve pathways for its mediation remain complex and obscure.

The common denominator for the definition of dyspnea is "an abnormally uncomfortable awareness of breathing that results from the increased work of breathing." This sensation is to be distinguished from the rapid and deep breathing brought on by exercise in normal individuals.

Patients describe this uncomfortable feeling in a variety of ways. Usually, they refer to being "short of breath." Others say they cannot get enough air, or the air does not go all the way down—perhaps they experience a choking sensation, a smothering feeling, or tightness in the chest.

MECHANISMS OF DYSPNEA There are numerous pathophysiologic mechanisms that may induce dyspnea, acting either singly or in concert. Because the brain and spinal cord are the receiving and sending stations for signals of distress from the cardiopulmonary system, it is to be expected that diseases involving various parts of the nervous system might give rise to dyspnea. Whereas a great deal of work has been done to elicit the precise mechanisms and reflex pathways through which these signals are sent, much is still shrouded in mystery; neural connections are not well-defined, and stimuli coming from many different sources can give rise to a similar symptom.

Where in the central nervous system these stimuli are collected and how they result in a sensation that reaches the conscious level is unknown.

Deformities and diseases affecting the structure and movement of the thoracic cage can give rise to dyspnea, sometimes out of proportion to the degree of apparent imperfection. Included in this category are paralysis of the diaphragm, restriction of rib motion by forms of arthritis, pectus excavatum (funnel breast), pectus carinatum (pigeon breast), and severe kyphoscoliosis.

Airways obstruction is another mechanism that may cause dyspnea in that there may be difficulty in getting air into or out of the lungs. Vocal cord paralysis, acute epiglottitis, foreign body aspiration, acute severe laryngotracheobronchitis, and intratracheal or extratracheal tumor may interfere with the ingress or egress of air. Bronchial asthma, chronic bronchitis, and chronic obstructive lung disease are notable examples wherein bronchiolar constriction interferes with the exhalation of air from the alveoli.

Diseases within the lung parenchyma are notable causes of dyspnea. They do so by encroaching upon the volume of functioning lung tissue; interfering with ventilation, perfusion or diffusion; or altering the elasticity and compliance of the lungs.

Notable for interfering with pulmonary perfusion is pulmonary thromboembolism. Pulmonary ventilation is impaired by obstructed airways, thoracic deformities, and atelectasis. Diffusion involves the exchange of carbon dioxide and oxygen across the alveolar-capillary membrane; it may be impaired in interstitial fibrosis and sarcoidosis. Defects such as these may result in ventilation-perfusion mismatches and incomplete arterialization of venous blood (Fig. 1.5).

Diseases that cause dyspnea by the destruction and infiltration of lung parenchyma as well as by decreasing the volume of functioning lung tissue include the pneumoconioses, pneumonia, primary or metastatic cancer, pulmonary congestion from left ventricular failure, chronic obstructive pulmonary disease, and a large pleural effusion.

Alterations in the composition of blood cause dyspnea, but the precise mechanisms remain obscure. Metabolic acidosis, hypercapnia, and hypoxia may be detected by central and vascular chemoreceptors (carotid and aortic bodies); these

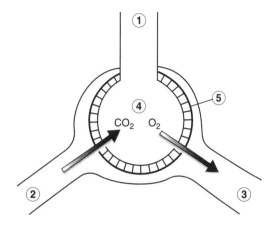

Anatomy	Physiology
1 Bronchiole	$1 \rightarrow 4$ ventilation
2 Pulmonary artery	2 perfusion
3 Pulmonary vein	$2 \rightarrow 5 \rightarrow 4$ ⎤
4 Alveolus	$4 \rightarrow 5 \rightarrow 3$ ⎦ diffusion
5 Alveolar-capillary membrane	

▶ **Figure 1.5.** Physiology of pulmonary gas exchange: ventilation, perfusion, diffusion.

in turn increase the respiratory drive, and indirectly cause dyspnea to occur by increasing the effort to breathe.

Severe anemia from any cause may be associated with dyspnea because of the decrease in the hemoglobin's oxygen-carrying capacity. But the exact way in which anemia does so is not clear. Indeed, why breathing becomes rapid and deep after exercise is equally shrouded.

It is important to note that *more than one mechanism for dyspnea may often be present* in one patient with a single illness. For example, in left ventricular failure, there is a ventilation defect that results from fluid filling many alveoli, a decrease in lung compliance because the bases are fluid-laden, and perhaps compression of lung tissue by associated pleural effusions. In COPD, there is airways obstruction, destruction of lung tissue, and restriction of chest motion.

In seeking the cause for the patient's dyspnea, it is most important to determine: (1) how and when it began; (2) what has been its progression since its onset; (3) whether it is continuous or intermittent; (4) whether it relates to body position; (5) what makes it better and worse; (6) what are the associated symptoms; and (7) whether it occurs at rest, on exertion, or both.

ONSET OF DYSPNEA The sudden onset of dyspnea is usually associated with a serious cardiopulmonary event such as acute myocardial infarction, pulmonary embolus, or spontaneous pneumothorax. The gradual onset over a period of days to weeks points to a chronic pulmonary disease, left ventricular failure, or pleural effusion.

Most patients who have illnesses associated with dyspnea at first manifest dyspnea only on exertion when the respiratory drive increases; later on in the course of the illness, dyspnea may also be present when at rest. If it first occurs at rest, it may well be part of the hyperventilation syndrome. This is especially apt to be true if the symptoms are intermittent.

Position, too, is important. The dyspnea of pleural effusion is worse when the patient lies on the unaffected side. The dyspnea on exertion that occurs in left ventricular failure is associated with dyspnea on recumbency so that sleep on two or more pillows is required (orthopnea). Patients who have chronic obstructive pulmonary disease often also have orthopnea, because of restriction of chest movement and diaphragmatic excursion when lying flat.

Associated Symptoms

It is to be appreciated that a chief complaint of dyspnea can occur in a wide variety of pathophysiologic states. These range from congestive heart failure to chronic obstructive pulmonary disease to bronchial asthma, and include such diverse causes as foreign body inhalation, hyperventilation syndrome, pleural effusion, spontaneous pneumothorax, and pulmonary embolus.

As a problem solver, not only must you know and understand the variable circumstances in which the dyspnea occurs in each instance, such as how it started, when it occurs, and whether it is related to exertion—you must also be familiar with the associated clinical features. The presence or absence of coexistent symptoms may point this way or that.

For example, if the dyspnea seems to be *cardiac in origin,* you might seek to find a cause for congestive failure, such as a history of heart murmur, rheumatic fever, hypertension, angina, or previ-

ous heart attack. Frequently, the patient with cardiac failure also has orthopnea, paroxysmal nocturnal dyspnea, night cough, palpitations, and peripheral edema as well, if right ventricular failure has supervened. If none of these features is present, cardiac failure is much less likely to be the cause of the presenting symptom.

For dyspnea that is *pulmonary in origin,* fellow travelers include chronic cough, expectoration, and wheeze. If asthma enters the picture, you seek a history compatible with allergy, such as childhood eczema, urticaria, or hay fever. The presence of leg pain or swelling suggests pulmonary embolus, and cigarette smoking or previous mastectomy hints at the possibility of carcinoma. In the absence of any of these clinical clues, the lungs are less likely to be at fault.

Fortunately for the diagnostician, especially for the budding young problem solver, the usual presenting symptom or clinical picture in most other patients does not conjure up a formidable list of diagnostic possibilities such as that created by dyspnea. The usual clinical presentation suggests only one, two, or three possibilities, one being most likely and another least likely. Perhaps there are two or three equally leading contenders.

Associated Signs

Because dyspnea may have its origin in a wide variety of disease states, a physical examination that focuses only on areas that may be concerned approaches what is essentially almost a complete

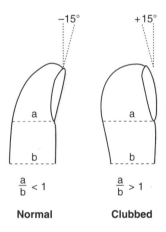

▶ **Figure 1.6.** Clubbed finger. Note shape of distal phalanx, angle of nail bed, and altered a/b ratio. *a* is diameter of finger at base of nail; *b* is diameter of finger at the distal joint.

Mechanisms for Dyspnea in Common Pulmonary Disorders

1 Interference with ventilation (V)
2 Interference with perfusion (P)
3 Interference with diffusion (D)
4 V-P-D mismatch
5 Anoxemia or hypercarbia
6 Decreased elasticity
7 Decreased compliance
8 Increased work of breathing
9 Decrease in amount of functioning
  lung tissue

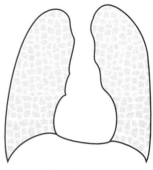

Normal chest

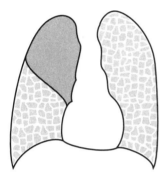

Right upper lobe pneumonia
1,4,5,7

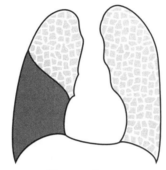

Pleural effusion
1,4,5,9

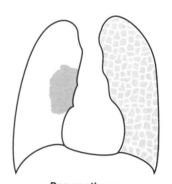

Pneumothorax
(collapsed right lung)
1,4,5,8,9

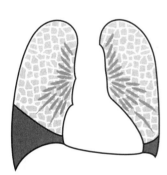

Congestive heart failure
(cardiomegaly, congestion,
effusions)
1,4,5,7,8,9

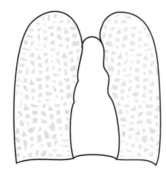

Emphysema
(vertical heart, low diaphragm,
hyperinflated lungs)
1,4,5,6,8,9

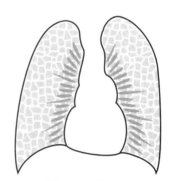

Pulmonary fibrosis
(prominent pulmonary artery)
3,5,7,8,9

▶ **Figure 1.7.** The numbered mechanisms for the production of dyspnea are stated under each common disorder.

physical examination. But certain parts of the examination are more critical than others.

In the *vital signs,* fever points to infection, rapid heart rate suggests distress or anxiety, and the rate and depth of respirations, as well as prolonged expiratory effort, help in determining the degree and type of respiratory distress.

Distention of neck veins may indicate the presence of congestive failure or the increased intrapleural pressure of COPD or asthma. In the neck, you feel for large, hardened lymph nodes that could result from an intrathoracic malignancy. The trachea may be deviated toward the side of the lesion if there is atelectasis, or away from the side of the lesion if a large pleural effusion or tension pneumothorax is present.

Clubbing of the fingers may be found in the presence of bronchiectasis, chronic pulmonary suppuration, or lung cancer, and there may be cyanosis of the lips and fingernail beds if hypoxemia and an increase in the amount of reduced hemoglobin exist (Fig. 1.6).

Key findings in the lungs include wheezes if bronchiolar constriction is present, as in asthma, and rales if there is fluid or pus in the alveoli. The signs of a pleural effusion—absent fremitus, absent breath sounds, and flatness on percussion—should be easily verifiable.

A careful examination of the heart is critical in the evaluation of any patient complaining of shortness of breath. If dyspnea results from *heart failure,* cardiac enlargement may be detected by an apex beat that is displaced downward and to the left. Often, too, there is a systolic mitral or aortic murmur. A third or fourth heart sound may be present. There may be a mitral diastolic rumble if mitral stenosis is causing the problem. A loud pulmonic component of the second heart sound may point to increased pulmonary artery pressure in the presence of a pulmonary embolus. The neck veins may be distended. And if the cardiac failure is prolonged or severe enough, there may be an enlarged, tender liver and peripheral edema. In the presence of a completely normal cardiac examination, it is most unlikely that heart disease is the cause of the dyspnea.

A much more focused initial examination can be done if, on the basis of the history, one diagnostic impression seems reasonably certain. For example, if the aggregate symptoms suggest congestive heart failure, examination of the lung bases and heart should suffice. If the dyspnea is accompanied by chest pain and a history of a recently swollen and painful leg, you would direct your examination to the lungs and legs, looking for evidence of pulmonary thromboembolus. If the patient has had a mastectomy for breast cancer in the past, you would check for pleural effusion.

On the grounds of the chief complaint and the associated symptoms and physical signs, the examiner should now be reasonably certain of the diagnosis. But if uncertainty still exists, or if it is necessary to achieve a higher degree of certainty in order to offer a prognosis or initiate treatment, the health care provider may request that *high-yield tests* be done. These may include arterial blood gases, sputum cultures, a chest radiograph, an ECG, perhaps a ventilation–perfusion scan, pulmonary function tests, imaging techniques, or biopsies.

Various common disorders associated with shortness of breath are portrayed on the chest diagrams in Figure 1.7. The pathophysiologic mechanisms that are operative in each instance are noted.

It should be reassuring to know that the vast majority of patients have chief complaints that are simply solved and do not require consideration of the wide range of pathophysiologic mechanisms that those patients who have shortness of breath require. Usually the single diagnosis is quickly evident, or at most the differential diagnosis consists of two or three diseases. But in all cases, the clinical reasoning process should be similar to the tactics described in this chapter.

Data Collection, Data Processing, Problem Lists

Paul Cutler

The principal initial steps in the problem-solving process are: the collection of patient data, the evaluation of this data, and the formation of a differential diagnosis or problem list. It is difficult to separate these three into sequential steps because they usually proceed simultaneously.

Information about the patient is evaluated piecemeal as soon as it is obtained. The gait, clothing, general appearance, hand shake, age, and gender register in the problem solver's mind even before a single word is spoken. Then, as you wind your way through the chief complaint and the history of the present illness, you should be well on the road to the diagnosis.

Each bit of information collected is interpreted as being relevant or irrelevant to the chief complaint, important or unimportant, perhaps a separate problem, then relegated to short-term memory or discarded—always in light of the information and impressions that came before.

Thus, clinical reasoning begins with or even before the history and continues throughout the collection of data. In fact, it is the clinical reasoning process that directs the flow of traffic through the circuitry of data acquisition during the doctor-patient encounter.

DATA COLLECTION

This represents all information obtained from and about the patient. Only a few points will be made here, because this subject is amply covered in many good textbooks where the rigid formats and formal outlines of the patient data base may be obtained.

Included in this data base are: (a) the history; (b) the physical examination; and (c) tests that include blood chemistries, complete blood count, urinalysis, chest radiograph, and electrocardiogram.

What is the relative importance of each? Certainly a diagnosis can be strongly suspected or definitely made during any one of the data-gathering processes. Sometimes a chest radiograph is the determining factor, as in the patient with low-grade fever and fatigue who has an infiltrate in the right apex. At other times a single physical finding may be the concluding factor, as in the 56-year-old man who complains of weakness and weight loss and in whom a hard nodular prostate gland is found. An elevated serum amylase level may be the key point in the diagnosis and therapy of the patient with severe pain, tenderness, and rigidity in the upper abdomen.

But in the great majority of cases the *history is the most important* and most revealing portion of the data base. By dialogue alone you can usually be reasonably certain of what is wrong. If it were possible to quantitate the relative importance of each portion of the data base in arriving at a diagnosis, it would probably be in the range of: history, 70%; physical examination, 20%; and laboratory tests and other procedures, 10%.

History Taking

A NEGLECTED SKILL Unfortunately, history taking has always been, and probably still is, the student's and physician's least perfected and most neglected skill. There are few poor historians but many poor history takers. Too often we ask a few questions, do a cursory examination, then order a huge array of studies, hoping to find the answer there.

But nowhere in the practice of medicine are interpersonal skills needed more than in taking a history. When patients give reasons why they change doctors, over half do so because the doctor is cold, abrupt, and impersonal. Most of the others switch because the doctor is evasive and gives "inadequate treatment." Common criticisms of a doctor's demeanor include statements that the doctor is arrogant, bored, impatient, aloof, seems rushed, explains too little, or confuses the patient.

On the other hand, patients seem satisfied with doctors who are relaxed, take time, explain things and answer questions, have patience, are cordial, and seem interested in them.

What It Takes As a student, you begin by learning how to approach a patient with sympathy, politeness, humility, and a smile. Extend your hand, introduce yourself, and tell the patient why you are there. And then begin with a kind introductory comment. Be informal and conversational but never familiar. You should not have to follow printed forms.

Above all, encourage the patient to talk, and do not dominate the conversation. Do not forget that the patient is trying to tell you what is wrong. Therefore, a good history taker must be a good listener.

At the beginning ask mainly open-ended questions that allow and encourage the patient to talk. For example, "tell me more,"; "what about that?"; "and then?"; "yes?"; and "you had pain?" are all invitations for the patient to continue. Specific closed-ended questions come later. For example, "did the pain make you vomit?" and "what was the color of your stools?" require simple answers.

Unspoken Language Silence can be golden or awkward depending on its use. It may indicate interest and spur dialogue if it is accompanied by a nod, a postural shift forward, eye contact, a "yes", or "uh-huh." On the other hand, if the interviewer looks elsewhere, sighs heavily, or looks evaluatively at the patient, the silence can be counterproductive.

Body language is almost as important as what you say. A head scratch, a tongue in the cheek, a shake of the head, or a sudden widening of the eyes can be disconcerting, whereas a smile, a sympathetic expression, or properly timed nods may be encouraging. The same expression used differently can mean vastly different things to the patient. Consider the use of "oh?"; "oh!"; "oh, oh!"; and "oh-HO!".

Getting at the Truth Some difficulties inevitably arise in trying to get at the facts. Truth is often colored by the patient's personality and attitudes; he or she may minimize; exaggerate; hide the truth; or be fearful, angry, quiet, or shy. There may be reluctance to be honest because of alcoholism, drug addiction, excessive eating, malingering, sexual difficulty, venereal disease, marital problems, criminal record, unstable job history, contact with a previous physician, or lack of adherence to a previous treatment program.

Do not forget that you are interviewing a patient who is not only sick but is experiencing all of life's events, such as disability, divorce, separation, retirement, parenthood, terminal illness, suffering, despondency, and perhaps responsibility. Some issues may be incompletely or inaccurately addressed if family members are present.

Because the purpose of getting a history is to elicit accurate bits of information that contribute to the problem-solving process, all the factors that may inhibit or expedite this process must be considered.

Rigid and Flexible Formats While we teach students to be rote in gathering data, physicians are fluid and freewheeling when they take histories. Why is there such a difference, and where does the change take place?

Of necessity, students who are just beginning to take histories must learn the time-honored, well-defined plan and sequence of questions. First come the identification data, next is the chief complaint, then the history of present illness, the family history, systems review, and so forth. Beginners need a format.

But the sooner the student learns to take histories like the physician, the better. The physician uses a flexible approach and a conversational style that seems to change order, bypassing some questions and asking others that are not in the traditional sequence. But this is always done for good reasons. The problem solver forms one or more early provisional diagnoses and asks questions with high sensitivity (to exclude a diagnosis if negative and to build a pattern of support for a diagnosis if positive) and questions with high specificity (to confirm a diagnosis if positive and to build evidence for rejection of a diagnosis if negative).

For example, if the patient complains of angina-like chest pain, the physician might go directly to selected questions from various parts of the patient data base that might guide him or her to quickly solve the problem. Does the patient have diabetes or hypertension? Does the patient smoke? The responses would support a diagnosis of coronary artery disease if positive and weigh somewhat against it if negative. A question with high specificity might be "tell me about the chest pain; when does it come and what does it feel like?" If the pain comes on exertion, feels like a constricting vise, and radiates down the inner aspect of the left arm—a pain that is virtually specific for myocardial ischemia—the diagnosis of angina is confirmed by history alone.

If the patient with angina claimed to have diabetes too, the physician might tangentially at this point ask all about the diabetes. This would include its onset; a family history; its course; its current state of control; information about diet, exercise, and medication; and questions that might aim to elicit other diabetes complications. After this avenue had been explored, the physician would return to the original line of conversation.

The more the student understands about disease processes and the greater his or her knowledge base, the more readily he or she can detour from traditional pathways and quickly get to the root and heart of the issues.

TWO MINUTES IN Very often the correct diagnosis is reached by the time the physician is only 2 minutes into the history. First, the history taker generates an *initial concept* that is based on the patient's age, gender, chief complaint, and perhaps one or two additional bits of information. Examples of initial concepts are: "28-year-old woman with recurrent polyarthritis"; "64-year-old man with a 6-month history of worsening cough, expectoration, and dyspnea on exertion."

The first example would generate *initial hypotheses* of rheumatoid arthritis, systemic lupus erythematosus, and perhaps sarcoidosis or Lyme disease. The second would warrant the consideration of chronic obstructive pulmonary disease (COPD), lung cancer, tuberculosis, and other diffuse parenchymal lung diseases.

A *hypothesis* is a presumptive diagnosis that the problem solver thinks may be the explanation for the patient's complaints, and it follows upon a consideration of the initial concept. There may be more than one hypothesis; there may be many. They can vary in their sophistication and precision from items as vague as "trouble in the gastrointestinal tract" to one as specific as Whipple's disease. They can include diseases, syndromes, and pathophysiologic states such as chronic renal failure, malabsorption syndrome, and inappropriate antidiuretic hormone secretion.

TO EXCLUDE OR CONFIRM Having formed initial hypotheses, the history taker then moves into areas of the interview that will gather information tending to exclude most possibilities and confirm one. This is called the *hypothetico-deductive method*. To use it, the interview must be highly directed and hypothesis-driven, so that shortcuts can be taken and hours not be spent gathering high-volume, low-value information. The interviewer searches for *clues* that are usually present if a hypothesis is correct; if these are present or positive, the hypothesis is more likely to be correct. If these clues are absent, then the hypothesis is likely to be incorrect, especially if these clues have a high incidence of positivity (sensitivity) in this disease.

A "clue" may be defined as any bit of information in the patient's data base that aids in the solution of a problem. It includes items in the history, physical examination, and ancillary tests and studies.

Suppose a historical clue is *always* present in a certain disease; if it is not present in the patient under investigation, the disease is ruled out. For example, edema is always present in the nephrotic syndrome; *its absence excludes* this hypothesis. On the other hand, a history of greasy, foul, floating stools is specific for the malabsorption syndrome; *its presence confirms* such a clinical impression.

STRENGTHENING YOUR IMPRESSIONS As the history is expanded with more conversation and questions, the physician sorts, extracts, subtracts, and adds bits of information into meaningful groups. He or she may enlarge on all aspects of a positive response, for example, when, where, how, and why an abdominal pain is manifested; what brings it on; and what relieves it. Negative responses are evaluated in the light of how strongly they militate against a hypothesis. Those hypotheses being considered undergo probability revision and reranking as the dynamic search for helpful information proceeds.

The term *rule out* is frequently used in medical circles. It means that a diagnosis or hypothesis has been eliminated from the list of possibilities by requesting data which, if negative or absent, more or less excludes the hypothesis under consideration. For example, for a patient who has chronic cough, the existence of congestive heart failure can be ruled out by the absence of dyspnea on exertion, orthopnea, basal rales, enlarged heart, and edema. The cough must therefore have a different cause.

Imagine a 38-year-old woman who consults you because of a swollen abdomen. The question arises as to whether she may be pregnant. You conclude that she is not pregnant on the basis of many bits of historical evidence, but each bit has only comparative strength and must be carefully weighed: (a) she is not married; (b) she is not concerned about pregnancy; (c) she says she has not had sexual relations; (d) she has never been pregnant before; (e) she had a pelvic operation 1 year ago; (f) she has irregular menses; (g) she uses oral contraceptives; (h) she says her breasts have not enlarged; and (i) she has anorexia and has lost weight but has no nausea or vomiting. You can see how some of these statements might raise an eyebrow, whereas others would make you reasonably certain she is not pregnant. Each item requires thought, consideration of psychosocial and pathophysiologic factors, and the application of logic. And each item tends to rule out pregnancy with varying degrees of certainty.

COMPLETE HISTORIES While espousing the philosophy of shortcuts in history taking, it is not implied that complete detailed histories are archaic. They must be done even though you may have decided on the major problems early in the anamnesis. In so doing, you confirm or reject these problems, uncover new ones, or find isolated historical facts that fit nowhere. Moreover, you may realize that what was thought to be a simple problem is really complex or involves more systems than had been suspected.

WHO TAKES THE HISTORY Today many other persons gather data for the busy physician. But the patient's history—the most important part of the patient data base—should be taken only by the physician, the physician's assistant, or the nurse practitioner, all of whom have been specially trained to do so. It should not be taken by an untrained person, nor is it acceptable to have the patient fill out a form or enter information into a computer. For it is primarily in the taking of the history that rapport is established and the patient's personality is noted. It is important to observe the patient's reaction to a question, the words chosen, what is emphasized, and his or her facial expressions. The history taker must be able to change the focus or direction of questions, to deduce simultaneously, to elaborate, and to discern fine shades of meaning. It is here where depression, anxiety, fear, exaggeration, and denial are detected, facial nuances can be weighed, and problem solving begins. What computer or paper form can do all of these things?

Any simplistic approach that attempts to add clues together in a machine that prints out the answers is probably naive. Such an approach completely ignores the critical value of the human intellect and is not a substitute for human thinking and patient-physician interaction.

Physical Examination

THE TWO TYPES If, after taking a history, the problem solver already has a good idea of what may be wrong with the patient, he or she may proceed to a selective or *ad hoc* type of examination in which specific physical findings that confirm the clinical impression are sought.

For example, if the patient complains of chronic indigestion, anorexia, and weight loss, and the physician suspects cancer of the upper digestive tract, he or she may then search specifically for signs of anemia, a pathologic left supraclavicular lymph node, an epigastric mass, or an enlarged nodular liver.

But if the history is vague and suggests no specific area for further search, or if the history is so complex that the problem solver is unable to select a hypothesis-driven subset for examination, then a complete, orderly, head-to-toe physical examination is in order. There, the examiner may uncover findings that: help in the formulation of a hypothesis; may confirm a previously held vague impression; or may suggest the presence of additional unexpected problems.

In the event that the problem solver opts for

an ad hoc examination and discovers physical findings that confirm the initial hypothesis, a complete physical examination is still mandatory in order to uncover further complications of the primary problem or to stumble upon unexpected evidence of coexisting problems.

PITFALLS In doing *complete* physical examinations, there are no substitutes for orderliness, thoroughness, and attention to one thing at a time. Most errors are due to lack of thoroughness, not lack of knowledge, for often the solution is found in the fundi, the supraclavicular nodes, the rectum, testes, or pelvis, which are much neglected or poorly examined areas.

The examination portion of the data-gathering process should require only 10 or 15 minutes. But too often the examiner falls into the slovenly habit of doing an abbreviated helter-skelter examination that includes a look at the tongue and conjunctiva, a tap or two on the chest, a quick listen to the heart, and a pat on the abdomen.

The general inspection of the patient should be thoroughly done first. Here important findings are often missed. The examination must be done in a programmed, systematic manner. Look successively for deformities, status of nutrition, and hydration, tremors and movements, body type, hair distribution, skin pigmentations and rashes, nodules, xanthomas, edema, venous distentions, pallor, jaundice, cyanosis, and plethora.

Pallor and jaundice are often overlooked because they were not specifically sought; the next day, the laboratory results will send you back to the patient for a second look. Endocrine disorders such as myxedema, hyperthyroidism, acromegaly, and Cushing's syndrome can often be diagnosed at a glance, but only if you are looking for them. Otherwise, they may be missed. Your patient, who gradually develops hypothyroidism while under your care, may remain undiagnosed until seen by another physician who inspects carefully at the first visit.

In examining the eyes, there are some 15 separate items to be checked; a single glance does not take them all in. Check for symmetry, protrusion, conjunctiva with eversion, and check the eyelids, eyebrows, cornea, sclera, pupillary reactions, lacrimal apparatus, tonometry, visual acuity, visual fields, extraocular movements, and the fundi (Fig. 2.1).

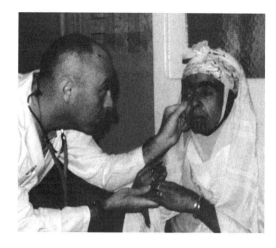

▶ **Figure 2.1.** Examining the eyes. It's not simply a glance at the conjunctiva.

On listening to the heart, do not listen for 15 seconds, then stop. Instead, concentrate first on S_1 at the apex, then S_2 at the base, systolic sounds, diastolic sounds, individual valve areas, and so forth. Allow the ears and brain to focus on one item at a time, blocking out all other sounds (Fig. 2.2).

The cavil to pay attention to one thing at a time sounds simple, but it is not. The examiner must look for only one item to the exclusion of others. The mouth is not examined by a glance at the tongue; many parts must be individually

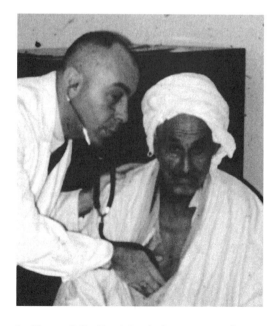

▶ **Figure 2.2.** Examining the heart. It's more than just a listen.

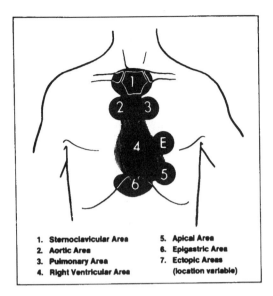

1. Sternoclavicular Area
2. Aortic Area
3. Pulmonary Area
4. Right Ventricular Area
5. Apical Area
6. Epigastric Area
7. Ectopic Areas
   (location variable)

▶ **Figure 2.3.** Areas of the chest to be palpated in patients who have cardiovascular diseases.

inspected—teeth, gums, tonsils, buccal mucosa, palate, uvula, salivary duct openings, oropharynx, floor—and say "ah!"

Palpation is an underused skill. An amazing amount of information can be obtained by simply touching and feeling, and students are often unaware of such multiple utilities. For example, light palpation with the fingertips can detect texture, moisture, crepitus, tenderness, fluctuation, and masses. Slightly firmer palpation with the distal phalanges elicits deep tenderness, rigidity, ballottement, thrust, and pulsation, and may further delineate and characterize masses. The dorsum of the hand is best for temperature change, and the thenar eminence and palmar aspect of the metacarpophalangeal joints is best for the vibrations of tactile fremitus, vascular thrills, and friction rubs.

Examiners will often be satisfied with only the detection of the apex beat, but there are many areas of the precordium to be palpated. These include: (1) the sternoclavicular areas for aneurysmal pulsation; (2) the aortic valve area for the thrill of aortic stenosis or aortic pulsation; (3) the pulmonic valve area for the palpable P_2 of pulmonary hypertension; (4) the precordial area for a right ventricular lift; (5) the apical area for the apex beat and the thrill of mitral stenosis; (6) the epigastric area for abdominal aortic aneurysm or right ventricular hypertrophy; and (7) the ec-

topic area for the pulsation of a ventricular aneurysm. And do not forget to feel over the liver for the presystolic or systolic pulsation of tricuspid valve disease (Fig. 2.3).

NORMAL OR ABNORMAL? You cannot be sure that a finding is abnormal unless you know what is normal. Although this statement may seem to go without saying, you often meet students or house officers who present physical findings without knowing for sure whether they are normal or abnormal.

Take a case of suspected male hypogonadism. To confirm the presence of testicular atrophy, you must first know the average volume of the normal adult testicle. Careful measurements must be made; just a feel is not sufficient. Similarly, you must know the size and shape of the normal liver, the distance the diaphragm moves on inspiration, the normal arterial-venous diameter ratio in the fundus, the exact location of the normal apex beat, and so forth.

It is important to know that the systolic blood pressure does not change more than 10 mm Hg on shifting from the supine to the erect position or on breathing in and out, and that the pressure should not normally vary more than 10 mm Hg from one arm to the other.

The distinction between normal and abnormal is critical in the evaluation of the patient with palpable lymph nodes, the female patient with some facial hair, the tall patient who has a heart murmur and in whom you seek to evaluate the palatal arch, as well as the numerous other examples seen every day. These are instances where you must decide whether or not a finding is an indication of disease.

CLINICAL MEASUREMENT Recent studies have documented the inaccuracies of measuring liver size and diaphragmatic motion by percussion as well as the presence of ascites by traditional techniques. Measurements made by radiograph, isotope scans, and ultrasound were compared to those made by groups of clinicians, and it was shown that clinicians were frequently wrong. Percussion of liver size had an overall accuracy of 50%—information that could have been gotten by the flip of a coin. The results of percussion for diaphragmatic excursion showed poor correlation with technical tests.

In a series of patients with *questionable* ascites, various physical signs such as bulging flanks, shifting dullness, fluid wave, and puddle sign had an overall accuracy of 58% compared with 100% accuracy for ultrasound studies.

It seems that many examining skills need careful reappraisals of this sort, and hopefully such studies will result in the more critical evaluation of data.

ONE SKILL DISSECTED On the surface, it might seem that a single examining skill would be simple. But most are not; they require many separate actions in order to be properly executed. Take, for example, the location and description of the cardiac apex beat. *First,* try to locate the apex beat by inspection; perhaps only 25% are visible. *Second,* place the palm of the right hand over the precordium and feel the apex beat; perhaps only 50% are palpable. If you cannot feel it, have the patient gently exercise and then lean forward; this maneuver may make the apex beat more palpable. *Third,* place your index finger where the apex beat was felt and mark the location. *Fourth,* locate the sternal angle and the second rib on the left. *Fifth,* count downward one rib at a time until you reach the interspace where you felt the apex beat. *Sixth,* measure the distance tangentially and horizontally from the midsternal line to the apex beat. You have precisely located the apex beat. *Seventh,* again feel the apex beat, noting its strength, shape, duration, and diameter, and whether there are associated impulses preceding or following it.

You are now ready to describe the normal apex beat. "The apex beat is in the fifth left intercostal space, 8 cm tangentially from the midsternal line. It is of normal force, lasts less than 0.1 second, occupies an area with a 2-cm diameter, has a normal shape, and is not associated with any other impulses."

Almost every examining skill can be broken down into its component parts in a similar manner. This enables the student to learn, do, and report his or her examination with accuracy and precision. Any student describing the apex beat as was just done would be regarded with awe and respect.

GETTING READY Other aspects of the physical examination almost too basic and simple to mention—yet often ignored—include the presence of proper light, having all necessary instruments, the comfort of patient and examiner, informing the patient of certain sensitive areas to be examined, gentleness, and disrobing and proper draping of the patient. You cannot possibly examine a female's heart while her brassiere is on, nor can you examine her abdomen through her clothes. Yet how often this is done! Frequently, jaundice or anemia is missed because the light is poor.

PROPER POSITIONS The novice examiner often has difficulty deciding on the proper sequence of examination vis-à-vis patient-doctor positioning. A good routine should be established. This will depend on whether the patient is ambulatory, in bed but mobile, or in bed and too sick to move about. In general, the patient has three positions during the examination—*lying, sitting,* and *standing.* The examiner stands either in front, behind, or to the right of the patient, and should aim for a minimum number of changes of patient position, thus sparing the patient the inconvenience and discomfort of an up-and-down disordered examination.

Because almost all patients can sit, the ambulatory patient should sit over the side of an examining table, and the hospitalized patient should sit over the side of the bed. With the patient in this position, the examiner can now complete the general inspection, obtain the vital signs, and study the head and neck, eyes, ears, nose, mouth, throat, back and front of the chest, heart, breasts, and axillae. The patient then lies down, and the heart, breasts, and axillae are re-examined. In this position, the abdomen, external genitalia, rectum, extremities, and peripheral circulation are reviewed.

A few selected parts of the examination can then be done in the standing position. These include a search for hernias and inspection of the leg veins.

As for the neurologic examination, the cranial nerves, reflexes, motor power, and sensation could have been tested while the patient was sitting. Cerebellar function is tested while sitting and standing. The pelvic examination occupies a position by itself, probably best at the end of the examination; the rectum can be examined at the same time in the female. The musculoskeletal system is examined in the sitting and standing positions.

A well-programmed examiner can intermingle the somatic, neurologic, and musculoskeletal examinations so as to minimize the changes in position. A simple sit-lie-stand sequence done only once should suffice. Bear in mind that the cardiovascular and abdominal examinations sometimes entail special positions to clarify murmurs or the presence of ascites. The foregoing orderly routine is for the patient who requires a complete traditional examination. If the diagnosis is already suspected on the basis of the history, any positional order may be followed, depending on what the examiner seeks.

For the patient who is very sick and cannot sit or stand, the examination must be done with the patient lying in bed at 30 to 45 degrees. Some parts may have to be omitted. The back of the chest presents a difficulty that can be partially resolved by an attendant who turns the patient from side to side or helps him or her to sit by pulling on the arms.

Paraclinical Studies

A tremendous array of tests and procedures is available to today's problem solvers. In addition to the traditional radiologic, serologic, immunologic, hematologic, microbiologic, and blood chemical tests, the recent technologic explosion has provided the physician with additional exquisite menus of diagnostic procedures.

Foremost among these are the various types of imaging procedures. New dimensions have been added to the diagnostic process by the introduction of computed tomography, ultrasound, magnetic resonance, and positron emission tomography. With the subsequent modification of these techniques by contrast enhancement, single photon emission, and color Doppler, the horizon for the application of these remarkable procedures seems boundless.

Catheters with dyes and drugs are insinuated into the cerebral, coronary, renal, adrenal, pulmonary, intestinal, and peripheral circulations. Isotopes define organs, detect defects within them, measure cardiac function, delineate ischemic areas, assess blood supply to the heart and brain, and locate metastases and occult infected areas.

Intrepid testers can perform biopsies on the heart, brain, liver, pancreas, kidney, and prostate, often guided by a simultaneous imaging procedure. Highly sensitive analytic techniques measure drug and hormone concentrations in ultra-minute nanograms or picograms, a process that allows microminiaturized assays in the one billionth (10^{-9}) or one trillionth (10^{-12}) range. Thus, the serum concentration of almost every known hormone is now assayable.

But just as a gourmet diet may be delicious but unhealthful, the formidable array of diagnostic studies now available to the clinician may be a mixed blessing. Although these studies are awe-inspiring, even mind-boggling, and usually very helpful, they are expensive and often risky, and sometimes are not in the best interest of the patient, the public policy, or the pocketbook of the patient or the health maintenance organization.

RESORTING TO TESTS The history and physical examination should provide the problem solver with either a definite diagnosis, a tentative diagnosis, or a list of ranked hypotheses. If additional information is needed to make the diagnosis more certain, tests and studies may be done. Bear in mind that a test is just another bit of patient data, another clue to help evaluate a hypothesis; and like any other clue, it may not be completely reliable.

But there can be no doubt that tests often provide crucial information. The protein electrophoresis may be the test needed to diagnose multiple myeloma in a 70-year-old woman who has back pain. Elevated ST segments in the electrocardiogram may serve to diagnose acute myocardial infarction in the 50-year-old man who has chest pain. A markedly elevated serum creatinine level may explain the reason for progressive weakness, nausea, and pallor in a uremic patient. But if their results are normal or negative, these tests tend to exclude the stated diagnoses.

ROUTINE STUDIES Remarkable advances in automation, computers, and laboratory management have permitted a large increase in tests at only a modest increase in cost. A battery of 12 to 20 tests is seen on most charts because they are done for only a small additional cost. So whether or not they are needed, the patient is tested for levels of serum bilirubin, creatinine, glucose, protein, albumin, calcium, phosphorus, uric acid, lactate dehydrogenase, aminotransferases, alkaline phosphatase, and cholesterol. Some of these tests may have been germane to the predicted problem, but most are valueless and sometimes misleading.

Currently, the serum sodium, potassium, chloride, and bicarbonate levels are routinely determined for each patient. Yet electrolytes are rarely helpful for screening purposes, except for patients in whom derangements might be expected; for example, the patient taking a diuretic, the patient who has cardiac or renal failure, or the patient who has severe fluid loss.

On the other side of the coin is the fact that the reflexive ordering of batteries of tests may uncover problems not suggested by the rest of the data base—for example, hypercalcemia, hypercholesterolemia, and diabetes mellitus.

WHAT TESTS TO ORDER Although routine tests may give you all of the additional information you need, there are many other special tests that may give yet more vital support to your provisional hypotheses. If liver disease is suspected, measurement of liver cell enzymes, coagulation tests, serum proteins, serum bilirubin, and immunologic markers for hepatitis may be requested.

For patients suspected of having a coagulation disorder, you may order only a platelet count if the clinical picture suggests thrombocytopenic purpura; and platelets, prothrombin time, and partial thromboplastin time if the clinical picture is less specific. On the other hand, for those who do not wish to think, check the item marked "coagulation studies," and the results of 10 or 12 tests will appear in a day or two, sometimes neatly labeled with a diagnosis.

Consider a patient who has an undiagnosed anemia. Your laboratory can perform 20 to 30 tests—all tests for anemias. Just imagine! You need not talk, think, examine, or read. The results may or may not give the correct answer. But on the other hand, a few questions, a brief examination, and perhaps only two or three carefully selected tests may be all that you need. Stool test findings that are negative for occult blood assure you that the problem lies in the womb of a 42-year-old woman with profuse menses and a hypochromic microcytic anemia. High levels of reticulocytes and indirect bilirubin

and the absence of sickle cells in a 24-year-old black man suggest that the problem lies in the genetic coding of glucose-6-phosphate dehydrogenase.

Many ethical, moral, and financial considerations enter into the selection of tests. Which is better: to cast a nylon line with a specific bait for only one kind of fish, or to throw out a large net that catches all? Should the procedure that quickly solves the problem be done first, no matter what the cost and risk, or should the less invasive, less risky, and less costly, although somewhat less informative, tests be done first?

Clearly, for emergent reasons, it may at times be necessary to opt for the procedure most able to provide an immediate answer, no matter what the cost and risk. If a myocardial infarction is imminent, angiography and consequent treatment are indicated at once; this is not the time for a treadmill test.

SHOULD THIS TEST BE DONE? In our procedure-oriented medical community, physicians are turning more and more to diagnostic studies that are complicated, discomforting, costly, or bear risk. A common situation is the case of a patient with chest pain for whom coronary arteriography and possibly eventual surgery are being considered. Many questions need to be answered first:

- From the clinical picture, what is the numerical likelihood that the patient indeed has coronary artery disease needing treatment?
- What are the sensitivity and specificity of the procedure, and how often may the test yield false-negative and false-positive results?
- Will arteriography establish the diagnosis with the degree of certainty that is required?
- What are the morbidity and mortality of the procedure?
- If arteriography reveals clinically significant coronary disease, will treatment be altered?
- Would the patient's general medical condition preclude surgery even if a surgically remediable lesion is found?
- What are the risks of surgery (of bypass graft and angioplasty)?
- What benefits can surgical treatment offer?
- Might medical therapy be of choice in this case no matter what the anatomy?
- Would the patient refuse surgery if offered?

- Are the patient's life-style and psychosocial conditions such that an improved coronary circulation does not really matter?
- Will the costs of the procedure and surgery be covered?

Numerous other questions could be asked, and they vary from patient to patient and, of course, from one medical situation to another. Decisions of such a critical nature should not depend solely on whether a diagnosis will be made, but, more important, on whether the procedure will benefit the patient.

DATA PROCESSING

What It Is

Data processing in medicine is the step by which the patient's data base is transformed into a problem list. Throughout the collection of patient data, every item in the history, physical examination, and paraclinical studies is evaluated in terms of its relevance to the chief complaint and to the various initial hypotheses. Positive clues are grouped into meaningful and related clusters that suggest ultimate diagnoses. The absence of certain clues may tend to negate one or more provisional hypotheses.

Perceiving the Problem

The chief complaint, its allied symptoms, and related physical signs can usually be grouped into a single diagnosis. If the underlying disease is in one organ, a knowledge of the symptoms and signs of diseases of that organ is most helpful; these signs and symptoms of disease usually relate to altered structure or function.

Not all of the classical symptoms and signs need be present; there may be only a few. The patient with early congestive heart failure may have only dyspnea on exertion, orthopnea, and basal rales. On the other hand, a full-blown picture may be present if the patient has not received proper treatment or is in the end-stage of long-standing disease.

Data acquisition and data processing usually proceed simultaneously as experience and confidence are gained. If the patient's chief complaint resembles angina pectoris, the problem solver seeks clues that may relate to the causes of coronary disease, such as a history of smoking, hypertension, and diabetes, or the presence of xanthelasma and evidence of vascular disease elsewhere in the neck and leg vessels.

Often, a few clues can be grouped with confidence into a single problem. At times, more clues are needed.

Does the Clue Relate?

Deciding on relevance between a clue and a diagnosis may not be an easy task. What seems relevant to one data retriever may not be considered so by another; the reverse also holds true. Sometimes a student will fail to see an obvious correlation; at other times, he or she may ingeniously relate two clues in a roundabout way even though the clues are truly unrelated.

You must know how to select clues that relate. A patient has chest pain, dyspnea on exertion, and hemorrhoids. The first two symptoms probably relate, but the third is no doubt an independent problem. It is difficult to pathophysiologically connect hemorrhoids to the two other clues that are probably cardiac in origin.

The next patient has angina pectoris, a recent myocardial infarction, and pain in the left big toe. The latter clue may or may not relate to the main problem. If the pain is chronic and antedated the cardiac episode, it is unrelated. If the pain followed the cardiac episode, it may be caused by thromboembolism, and therefore it may be related. But the pain could follow and still not be related: the patient may have gout, a bunion, or peripheral vascular disease, and further discerning evidence is needed.

Irrelevant material must be weeded out but not altogether disregarded, for it may relate to another problem. A chronic headache is probably not related to a chief complaint of tarry stools and syncope unless the excessive use of analgesics has caused gastric bleeding. Conversely, a recent backache may well be related to the presenting problem of nocturia, frequency of urination, and hematuria if you find carcinoma of the prostate on rectal examination.

Often it is easy to note relevance, especially if the clues come from the same system (e.g., cough and dyspnea). However, if this same patient also has a breast lump, the cough and dyspnea may be related by virtue of metastasis or may simply denote the presence of breast cancer in a patient who also has COPD. Your logic is frequently taxed in making decisions of this sort, and you may have to label a clue as *possibly* relevant.

Consider a patient with weakness and pallor who has hemorrhoids—possibly related if bleeding is present, but probably not related if bleeding is absent. The same patient has an inguinal hernia—not related. Suppose he or she also has chronic indigestion and a stool guaiac test result of 4+ for occult blood—almost certainly related.

Fitting Clues Together

The clustering of clues into meaningful groups is an integral part of data processing. Symptoms and abnormal physical signs in the same system usually can be pooled. For example, nausea, vomiting, diarrhea, fever, and diffuse abdominal tenderness are related. So are weakness, weight loss, anorexia, abdominal pain, and black stools.

Cough, expectoration, dyspnea, and sharp chest pain cluster quite nicely with signs of right lower lobe consolidation and fever to suggest the diagnosis of pneumonia or pulmonary infarction. Leg pain may or may not be related; leg pain with a tender calf probably *is* related. Additional information needs processing: the family pet is a healthy cat; the family pet is a sick cat; the family pet is a newly acquired parrot; the patient is an alcoholic; the patient's spouse had a similar illness last week; the patient is a male homosexual; and on and on. Each piece of information needs evaluation in light of what is already known.

Students often feel that only positive information is of value. But negative information may sometimes be even more helpful. The absence of a clue may be as important as its presence in helping you to decide. Patients with sarcoidosis usually have enlarged lymph nodes and an abnormal chest radiograph. If these two features are absent, you lean away from diagnosing sarcoidosis. The absence of thyromegaly, no abnormal eye signs, and a normal pulse rate militate against a hypothesis of hyperthyroidism, even if the patient is nervous and has sweaty palms and a tremor.

Choosing the Subsets

Do not forget that the processing of data is in some measure dependent on the acquisition of data; data acquisition in turn is a reflection of the data collector's ability to selectively pursue only certain subsets of information.

Given a 56-year-old man with chronic hoarseness of 3 weeks' duration, you can immediately form your initial concept and hypotheses. These include chronic laryngitis, laryngeal cancer, or recurrent laryngeal nerve paralysis from lung cancer, aneurysm, and so on. Your quest for additional data stems from these initial impressions, and data processing must of necessity follow the same course.

The information you selectively seek in this case includes the patient's occupation, hobbies, smoking history, pulmonary symptoms, chest examination, neck palpation, inspection for Horner's syndrome, chest radiograph, and vocal cord visualization, just as is done in Case 1 of Chapter 10.

As the student evolves into a clinician, he or she soon learns which data set to pursue for each inquiry departure point and develops his or her own scheme of data acquisition that is invariant for each problem or subproblem.

Every Bit Helps

Note how many pieces of meaningful information the brain and the computer can process from a simple presentation. Suppose you see a *35-year-old woman whose only problem is recurrent symmetrical polyarthritis for several years.* Eight items are almost simultaneously evaluated:

1. The patient is a woman.
2. The patient is 35 years old.
3. The patient has arthritis.
4. The patient's arthritis affects many joints.
5. The patient's arthritis has been present for several years.
6. The patient's arthritis recurs and remits.
7. The patient's arthritis was not present when she was young.
8. The patient has no extra-articular manifestations of disease, because the arthritis is stated to be her only problem.

Polyarthritis by itself can mean acute rheumatic fever, rheumatoid arthritis, systemic lupus erythematosus, gout, pseudogout, Lyme disease, sarcoidosis, and so forth. But given the eight modifying factors stated in this patient's 14-word presentation, many inferences concerning exclusions, probabilities, and likelihoods can now be made.

The fact that she is only 35 years old weighs heavily against pseudogout; the fact that she is 35 and a woman also weighs against gout; being sick for several years at 35 tends to exclude acute rheumatic fever, which begins at an earlier age; the absence of other manifestations points away from Lyme disease, sarcoidosis, rheumatoid variants, and lupus. More questions must follow, but the broad diagnostic field has already been considerably narrowed.

PROBLEM LISTS

What They Are

The data base you have acquired is processed into a list of problems that tells you what is wrong with the patient. The first problem list is usually derived within 24 hours and is placed at the beginning of the chart. It serves as a table of contents and quick reference source for all of the patient's afflictions. This list should represent the highest possible resolution of the patient's problems based on the data accumulated thus far.

Often a *diagnosis* may be clearly stated. At other times only a *syndrome* (such as hepatomegaly, ascites, and jaundice) may be listed because at this stage the physician may not yet be sure whether the patient has cirrhosis of the liver or metastatic carcinoma. Syndromes can also include pathophysiologic states or recognized entities, such as hepatorenal syndrome, inappropriate antidiuretic hormone secretion, and respiratory acidosis. A *cluster* of clues that seem to belong together may be stated as a problem if you do not yet have enough evidence to make a diagnosis; for example, nausea, vomiting, diarrhea, and fever—or dyspnea on exertion, night cough, basal rales, and an enlarged heart.

Also contained in the problem list are *isolated abnormalities* in the data base that do not seem to fit any of the other stated problems and were discovered in the course of routine data accumula-

tion. These may come from the history, physical examination, or laboratory information and often consist of uncategorized items, such as headaches, blurred vision, recurrent heartburn, rectal bleeding, internal hemorrhoids, a heart murmur, eosinophilia, or azotemia.

Psychosocial and *socioeconomic* problems constitute a last category to be included in the problem list; for example, unemployment, poverty, recent divorce, alcohol abuse, and heavy smoking.

To summarize, a problem list can contain a:

1. Diagnosis
2. Syndrome
3. Pathophysiologic state
4. Cluster of clues
5. Isolated abnormality
6. Psychosocioeconomic issue

Level of Resolution

Each diagnosis or problem on the problem list must be raised to the highest level of resolution with the information on hand. Examiners, especially students, will vary in their levels of confidence and amounts of basic knowledge.

Thus, the constellation of nausea, vomiting, diarrhea, and fever may be listed by some as "nausea, vomiting, diarrhea, fever"; others may describe the symptoms as "acute gastrointestinal disorder," and those with more confidence may refer to "viral or bacterial gastroenteritis." It is true that the third group may be settling for less than 100% certainty, but diagnostic infallibility may not be necessary in what is most likely a mild, self-limited illness. The more cautious examiner wants to see the results of a blood count and stool culture and wishes to observe the patient for 24 hours before attaching a definite diagnostic label. Each of the examiners is correct. But they vary in confidence and in the degree of diagnostic accuracy that they require.

In this regard, students commonly make one of three errors. *First,* they may fail to assemble clues properly into one recognizable group and thus list each symptom and sign as a separate problem. *Second,* they may cluster clues properly, list them as a single problem, but fail to raise the problem to as high a resolution as possible because of timidity. And *third,* they may make premature closure of a diagnosis and unjustified decisions before adequate information is available. Obviously, there is a twilight zone where the level of resolution is not clear-cut and is debatable.

How to Derive a List

A 52-year-old alcoholic male patient who has cirrhosis of the liver is admitted to the hospital with a massive upper gastrointestinal hemorrhage. After a 24-hour work-up concomitant with his emergency treatment, he is found to have the following problems:

1. Chronic alcoholism
2. Cirrhosis of the liver secondary to problem 1
3. Gastrointestinal hemorrhage
4. Benign prostatic hypertrophy
5. Hyperglycemia
6. Infiltrate right upper lobe
7. Unemployed
8. Divorced

Problems 1, 2, and 3 are quickly apparent. Note that problem 3 does not specify whether the bleeding is due to varices, ulcer, or gastritis, because at this stage it has not yet been clearly determined. Immediate gastroscopy was unsuccessfully attempted. Each problem must be formulated at a level that you can defend.

The prostatic condition is being recorded for the first time based on symptoms that have existed for 3 years plus the finding of a markedly enlarged prostate on rectal examination. It may or may not require attention in the near future and must be watched.

Problem 5, the hyperglycemia, was found on routine blood studies. It may be related to the intravenous glucose that the patient received while waiting for blood to be cross-matched; blood was drawn for chemical analysis at that time. But the glucose level was 300 mg/dL, which is higher than one would ordinarily expect from a slow intravenous drip. Listing it as a problem reminds you that it needs to be rechecked, especially after the patient is well. It may or may not indicate diabetes mellitus.

Problem 6, an asymptomatic finding noted on chest radiograph, is probably a separate problem, but it too will require present and future investigation. Problems 7 and 8 may relate to problem

1. In general, the problem list will increase in complexity with the patient's age.

Initial and Final Lists

The *initial problem list* is based on the first 24 hours of information and may need considerable adjustment as the case develops. Each problem is assigned a number that remains permanent. The order of number assignment may be determined by the sequence of pathophysiologic events, as in the case just described. Another way, preferred by many, is the assignment of numbers based on the importance or seriousness of each problem. In that event, gastrointestinal hemorrhage (problem 3) would have been listed as problem 1.

After the initial problem list is formed, each item in the list must be assessed, and a plan should be offered. The assessment may be written separately from the plan, or the assessment and plan may be written together, but each problem should be dealt with separately (as done in Chapter 11).

Included in the *assessment* of each problem should be the items in the data base that led you to label the problem as such, the urgency or seriousness of each problem, the pathophysiology of each problem, and the possible pathophysiologic relationship between problems. A differential diagnosis for a problem may be stated here—not in the problem list. By reading a student's assessment, you can easily measure his or her understanding of the entire case.

The *plan* is the proposed management for each problem. It includes the diagnostic studies and why you want them done; the proposed treatment for each problem, including medication, nursing care, surgery, diet, consultations, and so on; and what you aim to accomplish along the line of patient education.

The *final problem list* is completed when the patient is ready for discharge from the hospital, sometimes even sooner if satisfactory closure can be obtained for all problems. This may involve combining two or more problems into one, changes in diagnosis, or erasure of problems that were proved not to exist. Most important, the final diagnoses may now be stated at a higher level of resolution because more definitive and more diagnostic data have been obtained. The final problem list in the case previously discussed is as follows:

1. Chronic alcoholism
2. Cirrhosis of the liver
3. Gastrointestinal hemorrhage secondary to bleeding esophageal varices—resolved
4. Carcinoma of the prostate gland (established by elevated prostate specific antigen levels, ultrasound, and biopsy)
5. (No problem—subsequent glucose determinations normal; the problem and its number no longer exist)
6. (No problem—subsequent chest radiograph was normal; the problem and its number no longer exist)
7. Unemployed
8. Divorced

CONCLUSIONS

This chapter has taken you through the processes of acquiring information about the patient (history, physical examination, and paraclinical studies); evaluation of all the derived data; and their grouping into fairly well-defined problems. Chapter 3 will take you more deeply into the recesses of the various clinical reasoning processes that guide the problem solver in the formulation of a diagnosis. Chapter 4 tells you all about clues, whereas Chapter 5 aims to sharpen your data resolution skills through the use of many exercises (with answers) that demonstrate the selection of data subsets and the determination of a clue's relevance.

Problem-Solving Methods

Paul Cutler

WHAT PROBLEM SOLVING IS

Problem solving in clinical medicine is the process whereby the doctor finds out what is wrong with the patient. Given a chief complaint that may be as vague as " . . . not feeling well" or as specific as " . . . a painful, swollen big toe," the doctor then gathers additional information that guides him or her toward a solution.

How It's Done

Usually it's quite easy. Most patients have simple, common problems that are solved with a glance and a question. Sometimes, additional bits of information must be harvested from the history and/or physical examination. Less often, the patient presentation is vague or complex, and the problem solver must go more deeply into the patient's data base.

In that case, on the basis of the chief complaint and the patient's gender, age, and occupation, the doctor establishes a list of possible diagnoses (hypotheses) in his or her mind and then asks additional questions whose answers if positive tend to support one diagnosis, and if negative tend to exclude it.

After only 2 minutes of dialogue, one diagnosis usually emerges as a leading contender, and the doctor then proceeds to a selected hypothesis-driven subset of the physical examination, aiming to raise the most likely diagnosis to a level of virtual certainty.

What to Ask

In order to know what questions to ask and what parts to examine, the problem solver must have some knowledge of diseases, their pathophysiol-

ogy, and their symptoms and signs. The sooner the student acquires a knowledge base consisting of the cardinal manifestations of various diseases, the better he or she will be able to tackle the task of asking the correct questions and knowing where to search for additional clues.

For example, in a young male patient who has a "lump in the groin," the student should know that this may represent a hernia, an undescended testicle, or a pathologic lymph node. Questions should revolve around the presence of pain or tenderness; the effect of reclining, standing, or straining; whether the lump has increased in size; and the presence of systemic manifestations that might occur with a lymphoma, such as fever or weight loss. The student knows the anatomy of the area and is well-versed on how to check for the presence of hernia, palpate the scrotal sac, and examine for splenomegaly and nodes elsewhere.

Based on the answers to the problem solver's questions and the focus of the examination, the diagnosis becomes apparent.

Tradition

For generations, students have been taught to gather a data base and solve problems in separate, inviolate, orderly blocks. First, get a complete history. Second, do a complete physical examination. Then order routine laboratory tests, chest radiograph, and electrocardiogram (ECG). When these are completed, select the important clues from each of the three sources; then put them together so that they fit a known diagnostic pattern as closely as possible. It may be necessary to elongate the problem list for a leftover clue or a clue that doesn't fit. This method is tedious and time-consuming, although frequently necessary in obscure cases, in complicated or multisystem diseases, or when multiple diseases exist in one patient. It is especially helpful for the beginner who may feel uncomfortable about forming early hypotheses and may hesitate to depart from time-honored sequences. Even the seasoned clinician may find this method necessary at times.

Real Life

But this is not usually the way it's done in real life by experienced clinicians who begin to solve problems with their first questions in an almost subconscious manner, using maneuvers that they haven't clearly conceptualized. Studies have shown that the physician forms early hypotheses, tracks a key clue, forms a cluster, spots a triad or tetrad, considers a differential diagnosis, pursues only one subset of the data base, and zeroes in rapidly on a diagnosis.

Be Careful

It is important for the physician and student to know that even if the main problem is neatly and quickly solved with a few bits of information, a complete data base must usually still be fleshed out. The purpose is not only to make sure the original impression is correct and to discover the possible coexistence of other diseases, but to stumble on clues that don't fit, perhaps to rework the order of likelihoods, and last, to establish a baseline of normality for future comparison. Nobody wants to be locked into a wrong hypothesis.

Clinical Skills

To simulate the clinician who solves problems, the student must acquire and master many skills. These include:

- Facility for relating to people (interpersonal skills)
- Ability to take a history and perform a physical examination
- Knowing how to evaluate and process incoming information and put it all together
- Formulation of a problem list
- Skill at assessing the problem list and devising a diagnostic game plan

- Ability to transform all of the data into a written record
- Knowing how to access the information highway
- Ability to present the case to others in a nutshell

Some of these clinical skills will be detailed in subsequent chapters.

Diagnostic Criteria

What are the features of a disease that must be present before establishing its diagnosis in a particular case? Certainly not all of those that are listed in a textbook need be present. But how many are needed, and which ones? Must the diagnosis be clinical, chemical, or histologic?

The sad truth is that, except for acute rheumatic fever, rheumatoid arthritis, systemic lupus erythematosus, and perhaps a very few others, precise criteria for diagnosing diseases do not exist. And even the criteria for the three diseases just mentioned undergo revision from time to time. Diseases cannot be *diagnosed* with certainty because they cannot be *defined*. It is easy to list the many clinical features of a disease. We may be able to attach a number to each feature indicating the frequency with which it occurs; moreover, the number may be accurate. But that is *description,* not *definition*.

To define a disease, you must outline its borders, clearly identify and describe it, and exclude all other possibilities. You must establish a set of criteria that are fulfilled by *all* patients who are alleged to have a particular disease and fulfilled by *no* patients who do not have it.

Textbooks describe diseases but do not define them. Clinicians do the same. However, computers that demand definitions should serve as a further stimulus toward the delineation of diseases—not an impossible task, and certainly a worthy one. Such an accomplishment would go far in distinguishing between diagnostic look-alikes.

A Textbook Case

It must be said that textbook cases are rare and probably exist only in textbooks. Two patients with the same disease may present differently and often do not have the same manifestations. Books list all of the manifestations of a disease; sometimes, they even describe a fairly "typical case." But patients do not conform to textbooks, and common features are often absent. In fact, with few exceptions, no two patients with the same disease are identical; each has at least one feature that is peculiar to that particular patient and absent in others. Diseases differ as do people. And this concept is easier to grasp if you appreciate that a symptom or sign that is present in 50% of patients with disease A is not present in the other 50%. The textbook that describes disease A may present some 20 or 30 features of the disease, all of which are present in varying percentages of cases.

Diagnostic Certainty

Establishing the degree of diagnostic certainty needed in a particular case may be difficult. One hundred percent certainty is seldom attainable, and therapeutic decisions must often be made even if you are less than sure.

Diagnosis and treatment may proceed simultaneously. Chest pain needs treatment even before diagnosis. Diarrhea can be treated symptomatically before determining the underlying disease. So can urinary frequency and dysuria. Such decisions are determined by the seriousness of the case, the time required for more and more studies, the urgency for needed action, and the level of certainty humanly possible in each instance.

If coronary artery surgery is contemplated, you seek as close to 100% certainty as is possible with today's diagnostic armamentarium.

Simple or Complex Cases

Often, only minimal problem solving is needed. Nosebleeds, sore feet, and simple infections of the skin, fingers, toes, and upper respiratory tract are not usually problems requiring diagnostic skills. Nose picking, poor shoes, wounds, and transmitted nasopharyngeal secretions are common underlying causes.

But such seemingly simple problems can turn into riddles. Nosebleeds may result from multiple myeloma; repeated infections may presage diabetes mellitus or immunodeficiency; sore feet may result from neuropathy or vascular diseases. Hypertension may present no diagnostic prob-lem, but not if it results from kidney disease, an endocrine disorder, or renal artery stenosis. Beware of complacency in what seems like a simple matter.

One Organ, One System

One of the first things to decide in the course of harvesting patient data is whether the principal problem is limited to one organ or one system, involves several systems, or if indeed more than one disease exists. The decision about one organ or one system is usually easy because the symptoms and physical signs are apt to be thus confined. But the distinction between a multisystem disease and multiple diseases is not simple and requires added information and skill.

Duodenal ulcer is a one-organ disease in most cases; occasionally, it is associated with an endocrinopathy. Systemic lupus erythematosus and sarcoidosis are multiple-system diseases. Diabetes mellitus, essential hypertension, and cerebral thrombosis are multiple diseases that may often occur in the same person.

Prevalence and Probability

The *prevalence* of a particular disease is represented by the number of cases of the disease per population unit at any particular time. Thus, the prevalence of diabetes mellitus is .05 or 5%, of hypertension in adults is .20 or 20%, and of breast cancer in women over 50 years of age is .003 or 0.3% (3 cases per 1000 women).

The *probability* that a disease exists in a particular patient is a decimal or percentage estimate based on available data. For example, the clinical picture may suggest a .25 or 25% probability that the patient has coronary heart disease. This also means that in a cohort of 100 similar patients with the identical clinical picture, 25 would have coronary heart disease and 75 would not.

Both the prevalence and probability of disease are expressed by the Bayesian symbol $P(D)$.

Probability Revision

Given a patient whose clinical picture suggests that the likelihood of having a certain disease is 50:50 or one chance in two—$P(D) = .50$—you may wish to increase the likelihood before embarking on a special course of treatment.

To do so, more clinical information is needed, or tests must be done. A revised $P(D)$ may be calculated after each additional clue is added or a test is done, provided the sensitivity and specificity of the new information is known. The way in which this mathematical operation can be done is fully described in Chapter 7.

But the problem solver revises probabilities by simply adding clinical information. Precise computations are not practical at the bedside or in the clinic.

Suppose you see a 65-year-old man who has long-standing hypertension and, more recently, he has experienced dyspnea on exertion. On the basis of this scant information, you estimate the likelihood of having left ventricular failure to be .50. Then, add the fact that there are no pulmonary symptoms or history of smoking; the $P(D)$ rises to .75. Next, you note grade 2 hypertensive fundi, blood pressure 210/20, basal rales, an enlarged heart, and a third heart sound; the $P(D)$ rises to .95—virtual certainty. Had the S_3 and rales not been present, and the heart not been enlarged, the $P(D)$ would have been very much lower, which would have left room for an alternate diagnosis.

THE WAYS AND MEANS

The subsequent discussions will conceptualize, describe, and simplify many techniques used by experienced clinicians to solve problems. Hopefully, much of the mystery surrounding these seemingly magical skills will be lifted so that the student can begin to use them with facility. The idea that experienced clinicians use arcane and indefinable strategies to unravel diagnostic problems is a romantic myth. Actually, the processes by which medical diagnoses are established can be fragmented into clearly described, recognizable, and duplicable heuristic maneuvers.

Early Hypothesis Generation

This is the single most commonly used and most effective method of solving medical problems. The problem solver forms tentative impressions (hypotheses) early in the patient encounter based on:

- Age, gender, and chief complaint
- Pairs or combinations of symptoms
- Mention of a cause or complication of a disease
- A string-together technique

When a patient suddenly develops double vision, you think of a third nerve palsy, so one of your postulates is diabetes mellitus. A 36-year-old woman experiences sudden onset of a painful cold leg; you postulate mitral stenosis with atrial fibrillation.

The string-together technique for hypothesis generation can be exemplified by a 36-year-old man with pyuria and fever who reports that he passed clumps of tissue as well as blood. You think of necrotizing papillitis, but because he is not diabetic, you consider analgesic abuse. This suggests that there may be another disorder causing him to take analgesics. There is—chronic worsening headaches. Eventually, you hypothesize and subsequently prove the existence of a brain tumor. Note how you have gone from one hypothesis to another by chain reaction.

Once hypotheses are formed, the various subsequent maneuvers that determine the acceptance or rejection of hypotheses include cluster formation, case building, template matching, weight of evidence, proof by exclusion—all of which are described later in this chapter.

Although the novice may have ill-defined plans for managing each hypothesis, the seasoned clinician develops fixed deductive patterns. These patterns are integrated as templates into his or her cognitive structure and can be recalled on demand for any predicated hypothesis. If disease A is suspected, there are five precise bits of evidence to be sought. For disease B, there are eight. To distinguish A from B, three studies must be done—and so forth.

Clusters

The experienced clinician often uses classical groups, triads, or tetrads of clues to generate hypotheses and make diagnoses. These are easily committed to memory.

Thyromegaly, tremor, tachycardia, and heat intolerance equals hyperthyroidism. Large liver, bronzed skin, and diabetes equals hemochromatosis. Polyuria, polydipsia, and polyphagia equals diabetes mellitus.

Errors may occur if more than one disease can cause a cluster. Although right *upper* quadrant pain, tenderness, rigidity, and fever are almost always caused by acute cholecystitis, the same tetrad in the right *lower* quadrant may signify acute appendicitis, acute pelvic inflammatory disease, perforated cecal carcinoma, or regional ileitis.

If you must formulate your own cluster in a particular patient, decide if all of the symptoms and signs in the cluster apply to a single diagnosis or to several. Make sure you are not dealing with two or more simultaneous diseases. The cluster components should be clearly related, if not by region or system, then by pathophysiologic or chronologic sequence.

Pattern Recognition

This method allows you to make a diagnosis with a single glance. If you were to see Abraham Lincoln on the street, you would know him at once. You would not analyze his eyes, hair, nose, and mouth separately. In the same way, you can instantly identify your friends without consciously knowing the color of their eyes or hair. It is the overall pattern that counts. This is recognition by *gestalt*.

Many diagnoses are made this way. For ex-

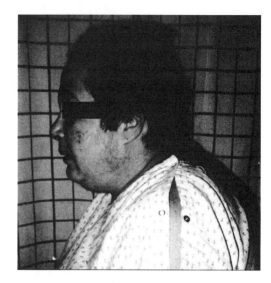

▶ **Figure 3.2.** Cushing's syndrome. Note central obesity, facial acne, hirsutism, and buffalo hump.

ample, an elderly man with an oily expressionless face and a coarse tremor shuffles into your office with small steps, bent over, his arms and legs slightly flexed. You recognize Parkinson's disease by one look. There is no mistaking it, provided you have seen it before and have the picture in your mind. The recognition of myxedema, acromegaly, Cushing's syndrome, and Turner's syndrome occurs in the same way (Figs. 3.1, 3.2).

Mitral stenosis can be diagnosed similarly by a single "listen." You do not have to analyze each of the six or seven separate auscultatory findings and put them together. Just place the bell of your stethoscope over the apex and listen to the song of mitral stenosis. It's diagnostic. You should know it and recognize it as readily as the "Star-Spangled Banner." The gestalt of a melody is distinct from its separate notes.

Syndromes

A syndrome is a concurrence of manifestations seen together often enough to be more than a chance relationship. This group of clues may simply be part of a disease, may be seen in a number of diseases, or may be a disease itself. There are well in excess of a hundred syndromes, and if you spot one, you may be well on your way to the final diagnosis.

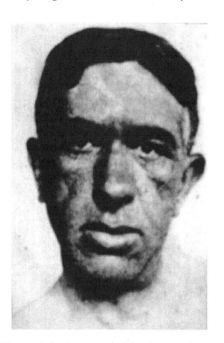

▶ **Figure 3.1.** Acromegaly. Note large and coarse facial features.

Let's describe three well-known syndromes. The first—**Kartagener's syndrome**—is a rare embryologic anomaly of unknown cause. It consists of sinusitis, bronchiectasis, and situs inversus. The **nephrotic** syndrome consists of a triad of edema; at least 3.5 g of albumin per 24-hour urine collection, and hypoalbuminemia (serum albumin of 3.0 g/dL or less); and hyperlipidemia. This syndrome is relatively common and is seen in association with many types of kidney disease as well as with some generalized diseases (see Case 58, Chapter 17). **Horner's** syndrome results from destruction of or infringement on the superior cervical sympathetic chain by a spinal cord lesion, an aortic aneurysm, or lung cancer. It consists of ptosis, myosis, enophthalmos, and anhidrosis on one side of the face.

The Key Clue

When various clues do not form a definite cluster, do not seem to relate, or are nonspecific in nature, you may not know where to begin. You must look for a *key clue* that is known to occur in a specified variety of clinical situations and track it down by seeking further information.

For example, if the patient has weakness, fatigability, nausea, and weight loss, all symptoms are so nonspecific as to be unsuitable for the focus of a search. However, if the same patient also has an enlarged abdomen caused by ascites, you can begin to search for the causes of ascites—cirrhosis, nephrosis, and metastatic cancer. More will be said about key clues in Chapter 4.

A *pivotal clue* is the linchpin around which hypotheses are formed and diagnoses are made in very complicated cases. The case may present hundreds of bits of information that need evaluation and aggregation, but from these you may be able to select a few that add up to a tableau, such as:

- Diffuse lung disease characterized mainly by a diffusion defect in a 48-year-old man
- Diabetes insipidus in a 58-year-old woman who has anorexia and weight loss
- Coagulopathy in a 48-year-old woman who is receiving treatment for breast cancer
- Malabsorption syndrome in a 60-year-old man who has had previous abdominal surgery

Each of these patterns serves as a pivot across which the problem solver can move from a large group of symptoms and signs to a manageable list of possible diagnoses.

Forming a Differential

Whether you start with an initial concept, a key clue, a cluster of clues, or a pivotal point, you must eventually form a list of possible causes for the patient's chief complaint—the *differential diagnosis*.

This list is similar to, although different from, the problem list. Whereas the problem list includes all of the medical, social, and psychologic problems the patient has or may have, the differential diagnosis includes all of the medical diseases that may possibly explain the patient's chief complaint or principal problem.

For example, in a patient who is vomiting blood and is known to have migraine and to be diabetic, the problem list might read: (1) hematemesis, (2) diabetes mellitus, (3) migraine, (4) recent divorce, and (5) poverty. On the other hand, the differential diagnosis for the chief complaint might read: (1) peptic ulcer; (2) cirrhosis with bleeding esophageal varices; and (3) acute hemorrhagic gastritis, and so on.

Most of the time, a differential diagnosis is simple and easy to form; it may include only two or three possibilities. Often it is more lengthy, and as you acquire more knowledge and gain more experience, you can generate a diagnostic list for each complaint, key clue, or cluster. You can consult one of numerous textbooks that are symptom-oriented, or you can read the differential diagnosis subheads in textbooks that are disease-oriented.

Usually, the differential diagnosis includes diseases that are limited to one organ or one system—sometimes to two. But if the problem is such as to implicate diseases from one of many possible organs or systems, the medical novice may not be able to form an *all-inclusive list*. The illness may remain undiagnosed because it wasn't considered. An effective system for avoiding such an oversight is to construct a differential diagnosis that has been selected out of the classification of disease categories that follows:

1. Infectious
2. Neoplastic
3. Endocrine-metabolic
4. Neuropsychiatric
5. Special organs (heart, lung, kidney, gastrointestinal)

6. Connective tissue and autoimmune
7. Hematologic
8. Genetic
9. Traumatic
10. Nutritional
11. Iatrogenic and drug-induced

Suppose you are confronted by a patient with long-standing fever and must formulate a list of diagnostic possibilities. By going through the previous categories one by one, you select tuberculosis, bacteremia, occult abscess, and enteric fevers from category 1; occult carcinoma from category 2; none from categories 3 or 4; infective endocarditis, cirrhosis, and regional enteritis from category 5; systemic lupus erythematosus from category 6; leukemia and lymphoma from category 7; none from categories 8, 9, or 10; and drug-induced fever from category 11. Each condition may cause fever with little else in the history. Now you have a good working list. Similar broad presentations can be managed in the same way.

After the differential diagnosis has been established, you must prove one diagnosis and eliminate the others, using the various other maneuvers described elsewhere in this chapter.

Suppression of Information

This diagnostic technique is used when a plethora of information is presented. The patient may offer excessive details, starting way back from early childhood. The story may be accurate, but the details can becloud the main issue, and the picture may be so smoggy that you cannot see the real clues. You must be able to separate pertinent data from unrelated information, just as you would tune out the rest of the orchestra if you wanted to concentrate only on the melody of the oboe.

Particular attention must be given to the psychoneurotic patient who often has a large number of positive symptoms and may answer yes to every question. Organic disease may be buried in a mound of affirmative answers, and it takes added skill to separate the psyche from the soma. In this case, suppression of unrelated information may be a required problem-solving technique.

Hunch and Intuition

At this point, the diagnostician becomes less than scientific. A *hunch* is a premonition or suspicion—a feeling—that something is so. It is not a stab in the dark or a mere guess. There is more to it than that. Usually, it is an educated deduction made almost subconsciously on the basis of a single observation—a bit of seemingly unimportant information mentioned by the patient, a facial expression, perhaps an odor—coupled with a case seen or read about the previous week. A hunch stands somewhere between a guess and intuition in degree of certainty. Hunches can often be wrong, but the more experience and knowledge the physician has, the more apt his or her hunches are to be right.

Intuition, on the other hand, is often regarded as a mystical process, but it is based on more solid evidence than is a hunch. The dictionary defines intuition as the "direct perception of a truth or fact independent of any reasoning process." Or it is defined as a cognition obtained or conclusion reached without recourse to conscious inference, reasoning, or reflection, as if it were a magical insight or gifted instinct.

Medical intuition may not be so abstract as definers would have us believe. It is probably the product of multitudinous messages transmitted across the vast neurochemical network linking memory, thought, knowledge, experience, judgment, and horse sense. The intuitive process may be a complex, highly intellectual skill that arises from the finest assembly of microcomputers that ever was or ever will be built—the human brain.

One does not intuit a judgment, decision, diagnosis, or treatment by pulling a rabbit out of a hat, no matter how instinctive or spontaneous the action may seem. Instead, such performances result from many *conscious and subconscious* mathematical calculations and psychologic transactions.

The intuitive decision to perform a test depends on quick evaluations of the operating characteristics of the test, the need for elevating or lowering the disease probability, the cost-risk-benefit factors, time-emergency elements, and the availability and skill of the test performer. And on these bases, the physician may say "do the test."

Symptomless Disease

Today, when so many routine examinations are being done and when complete chemistry profiles are generated for no matter what illness, numerous situations exist wherein problems are discovered that are not yet causing symptoms. In many cases, the patient may be symptomatic for one illness, consult the physician for that reason, yet may be found to have other unrelated problems.

For instance, there may be an abnormality in the urine, blood, radiograph, ECG, or physical examination. No symptoms are present, yet serious disease may exist. A high serum uric acid warrants a second look at the history for joint pains, kidney stones, or a family history of gout. Or a small infiltrate is noted on the annual chest radiograph. The blood count discloses marked lymphocytosis. A murmur is discovered by the school physician. Each of these findings deserves investigation.

More and more, asymptomatic problems are being encountered in practice. Common examples include albuminuria, glycosuria, pyuria, leukocytosis, anemia, polycythemia, hyperglycemia, hepatomegaly, splenomegaly, hyperglycemia, hypercalcemia, increased alkaline phosphatase levels, and radiographic or electrocardiographic abnormalities. Several examples of such presentations and their solutions are portrayed in Cases 2 and 8 (Chapter 12); Case 18 (Chapter 13); Case 23 (Chapter 14); and Case 33 (Chapter 15) of Section 2. How to solve them? Each presents its own challenge—no symptoms, possibly some physical findings, yet a definite abnormality! The physician must know or look up the various causes of the abnormality and proceed from there, using any or many solving techniques. Usually he or she eliminates the possibilities one by one and proves the existence of only one. Then again, he or she may remain in doubt, choose to wait and observe, or opt for a consultation as with any problem.

Rashes, Lumps, and Bumps

Here the patient consults the doctor because of a discrete abnormality that is seen or felt. A rash may be simply solved, yet may be an omen of an underlying disease. Often the patient notices a lump or bump under the skin, in the neck, or in the breast. Sometimes a mass or protrusion is felt in the abdomen.

Each finding presents its own differential di-

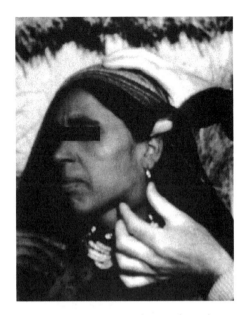

▶ **Figure 3.3.** Examining a lump in the neck.

agnosis. In all cases, the abnormality must be carefully examined, and associated symptoms must be sought. Ultimately, the diagnosis may depend on biopsy and imaging procedures.

Neck lumps require especially careful examination because they may represent congenital rests, cysts, tumors, metastatic cancer, or lymph nodes that could be tuberculous (Fig. 3.3). Most lumps will require a meticulous examination and evaluation as was done in Case 7 (Chapter 12); Case 12 (Chapter 13); and Case 66 (Chapter 18) in Section 2.

In the abdomen, serious consideration must be given to cysts, tumors, cancers, and enlarged or displaced organs such as the liver, spleen, kidney, pancreas, and colon.

Tactics with Clues

In order to prove or disprove a hypothesis, additional clues from the history, physical examination, and ancillary studies must be entered into the clinical setting by a series of maneuvers.

Pattern building is a device whereby positive clues are added until a picture that is suggestive of the suspected disease is constructed. If highly sensitive clues are present, the disease is likely; if highly specific clues are present, the disease is virtually certain to be present.

Template matching is another similar tactic. You must know the entire clinical picture of the suspected diagnosis and the features of the patient's data base, then build the clues into an architectural pattern that coincides with the textbook template as closely as possible. The match does not have to be perfect. There may be only a family resemblance.

When you are not sure that a diagnosis is correct, yet many clues point in that direction, you might say that the *weight of evidence* is in favor of the diagnosis. As more positive clues are found, the weight increases. Five positives are heavier than three. Also, the more sensitive the clues, the heavier the combined weight. If a highly specific clue is present, no additional weight is needed, and the diagnosis is confirmed.

On the other hand, a contending diagnosis may be excluded or ruled out if highly sensitive clues are absent or if the results of a highly sensitive test are negative. A normal pulse rate virtually excludes hyperthyroidism. A normal urinalysis rules out acute glomerulonephritis. The absence of anorexia and abdominal tenderness tends to exclude acute appendicitis.

Algorithms

An algorithm is a printed format that uses a branching pattern to solve problems. Given a chief complaint or key clue, the graphic structure of the algorithm represents a plan for the collection of data. From these data, the user is guided logically through a predetermined branching sequence of steps needed to make a decision. A characteristic feature of the algorithm is that the result of one test or one piece of information allows you to eliminate large chunks of the overall structure and directs you to follow only one path. Thus, your line of inquiry is diverted to one pathway as if by a switch at a railway junction point (Fig. 3.4).

Algorithms substitute symbols, lines, directions, and strategies for detailed language, thereby acting like a Michelin guide that methodically tells you where to stay, where to go, and what to do.

Should it be determined at the first decision

Algorithm

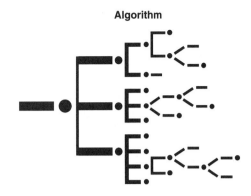

▶ **Figure 3.4.** Prototype algorithm.

point that a patient with anemia has a hypochromic microcytic anemia, you need only pursue the diagnostic plan for that type of anemia, and you may exclude all other lines of inquiry. Follow the track that obtains data referable to blood in the stool and abnormal vaginal bleeding. On the other hand, knowing the type of anemia that exists, you would not steer the course for macrocytic anemias, nor would you seek information referable to malnutrition, malabsorption, gastric acidity, vitamin B_{12} absorption, and B_{12}/folate blood levels (Fig. 3.5).

In time, algorithmic pathways become indelibly imprinted in the minds of good clinicians, and a medical problem immediately conjures up a seemingly instantaneous plan.

The principal values of algorithms are that they teach the student, help the practitioner to think and decide, improve patient care, decrease the cost of medical care, act as consultants, and make chart audit easier. Students read and understand algorithms better and faster than prose.

Although physicians should be able to collect information properly, act logically, and make appropriate decisions, this is not always the case, and algorithms may be of value there, too. There is abundant evidence that common conditions like diabetes, hypertension, and urinary tract infections are improperly handled; algorithmic guidelines might help. And in this era of computerized everything, algorithms are ideally structured for computerization and may thus be recalled for any of the aforementioned purposes.

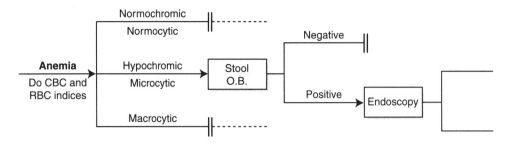

▶ **Figure 3.5.** Algorithm for the solution of an anemia. ‖ indicates no further need for tests.

Flowcharts

These printed aids guide the reader through a labyrinth of questions with "yes" or "no" answers until an endpoint is reached. You start with a presenting picture or key clue and go to *question 1.* Yes or no answers lead you along different lines of questioning. By following the *arrows* you should reach a conclusion that may vary from "*go to flowchart 2*" to "*re-examine in 1 month*" to "*consult surgeon*" to "*diagnosis A.*" (Fig. 3.6).

The same pros and cons are true for both flowcharts and algorithms. Although they may be of help in selected instances, they should not be relied on too heavily. Perhaps their greatest use lies in teaching. Printed flowcharts should not be regarded as a problem-solving panacea! They are little more than prefabricated dendrograms that serve as recipes for a mindless cook. They may inhibit independent thinking and are often so intricate as to require a road map and compass.

Good physicians generate their own flowchart every time they see a patient and solve a problem. They should not have to follow printed pathways. But for the physician who needs help, the student who seeks guidance, and the problem which is unusual, they may be of value.

Data Paths

This is a pathway that is constructed by the experienced problem solver. When facing a diagnostic problem, rather than collect information in a traditional way, it is often helpful to follow an efficient trail by asking a limited number of questions, examining a few areas, and getting a minimum number of tests. He or she must know in advance the specific bits of information that must be obtained to solve the particular problem.

Consider a 28-year-old man who develops acute nonarticular arthritis of the knee. The two dominant initial hypotheses are *gout* and *acute suppurative arthritis.* The clinician will acquire pertinent information in a sequence that is for him or her reasonably fixed for this problem. The order and line of inquiry is: (1) urethral discharge; (2) previous episodes; (3) history of new sexual contact; (4) examination of vital signs, ears (for tophi), joints (for inflammation), and urethra (for discharge); (5) obtaining serum uric acid level;

Chief Complaint

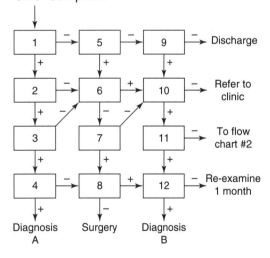

Simplified Flow Chart
question 1–12
answers   + (yes)   – (no)

▶ **Figure 3.6.** Sample flowchart.

(6) Gram's stain of urethral discharge, if present; and (7) examination of joint aspirate for bacteria, white blood cells, and urate crystals. These limited numbers of steps should establish a diagnosis (see Case 67, Chapter 19).

Decision Trees

A *decision tree* is a modified algorithm that depicts the various options and outcomes of a clinical situation that requires a decision. The decision tree tells you with *mathematical precision* what can happen if you go in one direction rather than in another. This sophisticated field aims to combine scientific, ethical, and personal considerations within a framework that permits the physician and patient to make a wise choice.

You can start with a clinical situation requiring a decision that usually revolves around (1) whether to test or treat, (2) which treatment has the best outcome, and (3) risk-cost-benefit analysis. In constructing the tree, you must deal with the probability that the disease exists, the treatment options, a test's sensitivity and specificity, and the morbidity and mortality for each option, as well as with a mathematical representation of expected outcomes.

For example, given a patient who has had what you think may be a pulmonary embolus—$P(D) = .50$—should anticoagulant drugs be given? What will be the outcome if you do or if you don't? Is there a test with known sensitivity and specificity that can raise the level of diagnostic certainty? Is there an alternate treatment, and what will be its outcome? Structure the risks and benefits into the tree. You may include branches that deal with the added risk of coincident hypertension and denote outcomes such as hemorrhage, re-embolization, success, and death (see Chapter 7 for a structure of a prototype decision tree).

Computers

The various roles for computers in medicine are well known. Here we are concerned only with those computer capabilities that enable us to solve medical problems, thus implicating the computer's functions in medical information storage, patient data processing, mathematical manipulations, and artificial intelligence.

To help the clinician find out what disease the patient has, the computer must be able to match the patient's symptoms and signs with its stored data base, and thereafter suggest diagnostic likelihoods, treatment, requests for additional information, and prognosis.

The question is whether or not computerized mathematical and statistical models manipulated by a machine can perform a better job than the human diagnostician.

It would seem on the surface that a computer system—with data acquisition, data display, instant recall, perfect memory, and arithmetical powers—should be an ideal tool for the application of high technology to diagnosis. But a computer has only one organ of communication; it cannot yet think, and it cannot mimic the sacred and subtle interaction between doctor and patient.

For the moment, although there are innumerable computer programs with meaningful acronyms, each covering a microcosm of medical diagnosis and management perhaps at least as well as an average clinician, there is as yet no effective program for the macrocosm of medical decisions that physicians can use on a regular basis.

CONCLUSIONS

Numerous problem-solving techniques have been described, and examples have been given. Many of these techniques are practical methods used daily by the physician. Some are variations on a single theme. Others have only limited value. Most decisions and diagnoses are straightforward and simple and require only a limited number of thought processes.

For the patient whose clues cannot be quickly clustered or in whom a key clue cannot be easily found, it is best to proceed in the traditional way. Gather a complete data base, block by block. Seek out the clues, synthesize them into diagnostic possibilities, and then prove your hypotheses. Although this method is lengthy, it is thorough and often necessary.

But for most cases, a key clue is easily identified, or the quick formation of a cluster, syndrome, or pattern is possible. Then a hypothesis is rapidly generated and proved via a selective search of the data base. This remains the most commonly used, speediest, and most practical method of problem solving.

Various styles of mathematical and schematic thinking such as Set Theory, Boolean algebra, and Venn diagrams are designed to help you think clearly and develop your logic, but these tools do not solve problems. Therefore, they are not included in this chapter. But Bayes' theorems are most helpful because playing the odds, probabilities, and statistics greatly influence our selection of the most likely diagnosis. These concepts were introduced in this chapter, but they will be more fully explained in Chapter 7. Algorithms and flowcharts offer help in selected instances. Computers have yet to find and establish their rightful place, but there is no doubt their role will increase.

Clues: The Building Blocks

Paul Cutler

A clue can be defined as a bit of information that seems to guide or direct in the solving of a mystery or in the solution of a problem. The principal clues you seek in a medical data base are found in the history, physical examination, and paraclinical studies. Mostly, clues reside in the history. And because clues are the basic elements upon which many of the subsequent diagnostic steps depend, their various types and properties will be reviewed.

TYPES OF CLUES

Positive Clues

A clue obtained from the history is *positive* if it is present and abnormal: "weakness." A clue found in the physical examination is positive if it is abnormal: "uremic frost." The result of a test or procedure is positive if it is abnormal: "serum creatinine, 6.0 mg/dL."

Positive clues in any history include such symptoms as chest pain, dyspnea, cough, chills, indigestion, abdominal pain, or anything of which a patient complains, as well as items excerpted from the rest of the history that may be related: "mother died of breast cancer at age 48." Positive clues in the physical examination include findings such as a carotid bruit, heart murmur, basal rales, enlarged liver, and a nodular prostate gland. Laboratory abnormalities are clearly flagged on the printed report—anemia, leukocytosis, hyperuricemia, and so forth.

The payoff of a positive clue can be dramatized by the following scenario for a patient who complains of repeated bilateral nosebleeds. There are thousands of known medical diseases, only 12 of which are characterized by such nosebleeds. A positive history directs you to only 12 diseases while it eliminates thousands. The absence of nosebleeds tends to exclude only 12 possibilities. Thus, the diagnostic power of a positive clue in this case is several hundred times greater than a negative clue. Every clinician knows this as he or she instinctively seeks positive data.

Of the 12 diseases with nosebleeds, large lymph nodes are present in only four. If these two clues are positive, the diagnostic field is considerably narrowed. Thousands of diseases in which these clues do not coexist are ruled out as you reduce the possibilities to a finger count.

You must always search for clues that are known to be positive in a suspected disease. The more positive clues there are, the more likely the disease. If most known positive clues are not present, the less likely it is that the particular disease is present.

Consider a clue that is positive in every case of a suspected disease (100% sensitivity); if the clue is not present, the disease is ruled. More commonly, a clue is present in 20, 50, or even 90% of cases, in which events it will be absent in 80, 50, or 10% of cases of the disease in question.

Negative Clues

Negative clues include items in the medical data base that are either not present or are normal. For example, the patient does not have any chest pain; there is no cough; the neck veins are not distended; there are no heart murmurs; the chest radiographic findings are normal; and the sequential multiple analysis-20 results are normal.

Negative clues may sometimes be as important as positive ones. Take the case of a patient who is complaining of shortness of breath on exertion and in whom you are trying to decide between chronic lung disease and congestive heart failure. The presence of cough and expectoration makes you lean toward the former, and the absence of both distended neck veins and an enlarged heart with murmurs tends to exclude the latter.

It seems that negative clues serve best to eliminate or rule out diagnostic possibilities. The fact that something is absent may be a strong indicator that a particular disease in question does not exist.

When a student or intern presents a case on rounds or reads a case report in a journal, a list of *pertinent negative findings* usually follows the chief complaint and history of present illness. These allegedly important negative findings may sometimes be stated in the systems review. Obviously, they are inserted for a very good and logical reason. On the basis of the chief complaint and history of present illness, certain provisional hypotheses have already been formed; the negative findings are stated in order to rule out or negate some of the competing hypotheses.

Take the case of a 64-year-old man who has had a cough, expectoration, and exertional dyspnea for 2 weeks. A long list of negatives follows, and each has special significance: there is no history of chills, fever, night sweats, weight loss, anorexia, chest pain, hemoptysis, leg pains, peripheral edema, recent travel, or exposure to industrial dusts or toxins. The patient does not smoke and never did, does not frequent caves for fun, and has no family pets.

This list provides a wealth of information. On the basis of the initial clinical picture, many diagnostic possibilities exist. Each negative statement tends to exclude one or more possibilities. The absence of chills, fever, and night sweats points away from pneumonia or tuberculosis. No anorexia, no weight loss, no chest pain, and no hemoptysis are all points against tuberculosis and direct you away from lung cancer. The fact that the patient has never smoked also goes a long way toward excluding lung cancer. No chest pain, no hemoptysis, no leg pains or leg edema, as well as no recent prolonged travel tend to exclude the possibility of pulmonary emboli. No recent travel also weighs against the presence of pulmonary fungal diseases, which are endemic to the Far West, the Southwest, and the Ohio-Mississippi basins (coccidioidomycosis and histoplasmosis). The statement that the patient does not frequent caves where the spores in bat droppings might spread similar diseases also weighs

against pulmonary disease. Furthermore, he has not worked in a coal mine, cotton mill, sugar cane mill, asbestos plant, and so on, where toxic inhalants can cause lung problems. The absence of family pets excludes the presence of sick or healthy psittacine birds and cats that may transmit lung infections.

When you read a list of pertinent negative findings on teaching rounds, you must be sure you understand the significance of each item, and not simply read a list that may have been written by a house officer. A similar list of pertinent negative findings may be extracted from the physical examination and laboratory data. These negative clues do not tell you what diseases the patient has, but they help tell you what diseases the patient does *not* have. You should always be prepared to defend and explain your list of pertinent negatives.

Negative clues may also tell you how far a disease has progressed. If carcinoma of the stomach is suspected from the history, it is important to note that there are no palpable supraclavicular lymph nodes, that the liver is not enlarged, and that the patient is not pale. In this instance, these negative clues denote that if stomach cancer does indeed exist, at least there is so far no physical evidence of metastases or much blood loss.

Key Clues

The principal or key clue may be a symptom, a sign, or a laboratory abnormality. Most of the cases in Chapters 12 to 22 revolve around the progressive steps that lead from a key clue to a diagnosis. Common key clues in the history include various visual disturbances, pain anywhere, shortness of breath, cough, difficulty in swallowing, indigestion, diarrhea, blood in the stool or urine, joint swelling, rash, itch, and so forth. Each clue prompts you to think of or look up a specific list of causes, and conjures up a unique approach to solving the problem.

Prominent physical findings that may serve as key clues include hemianopsia, large lymph nodes, large liver, large spleen, mass in the abdomen, pallor, jaundice, ascites, enlarged heart, murmur, rales, and so on.

Salient laboratory clues include anemia (see Cases 1, 2, 9 in Chapter 12); polycythemia (see

Case 8 in Chapter 12); leukocyte abnormality; low platelet count (see Case 3 in Chapter 12); elevated alkaline phosphatase level; eosinophilia; and many others. Each clue can serve as a departure point.

Decisive Clues

A clue that leads the problem solver directly and decisively to the correct diagnosis is often found in the family history, the social history, or the patient profile, and it is not uncommon to find this clue in the initial laboratory work-up.

The patient with a bleeding disorder may tell you of a similar illness in her mother (see Case 3, Chapter 12). A diagnosis of infective endocarditis may not be considered until the telltale needle tracks are noted over the veins of the forearm. The patient who has a poultry farm may have histoplasmosis as the cause of his diffuse pulmonary disease.

Although some tests, like the erythrocyte sedimentation rate and alkaline phosphatase, are not specific and merely tell you something is amiss, others point directly to the correct diagnosis. A blood glucose of 500 mg/dL completes the picture in a patient with polyuria and polydipsia—diabetes mellitus. A serum calcium of 13 mg/dL explains flank pain and hematuria in an otherwise healthy patient—parathyroid adenoma (see Case 19, Chapter 13). And a small apical infiltrate solves the problem of anorexia, cough, and low-grade fever—tuberculosis.

Primary and Secondary Clues

When trying to form a composite picture of a disease, you may be misled by clues that don't seem related but really are. *Primary clues* are those that are related to the disease process in situ. *Secondary clues* occur at a distant site and are pathophysiologically related.

For example, cough and hemoptysis are primary clues for carcinoma of the lung. Secondary clues might be hemiparesis from a cerebral metastasis, clubbing of the fingers, thrombophlebitis in the legs, or hyponatremia, as well as other bizarre and unexplained manifestations.

You may think that there are several problems when there is really only one.

False Clues

There are many instances in which a clue is found that could be related to the clinical picture, but is not. Because a substantial number of elderly patients have gallstones, the finding of stones on radiograph or ultrasound does not necessarily explain the patient's indigestion or abdominal pain. The symptoms may result from an occult carcinoma or another disease. No wonder so many gallbladders are removed, yet symptoms persist (see Case 43, Chapter 16).

A large heart seen on radiograph may not explain the patient's dyspnea if he or she is not in congestive failure, but the patient may also have coexistent chronic obstructive pulmonary disease (COPD) that does explain it.

Hypertrophic osteoarthritis of the spine seen on radiograph is a common finding in asymptomatic people. It cannot be assumed that this condition is the cause of every kind of pain or discomfort starting in the back and radiating to the sides, front, or legs.

A retroverted uterus is often unjustifiably blamed for many more symptoms than it should be, and "low blood pressure" is another common scapegoat.

ADVICE FOR THE CLUE SEEKER

Relationships Between Clues

Two clinical clues may be *independent, interdependent,* or *mutually exclusive.* For example, carcinoma of the lung can cause hemoptysis or chest pain, depending on whether the lesion is eroding a blood vessel or a rib. The two consequences are independent of each other.

Interdependence is noted in the case of patients having both diabetes and hypertension. Because diabetes is said to exist in 5% of adults, and hypertension in 20%, you would expect both to exist in 1% of adults—the product of the individual probabilities—if the two diseases were independent. But there must be a certain degree of interdependence, because more than double that number of adults have both diseases.

Certain clues may not ordinarily coexist. For example, good peripheral pulses and intermittent claudication are considered mutually exclusive. So, too, are loss of appetite and weight gain. Increased appetite and loss of weight might at first glance seem to be mutually exclusive, but remember that they may be seen together in hyperthyroidism where calories are rapidly used, in severe diabetes where calories are lost in the urine, and in malabsorption where calories are lost in the stool.

Pinpointing the Diseased Organ

Often a clue will point directly to the site of disease. Diarrhea implicates the intestines; jaundice points to the liver and biliary tract; pain usually locates the problem. But frequently the clue is not in a specific location, and symptoms like headache, fatigue, and anorexia are nonspecific and could result from a disorder in any one of many organs.

Chest pain can be caused by a handful of problems, but chest pain on exertion is a different story. Fatigue is nonspecific and can arise from psychosomatic as well as organic causes (see Case 61, Chapter 17). But, if in addition, the patient is pale and has epigastric tenderness, the problem localizes to the upper gastrointestinal tract—probably a duodenal ulcer. The presence of headache does not locate the problem, but if papilledema is also present, the lesion is in the brain.

When the Clue Does Not Fit

What about the case where one clue does not fit the picture or may even seem to negate your provisional hypothesis? How is this reconciled? First of all, the problem solver may be on the wrong track, and his or her supposition may be incorrect. Second, the clue may have been incorrectly obtained and must be rechecked for accuracy. Third, it may be part of a separate problem. And fourth, it could be "just one of those things."

For instance, suppose you have a patient with presumed hyperthyroidism who has, among other things, (1) a large thyroid and (2) evidence of hypermetabolism (tachycardia and tremor). He has a good appetite but has not lost weight as expected. The absence of weight loss does not fit the picture. Perhaps his appetite makes him eat so much that he has maintained or even gained

weight. On the other hand, he may have congestive heart failure too, and is therefore retaining fluid. Although weight loss is a prominent feature of hyperthyroidism, statistical studies show that it does not occur in all cases.

Even more perplexing, a single clue may be present that seems to contradict your diagnostic impression. This does not necessarily mean that you are wrong. All clinicians have seen occasional patients with congestive heart failure who can sleep flat; patients with duodenal ulcers that do not improve with alkali, antibiotics, or a histamine H_2-receptor antagonist; and patients who have endocarditis without murmurs. There may or may not be a good reason for these paradoxical situations. Diseases do not conform to textbook descriptions, patients react uniquely, and the combination of disease manifestations and patient responses is often unpredictable.

The Intersection of Clues

One more important issue. Suppose you have *two key clues that do not seem to relate,* and each has a separate list of causes. For instance, a 48-year-old woman has fatigue and chronic diarrhea plus peculiar weak, sweaty, nervous spells. Fatigue and diarrhea bring to mind six or seven different diseases. The weak, sweaty, nervous spells could be caused by hypoglycemia, menopause, pheochromocytoma, or simple anxiety. Are we dealing with two separate problems, or do both diagnostic lists have a common denominator resulting in one diagnosis? Careful thought and further data disclose that the patient has Addison's disease, which can cause weakness, diarrhea, and hypo-

TABLE 4.1. Intersection of Key Clues

FATIGUE AND DIARRHEA	WEAK, SWEATY NERVOUS SPELLS
Crohn's disease	Menopause
Ulcerative colitis	*Hypoglycemia
Amebiasis	Pheochromocytoma
Carcinoid	Anxiety-panic
*Addison's disease	Hyperthyroidism
Bacterial enteritis	Cocaine abuse
Malabsorption	

*Addison's disease causes both clusters.

glycemic episodes. One disease has caused both key clues. However, she could have had two separate diseases. Track down each key clue and determine if they intersect at a common diagnosis (Table 4.1).

Three Properties of Clues

It is critical to know three things about a clue: its sensitivity, its specificity, and its relative importance. All three factors count. The *sensitivity* of a clue in a disease is a quantitative statement of how often this clue is present in patients who have that disease. For example, the sensitivity of weight loss in hyperthyroidism is .96; this means that 96% of all patients with hyperthyroidism have weight loss; 4% of the patients don't. The more sensitive a clue is, the more its absence will exclude a disease. If the clue is always present, then its absence completely excludes the disease.

The *specificity* of a clue for a disease is a quantitative statement of the frequency with which that clue is *absent* in persons who do not have the disease. If a clue is 90% or .90 specific for a disease, it means that 90% of persons not having that disease do not exhibit the clue, and that the clue will be present (false-positive finding) in 10% of persons who do not have the disease. The more specific a clue, the more its presence will diagnose a disease, because false-positive findings would be rare.

Although weight loss is a highly sensitive clue for hyperthyroidism, it has very low specificity, because weight loss occurs frequently with many other diseases. On the other hand, Kayser-Fleischer rings are virtually 100% specific for Wilson's disease. They are also 100% sensitive. If present, the diagnosis is certain. If not present, the diagnosis is in grave doubt.

The *relative importance* of a clue is an indication of how significant a role the clue plays in the pathophysiology of the disease under consideration as well as the weight you attach to its presence or absence. For example, in hyperthyroidism, fine silky hair may not be important, but an enlarged thyroid and evidence of hypermetabolism are. In mitral stenosis, the malar flush and palpitations do not even remotely approach the significance of the auscultatory findings. If hepatitis is suspected, jaundice has more relative importance than anorexia or nausea because it points in the precise direction of the pathophysiology.

The *ideal clue* has an amalgam of high sensitivity, high specificity, and high relative importance. Such clues are rare.

Clues That Come and Go

The manifestations of a disease may be considerably altered by previous treatment. For instance, the patient who has severe congestive heart failure may have no edema because of the diuretics that have been given. On the other hand, the patient may have symptoms of hypokalemia imposed by those same diuretics.

The patient who has undiagnosed pernicious anemia may have received an injection of vitamin B_{12} in the recent past as part of indiscriminate therapy. The laboratory aspect of the clinical picture will change after only one injection of the vitamin.

The stage of the disease is important. In early chemical diabetes, the appetite is normal. If polyuria and thirst are present, the appetite is excessive. But when ketoacidosis supervenes, anorexia is the rule.

Sequential Clues

The relationship, timing, and sequence of events weights our logic. If two symptoms develop close together in time they are probably related. But the sequence is important. Consider the patient who becomes dyspneic on exertion and several weeks later has ankle edema. Congestive heart failure is likely, although COPD is possible. On the other hand, if edema precedes the dyspnea, you might think of cirrhosis or the nephrotic syndrome, where edema may occur first and pleural effusion perhaps later.

Leg pain followed by sharp chest pain suggests venous thromboembolism, whereas chest pain followed by leg pain suggests arterial thromboembolism—myocardial infarct with an embolus to the leg. The astute clinician, however, knows that the pain of pulmonary embolus may precede evidence of venous thrombosis in the lower extremity or that the latter may not be evident at all.

If a patient vomits blood, it is important to know if vomiting preceded or occurred simultaneously with the bleeding. If it preceded the bleeding, there may be an esophagogastric mucosal tear (Mallory-Weiss tear). If not, the vomited blood was probably from some other gastrointestinal source. Although one event followed by another often constitutes cause-and-effect relationship, beware of the *non sequitur*.

Three More Tips

First, symptoms occurring in the same system are apt to be related. If they occur in different systems, this may indicate the presence of two different diseases, a single multisystem disease, or diffuse spread of a single disease such as infection or cancer.

Second, the clinical picture of a single disease may be altered when another disease becomes superimposed. The diabetic patient who develops renal failure increases his or her glucose tolerance, which seems to cure the diabetes. Angina improves as claudication develops, because the patient cannot walk far enough to get chest pain. And the dyspnea and orthopnea of left ventricular failure improve when right ventricular failure supervenes and edema appears.

And third, there is the unusual situation where all clues point to a diagnosis that is statistically most likely and logically correct, yet the patient is found to have a diagnosis other than the expected one. Or the reverse happens; most clues point away from a particular diagnosis, which turns out to be the correct one. Unfortunately, this does occur from time to time and serves to humble even the most confident problem solver for whom it re-emphasizes that medicine and diagnosis are not precise sciences wherein mathematical problems can be solved by machines.

Quantitation of Clues

Not only may a clue be present or absent, but if present it may be necessary to determine to what degree the clue is present. Such quantitation may reflect directly on the diagnosis.

Just as systolic heart murmurs are graded on a scale from 1 to 6 and leg edema on a scale from 1 to 4, other clues need similar weights.

Claudication might be graded by the distance that can be walked before calf pain occurs—"one block claudication"—but the speed of walking, the length of steps, and different pain thresholds create immeasurable variables.

Angina is difficult to quantify. It is sometimes measured by occurrences per day or the number of nitroglycerine pills taken. But what about variables such as weather, emotional state, relationship to meals, duration, and severity of pain? And likewise, can the history taker attach numbers to the severity of abdominal pain, headache, insomnia, weakness, or anorexia?

Accurate quantitation of a clue—and qualitation, too—is usually of great value and is required not only for making the diagnosis, but also for determining the stage and severity of the disease, its prognosis, and its treatment.

SUMMARY

Because clues are the bedrock of the art and science of diagnosis, this chapter has aimed to present a detailed analysis of their various characteristics and properties. A clue may be positive, negative, contrary, organ-specific, primary, secondary, key, sensitive, specific, false, vanishing, sequential, or quantifiable.

Once a clue is completely evaluated, it may point immediately to the precise diagnosis; it may be attached to another clue or clues to form a workable cluster; or it may serve as a focal point for the formulation of a hypothesis or a differential diagnosis.

**Self-Evaluation Exercises
(Answers appear at the end of the exercises).**

1. Which *one* of the following has the greatest diagnostic weight in a single patient?
   (a) Splenomegaly
   (b) No splenomegaly
   (c) Enlarged lymph nodes
   (d) No enlarged lymph nodes
   (e) Neither spleen nor nodes enlarged
   (f) Both spleen and nodes enlarged
   (g) Fatigue and weakness
2. Two clues for a disease are 90 and 80% sensitive, respectively. Neither is highly specific. Which of the following has the greatest diagnostic significance?
   (a) Both clues present
   (b) Both clues absent

(c) One clue present

(d) One clue absent

3. Contrive such a clinical situation (see Question 2).

4. Select the *pertinent negative* clues: A 52-year-old man with a chronic cough and expectoration
   (a) Does not drink alcohol
   (b) Does not smoke
   (c) Does not drink coffee
   (d) Denies venereal disease
   (e) Has no shortness of breath
   (f) Has no hemoptysis
   (g) Has anorexia
   (h) Has weakness
   (i) Has weight loss
   (j) Has no contact history for tuberculosis
   (k) Has no family

5. A 42-year-old, extremely obese, 350-lb man has severe dyspnea on exertion, somnolence, and fatigue. The physical examination is normal except for obesity, a widely split S_2 with a very loud pulmonic component, and a presternal lift. What is the key pathophysiologic entity that will serve as a takeoff point for your diagnostic search? (Questions 6 and 7 refer to the same patient).

6. The patient has no cough or pulmonary abnormalities on examination. What kind of clues are these?

7. The PO_2 is low, and the PCO_2 is high. What does he have?

8. Select the *key clue* for a patient with weakness, weight loss, anorexia, and black stools. She stopped menstruating at 52 and now has dyspareunia and occasional burning on urination. She has had mild diabetes and hypertension for 10 years.

9. Select the *key clue:* A 60-year-old man has anorexia, weakness, weight loss, jaundice, and dark urine. The liver is enlarged as evidenced by percussion, but this enlargement cannot be confirmed by palpation. He smokes, takes medication for arthritis, eats raw seafood, and had an abdominal operation 1 year ago.

10. Select the *key clue:* For 3 weeks, a 28-year-old woman has had bloody diarrhea, weakness, easy fatigability, headaches, and feverish feelings. The abdomen is slightly distended and somewhat diffusely tender.

11. Form a pathophysiologic entity from which you may pursue a diagnostic quest: A 32-year-old woman delivers a child, has a severe postpartum hemorrhage, requires three blood transfusions, and over the next few days develops oliguria, nausea, weakness, and confusion.

12. Select the *key clue* for a patient who has mild nausea, anorexia, abdominal cramps, headaches, and irritability. Examination is normal, and laboratory results show normal electrolyte levels; blood glucose, 148 mg/dL; serum uric acid, 7.6 mg/dL; and 12000 white blood cells/mm³ of which 64% are polymorphonuclear leukocytes, 12% are lymphocytes, and 18% are eosinophils.

13. Which of the following is *not* a "scapegoat" clue (*false clue*)?
    (a) Retroverted uterus
    (b) Hypertrophic osteoarthritis of the spine
    (c) "Borderline anemia"
    (d) Blood pressure 90/60
    (e) Blood glucose at lower limit of normal
    (f) Serum calcium level 10% above upper limit of normal
    (g) "Calcium deficiency"

14. What is the sequence of pathophysiologic events?
    (a) Peritonitis
    (b) Albuminuria
    (c) Long-standing diabetes mellitus
    (d) Ascites
    (e) Hypoalbuminemia

15. What is the probable sequence of events in the following scrambled scenario?
    (a) Hemoptysis
    (b) Pneumothorax
    (c) Percutaneous lung biopsy
    (d) Chest radiograph
    (e) 60 pack-year cigarette history

Answers

1. (f)
2. (b): tends to exclude the disease
3. Many examples may be found. For instance, let the clues be dyspnea on exertion and rales, and the diagnostic consideration would be left ventricular failure.
4. (b), (e), (f), and (j)
5. Pulmonary hypertension
6. Pertinent negative clues. They tend to exclude chronic pulmonary disease as a cause of this patient's pulmonary hypertension.
7. Anoxia and hypercapnia—the pickwickian syndrome
8. Black stools
9. Jaundice
10. Bloody diarrhea
11. Acute renal failure
12. Eosinophilia
13. (f)
14. (c), (b), (e), (d), (a)
15. (e), (a), (d), (c), (b)

Data Resolution Skills

Paul Cutler

It is not an easy matter to decide whether two clues relate, whether a bit of information is relevant, or whether a finding should be ignored. To be an effective medical sleuth, you must be able to categorize every single item concerning the patient. For this, you need to have good *data resolution skills*.

Such skills include knowing:

- How to put things together
- Signs and symptoms of diseases
- Additional high-yield data needed to solve knotty problems
- Clues that exclude or confirm a diagnosis
- Subsets of data to be investigated for many common complaints

For example, you might need to know whether a single clue is evidence for, evidence against, or neither for nor against a suspected diagnosis. Also you might want to know if an additional piece of information is relevant, possibly relevant, or irrelevant to the chief complaint. Perhaps it is a pertinent negative clue. On the other hand, it may indicate the existence of a problem other than the principal one.

When you receive information about a patient, you must quickly decide what to do with it and where to categorize it. This chapter aims to sharpen your skills in this regard.

The methods to be used are: (1) the selection of data subsets for eight mini-cases, (2) the performance of relevance exercises involving three common medical presentations, and (3) the decoding of three problem sets.

In all instances, you will be asked to furnish the answers, then refer to the author's answers in the pages that follow, and compare your skills. Don't be surprised, disappointed, or chagrined if you disagree with the author. *Your answer* might be the correct one. At least the exercises will encourage you to think!

The numerous cases to be discussed in Section 2 give hundreds of examples of data evaluation. However, in the present chapter there are many small exercises that are designed to acquaint the reader with some special skills needed to process data, improve these skills, and prepare him or her for the more complex and detailed cases that follow in the next section.

Make sure that you try your own hand at the following exercises before seeking the author's answers. Course instructors may conceive additional mini-cases and ask their students to select special data subsets for each one. This type of exercise is particularly effective when students prepare such cases in small groups and then exchange their ideas in larger groups under instructor supervision.

SELECTING DATA SUBSETS

In the following exercises, only the initial statement is given. This includes the age, gender, and chief complaint. The reader will then be asked to: make a short list of the diagnostic contenders that could explain the initial statement; decide which questions might elicit the most valuable information; select the parts of the physical examination that will best further narrow the field; and choose the tests or procedures that are most likely to clinch the diagnosis.

Remember: first, do each case yourself, then read the author's logic!

Request only data that will be very productive and do not ask for useless information. Such exercises make you very selective in your search for clues and demand that you know exactly what you are looking for and how to find it. *The author's answer and his commentary follow at the end of the eight initial statements.* For each of the eight exercises, perform the following four steps:

1. List the differential diagnosis.
2. Ask three to seven questions.
3. Examine three to seven parts.
4. Decide which one to four tests will help the most.

CASE 1

*A 48-year-old woman who has had **swollen legs** for 2 weeks.*

CASE 2

*A 52-year-old woman who has noticed a **mass** in the left upper quadrant of 1 week's duration.*

CASE 3

*A 36-year-old woman who has just had her first **grand mal** seizure.*

CASE 4

*A 60-year-old man who has had **cough** and **expectoration** for 6 weeks.*

CASE 5

*A 46-year-old woman who has noticed an **enlarged thyroid** gland for the past 6 weeks.*

CASE 6

*A 68-year-old man with markedly **diminished vision** in his right eye.*

CASE 7

*A 58-year-old woman with a 2-week **discharge** from her left **nipple**.*

CASE 8

*A 12-year-old boy has noticed a **lump** in his right groin.*

ANSWERS TO SELECTING DATA SUBSETS

CASE 1

A 48-year-old woman who has had swollen legs for 2 weeks.

(1) *Differential diagnosis:* The differential diagnosis must include: (a) right ventricular failure and its various causes, (b) cirrhosis of the liver, (c) nephrotic syndrome, and (d) venous or lymphatic obstruction.

(2) *Questions to ask:* Productive questions will determine the presence or absence of (a) dyspnea on exertion, (b) heart disease or murmurs, (c) heavy alcohol ingestion, (d) previous hepatitis, (e) kidney disease, and/or (f) vein trouble.

(3) *Parts to examine:* Search for (a) cardiac enlargement or murmurs; (b) other evidence of right ventricular failure (distended neck veins, large tender liver, diffuse lung disease); (c) large, nontender liver and other stigmata of chronic liver disease; (d) an obstructing intrapelvic tumor; and (e) evidence of venous thrombosis (calf tenderness and positive Homans sign).

(4) *Tests to do:* Helpful studies include (a) chest radiograph for enlarged heart, pulmonary congestion, or chronic pulmonary disease that might cause right ventricular failure; (b) liver function tests (levels of serum albumin, transaminase, alkaline phosphatase, and bilirubin); (c) urinalysis for proteinuria; and (d) venogram or ultrasound of leg veins only if doubt exists.

Comment

It is important to note that the aforementioned list can be radically reduced if the answer to a question or the result of an examination leads you in one direction rather than another. For example, if this patient were a known severe alcoholic and had an enlarged liver, ascites, and palmar erythema, there would be no need for additional questions, examinations, and tests—except for completing the data base.

Or if the answers led you in the direction of heart failure, much less additional information would be needed. If there were no symptoms or signs of heart disease, this possibility could be excluded with a high degree of certainty. On the other hand, if the history and examination were fruitless, heavy albuminuria and hypoalbuminemia would point to the nephrotic syndrome, but not to the precise renal disease causing it.

But given a normal heart, liver, and kidneys, the pelvic examination and a variety of studies for deep vein patency are indicated.

The algorithmic principle by which we build on pieces of positive data to direct our further line of inquiry is a method commonly used by the problem solver.

CASE 2

A 52-year-old woman who has noticed a mass in the left upper quadrant of 1 week's duration.

(1) Possible causes are: (a) splenomegaly (lymphoma, leukemia, and so forth); (b) pancreatic pseudocyst; (c) kidney cyst, tumor, or hydronephrosis; (d) leiomyosarcoma of the stomach; and (e) carcinoma of the colon.

(2) High-yield questions revolve around: (a) how and when the mass was first noted (weight loss?); (b) general strength, fatigue, appetite; (c) history of recent severe abdominal pain suggestive of pancreatitis; (d) gallstone or alcohol ingestion history that may predispose the patient to pancreatitis; (e) bowel symptoms of colon cancer (blood in the stools, constipation, narrow stools); (f) urinary tract symptoms; and (g) easy satiety, hematemesis, or black stools that might correlate with a stomach mass.

(3) Examination should aim to: (a) locate, delineate, and characterize the mass, noting tenderness and mobility with respiration; (b) search for enlarged lymph nodes; and (c) detect anemia.

(4) Helpful studies include: (a) stool samples for occult blood; (b) complete blood count for anemia and leukocyte abnormalities; (c) urinalysis for renal disease; and (d) x-ray studies may be helpful and necessary; depending upon where previous data lead, you may need to order a plain abdominal radiograph, an intravenous pyelogram, a barium enema, a gastrointestinal series, a colonoscopy, a sonogram, and/or a computed

tomographic (CT) scan. A chest radiograph may detect metastases or hilar adenopathy.

Comment

Here, too, you may be immediately detoured into one line of reasoning by a single clue. If the mass moves with inspiration and is therefore thought to be the spleen, the patient is pale, and diffuse lymphadenopathy is present, a complete blood count alone may diagnose leukemia and conclude the search.

On the other hand, if the mass moves little and seems to arise in the kidney, and all of (2) and (3) are fruitless, a CT scan or sonogram might be the test to perform.

CASE 3

A 36-year-old woman who has just had her first grand mal seizure.

(1) Diagnoses should include: (a) idiopathic epilepsy, (b) drug withdrawal or overdose, (c) brain tumor, (d) insulinoma, and (e) meningitis.

(2) In the history, look for: (a) exact description of the preictal, ictal, and postictal state; (b) precise history of drug and alcohol ingestion; (c) headaches, visual disturbances, or other neurologic symptoms that suggest an expanding intracranial lesion; (d) fever; and (e) preceding trauma.

(3) Examinations include: (a) neurologic examination, including fundi; (b) temperature, nuchal rigidity, Kernig's and Brudzinski's signs for meningitis; (c) evidence of head trauma; and (d) track marks on arms.

(4) Tests include: (a) toxic drug screen, (b) electroencephalogram, (c) blood glucose levels, (d) insulin immunoassay, (e) lumbar puncture, and (f) x-ray skull and CT scan.

Comment

Most information and studies are not needed if a positive lead is obtained early. Track marks from stimulant drugs may obviate the need for further information. Fever and nuchal rigidity mandate a lumbar puncture, but little else. If there is suspicion of a brain tumor, even in the absence of any other positive clues, a dye-enhanced CT scan is the road to take.

But do not be trapped by fuzzy logic. For example, the fact that a sister has epilepsy does not exclude the patient from having meningitis. Diagnoses must be buttressed by harder evidence.

C A S E 4

A 60-year-old man who has had cough and expectoration for 6 weeks.

(1) Diagnoses to be considered are: (a) lung cancer, (b) tuberculosis, (c) chronic bronchitis, (d) chronic obstructive pulmonary disease, and (e) other parenchymal lung diseases.

(2) Historical data germane to the case include: (a) smoking history, (b) chronic exposure to toxic industrial pollutants, (c) occupational history, (d) recent respiratory tract infection that did not clear, (e) wheeze or dyspnea, (f) exposure to a tuberculous individual, and (g) description of sputum.

(3) Examine for: (a) clubbing of fingers, which would be suggestive of cancer; (b) detailed chest examination for rales, wheezes, consolidation, localized areas of disease, diaphragmatic excursion, and expiratory duration; and (c) supraclavicular hard lymph nodes.

(4) Essential studies include: (a) chest radiograph; (b) sputum examination for acid-fast bacilli and tumor cells; (c) fiberoptic bronchoscopy for washings and possible biopsy; and (d) pulmonary function tests for diagnosis.

Comment

The diagnosis should be clearly evident. If all findings in areas (3) and (4) are negative, suspect chronic bronchitis. Eschew conclusions like cancer on just the feeble evidence of a history of smoking. Don't be caught in a spider's web between tuberculosis and cancer unless biopsy results or bacteriologic proof is established. Evidence for serious disease must be robust. Detours that reach diagnoses quickly and eliminate the need for studies apply here, as in other cases.

C A S E 5

A 46-year-old woman who has noticed an enlarged thyroid gland for the past 6 weeks.

(1) Diagnostic considerations include: (a) simple goiter; (b) adenomatous thyroid hyperplasia (toxic or nontoxic); (c) subacute thyroiditis; (d) Hashimoto's disease (with or without hypothyroidism); and (e) carcinoma.

(2) Questions to be asked center around: (a) growth of the thyroid; (b) existence of pain, fever, or "sore throat"; (c) evidence of toxicity (heat intolerance, sweats, good appetite, weight loss, nervousness); and (d) clues for hypofunction (cold intolerance, sluggishness, skin changes, weight gain).

(3) Examine the: (a) thyroid for consistency, size, tenderness, and nodularity; (b) eyes for exophthalmos (and other related signs); (c) hands for fine tremor, skin for warmth and dampness, hair for fine silkiness; (d) facial features, hair, eyebrows, and skin for evidence of hypothyroidism; (e) pulse and blood pressure for indication of thyroid hypofunction or hyperfunction; and (f) reflexes for quick or late responses.

(4) From the supermarket of tests, you need choose only the thyroxine (T_4) and the thyroid-stimulating hormone (TSH) measurements to determine thyroid function. If medullary carcinoma is suspected, order a calcitonin radioimmunoassay as well as determination of levels of serum calcium and 24-hour urinary catecholamines to evaluate for possible multiple endocrine neoplasia (associated parathyroid adenoma and pheochromocytoma). Thyroid aspiration biopsy must be considered, too. High titers of antithyroglobulin antibodies confirm suspected Hashimoto's disease, and a very rapid erythrocyte sedimentation rate (ESR) goes along with subacute thyroiditis.

Comment

Thyroid palpation and patient inspection are paramount in diagnosis here. Cancer is usually a single mass, rarely diffuse. It would be a tour de force performance to find a Type II multiple endocrine adenomatosis; if medullary carcinoma is suspected, also look for other endocrine abnormalities. An enlarged thyroid without endocrine dysfunction most commonly signifies diffuse (possibly nodular) benign hyperplasia, simple goiter, or Hashimoto's disease. In all cases, a feel of the thyroid gland directs you to the correct line of inquiry.

C A S E 6

A 68-year-old man with markedly diminished vision in his right eye.

(1) One bit of information must precede all others, for it divides the tentative hypotheses into two separate groups. Did the poor vision come on slowly or rapidly? Because if the onset was slow, and the progression occurred over months to years, you should consider cataract, glaucoma, refractive error, retinitis pigmentosa, macular degeneration, and so forth. But if the vision diminished acutely over a time frame of seconds to days, you are in another ballpark. The latter situation occurred in this case. Therefore, consider: (a) retinal artery thrombosis or embolus; (b) retinal vein thrombosis; (c) retinal detachment; (d) cerebrovascular accident; (e) retinal or vitreous hemorrhage; (f) acute angle-closure glaucoma; and (g) optic neuritis (papillitis, retrobulbar).

(2) Other helpful historical hints are: (a) preceding flashing sensations indicative of retinal detachment; (b) pain with acute glaucoma; (c) history of previous vascular episodes; (d) other neurologic symptoms denoting a more widespread intracerebral vascular accident; (e) presence of diabetes or hypertension; and (f) painful eye movements, as seen in optic neuritis.

(3) Examination should be diagnostic. You may find: (a) high intraocular tension in a red eye if acute glaucoma exists; (b) characteristic ophthalmoscopic evidence of retinal artery occlusion, retinal vein thrombosis, detachment, or vitreous hemorrhage; (c) right carotid artery bruit or diminished right internal carotid pulsation if platelet aggregates have embolized to the retinal artery; (d) thickened tender temporal arteries if the retinal artery disease is part of the generalized arteritis of polymyalgia rheumatica; and (e) results of visual field studies that determine for certain whether the loss of vision is clearly in one eye or in one half of each eye (homonymous hemianopsia); in the latter instance, the lesion would be intracerebral.

(4) Other studies will be of little of value. Request an ESR determination if arteritis is suspected. Order a coagulation study if venous thrombosis has occurred. Visualize the carotid arteries with ultrasound, if warranted.

Comment

The crucial clues here are the rapidity of onset, presence or absence of pain, and visualization of the fundi. Because vision is poor, pupillary light reflexes will be sluggish, and the fundi will be easily seen. Optic neuritis is a diagnosis of exclusion and is unlikely at this age. Migraine can produce hemianopic prodromes. Although a presentation such as this is usually an ocular problem, it is important to recognize that it may be a local manifestation of a generalized disease.

CASE 7

A 58-year-old woman with a 2-week discharge from her left nipple.

(1) The possibilities are many; they include: (1) breast lesions, such as intraductal papilloma, carcinoma, and fibrocystic disease, as well as (2) a large number of endocrine problems. In the latter category belong prolactinomas, hypothalamic-pituitary disorders, hypothyroidism, ingestion of specific drugs, and the cessation of oral contraceptives.

(2) The type of discharge and involvement of one or both breasts are decisive bits of information. Inquire about or look at the discharge. If the discharge is watery, it may mean nothing. If it is *milky and bilateral,* the cause is endocrine. And if it is *bloody and unilateral,* the cause is neoplastic. Because this patient is 58, we need not inquire about oral contraceptives or menses, but do ask if the patient is taking reserpine, phenothiazines, or α-methyldopa—all of which are known lactogenics.

(3) Physical examination is directed primarily at the breast. Feel for fibrocystic disease. Search carefully for a breast lump, inspect the skin for dimpling or retraction, and meticulously feel the nipple and subareolar tissue. Then inspect the patient for stigmata of hypothyroidism or pituitary adenoma.

(4) Tests to be done depend on the direction that you are taking. If neoplastic disease is your prime choice because the discharge is unilateral and bloody, order mammography or computed tomography. Ductography may help, and open biopsy may be indicated. But if the discharge is bilateral and milky, and the above-mentioned obvious causes have been excluded, a search for intracranial or intrasellar tumor is indicated. This may necessitate a CT scan of the sella for a prolactinoma.

Comment

This is really a simple problem. The answers to two questions send you off on one quest or another.

C A S E   8

A 12-year-old boy has noticed a lump in his right groin.

(1) This could be a lymph node, an undescended testicle, or a hernia. It sounds simple.

(2) Questions to ask are: (a) How long has the lump been there? (b) Does it hurt? and (c) Does it go away when the paient is lying down and reappear when he is straining?

(3) Examine, locate, elicit, and describe the lump. Is there a testicle in the right scrotum? See if the lump disappears when the patient is lying down and reappears when he is standing or straining. Put your finger in the inguinal canal and have the boy cough. Search for other lymph nodes and splenomegaly.

(4) No studies should be necessary. If the possibility of a lymph node disorder exists, a complete blood count and biopsy may be indicated.

Comment

Most patients seen in the office or outpatient department are diagnosed as easily as the one just presented. A few questions and examination of one or two places will make the answer apparent. It may be necessary to exclude one or two unlikely contending diagnoses.

PERFORMING RELEVANCE EXERCISES

Initial statements about three different patients will be presented. Following each statement, a large number of individual bits of acquired information will be given. Decide whether each item per se, as it relates to the initial statement, is:

a. Relevant
b. Possibly relevant
c. Pertinent negative
d. Irrelevant
e. A separate problem

This is an exercise in data evaluation. After you have written your own answers and justified them in your mind, compare your thoughts with the author's logic that follows. Also compare your reasoning with the author's defense of each judgment. You may not be in agreement. If you can rationally relate a clue that the author could not, *you* may be correct. Give each item much thought and be able to justify your answer. *More than one answer may be applicable to each item.* Information derived from the history and physical examination will be stressed.

Your learning will be greatly enhanced if you do the exercises first yourself and then compare your reasoning with the author's. On an index card, make a list of relevance options (a)-(b)-(c)-(d)-(e). It will help you evaluate each bit of data without turning pages.

C A S E   1

Patient with Anemia

*A 66-year-old woman with **weakness** and **diffuse pallor** of 6 months' duration.*

This patient presents a common problem. You immediately consider a constellation of common causes that include primarily: malignancy somewhere, primary anemia, secondary anemia due to blood loss, diffuse granulomatous disease, and uremia from chronic renal failure.

You seek additional data to confirm or negate the tentative hypotheses. Although each separate item is considered here by itself, generally a bit of information is not evaluated in a vacuum. Its interpretation often hinges on previously collected data. For pedagogic reasons, this exercise deals only with the evaluation of single clues by themselves.

Evaluate the following pieces of data using the (a)-(b)-(c)-(d)-(e) scale just described (*see p. 50 for answers*).

1. Smokes 10 cigarettes daily
2. Drinks eight cups of coffee daily

3. Twenty-pound weight loss in last 3 months
4. No weight loss
5. Poor appetite
6. Good appetite
7. Considerable indigestion
8. Nonbleeding hemorrhoids
9. Bleeding hemorrhoids
10. Loose bowels for 2 months
11. Black stools noted occasionally
12. Menopause at age 48
13. No vaginal bleeding
14. Spleen palpable
15. Chronic worsening cough
16. Hemoglobin, 6 g/dL; red blood cell count, 3 million per mm^3
17. Slight jaundice present
18. Trachea in midline
19. Thyroid not palpable
20. Urinalysis normal
21. Aortic systolic grade 2 ejection murmur
22. Patient of Swedish extraction
23. Patient comes from California
24. Patient is black American
25. Does housework
26. Conjunctiva pale
27. Hematocrit, 35%; red blood cell count, 2.5 million per mm^3
28. Eats two trays of ice cubes daily
29. Severe backaches for 1 month
30. Backaches for 5 years
31. Very obese
32. Stools positive for occult blood
33. Stools negative for occult blood
34. Vaginal bleeding for 2 years
35. Vaginal bleeding after examination
36. Cholecystectomy 10 years ago
37. Frequent nosebleeds and bleeding gums
38. Lethargy and mental confusion
39. Mastectomy 1 year ago
40. Tongue pale but otherwise normal
41. Tongue red and sore
42. Blood pressure (BP) 130/80
43. BP 200/120
44. Sparse coarse hair
45. Albuminuria +4
46. Physical examination normal except for pallor
47. Fundi normal
48. Glycosuria +2
49. Leg paresthesias
50. No lymph nodes palpable

AUTHOR'S ANSWERS REGARDING THE PATIENT WITH ANEMIA

1. (d). Irrelevant
2. (d). Irrelevant
3. (a). This signifies underlying serious disease like cancer or lymphoma.
4. (c). This tends to deny malignancy.
5. (a), (b). This probably denotes serious disease, although anorexia is nonspecific.
6. (c). A good appetite speaks against serious disease.
7. (b). This might be related to a gastrointestinal ulcer or neoplasm that is slowly bleeding.
8. (d). This is not related unless it is the "sentinel pile" of colon cancer.
9. (a), (b), (e). This is possibly a separate problem, although it could be the cause of the patient's anemia.
10. (b), (e). This could signify colon cancer or malabsorption syndrome (not listed as a hypothesis), or it could be a separate problem.
11. (b). Truly black stools usually mean melena (blood in the stool) and testify to repeated episodes of gastrointestinal bleeding from a source above the midtransverse colon.
12. (d). Irrelevant
13. (c). This indicates there is no blood loss from the genital tract.
14. (a). A palpable spleen is an enlarged spleen, and when it occurs together with anemia, this finding strengthens the hypotheses of lymphoma or leukemia.
15. (a) or (b). Chronic pulmonary tuberculosis is possible, although its presentation is not primarily as an anemia.
16. (a). The anemia is hypochromic and suggests chronic blood loss.
17. (a), (b). Jaundice and anemia suggest hemolysis, or cancer with metastases to the liver.
18. (d). Irrelevant
19. (d). Irrelevant
20. (c). Uremia from renal failure almost invariably causes severe urine abnormalities (casts, albumin, and so forth).
21. (a), (e). The murmur could be a flow murmur resulting from chronic anemia, or it may be a separate problem.
22. (b), (d). Pernicious anemia is more common

in Scandinavians, but Swedes have other causes of anemia, too, so it may well be irrelevant.

23. (d). Irrelevant
24. (d). "Ethnic anemias" are not apt to appear at this age.
25. (c). Although weak and pale, she is still able to do housework.
26. (a). This merely confirms the visible pallor.
27. (a). The anemia is macrocytic, so pernicious anemia, folic acid deficiency, and so forth are suspected.
28. (b). Pagophagia is not uncommonly seen as a *result* of chronic iron deficiency anemia.
29. (b). This suggests a malignancy with spinal metastases.
30. (e). It is unlikely that backaches and anemia would be related for 5 years; myeloma or metastases would most likely have caused death before then.
31. (c), (d), (e). It is either unrelated, a separate problem, or may be considered a pertinent negative in that the patient seems not to have a disease that causes both weight loss and anemia.
32. (b). This very important finding, especially if persistent, suggests that the anemia results from chronic gastrointestinal blood loss.
33. (c). This negative finding weighs against chronic gastrointestinal blood loss, unless the lesion bleeds intermittently and you are testing only between bleeding episodes (an unlikely event).
34. (a), (b), (e). This very significant abnormality may well be the cause of the patient's anemia, but don't be lulled into complacency. There could be two unrelated problems here.
35. (d). Bleeding was probably caused by the examination, especially if no lesion was visualized.
36. (d). Irrelevant
37. (a), (b). This combination is highly suggestive of a bleeding disorder which, in turn, indicates a problem with red blood cell and platelet production (leukemia, myeloma, or bone marrow failure or replacement).
38. (a), (b), (e). Severe anemia can cause cerebral anoxia and mental symptoms. Pernicious anemia is notorious in this regard. This could be a separate problem resulting from one of many possible causes in a person of this age.

39. (b). The possibility of breast cancer metastases to the bone marrow must at least be considered.
40. (a), (c). This confirms evident pallor but weighs against primary anemias like pernicious anemia.
41. (a), (b). This finding suggests pernicious anemia, although it could also be a glossitis resulting from concomitant vitamin deficiencies (vitamin B or folic acid).
42. (c), (d). This finding is probably irrelevant, though it may be considered a pertinent negative if renal failure is a diagnostic consideration.
43. (b), (e). If uremia is the cause of the anemia, hypertension may well be part of the renal disease complex; on the other hand, it may be a separate problem.
44. (b). This finding suggests hypothyroidism (which is not one of the originally proposed diagnoses).
45. (b). Severe renal disease and uremia become possibilities; as always, this too could be a separate problem.
46. (c). This finding includes many highly pertinent negatives. The *absence* of splenomegaly, lymphadenopathy, evidence of weight loss, a rectal lesion, abnormal fundi, neurologic abnormalities, and uremic breath are all points against some of the speculative diagnoses.
47. (c). This normal finding weighs against severe chronic hypertension associated with chronic renal disease and also against primary anemias where fundal abnormalities are common.
48. (e). This problem is probably separate and unrelated to the anemia. Long-standing diabetes with its associated renal failure is a long shot.
49. (b), (e). Such paresthesias may be associated with the posterolateral sclerosis of pernicious anemia, although they may have other causes and could represent another problem, especially at this age.
50. (c). This finding makes chronic lymphatic leukemia unlikely and also signifies the absence of metastatic cervical lymphadenopathy.

Comment

Note that each bit of information is evaluated in its own context. Usually, however, we deal with entire clusters of data wherein individual clues tend to reinforce each other. For example, the presence of clues 3, 5, 7, 11, 16, 26, 28, 32, and 40 all together weigh very heavily in favor of gastrointestinal cancer. But clues 4, 6, 14, 17, 22, 26, 27, 33, 38, and 41 would be virtually conclusive for pernicious anemia.

In fact, only three or four of these clues in a patient would heighten your suspicion. And as each new clue is added, you are building a weight of evidence for the diagnosis. With the appearance of each positive clue, you increase the likelihood ratio of $D:\bar{D}$. (Recall that D signifies the probability that a suspected disease is present, and $\bar{D}$ represents the probability that the disease is not present.)

C A S E   2

Patient with Chest Pain

*A 52-year-old man who has had **severe substernal pain** for 3 hours.*

In a 52-year-old man who has had severe substernal pain for 3 hours, the first and foremost consideration is acute myocardial infarction. But also included in the differential diagnosis are acute pericarditis, dissecting aneurysm, and pulmonary embolus. Esophageal pain (spasm or esophagitis) and acute cholecystitis are more remote speculations.

Evaluate the following pieces of data using the (a)-(b)-(c)-(d)-(e) scale previously described (*see p. 52 for answers*).

1. Pain radiates to right arm
2. Never had pain before
3. Had same pain many times before, brought on by exertion
4. Has had similar shorter pains, but never on exertion
5. Chronic headaches
6. Recurrent nosebleeds
7. Father died at age 48
8. Mother has diabetes
9. Plays tennis daily
10. Had dental extraction 2 months ago
11. Has nausea and vomiting
12. Attends church regularly
13. On no dietary restrictions
14. Smokes two packs of cigarettes daily
15. Has had hypertension for 15 years
16. Drinks 12 beers daily
17. Is an attorney
18. Fundi normal
19. BP 180/100
20. BP 80/60
21. BP 130/80
22. BP equal in both arms
23. BP differs by 50 mm Hg in the arms
24. Skin cold and clammy
25. Skin warm and dry
26. Recent 24-hour bus trip
27. Inguinal hernias for 10 years
28. Jaundice present
29. Liver enlarged
30. S_4 present
31. Grade 3 mitral systolic murmur radiating to axilla
32. Rales in both bases
33. Atrophic left testicle
34. Temperature normal
35. Temperature 38.5°C
36. Pericardial friction rub on admission
37. Pericardial friction rub not present on admission
38. Legs swollen
39. Aortic diastolic murmur present
40. Prostate gland 2+ enlarged
41. Tender calves
42. Appears dyspneic
43. BP 140/30 both arms
44. No pulse in left dorsalis pedis artery
45. Varicose veins present
46. Chest radiograph normal
47. Stat creatine kinase–MB isomer normal
48. Initial electrocardiogram (ECG) normal
49. Initial ECG abnormal
50. ECG normal on 3 successive days

A U T H O R ' S   A N S W E R S   R E G A R D I N G   P A T I E N T   W I T H   C H E S T   P A I N

1. (a). Although this symptom is atypical for coronary chest pain radiation, it is highly specific when it occurs.
2. (a), (c). Usually coronary artery thrombosis is preceded by one or more shorter episodes of pain. No previous pain suggests possible other causes.

3. (a). This sounds very much like angina pectoris terminating in myocardial infarction.

4. (a), (b). Although not typical for angina pectoris, this finding may represent variant angina, which may also terminate in a myocardial infarction.

5. (d). There is no relationship. If you stretch hard, you might relate analgesic use to gastric hyperacidity and esophageal reflux.

6. (d). Even if there is associated hypertension, which can predispose to myocardial infarction or aortic dissection, nosebleeds are probably not related to hypertension.

7. (b). Early paternal death might signify hereditary coronary artery disease.

8. (b). Parental diabetes may indicate subclinical diabetes in the son or an increased incidence of coronary artery disease, even in the absence of diabetes in the son.

9. (c), (d). This is arguable. Playing daily tennis implies great exercise capacity without the production of angina. These implications may not be accurate. You might reasonably expect the patient to have had some prior angina on exertion if he were presently having a myocardial infarction. On the other hand, the absence of symptoms suggests that this is not an infarction and could be regarded as a pertinent negative.

10. (d). This is irrelevant unless we have discovered a "zebra" that has aortic valve endocarditis with coronary embolization.

11. (a), (b). Nausea and vomiting can occur with any severe visceral pain, but acute cholecystitis increases in likelihood.

12. (d). Irrelevant

13. (d). However, he may have diabetes, obesity, or hyperlipidemia but may not have received or heeded medical advice.

14. (b). This is a definite risk factor for coronary artery disease.

15. (b). This too is a risk factor for coronary artery disease, but it also contributes to aortic dissection.

16. (e). Separate problem

17. (d). This is irrelevant unless you subscribe to the theory that "high-pressure work" causes coronary disease or hypertension.

18. (c). This is a point that weighs against sustained severe hypertension.

19. (b). Not only is hypertension a risk factor for two possibilities, but the fact that it is still elevated bears diagnostic, prognostic, and therapeutic implications.

20. (a). Hypotension with a low pulse pressure indicates a potentially catastrophic illness (infarction or dissection).

21. (b), (c). This may represent a drop from a previously high pressure, or it may signify normal pressure and tend to discount but certainly not exclude infarction or dissection. Check both arms!

22. (c). This finding weighs against aortic dissection.

23. (a). This symptom is strongly suggestive of aortic dissection and signifies partial occlusion of blood supply to one arm (unless this differential pre-existed).

24. (a). This finding bespeaks a severe illness like infarction or dissection (or even pancreatitis).

25. (c). This symptom weighs against a catastrophic illness, but pulmonary embolization, myocardial infarction, and dissecting aneurysm may exist even though evidence of critical illness (shock, hypotension, clammy skin) is lacking.

26. (b), (d). This is probably irrelevant, although prolonged leg dependency predisposes to venous thromboembolism.

27. (e). Separate problem.

28. (b), (e). None of the mentioned hypotheses causes jaundice early. Acute cholecystitis with complications, pancreatitis (not hypothesized), and pulmonary embolism (with infarction) can all produce varying degrees of jaundice, but not within 3 hours.

29. (e). Separate problem

30. (a), (b). This is a sensitive clue in myocardial infarction.

31. (a), (b). If not present before, this symptom suggests infarction with papillary muscle dysfunction and mitral regurgitation.

32. (a), (b). This finding indicates probable myocardial infarction with left ventricular failure, unless the rales have been long present from smoking, chronic bronchitis, and so forth.

33. (d). Irrelevant

34. (c). This finding is a pertinent negative for pericarditis and cholecystitis but is consistent with other diagnostic possibilities.

35. (a), (c). Fever on admission suggests pericarditis or cholecystitis but weighs against

other predications. Fever occurs 12 to 24 hours later in myocardial infarction and often not at all in pulmonary infarction or aortic dissection.

36. (a). This finding indicates pericarditis. The friction rub of myocardial infarction occurs 1 or more days later.

37. (c). This finding weighs against pericarditis, although the clue does not have high sensitivity.

38. (b). Swelling may point to leg vein thrombosis with pulmonary embolization; otherwise, it is not related to the other possibilities.

39. (a), (b), (e). This finding can be seen with retrograde dissection causing aortic valve malfunction and regurgitation, but it may represent a pre-existing valvular problem.

40. (e). Separate problem.

41. (b). Most calves are tender if squeezed, but you must consider thromboembolism again (even though this is a low-sensitivity, low-specificity clue).

42. (a). Dyspnea argues for pulmonary embolism or myocardial infarction with left ventricular failure.

43. (a), (e). The wide pulse pressure hints at aortic regurgitation, which may be an old problem or, if new, may represent retrograde aortic dissection.

44. (b), (e). This finding represents peripheral vascular disease, which is a close cousin of coronary artery disease.

45. (d), (e). These are not related; emboli rarely come from varicose veins.

46. (c). There is no aortic widening, no evidence of congestive failure, and no evidence of pulmonary embolism; but more procedures may be needed to exclude the former and latter possibilities.

47. (d). This finding neither excludes nor confirms a myocardial infarction; more hours are needed before this enzyme increases.

48. (c). Electrocardiographic abnormalities are at most 50% sensitive for pulmonary embolism; although the sensitivity is higher for myocardial infarction pain that has existed for 3 hours, it is not uncommon to wait longer before electrocardiographic evidence is apparent.

49. (a), (b), (e). The abnormalities may have existed for a long time, but if new, myocardial infarction or pulmonary embolus is suspected (the changes may or may not permit you to distinguish one from the other).

50. (c). Under these circumstances, myocardial infarction is not likely, although small areas of necrosis may occur without electrocardiographic but with enzyme confirmation. Consider other possibilities more strongly.

Comment

If we were to consider clusters of clues rather than individual ones, the presence of clues 3, 7, 8, 14, 15, 20, 24, 30, 32, 42, and 49 virtually guarantees the diagnosis of acute myocardial infarction. Dissecting aneurysm is highly likely if clues 2, 15, 19, 23, 48, and 50 are present. And if findings 26, 38, 41, and 42 are present, the diagnostic pointer swings toward a pulmonary embolus. If only some of the mentioned clues exist, the respective diagnoses are less likely. Additionally, if only a few clues are positive, if there is considerable overlap of clues between two diagnoses, or if some clues are *unexpectedly* positive or negative, further information is needed. This may necessitate obtaining more data from the history and physical examination or ordering additional diagnostic tests.

C A S E   3

Patient with Jaundice

*A 46-year-old woman has had clearly visible **jaundice** and **dark urine** for 10 days.*

This brief clinical picture suggests the possibilities of hepatitis, bile duct obstruction from a stone or cancer (biliary tract or pancreas), metastatic carcinoma to the liver, and cirrhosis.

Evaluate the following pieces of data using the (a)-(b)-(c)-(d)-(e) scale previously described (*see p. 55 for answers*).

1. Bowel operation 3 years ago
2. Bowel operation 3 months ago
3. Favorite food is seafood

4. Is a nurse
5. Works in a restaurant kitchen
6. Recently returned from North Africa
7. Drinks coffee twice daily
8. Father died of heart attack
9. Has itching of skin
10. Gets weekly injections for "no pep"
11. Takes aspirin for headaches
12. Takes α-methyldopa for hypertension
13. Takes isoniazid after recently discovered positive findings of purified protein derivative skin test
14. Has no pain
15. Has diffuse abdominal pains
16. Has had recurrent severe right upper quadrant pains
17. Nausea for 2 weeks
18. Nausea for 2 months
19. Nausea for 2 years
20. Takes no narcotic injections
21. Feels well
22. Feels sick
23. Occasional ringing in the ears
24. Is being treated for diabetes
25. Stools black
26. Stools brown
27. Stools clay-colored
28. Has lump in breast
29. Drinks alcohol "socially"
30. Doesn't smoke
31. Does smoke
32. Stopped smoking 2 weeks ago
33. Poor appetite for 2 weeks
34. Poor appetite and weight loss for 2 months
35. Eyeballs yellow
36. Has seasonal hay fever
37. Liver not palpable
38. Liver enlarged and tender
39. Liver enlarged and nodular
40. Spleen not palpable
41. Abdomen not distended
42. Abdomen distended
43. No large veins on abdomen
44. No spider angiomata
45. Neck veins flat at 45 degrees
46. Palmar erythema present
47. Tender mass in right upper quadrant
48. Mass in right lower quadrant
49. Varicose veins present
50. Menses normal; pelvic examination normal

AUTHOR'S ANSWERS REGARDING PATIENT WITH JAUNDICE

1. (b). Surgery for possible colon cancer could result in liver metastases 3 years later.
2. (b). Recent surgery may relate to early liver metastases or to viral hepatitis (if transfusions were given).
3. (b), (d). This is probably not related, but inquire further about eating raw seafood (clams) from polluted waters. Hepatitis may result.
4. (b). Hepatitis is an occupational hazard of nursing.
5. (d). This fact is only a questionable risk for the patient but a definite risk for the diner if the patient has hepatitis.
6. (b). Hepatitis is rampant there.
7. (d). Irrelevant
8. (d). Irrelevant
9. (a). Cholestasis with retention of bile salts causes itching.
10. (b), (e). Injections can transmit hepatitis, but this is less likely with the use of disposable syringes; "no pep" may be a symptom of underlying serious disease resulting in jaundice.
11. (d), (e). Irrelevant or separate problem
12. (b). This drug can cause hepatitis.
13. (b). This drug also can cause hepatitis.
14. (c). Absence of pain weighs strongly against common duct stone and favors other considerations, such as cirrhosis, pancreatic cancer, and hepatitis—although the latter two may also be characterized by abdominal pain.
15. (b). This finding suggests diffuse abdominal carcinomatosis.
16. (b). This symptom implies cholelithiasis with recurrent cystic duct obstruction and subsequent common bile duct stone.
17. (b). This finding points to recent onset of hepatitis.
18. (a). This symptom argues for a longer illness such as upper gastrointestinal tract carcinoma with liver metastases.
19. (d), (e). This finding is hardly consistent with a present illness of jaundice.
20. (c). This symptom argues against needle-spread hepatitis.
21. (c). This finding suggests that widespread cancer is not present; it also tends to negate hepatitis, whose victims usually feel sick. It

does not rule out an early small cancer obstructing the common bile duct.

22. (a). Patients with acute hepatitis or metastatic cancer usually feel sick.

23. (e). Separate problem

24. (b), (d), (e). Diabetes is probably another problem and is irrelevant; but remember that pancreatic cancer can present as diabetes, and that oral hypoglycemic agents rarely do cause hepatitis.

25. (b). Black stools suggest a bleeding gastrointestinal malignancy with associated liver metastases (stomach, ampulla of Vater).

26. (c). Brown stools deny melena and complete biliary duct obstruction.

27. (a). This finding typifies complete obstructive jaundice (stone or cancer or severe hepatitis at its peak).

28. (b), (e). The lump may be a separate problem, or it may be the cause of liver metastases.

29. (b). "Social drinking" often means heavy alcohol intake and may therefore hint at cirrhosis.

30. (d). Irrelevant

31. (e). This is irrelevant unless the patient has lung cancer with metastases. Anyway, it's a separate problem.

32. (b). Abrupt cessation of smoking may be related to a sudden distaste for cigarettes, which is often an early symptom of viral hepatitis.

33. (b). Recent anorexia is often the first symptom of hepatitis.

34. (a). This sinister combination argues for widespread cancer.

35. (a). This finding confirms the chief complaint.

36. (e). Separate problem

37. (c). In hepatitis, the liver is usually enlarged and tender; in cirrhosis, it is usually enlarged; in metastatic cancer, the liver may be enlarged and nodular. But in any of these cases it may *not* be palpable. Bear in mind that liver size as judged by palpation is neither highly sensitive nor specific. Percussion may be preferable.

38. (a). This finding speaks for viral hepatitis.

39. (a). This finding indicates metastatic cancer or posthepatitic cirrhosis; the nodules of alcoholic cirrhosis are small and usually not felt.

40. (c). The spleen may be enlarged yet not palpable; if it is palpable and therefore much enlarged, cirrhosis with portal hypertension must be considered.

41. (c). This finding argues against cirrhosis with ascites.

42. (b). Although there are many causes of abdominal distention, in this case ascites from cirrhosis and metastatic cancer are considerations.

43. (c). This finding weighs against cirrhosis with portal hypertension.

44. (c). This finding weighs against alcoholic cirrhosis; spider nevi are uncommon in patients who have posthepatitic cirrhosis.

45. (d). This is a normal finding.

46. (b). This symptom suggests cirrhosis, although it is nonspecific; remember that cirrhosis can exist with cancer being superimposed.

47. (a). This finding speaks for cholelithiasis with a cystic duct stone obstructing the gallbladder and perhaps another stone in the common bile duct.

48. (a). This picture is suggestive of cecal carcinoma with liver metastases.

49. (e). Separate problem

50. (d). Irrelevant

Comment

Again, if the order of data accumulation were such that findings 4, 17, 22, 33, and 38 were elicited in rapid sequence, hepatitis would be the leading contender. On the other hand, in the event that findings 15, 22, 25, 34, and 39 were present, metastatic cancer would be most likely. This is how clues are aggregated to form likely diagnoses which, in turn, are confirmed by additional information.

SUMMATION

The three patients just discussed—one with anemia, one with chest pain, and one with jaundice—will be presented in Section 2 in a more typical way. There, findings will be evaluated in chunks or in the light of previously acquired data. So rather than regard bits of information separately, the patient–problem will be approached in a more realistic style. I believe that the elementary exercises just presented in this chapter are good preparation for real-life patient encounters that come later.

DECODING PROBLEM SETS

Here is another way to improve your data management skills. The same set of clues occurring in dissimilar population subsets can have vastly different diagnostic and therapeutic implications.

P R O B L E M   S E T   1

Consider first the problem of *headache, confusion, stiff neck, and fever* in a:

1. Two-year-old child who has been sick for 3 days
2. Fifty-three-year-old healthy woman who suddenly became sick 24 hours ago
3. Forty-eight-year-old man being treated for Hodgkin's disease
4. Nineteen-year-old recent Army recruit
5. Thirty-two-year-old woman who has known polycystic kidney disease
6. Twenty-six-year-old male sewer worker
7. Thirty-eight-year-old horse rancher in Texas
8. Fifty-two-year-old man 5 days after craniotomy
9. Eight-year-old child with running left ear
10. Four-year-old child recovering from measles
11. Eighteen-year-old girl with sore throat and diffuse lymphadenopathy
12. Sixteen-year-old boy who has had a lengthy upper respiratory tract infection and lives in a mouse-infested home

D I A G N O S E S   F O R   P R O B L E M   S E T   1

Clearly, we are dealing with three possible diseases, each of which has diverse etiologic agents. Yet all can have a similar presentation. *Meningitis, encephalitis, and subarachnoid hemorrhage are under consideration.* But each of the 12 initial statements has certain features that seem to set it apart from the others by virtue of age, occupation, and clinical background. Be cautious! Things are not always what they seem, and one type of meningitis may

exist even when you suspect another. However, based on the information given, venture an educated guess of the diagnosis and the specific etiologic agent. Whatever you think, a lumbar puncture will probably be needed in almost all cases.

The diagnoses that initially occur to the author are:

1. *Haemophilus influenzae* type B meningitis—common at this age
2. Subarachnoid hemorrhage from a berry aneurysm
3. *Enterobacter, Pseudomonas, Listeria,* or other types of meningitis—patient is immunosuppressed
4. Meningococcal meningitis
5. Subarachnoid hemorrhage—aneurysms are common in patients who have polycystic renal disease
6. Leptospirosis—contact with excreta of infected rodents
7. Equine encephalitis—even though uncommon
8. *Staphylococcus aureus* meningitis
9. Pneumococcal meningitis
10. Encephalitis
11. Infectious mononucleosis—Epstein-Barr virus
12. Lymphocytic choriomeningitis—RNA virion

When given hints, you are immediately directed toward a specific microbial diagnosis, but this type of logic, although perhaps most often correct, can lead you astray. The sewer worker can have meningococcal meningitis. The boy living in the mouse-infested home may contract a bacterial meningitis. The suspected subarachnoid hemorrhage may be meningitis, and vice versa. And the horse rancher is statistically more apt to have a bacterial meningitis than equine encephalitis, despite his occupation.

P R O B L E M   S E T   2

Now, ponder another cluster—*flank pain, fever, and dysuria*—in a:

1. Recently married young woman
2. Sixty-eight-year-old man who has 3 years of worsening nocturia and frequency of urination
3. Two-year-old girl

4. Vietnam veteran who has paraplegia
5. Thirty-six-year-old football player immobilized for months with a body cast
6. Twenty-eight-year-old woman who is 6 months pregnant
7. Thirty-eight-year-old executive taking large quantities of milk and absorbable alkali for chronic indigestion
8. Fifty-two-year-old woman with bone pains, constipation, and known bilateral renal calculi

DIAGNOSES FOR PROBLEM SET 2

The small amount of critical clinical information given in each circumstance enables you to predict the diagnosis and underlying pathophysiology with reasonable accuracy. Additional particulars are needed to confirm your impression and guide your treatment in each case. Urinary tract infections (acute cystitis and acute pyelonephritis) exist in all of these patients, but the causes vary:

1. Possibly related to excessive sexual activity
2. Enlarged prostate gland with obstruction and retention
3. Ureterovesical reflux or other congenital defect
4. Neurogenic bladder or nephrolithiasis (immobilization)
5. Renal calculi resulting from prolonged immobilization and bone resorption
6. Ureterectasis and pyelectasis of pregnancy
7. Calculi caused by excessive intake of milk and alkali for possible duodenal ulcer
8. Calculi in a patient with probable hyperparathyroidism (stones may predispose the patient to infection)

In each instance, you must analyze the presentation. See if the age, gender, occupation, geography, or other demographic features influence your impression. Occasionally, an additionally stated clue will help you draw a conclusion, and you must therefore seek more data to confirm or reject your hypothesis.

PROBLEM SET 3

A third problem set concerns a patient with *fever, malaise, anemia, and a heart murmur.* Suppose it occurs in a:

1. Forty-two-year-old woman who had mitral valve replacement 2 months ago
2. Twenty-eight-year-old woman who has a papular rash, diffuse lymphadenopathy, and mild polyarthritis
3. Twenty-one-year-old male heroin addict
4. Sixty-four-year-old woman who has a sore tongue and leg paresthesias
5. Five-year-old child who has a large spleen
6. Forty-six-year-old woman who has a long-standing mitral diastolic rumble
7. Fifty-two-year-old man who has large glands in the neck and left axilla
8. Sixty-eight-year-old man who has had weakness, weight loss, and indigestion for several months
9. Sixteen-year-old Haitian girl who has chronic cough and expectoration
10. Four-year-old underdeveloped cyanotic child

DIAGNOSES FOR PROBLEM SET 3

Although all four clues in the stated cluster may be present in each of the 10 presentations, in some cases one clue may not be prominent. For example, the fever may be low grade, or the murmur may be slight. Sometimes, the murmur may be secondary to the anemia and not to the disease. In fact, the murmur may represent an added problem. You must be able to deal with: the varied degrees of expression of a clue, the fact that a clue may not be part of the pathophysiologic cluster, and even a discrepant clue.

The initial hypothesis for each presentation follows:

1. Infective endocarditis on a valve prosthesis
2. Sarcoidosis or systemic lupus erythematosus
3. Infective endocarditis—*Staphylococcus aureus* likely
4. Pernicious anemia—usually mild fever, and murmur secondary to the chronic anemia
5. Acute leukemia—murmur secondary to anemia, fever, and/or high flow state
6. Infective endocarditis—*Streptococcus viridans* likely to be imposed on a stenotic mitral

valve; atrial myxoma is another consideration

7. Lymphoma is likely—murmur not explained
8. Gastrointestinal carcinoma with metastases—
   murmur not clearly explained
9. Pulmonary tuberculosis—murmur may represent another problem
10. Infective endocarditis—superimposed on a
    serious congenital heart defect

Comment

It is a simple matter to create many other problem sets revolving around such clusters as cough,
expectoration, and chest pain; enlarged liver and
jaundice; polyuria and polydipsia; and so forth.
Then, postulate the various brief clinical settings
in which such groups of clues may occur, and you
have organized *a lively medical rap session.*

More Clinical Tools

Paul Cutler

There is no field in medicine more important than diagnosis, for without it we are charlatans and witch doctors treating patients in the dark with potions and prayers. Yet there are few fields more difficult to explicate and teach.

When you see a patient, how do you decide what's wrong, and how do you explain how you did it? You may use terms such as hunch, intuition, judgment, experience, deduction, and so forth. You may be able to explain the individual cases, but have difficulty with general rules and principles. This poses problems for the educator, too.

Despite attempts to make a precise science of the skill of medical problem-solving, the problem solver is frequently left with indefinable although universally used techniques. In part, the clinician uses the axioms, postulates, and syllogisms first propounded by Euclid and Aristotle. At times a glance, a simple addition, a smell, a hunch—and out comes a possibly correct hypothesis. To this the clinician adds a careful consideration of cause and effect, especially insofar as temporal and pathophysiologic sequence are concerned, and out comes a correct diagnosis.

The making of a masterful diagnosis, often on the basis of scant or incomplete data, is not an art, not a science, but a disciplined amalgam of both. The successful problem solver is able to interlace the patient's data base with his or her own knowledge base in order to arrive at a sensible problem list.

The sequence of gathering a complete data base, then diagnosing, then acting, is the one that is traditionally taught. However, this route is less traveled than the one by which a provisional diagnosis is based on the first few bits of information, and evidence for and against this diagnosis is then sought via a branching technique. The latter course pursues a single line and gathers sup-

portive data until confidence in a diagnosis has been attained—then action can proceed.

Previous chapters dwelt on the selection of clues from the data base and how these clues are used as building blocks in the problem-solving process. Subsequent chapters will enlarge on the mathematics of problem solving and how to use tests and new technology. This chapter aims to expand upon some clinical tools that were touched upon in previous chapters, but were not fully developed because they might have diverted the reader and interfered with the chapter's flow.

HOW THE MIND WORKS

It is difficult to teach somebody how to think. You cannot give precise instructions on how to use the interneuronal processes involved in memory, thought, reasoning, and logic. Yet there are certain basic principles and maxims that can help you arrive at reasonable or logical conclusions.

For example, the problem solver must always consider the patient's age, gender, race, habitat, and the natural history of the disorder when weighing the various contenders for the diagnosis.

ON THE BASIS OF AGE

For instance, a 21-year-old patient with certain symptoms is much less likely to have cancer than is a 65-year-old patient. Some diseases are more common in young persons, whereas others are more common in old persons. Urinary tract symptoms in the 21-year-old male patient are commonly caused by venereal infection, whereas similar symptoms in a 71-year-old man suggest prostatic enlargement. Abnormal vaginal bleeding at age 21 is probably functional; at 61 it is probably neoplastic. Hypochromic microcytic anemia in an elderly person leads you to think seriously of a gastrointestinal malignancy, but in the 28-year-old multigravid patient, excessive vaginal bleeding is the likely cause.

THE CASE FOR SEX, RACE, AND PLACE

The patient's *gender* is an important factor in the physician's diagnostic logic. Certain diseases are more common in one sex—for instance, systemic lupus erythematosus (SLE) in women and coronary disease in men. Although statistics like these always influence our reasoning, a disease should not be ruled out solely on this basis.

Race, too, is important. Sarcoidosis is far more common in a young black woman than in a white woman of similar age. If you see a 28-year-old black woman with hilar adenopathy, sarcoidosis would be your first thought; for members of other races, you might give more serious consideration to lymphoma. The predilection of certain anemias for ethnic or geographic origins is well known—pernicious anemia in the Scandinavian, sickle cell anemia in the black, thalassemia in the person of Mediterranean origin, and fish tapeworm in the Finn. Furthermore, carcinoma of the liver is more common in the Chinese; carcinoma of the stomach has a strikingly high incidence in Iceland and Japan; and diabetes is almost universal in some American Indian tribes.

Geography might weight your logic. In the southwest United States, certain clues for pulmonary disease suggest coccidioidomycosis. The same clues signify histoplasmosis if the patient lives in the Ohio or Mississippi valleys. Hematuria in the United States warrants a detailed study for tumor and stone, whereas in Egypt schistosomiasis of the urinary bladder would be your first choice. In Afghanistan a mass in the liver is considered to be an echinococcus cyst, whereas in the United States cancer is primarily thought of.

HELP FROM THE NATURAL HISTORY

The clinical course of an illness is helpful in making a diagnosis, because many diseases have courses that fit specific patterns. For example, multiple sclerosis has exacerbations of varying symptoms, with long remissions at first and shorter ones later on; the illness eventually becomes continuous. A stroke has an acute picture from which it derives its apoplectic name; it may gradually improve. But a brain tumor begins gradually and becomes progressively worse. Cancer, too, gets progressively worse, as do its accompanying symptoms. Duodenal ulcer has its ups and downs, is often symptom free, and may recur for many years. Asthma displays intermittent attacks of variable severity with symptom-free intervals; the disease may eventually become almost continuous. The same holds true for untreated gout or rheumatoid arthritis. The pattern, progression, and intermittency of the disease process must be documented in the history of the present illness; this information is helpful in the formulation of a diagnosis.

A gastric problem that has been present intermittently for many years is not likely to be a result of gastric cancer, but if symptoms have existed for only 6 months and are unremitting and progressive, cancer becomes a more serious consideration. A 46-year-old man who has had recurrent chest pain for 20 years is not apt to have coronary disease as the cause of his pain, but be wary of the chest pains he has had for only 1 or 2 weeks, especially if the character of the pain is suggestive. Cough and fever for 1 month may well be tuberculosis; for 2 days, pneumonia is more likely. The abrupt onset of a relentless progressive wheeze and dyspnea does not sound like bronchial asthma. Other considerations are more likely.

You should be able to match the patient's history of present illness to the known clinical courses of suspected diagnoses.

THREE MAXIMS

(1) "Common diseases occur commonly" may seem elementary and redundant, but the phrase contains much wisdom. If you base your diagnostic reasoning on what is common, you will be right most of the time. Do not diagnose a rare disease when a common one fits the picture just as well. Three birds sitting in a row on a branch are more apt to be sparrows than canaries—unless you are in a pet shop. And if you hear the galloping of hooves, think of horses, not camels—unless you are in the Sahara desert (Fig. 6.1).

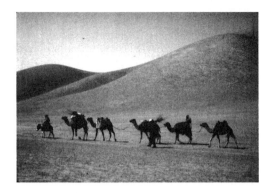

▶ **Figure 6.1.** The Sahara desert.

(2) "Uncommon manifestations of common diseases are more common than common manifestations of uncommon diseases." For instance, a 56-year-old man who has manifestations of superior vena cava obstruction is more apt to have lung cancer than Concato's disease or primary thrombosis of the vein. Although it is uncommon for cancer and common for the latter two possibilities to have this type of presentation, lung cancer is by far the leading diagnostic contender in this case because it is much more prevalent than the other choices.

And an atypical presentation of coronary disease in a 56-year-old man with vague chest pain is far more common than a typical presentation of mesothelioma of the pericardium.

(3) And do not forget this maxim: "No disease is rare to the patient who has it." In our zeal to stay common, let us not overlook the rare possibilities. Think common—but remember rare.

Although the combination of hypertension, diabetes, obesity, and hirsutism is far more apt to occur in a middle-aged woman with four separate problems, do not overlook that once in your lifetime you may be seeing a patient with Cushing's disease (see Case 15, Chapter 13). Your next patient with gastrointestinal problems may have Whipple's disease; your next endocrine problem may be a case of Sipple's syndrome.

For the tertiary care specialist, common simpler problems have already been weeded out, and rare diseases have a higher prevalence. The same can be said for certain diagnostic conferences in teaching centers where only unusual cases are presented to confound the discusser and amuse the listeners.

IN REVERSE GEAR

The principle of reverse logic merits some additional words. Medical teaching and textbooks generally conform to a format whereby disease manifestations are emphasized. You learn separately about eight different diseases that cause hypertension. When confronted by a patient with high blood pressure, you must comb your knowledge base for all of the causes—not an easy task.

A patient hospitalized with acidotic coma could have one of four conditions: uremia, diabetic ketoacidosis, lactic acidosis, or respiratory failure. Before attacking the problem, you must know these possibilities; however, human retrieval mechanisms are neither perfect nor complete. Many students find it difficult to use this approach. Although they may know diseases, they do not know much about patient presentations.

For the student who may need to know the many diseases associated with a symptom or sign, it may be necessary to search the index of a standard disease-oriented textbook. If not found there, the student may consult less common textbooks that are categorized according to isolated symptoms, signs, and laboratory abnormalities. In time, these lists become fixed in the mind of the student, who by this time has already become a house officer.

THE PRESENTING SYMPTOM

If you were to look up the cause of *dyspnea* in any modern textbook of differential diagnosis, you would find a list of between 20 and 100 causes. This does not mean that a patient who comes to a physician with shortness of breath as the chief complaint can have that many possible causes of the symptom. There are far fewer diseases whose *presenting symptom* is dyspnea.

For example, a patient with lobar pneumonia will have cough, fever, chills, expectoration, chest pain, and possibly even shortness of breath. But his chief complaint or presenting symptoms will in all probability be cough and fever. He may be dyspneic as well, but that is not the complaint.

The male patient with secondary hypogonadism is seen with complaints of loss of libido and impotence, not with loss of body hair, even though that may be present also. It is helpful to know how patients with certain diseases present themselves to a physician for care.

DEPTH OF STUDY

A patient comes to you with a problem. Your job is to find out what is wrong and do something about it. Often this may require only one or two questions and a brief glance. At other times, you need an exhaustive history, a complete physical examination, extensive laboratory work-up, radiographs and other special studies, consultations, and at least 1 or 2 weeks before arriving at a solution. Between these two extremes, various gradations and complexities of work-ups are needed.

Short Cases

The patient who has an obvious head cold needs only meager problem solving. He has had a stuffed runny nose, watering eyes, and a sore throat for 2 days. Quick examination confirms the nasopharyngitis, and symptomatic therapy is given. Most patients fall into the category of those problems that can be solved in a few minutes— gastroenteritis, infected finger, nasopharyngitis.

Revisits

In working with ambulatory patients in the office and outpatient department, speed is generally required. Monthly revisits by patients with known chronic diseases should take no more than 10 or 15 minutes. Inquire about old and new symptoms, examine the few pertinent areas, and check one or two laboratory tests—allowing a minute or two for a chat about the patient's progress and treatment. Angina, hypertension, diabetes, asthma, and arthritis—among the most common diseases seen in the office—can be so managed.

Ambulatory patients can usually be treated at an acceptable standard in the context of the realities and pressures of practice. You must learn to focus on the economy of time and money in patient encounters, bearing in mind that shortcuts have legitimate trade-offs and are not necessarily bad.

Puzzling Cases

Consider the case of a patient with fever of 4 weeks' duration who has been treated with antibiotics by two previous physicians. No better, the patient comes to see you. A complete data base is obtained, and numerous laboratory studies reveal nothing. Consultants didn't help, either. After a variety of noninvasive studies, a liver biopsy reveals miliary tuberculosis. The process took 10 days, but treatment is now simple (see Case 86, Chapter 22).

Hospital Cases

All hospitalized patients should have a complete work-up. This includes obstetric, gynecologic, and surgical as well as medical and pediatric cases. The price you may pay for treating only the principal illness is that, for example, 3 months after the cholecystectomy, the patient may be found to have carcinoma of the breast—now too advanced for cure. Or, 6 months after treatment of acute myocardial infarction, the patient may be found to have inoperable carcinoma of the prostate.

Midlong Cases

Somewhere between the short case that takes only several minutes and the long case involving hospitalization lies the patient who is too sick or whose problem is too emergent to permit a complete history and examination. Included might be patients with acute myocardial infarction, gastrointestinal hemorrhage, and acute renal or respiratory failure. Here, the problem solver does only what is needed to diagnose and treat the primary disease. But in all such cases, a complete data base must eventually be fleshed out.

The Complete Work-up

Those who definitely need a complete work-up include:

- New patients who are coming under your general care either de novo or from another physician, and for whom you should establish a baseline;

- New patients who have a variety or complexity of illnesses, or those who have illnesses that are difficult to diagnose easily;

- Patients whose mosaic does not add up to a definite somatic problem and whose symptoms may possibly be functional or psychosomatic;

- Patients desiring or needing annual complete examinations, including the healthy patient who wishes to remain well or seeks reassurance that he or she is well, and the ill patient who should probably receive a complete re-evaluation at least once a year (you want to know if the situation is stable, if complications have occurred, or if new problems have developed);

- The patient with a chronic disease whom you have not seen for the previous 6 to 12 months and who needs a new baseline for continuing care;

- Patients with seemingly minor illnesses who don't get well in the expected time and in whom you may be concerned about an underlying more serious disease—for example, "flu" lasting beyond a week, headaches that don't go away, and unexplained pain anywhere that persists; and

- All hospitalized patients (as stated earlier).

SHORTCUTS

Although much of Chapters 3 and 4 were devoted to problem-solving methods, some of the methods, especially those that permit the job to be done more efficiently and in less time, are so important as to need reinforcement. Here are some shortcuts—frequently used by the experienced clinician—that the beginner may try now and solidify in time and with experience.

Diagnosis at a Glance

This tactic is popular with clinicians. One glance can spot myxedema, exophthalmic goiter, acromegaly, Cushing's disease, and Parkinson's disease (Figs. 6.2 and 6.3).

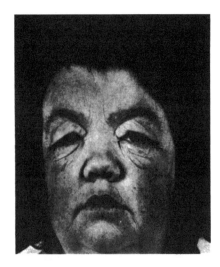

▶ **Figure 6.2.** Myxedema. The coarse features, dull expression, and baggy skin are characteristic.

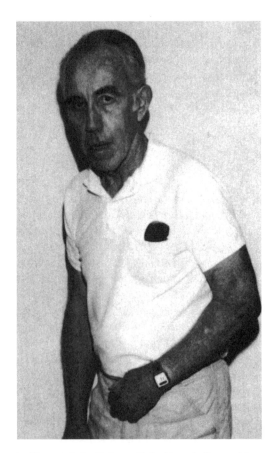

▶ **Figure 6.3.** Patient with Parkinson's disease. Note loss of facial expression and flexed posture.

How Inspection Helps

Simple inspection of the patient during the taking of the history and at the beginning of the physical examination may often furnish the diagnosis. However, this inspection is usually sketchy, poorly done, and is where many oversights or errors occur. You must set aside enough time to look at the undressed patient—front, back, top, and bottom—programming your mind to look for a certain number of items in a definite order, as noted in Chapter 2. It is here where you will either note or overlook jaundice, anemia, edema, rashes, and other items, each of which may either tell you the diagnosis or offer a key clue.

Zeroing In

This is the process whereby you piece together two or three clues, formulate a provisional hypothesis or two, then seek out an additional bit of information that confirms one contender and eliminates the other(s). It's the most commonly used method to solve problems.

You greet a 46-year-old bartender who tells you that his eyeballs appear yellow and his urine is dark. He has palmar erythema and spider angiomas on his face. Laënnec's cirrhosis is the prime contender.

A 52-year-old comatose patient is brought to the emergency department. She appears dehydrated, and you smell acetone on her breath. An additional test confirms diabetic ketoacidosis.

The next patient complains of fatigue and lumps in the neck. Palpation for enlarged lymph nodes and an enlarged spleen may limit the diagnostic choices to two or three contenders.

A strongly positive antinuclear antibody confirms SLE in a febrile 36-year-old woman who has arthritis and a butterfly rash.

Be Freewheeling

Patient information need not be collected in separate, orderly, inviolable blocks. Once the student has become more proficient in doing a history and physical examination, he or she can shift rapidly to a more selective search of the patient's data base. Based on the chief complaint of shortness of breath, the clinician may first inquire about its details, limit questions to, for example,

the cardiovascular system, and then examine only the heart and lungs. The diagnosis may be immediately apparent.

Another example of quick problem solving is examination of a 60-year-old man who has pains in both legs for several months. You think of arterial insufficiency, venous insufficiency, peripheral neuropathy, and arthritis. The latter is ruled out by examining the joints. Venous insufficiency is unlikely because the legs are not swollen, there are no varicose veins, and the pain does not come on after the patient has been standing for a long time. Neuropathy is excluded because reflexes and sensory perceptions are normal. However, the pain comes on walking, is relieved by stopping, and pulses are not felt in the lower extremities. It takes no longer than 1 or 2 minutes to decide that this patient has severe peripheral vascular disease.

Symptoms and Signs Together

When doing a complete examination, another time-saver is to ask questions at the same time as you examine each system. Ask about the usual gastrointestinal system symptoms while you examine the abdomen, pulmonary symptoms while examining the lungs, and so forth—elaborating only when you get a positive response.

In trying to achieve a correct balance between taking shortcuts and being complete, the problem solver must often ride the straits between Scylla and Charybdis and not steer too close to either shore. If the examination is too short and too quick, a crucial clue may be missed. Yet if the examination is complete and orderly, the main thread may be lost.

COMING TO TERMS

Word Definition

One of the most common shortcomings and causes of misunderstanding among physicians, and especially among students, is the failure to use simple quantitative terms properly. Few of us understand exactly what others mean when they say, "most of the time," "almost always," or "rarely." Students taking examinations often ask what the examiner means in terms of percentages when such words are used in questions—because their answers depend on this interpretation. Dialogue between physician and patient can be a similar source of misunderstanding. Unfortunately, there is no uniformity of meaning of such terms for all persons. What may signify 60% to one person may be 95% to another.

Communication would be markedly enhanced if likelihoods and probabilities were expressed in percentages rather than in words—just as in the weather report. The statement that a patient *probably* has a disease would be more meaningful if "probably" were assigned a 75% value by general agreement. Similarly, there is no doubt in the patient's mind when he or she is told there is a 10% chance of postoperative complications. But the statement that "complications are uncommon" makes him or her wonder.

Causes for Confusion

Always have your patient quantify the symptoms, if possible. If you ask a patient how frequently the headaches occur, the answer may be, "All the time." The patient probably means "often," so you ask, "Are you having one now?" And the answer may be "no," which further indicates that "all the time" really means "some of the time." And "frequent" to the patient means three or four times per day. "Now and then" to one patient may mean once a month, but to another it means two or three times daily. It behooves the history taker to nail down exactly what the patient means.

On Being Precise

Quantitative ambiguities should be avoided whenever possible. Movements of the diaphragm and size of the liver, even though perhaps of questionable reliability, should be recorded in centimeters rather than finger breadths or rib interspaces. Centimeters never vary, but the width of fingers does. An apex beat should be located in terms of centimeters tangentially from the midsternal line rather than at

an often ill-defined place, such as the midclavicular or anterior axillary line. Above all, the size of masses, tumors, or organs should be measured in centimeters rather than compared to fruit, nuts, and sporting goods.

DIAGNOSTIC CERTAINTY

A diagnosis can only rarely be made with 100% certainty. The physician usually works with probability, likelihood, and weight of evidence. He or she can be certain only if a biopsy is 100% unequivocal or a test is unquestionably diagnostic.

How Certain To Be

The degree of diagnostic certainty that must be obtained in any particular case is arguable. Even in a court of law, proof beyond a reasonable doubt does not require 100% certainty. When do you decide that enough investigation has already taken place so that you can proceed with management? The threshold for arriving at diagnostic conclusions is an important part of clinical judgment.

To be considered are the seriousness of the disease; the age and otherwise general condition of the patient; the risks of further study; the already existing disease probability; and the costs to the patient and society in terms of inconvenience, money, and delayed treatment.

A search for evidence of a second diagnosis might be less diligent in an 85-year-old man with congestive heart failure than in a healthy 45-year-old wage earner. When contemplating a coronary artery bypass graft, 80% certainty is not enough. But if a patient wants to have coronary heart disease ruled out because of a contemplated vigorous adventure, a 10% likelihood does not yet give sufficient exclusion.

Chapter 7 will show you how the degree of diagnostic certainty can be revised upward by the addition of positive clues, the elimination of contending hypotheses, and confirmatory positive tests or procedures. In like manner, the degree of diagnostic certainty can be revised downward if there are no additional positive clues, if a contending hypothesis increases its own likelihood, and if the findings of supposedly confirmatory tests or procedures are normal or negative.

A Wrong Label

Before making a diagnosis, you may sometimes have to *undiagnose* a patient. Such patients may have been given labels on the basis of inadequate or inaccurate data and are then treated for those labels—sometimes for life.

Included are some who take digitalis for alleged heart failure but who may be dyspneic only from hyperventilation. The obese person is often given thyroid preparations for supposed hypothyroidism when thyroid function tests are borderline. Others who are nervous, shaky, and sweaty from simple anxiety may be treated for hyperthyroidism for years. Perhaps the most common false label is the "mild anemia" attached to psychoneurotic individuals whose blood counts are near the lower limits of normal and who complain of chronic fatigue. Vitamin B_{12} injections may be improperly given in these instances. The tragedy of this latter situation is that if mild anemia truly exists, the anemia may arise from a serious disorder that is unresponsive to vitamin injections.

In general, when wrong labels are applied, patients are treated for illnesses that are more serious than the ones they actually have. But the reverse can occur, and a very serious yet treatable disease may be overlooked. Such situations must be managed with skill and diplomacy. Patients are often reluctant to relinquish their designer labels!

So what do you do? If you suspect that this situation may exist because the patient is not getting better or for some other reason, take the label off. Begin the diagnostic process over again. You may even tactfully have to discontinue the former treatment, cautiously observing the patient while you rediagnose—it may be *you* who is wrong.

WHY CLINICAL PICTURES DIFFER

Action and Reaction

It is no surprise that the signs and symptoms of a disease vary from person to person, that patients with the same disease can have different presentations, and that the usual clues for a disease may be present or absent. The disease *inoculum* may vary with the quantity and virulence of the bacterium, the aggressiveness of the cancer cell, or the genetic penetrance. Hosts may respond with their own pattern of behavior. They may be frightened, anxious, calm, stoic, dramatic, or have a different level of perception. Patient response may be to procrastinate, deny, or report promptly at the first abnormal feeling. The patient may react organically with low or high fever; his or her renin-angiotensin-aldosterone mechanism may be sluggish or hyperactive.

Patients seen in office practice differ in their clinical manifestations from those seen in the hospital. The office patient is seen earlier, is usually in a less serious stage, and has fewer disease manifestations. Only later, when the patient is sicker, exhibits more clues, or perhaps has had a delay in diagnosis, does he or she reach the hospital.

Symptom threshold is another factor. Some patients who have cirrhosis see the doctor when their abdomens enlarge. Others attribute this enlargement to beer drinking and see you later for sexual problems related to testicular atrophy. It requires massive vomiting of blood or impending hepatic failure to get some cirrhotic patients into the medical care system. Obviously, the clues and clinical picture will vary at each stage and depend upon the cause and time of presentation. This accounts in part for the many faces of cirrhosis of the liver.

The patient's intelligence and intellect may be a factor. Would you expect both Einstein and an individual of low intelligence to have the same presentation even if they had the same disease? You can easily see, then, why two patients with the same disease can present vastly different clinical pictures when they are first seen by a physician.

Unanswered Questions

The foregoing reasoning notwithstanding, we are still perplexed in many instances as to why pictures differ from patient to patient. Why are some diabetic patients who have had the disease for 20 years free of retinopathy, whereas others are blind after only 10 years? Why do some diabetic patients develop neuropathy almost at or even before disease onset, whereas others never do?

The same can be said of patients who have cirrhosis. Portal hypertension, hyperestrogenism, hyperaldosteronism, ascites, bleeding tendencies, anemia, and hepatic coma are some of the different groups of manifestations that may occur all together or in any combination. Only one or two may dominate the picture, and the others may be absent. The presence or absence of clues can be extremely chancy.

The fact that the many symptoms, physical signs, and laboratory tests for a particular disease have different sensitivities tells you that not every clue need be present in the patient who has the disease. Therefore, the clinical picture of a disease will differ from patient to patient.

Osler expressed this concept well: "Variability is the law of life, and as no two faces are the same, so no two bodies are alike, and no two individuals react alike, and behave alike under abnormal conditions that we know as disease. This is the fundamental difficulty in the education of the physician."

TIME WILL TELL

It seems appropriate to close this chapter with a reminder that physicians are not omniscient, that humbleness is a virtue, and that there is inevitably a certain percentage of patient problems we are unable to solve without prescriptions for *essence of patience, tincture of time, and long-acting capsules of observation.* If you do not know what is wrong, consultants may be helpful. And if you are pressed to treat, you can always resort to a therapeutic trial and treat "as if"—bearing in mind that this action is to be regarded only as a desperate measure.

The Bible speaks of man living three score years and ten. Public health measures and preventive medicine deserve the bulk of credit for man's present life span matching this expectation. If one considers the life expectancy of a 60-year-old today, not much has changed since biblical times. Occasionally, we do save a life with antibiotics or surgery. We may even prolong life a year or two with good care. But a life expectancy of 70 years still stands, give or take 10 years, depending on whether the genetic background does or does not include diabetes, hypertension, or atherosclerosis.

Digits, Decimals, and Doctors

Paul Cutler

WHO NEEDS MATH ANYWAY?

Most students of medicine are repelled by discussions of complicated mathematical concepts. Physicians are too. Such antipathy is both understandable and justifiable because medicine deals with people, not numbers.

However, the proposition that doctors don't need "math" is not valid.

Modern medical economics, the rising importance of demographics, mathematical models of the diagnostic process, cost-benefit analysis, informed consent, scientific decision making, managed care, and the increasing use of computers in medicine—all mandate that the physician of the 21st century know more about percentages, numbers, statistics, and mathematical methods.

How, then, does one make palatable the minimal amount of mathematics that *is necessary* for the 99% of students who will spend their lives treating patients? Over the past 10 years it has become increasingly evident that physicians must be familiar with some basic equations, theorems, and simple mathematical concepts in order to be able to:

- Calculate the probability that a disease exists
- Alter the probability of a disease by the performance of a test
- Interpret test results
- Construct decision trees that measure the outcomes of alternate pathways
- Perform cost/risk/benefit analyses
- Decide which form of patient management is best
- Solve problems with precision
- And much, much more

In large measure, reason, logic, intuition, and decisions are based on nonintellectualized inter-nal mathematical operations. The text that follows includes the arithmetic essentials that a non-mathematical clinician-teacher thinks medical students need to know in order to be better physicians.

The Prototype Problem

You see a 65-year-old man who is being treated for chronic congestive heart failure with mild salt restriction, decreased activity, and .25 mg of digoxin and 40 mg of furosemide daily. He had been doing fairly well for the past 6 months on this regimen, but for the preceding few weeks he has complained of nausea, anorexia, and occasional palpitations. These symptoms had occurred from time to time in the past and were usually associated with clinically evident mild cardiac decompensation. Now, however, he has only mild dyspnea, but no orthopnea; there is no evidence of basal rales, jugular venous distention, enlarged liver, or ankle edema. The patient has lost weight. Cardiac abnormalities associated with his heart disease are present as before, but the first heart sound seems more faint than usual. The electrocardiogram (ECG) shows no change from the one taken 6 months ago, except for occasional ventricular premature depolarizations and a PR interval of .23 second, which was .18 second when last recorded.

The questions: Are the patient's complaints caused by his heart disease, by digitalis intoxication, or by something else? Does he need more or less digitalis? Does he need more or less diuretic? Does he need a search for another disease? Does he have occult cancer? Is the first-degree heart block caused by his heart disease or the digitalis?

The patient's serum electrolyte and creatinine levels are normal. He has no other symptoms. You predict that he has digitalis intoxication with an estimated probability of 50%. Now you wish to obtain a serum digoxin assay in order to revise the probability upward.

Assume that the cutoff point for this test that designates toxicity is 2.0 ng/mL in your laboratory. Moreover, you understand that in using any cutoff point, you inevitably create false-positive and false-negative results. If the test result is normal (e.g., 1.5 ng/mL), how far down has the probability estimate of 50% fallen? If the test result is abnormal (2.5 ng/mL), how much more certain are you that the patient has digitalis intoxication? The decision on further management hinges on this issue.

After exploring the mathematical processes needed to deal with this prototype problem, a decision on further management is made in "The Prototype Problem Revisited" section discussed later in this chapter.

A Pause for Orientation

The subjects of sensitivity, specificity, probability, predictive value, probability revision—and how these mathematical concepts may be expressed by words, symbolized by algebraic notation, and diagrammed by tables, are what this chapter is all about. You can easily see how these concepts relate to the common problem just presented and how comprehension of these concepts establishes a firm basis for the numerous clinical decisions made daily.

Questions That Arise Daily

Hundreds of times each day physicians ask themselves questions that need quantitative answers. For example, how certain am I that patient 1 has cancer? Does this test prove that patient 2 has coronary artery disease? Should I recommend surgery when I am only 75% sure of the diagnosis? The next patient has a sore throat; what are the chances it is streptococcal, and should I therefore give penicillin? Will further tests help, and how much? Here's an 18-year-old female who has a positive serologic test for syphilis; her mother has lupus. What is the likelihood of a false-positive test, and should she receive antibiotic treatment? And on and on each day.

The physician proceeds to answer one question after another without precision. Not knowing the numbers game, he or she must usually make decisions that are based on imprecise premises. But an understanding of the application of *old* mathematical concepts to *new* medical information can give added dimension to diagnostic precision.

BAYES' THEOREMS

In 1763, Sir Thomas Bayes, a British minister and mathematician, devised a set of theorems that are mathematical expressions of statistical probabilities. His theorems relate disease prevalence and disease probability to the sensitivity, specificity, and predictive values of a test or clue. These theorems are of great help and have done much to quantify medical judgment, but they also have serious limitations; both factors must be appreciated.

These precise old arithmetic methods have been resurrected in the past two decades and applied to new methods of medical problem solving. Physicians deal with Bayes' theorems when they consider: (1) the incidence of a disease in a population, (2) the incidence of a specific clue in a disease, and (3) the incidence of this clue in persons who do not have the disease. Thus, the physician aims to relate individual clues or combinations of clues in order to make a specific diagnosis in a precise mathematical probabilistic fashion.

Prevalence and Probability

Simple Bayesian terminology must be understood before proceeding. D represents the presence of a disease, whereas $\bar{D}$ signifies the absence of a disease. C represents the presence of a clue (or the positivity of a test), whereas $\bar{C}$ signifies the absence of a clue (or the negativity of a test). $P(D)$ symbolizes the prevalence of a disease or the probability that a disease exists in a particular patient.

For example, if one person in 1000 has a disease, the $P(D)$ or *prevalence* of the disease is .001. Diabetes mellitus has a 5% or .05 prevalence; essential hypertension has a 20% or .20 prevalence in adults.

The *prevalence* differs from the *incidence* in that the former represents the number of cases per unit of population that exists at any one time; the latter tells the number of cases per unit of population over a given period of time. They are not the same. At any one time, there may be 10 cases of influenza per 1000 persons (prevalence .01), but the annual incidence of influenza may be 100 cases per 1000 persons (incidence .10).

Not only does $P(D)$ represent the prevalence of disease, but it has also come to signify the *probability* that a disease exists in an individual patient or in a cohort of identical patients. When we say that the $P(D)$ in a patient is .20, we also mean that in a cohort of 100 identical patients, 20 patients will have the disease, and 80 patients will not. Given a lean patient with hypertension and dyspnea on exertion, the probability that he has left ventricular failure can be estimated at .40; the same $P(D)$ would hold true for 100 similar patients.

Sensitivity and Specificity

Consider the following four statements about a disease and a related clue:

1. $P(C/D) = .85$
2. $P(\bar{C}/D) = .15$
3. $P(\bar{C}/\bar{D}) = .95$
4. $P(C/\bar{D}) = .05$

The first statement says that 85% of persons with a certain disease will exhibit a given clue. Stated differently, the clue has a *true positive (TP) rate* of .85, and the *sensitivity* of the clue (positivity in disease) is .85.

The second statement says that given the same disease, the clue under discussion will be absent in 15% of cases; the *false-negative (FN) rate* is therefore .15, and this is equal to 1 minus the sensitivity. Because a clue is either present or absent, the *"rule of ones"* can be readily understood.

The third statement says that 95% of persons who do not have the disease under discussion do not have the clue. Those persons who do not have the disease in question may be healthy or have a different disease. Therefore, in 95% of those persons without the disease, the clue is *truly negative (TN);* and the *specificity* of the clue, which is the TN rate, is .95.

The fourth statement falls quite naturally into place. If 95% of persons who do not have the disease do not have the clue, it follows that 5% of

those without the disease *do* have the clue. In these persons, the clue is *falsely positive* (FP), and you may conclude that even in the absence of that disease, 5% of persons do exhibit the clue. Note that the false-positive rate also follows the "rule of ones"; even in the absence of the disease, the clue may or may not be present, and the *FP rate equals 1 minus the specificity.*

It follows that the TP rate plus the FN rate equals 1, and the TN rate plus the FP rate also equals 1. In the consideration just cited, if the disease is *tuberculosis* and the clue is *cough,* 85% of persons with tuberculosis cough, and 15% do not; 95% of persons without tuberculosis do not cough, and 5% do.

Predictive Value

But in medicine we are less interested in how many persons with tuberculosis will cough than in how many persons who cough have tuberculosis. Put more dramatically, it is more helpful to know how likely is a person with hemoptysis to have lung cancer than to know how likely is a person with lung cancer to have hemoptysis. And how likely is a lesion to be not malignant if there is no associated hemoptysis. The doctor at the bedside wants to be able to prove a suspected diagnosis.

Clearly, we are now dealing with *the probability of a diagnosis given a clue* and the probability of the absence of a diagnosis given the absence of a clue—$P(D/C)$ and $P(\bar{D}/\bar{C})$. These are also called the *positive predictive value* (PV+) and the *negative predictive value* (PV−) of a clue.

For example, if 10% of patients with hemoptysis have cancer of the lung, 90% of those with hemoptysis do not have cancer. The positive predictive value of hemoptysis for lung cancer is therefore .10 ($P[D/C] = .10$). The probability that cancer does not exist is .90 ($P[\bar{D}/C] = .90$). The calculation of predictive values is made from the prevalence (or clinical probability) and the sensitivity-specificity of the clue being considered.

Two-By-Two Tables

The relationships between clues and diagnoses can be expressed by language, two-by-two (2×2) tables, Bayes' theorems, or stick diagrams. Language was the method just used. Although Bayes' theorems and stick diagrams are frequently seen in medical literature, 2 × 2 tables are probably the easiest to understand, learn, and apply.

To start, the reader must understand that *"test"* and *"clue"* are used interchangeably for this and subsequent related discussions. The same mathematical models may be applied to any feature in the history or physical examination, to laboratory tests, and to diagnostic procedures.

Figure 7.1 shows the results obtained in each cell of a 2 × 2 table where a clue is either positive or negative in the presence or absence of a disease. Inspect the left half of the diagram and note the derivation of TP, FN, TN, and FP (true positive, false negative, true negative, and false positive). Then study the right side of the diagram, where numbers are substituted for symbols. This represents a hypothetical case where the disease probability is .10 and the clue's sensitivity and specificity for that disease are both .90. A patient with a 10% likelihood of having a disease is represented schematically by 100 identical cases of whom 10 will have the disease, and 90 will not. Calculations of the exact TP, FN, TN, and FP values are made on this basis. Of the 10 patients with the disease, 90% will evidence a positive clue; thus, there will be 9 TPs and 1 FN. Of the 90 patients who do not have the disease, the clue will be absent or negative in all; therefore, there will be 81 TNs and 9 FPs.

Note also that there are 18 positive results in 100 patients; 9 of the 18 are truly positive. This means that the predictive value of a positive clue (PV+) is .50, and that a positive clue in this case raises the likelihood of disease from .10 to .50. In

addition, note that there are 82 negative results, of which 81 are truly negative. This means that the predictive value of a negative clue (PV−) is approximately .99, and a negative clue in this case reduces the likelihood of disease from .10 to .01 (or increases the *unlikelihood* from .90 to .99).

Note that the PV+ equals the ratio of TPs to the total number of positive tests (TPs plus FPs); the PV− equals the ratio of TNs to the total number of negative tests (TNs plus FNs). It can readily be seen that the higher the $P(D)$, the higher will be the resulting PV+, and the lower will be the resulting PV−.

When a test is performed on a patient with an estimated pretest $P(D)$, *the resultant PV becomes the post-test P(D)*. The difference between the pretest $P(D)$ and the post-test $P(D)$ is equal to the incremental gain (or loss) in the probability that the disease is present.

THE OPERATING CHARACTERISTICS

The operating characteristics of a clue, test, or diagnostic procedure are its two most important features—*sensitivity* and *specificity*. They have a profound influence on the overall usefulness and predictive value of the clue, test, or procedure.

The higher the sensitivity and specificity, the better the procedure, and the more effect it will have on the diagnostic probability. *Test efficiency* is measured by the sum of the sensitivity and specificity divided by 2. If the sensitivity is .90 and the specificity is .90, then the test efficiency is 1.8/2.0, or 90%. This is a "decent" test, clue, or procedure. If the sensitivity and specificity total 1.0, the efficiency is 1.0/2.0, or 50%; this is a worthless test, and it will not alter the initial probability.

But if a test raises the probability of a disease from .10 to .60, or from .30 to .90, it is a good test. Likewise, if the test reduces the probability from .30 to .01 or from .60 to .01 by virtue of its results being negative, it is also very helpful. The matter boils down to the degree of positivity and negativity you seek before making a further decision.

How to Derive the S and S

Select a population known with absolute certainty to *have* a disease, and a population known

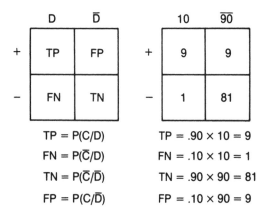

> **Figure 7.1.** Two-by-two tables relating a clue to a disease.

with absolute certainty to *not have* that disease. This degree of certainty can be attained only by a biopsy, surgery, or arteriography, although there is some doubt as to the absoluteness of even these tests.

Assume then that coronary arteriography was performed upon 1000 men with chest pain of various types. Assume further that arteriography was able to separate those persons with and those without "significant" coronary disease according to predetermined criteria of cross-sectional narrowing. Such a perfect test is commonly called a "gold standard test." As a result of these tests, it was determined that 600 men do and 400 men do not have significant coronary disease.

Now, apply a *new test* to this cohort so that you may evaluate its performance and determine its sensitivity and specificity. The test is inexpensive, noninvasive, seems fairly reliable, and you wish to establish its operating characteristics for future clinical use. Criteria for positivity and negativity are decided, and the test is performed on both groups. Results are seen in Figure 7.2. Of those persons with proven coronary disease, 540 had a positive test (TP) and 60 had a negative test (FN). Therefore, the sensitivity of the test is 540 divided by 600, or .90. In men without coronary disease, there were 320 negative results (TN) and 80 positive results (FP). Therefore, the specificity of the test is 320 divided by 400, or .80. Knowing the operating characteristics of the test, you can now apply it to any individual who needs further study and for whom you can form a fairly reliable clinical estimate of disease probability.

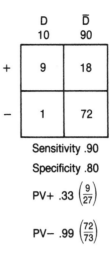

Sensitivity .90
Specificity .80
PV+ .33 $\left(\frac{9}{27}\right)$
PV− .99 $\left(\frac{72}{73}\right)$

▶ **Figure 7.3.** Changing the probabilities by using a test with known operating characteristics.

Applying the S and S

A 36-year-old man consults you for vague chest pain that has been intermittently present for 3 days. He smokes heavily; his father died of a heart condition at age 42; and the patient is most apprehensive. The pain does not sound like coronary pain, but you're not sure. Aside from the blood pressure of 160/94, his examination is normal. So is the ECG. You assign him a clinical $P(D)$ of only .10 and perform the special new test. Executing the test on a cohort of 100 patients with the same picture would produce the 2×2 table seen in Figure 7.3. The PV+ is .33, less than you might think, because the original $P(D)$ was low. A positive test would increase the likelihood

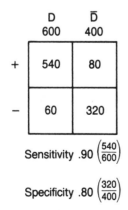

Sensitivity .90 $\left(\frac{540}{600}\right)$

Specificity .80 $\left(\frac{320}{400}\right)$

▶ **Figure 7.2.** Determining the operating characteristics of a new test.

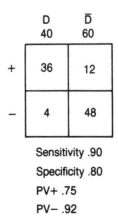

Sensitivity .90
Specificity .80
PV+ .75
PV− .92

▶ **Figure 7.4.** Alteration of probabilities when the $P(D)$ is more likely.

only a little, but a negative test would rule out the disease with 99% certainty. The test is negative.

The same man consults you 10 years later. His pain is different and more closely resembles angina, although it is still not typical. Everything else is the same. A serum cholesterol is 350 mg/dL. You revise the $P(D)$ to .40 and do another test. A positive test increases the $P(D)$ to .75, and a negative test reduces it to .08 (Fig. 7.4). Depending on the results in either instance, you might give reassurance with caution, treat medically, or do arteriography in contemplation of surgery, considering all of the other factors that go into the decision.

Pas de Deux

There are basically four relationships that can exist between a clue and a disease:

1. A clue that is *100% sensitive* is seen in all cases of the disease. If the clue is absent or negative, the disease is absolutely ruled out. It may, however, be present in other conditions. Albuminuria in the nephrotic syndrome and tachycardia in hyperthyroidism are examples of such clues.
2. A clue that is *100% specific* is seen only in the disease. If present or positive, the disease is definitely diagnosed. However, it is not necessarily present in all patients who have the disease. A tophus in gout (Fig. 7.5), the Kayser-Fleischer ring in Wilson's disease, and free air under the diaphragm in the case of a perforated viscus are examples of such clues.
3. A clue that is *100% sensitive and 100% specific* is present or positive in all cases of the disease and never occurs in patients who do not have the disease. When the clue is present or positive, the patient has the disease; when the clue is absent or negative, the patient does not have the disease. Such clues are indeed rare.
4. The fourth relationship is the usual situation seen in medicine. Here, the clue is *often* but *not always* present or positive if the disease exists, and is *sometimes* but not often present or positive if the disease does not exist (false positive).

It is important that patients as well as doctors understand the *concept of imperfect information,* and that they do not have the false perception that a clue or test that is positive or negative concludes the story.

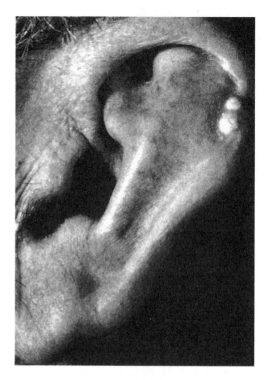

▶ **Figure 7.5.** Gouty tophus. The two white lesions on the helix of this patient's ear were hard and nontender.

Where to Draw the Line

Until now we have dealt only with dichotomous tests and clues that are either positive or negative, or present or absent. But other tests show a linear distribution of values, and a cutoff point between normality and abnormality must be established. An ideal test of this type clearly separates health from disease and is illustrated by Figure 7.6, where there is no overlap of values; consequently, there are neither false-positive nor false-negative results.

Unfortunately, such tests are rare or nonexistent. The usual situation is depicted in Figure 7.7, where there is an overlap of values between healthy persons and those persons who have a disease. In fact, this diagram aptly describes the situation that is seen with serum uric acid levels in normal persons and in those persons with gout. The overlap of values between 5 and 8 mg/dL determines that some normal persons have what is regarded as elevated serum uric acid (FP), whereas some patients who have gout have normal serum uric acid (FN). The cutoff point determines the incidence of false negativity and

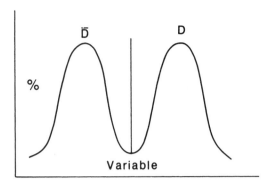

▶ **Figure 7.6.** Distribution of values for the ideal test. No overlap is present, and there are no false-positive results.

false positivity. If the separator is set at 6.5 mg/dL (*c*), the FN and FP rates are approximately equal.

However, by moving the cutoff point to the left (from *c* to *b* to *a*), all patients with gout will have a positive or abnormal test result. In so doing, the sensitivity of the test has been markedly increased; but this was done at the expense of decreasing the specificity, because many normal persons will now have "abnormal" serum uric acid levels.

Similarly, if the cutoff point is moved to the right (from *c* to *d* to *e*), normal persons will almost always have normal test results. The specificity of the test has been markedly increased, but the sensitivity is diminished, because many more patients with gout will have normal serum uric acid levels, according to the new separator. There are obvious trade-offs when moving in either direction. This generalization holds for all tests.

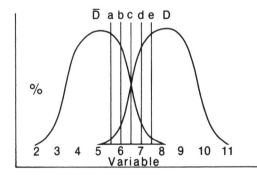

▶ **Figure 7.7.** Distribution of values for the usual test. Overlap is present, and false-positive and false-negative results exist. Operating characteristics vary with the location of the cutoff point.

TABLE 7.1. Test Results

DISEASE	NONDISEASE
Dichotomous Tests	
Clue present	Clue absent
Test results positive	Test results negative
Linear Variable	
Abnormal	Normal

To summarize, in deciding on a separator point, consider the consequences of false-negative and false-positive results. The trade-offs revolve around two questions. Is it serious if the disease is missed and left untreated? Is it serious if the disease is overdiagnosed? In the final analysis, it depends on whether you wish to minimize the FP results or the FN results.

At this point, we must clarify the confusion resulting from the use of antonymous terms under varying circumstances. For example, a clue in the history or physical examination is either *present* or *absent*. A test or procedure is either *positive* or *negative* if the test result is dichotomous, or the test is *abnormal* or *normal* if the test result is measured by continuous variables.

For example, you may say that cough is present but hemoptysis is absent. The results of a test for occult blood in the stool are either positive or negative. But the results of a chest radiograph, ECG, serum glucose, serum bilirubin, or computed tomographic liver scan is either abnormal or normal. In the interpretation of some procedures, *positive* and *abnormal*—or *negative* and *normal*—may be used interchangeably (Table 7.1).

As ill luck would have it, some tests and procedures needing expert interpretation may yield equivocal results. They are neither positive nor negative for sure. This all-too-common occurrence causes doubt and concern for the diagnostician and compels decisions that require further actions.

SIMPLE CLINICAL USES

The principles just discussed are very commonly used by problem solvers as they obtain and process information. Take the case of a 42-year-old white man who has backaches, generalized aches and pains, and a rapid erythrocyte sedimentation rate. You estimate that he has a 50% likelihood of having ankylosing spondylitis, and therefore you order a test for the HLA-B27 molecule to increase the diagnostic probability. For white men, the test is 92% sensitive and 93% specific. If the test results are positive, the revised probability is now greater than 90%, and you have achieved reasonable diagnostic certainty (Fig. 7.8).

This test could not be used as a general screening test because of the high (7%) incidence of false-positive results. Also, the test is less useful in black men for whom the operating characteristics are different.

Contemplate the use of the fluorescent antinuclear antibody test. Its sensitivity in systemic lupus erythematosus is 98%; its specificity is 90%. When applied to any individual for whom the $P(D)$ is extremely low, the test is of little value because of the high number of FPs that might occur. The test has its maximal value when five clinical criteria are already present, and the $P(D)$ is moderately high.

The marginal benefit of a test is the difference between the pretest and post-test $P(D)$s. When the $P(D)$ is very low or very high, the marginal benefit (incremental gain) is small; when the $P(D)$ is intermediate, the marginal benefit (incremental gain) is greatest. This is readily demonstrable by graphing techniques that tell us that the greatest value of a test is obtained when it is ordered with a *diagnosis already in mind.*

Consider mammography for the routine screening for breast cancer (Fig. 7.9). Assume that the prevalence of breast cancer in women over 50 is .003, or 3 cases per 1000 women, and that the mammogram is 66⅔% sensitive and 99% specific.

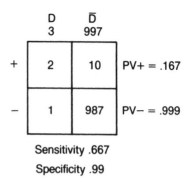

▶ **Figure 7.9.** Mammography and breast cancer.

Now, fill the cells of the 2 × 2 diagram. Should a patient ask you for the significance of a positive mammogram result found on a routine survey, you can calm her somewhat by telling her that the chance of having cancer is only 16⅔%. If the test results are negative, she can be 99.9% sure that she doesn't have the disease. On the other hand, if her mother and sister had breast cancer, she is in a different subset, and her $P(D)$ is more likely to be .012 than .003. In this case, a positive mammogram result would have a PV+ of approximately .50. Note how these calculations translate into the practicalities of doctor-patient interaction.

The Prototype Problem Revisited

Now let's get back to the problem presented at the beginning of this chapter and apply the mathematical logic that has just been learned.

The clinical estimate of digitalis toxicity is .50. It has already been determined in your laboratory that with a cutoff point of 2.0 ng/mL the digoxin assay is 90% sensitive and 80% specific for toxicity. The 2 × 2 table (Fig. 7.10) tells us that the PV+ is .82, and the PV− is .89. The assay reports 2.5 ng/mL; this is abnormal. At this level, the test offers even higher predictive values (see page 84). Therefore, the probability of digitalis toxicity has risen to more than .82; digoxin administration is stopped, and the patient should improve in several days, at which time he will be started on a smaller dose of the drug. Had the digoxin assay shown normal values (e.g., 1.5 ng/mL), the probability of digitalis toxicity would have fallen to less than .11 (i.e., $P[D] = .89$). In this instance, you would consider the progressive worsening of

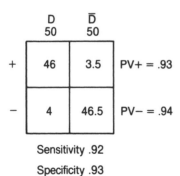

▶ **Figure 7.8.** Relationship between HLA-B27 and ankylosing spondylitis in white men.

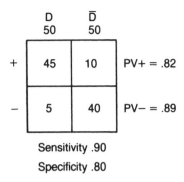

Sensitivity .90

Specificity .80

▶ **Figure 7.10.** Solving the prototype problem of digitalis toxicity.

his heart disease or the presence of another underlying disease, such as cancer.

The preceding information in this chapter and an appreciation of the prototype problem should leave you with the important conclusion that most information you receive about patients is imperfect in some respects, and that the *concept of imperfect information* applies to items in the history, the physical examination, and to almost all tests and procedures.

Revision of Probability

So far you have seen how a positive or negative clue can revise the likelihood that a disease is present. But revisions can also be made if there are *two* primary contenders for the diagnosis, and the test has different operating characteristics for each contender.

Assume that clue C—a major diagnostic determinant—is being applied to two diseases D_1 and D_2. Assume also that clue C is present in *only* these two diseases. D_1 is common and occurs in 20% of a given set of 1000 persons. D_2 is uncommon and occurs in only 1% of that set. Clue C is 10% sensitive in D_1 and 50% sensitive in D_2. Table 7.2 demonstrates that if clue C is present or positive, D_1 is now four times as likely as D_2.

TABLE 7.2. Revision of Disease Likelihood by a Positive Clue

DISEASE	P(D)	P(C/D)	P(D/C)
D_1	0.20 (200 pts)	0.10 (20 pts)	0.80
D_2	0.01 (10 pts)	0.50 (5 pts)	0.20

Key: pts = patients.

This is an example of the situation wherein the uncommon manifestations of a common disease are more common than the common manifestations of an uncommon disease.

A revision of probabilities may also be accomplished by a normal test result or the absence of a clue. Suppose a clinician decides that a patient with a given cluster has a 75% likelihood of having disease D_1 and a 25% likelihood of having disease D_2. A further diagnostic procedure (radiograph, scan, laboratory test) is done, and the test result is negative. The fact that it is negative may give much useful information.

The pathologist or radiologist (the test expert) tells us that this test is negative in 20% of patients with D_1 and in 60% of patients with D_2. In a cohort of 100 patients with this given cluster, there will be 30 negative results: 15 in D_1 and 15 in D_2. Therefore, given a negative result, the revised likelihoods of D_1 and D_2 are 50% and 50% (Table 7.3).

For example, on the basis of clinical evidence, you decide that a patient has a 50%, 25%, 25% chance of having pulmonary tuberculosis, cancer, or sarcoidosis, in that order. The results of a purified protein derivative skin test, fiberoptic bronchoscopy, and computed tomography alter the computed likelihoods to 5%, 5%, 90%. A good physician performs these calculations many times daily, although he uses quick mental maneuvers instead of precise figures and formulas.

Given correct statistical data, formulas and equations can be written for all combinations and probabilities. For instance, in the presence of three clues and the absence of a fourth, how likely is a diagnosis? Physicians approximate such statis-

TABLE 7.3. Revision of Disease Likelihood by a Negative Clue

DISEASE	INITIAL LIKELIHOOD (%)	NEGATIVE TEST PER COHORT OF 100 PTS	REVISED LIKELIHOOD (%)
D_1	75	20% = 15 pts	50
D_2	25	60% = 15 pts	50

Key: pts = patients.

tics and probabilities many times daily as they solve their patients' problems, without writing equations for Bayes' theorems—indeed, without being aware of their existence.

Estimating the Likelihood

As has been previously discussed, $P(D)$ means the *prevalence* of a disease or the probability that it is present in a particular patient based on the clinical evidence on hand. The $P(D)$ changes as each new bit of evidence is added.

It is surprising to note that various physicians, given only the barest of clues, show only little or modest differences in their original estimates of disease likelihood. Consider a 34-year-old woman with polyarthritis, a 26-year-old woman with periodic dyspnea at rest, a 56-year-old man with severe substernal pain, or a 3-year-old child with a large tumor in the left abdomen. Most would agree that the respective likelihoods are in the vicinity of rheumatoid arthritis .80, hyperventilation .90, coronary heart disease .50, and Wilms' tumor .50. Then, as additional data are gathered, the likelihood increases or decreases, especially in comparison with a competing diagnosis.

If you see a youngish woman with recurrent polyarthritis, the differential diagnosis rests almost entirely between rheumatoid arthritis and systemic lupus erythematosus. Knowing that the former disease is 20 times more common than the latter, you can begin with these relative likelihoods (Table 7.4). Each additional clue alters the relative likelihoods so that in this case, you may end with a reversed ratio. The values stated are approximations. More exact figures can be determined if the operating characteristics of each clue are known for each of the two diseases. Each $P(D)$ is revised by a clue, and the resultant positive predictive value turns out to be the $P(D)$ for subsequent testing ($P_1 \rightarrow P_2 \rightarrow P_3 \rightarrow P_4$, and so forth).

A second example concerns a 68-year-old

TABLE 7.4. Alteration of Likelihoods by Adding Clues

ADDITION OF CLUES TO INITIAL $P(D)$	RA	SUBSEQUENT $P(D)$	SLE
Initial $P(D)$	.95	P_1	.05
Pleurisy	.70	P_2	.30
Rash	.50	P_3	.50
Albuminuria	.30	P_4	.70
RF test +	.50	P_5	.50
ANA test +	.05	P_6	.95

RA = rheumatoid arthritis, SLE = systemic lupus erythematosus, ANA = antinuclear antibody, RF = rheumatoid factor, P = probability.

TABLE 7.5. Fluctuation of Likelihoods in an Obese Woman with Dyspnea on Exertion

ADDITION OF CLUES TO INITIAL $P(D)$	LVF	SUBSEQUENT $P(D)$	OTHER DISEASES
1. Initial $P(D)$	.30	P_1	.70
2. Chronic hypertension	.50	P_2	.50
3. Chronic cough—2 packs/day	.30	P_3	.70
4. Orthopnea	.50	P_4	.50
5. Basal rales, no wheezes	.60	P_5	.40
6. S_3 at apex	.80	P_6	.20
7. Large heart, Kerley's B lines	.95	P_7	.05

LVF = left ventricular failure, P = probability.

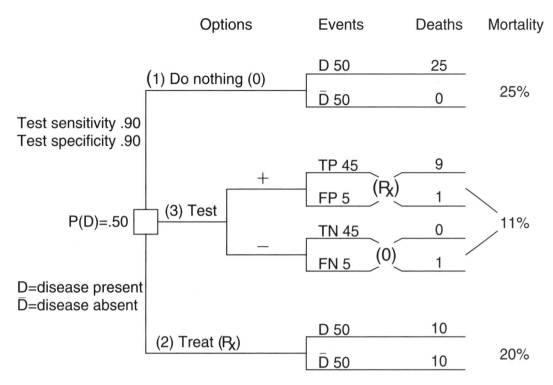

▶ **Figure 7.11.** Decision tree for a cohort of 100 identical patients with a disease probability of .50

obese woman who complains of dyspnea on exertion. You estimate that the $P(D)$ for left ventricular failure is .30; but other conditions may exist. Note in Table 7.5 how the probabilities fluctuate up and down with each additional clue. Eventually, left ventricular failure becomes almost certain.

To Test or Treat

Sometimes it is difficult to decide whether to give or withhold treatment because you're not very sure of the diagnosis. For example, based on your clinical evaluation, you think a patient has a 50% chance of having a serious disease whose mortality is 50%, if untreated. The proposed treatment reduces the mortality from the disease to 20%, but it is such that the treatment itself causes the death of 20% of persons who don't have the disease.

You construct a decision tree (Fig. 7.11) that has three alternative pathways and calculate the mortality resulting from each one—(1) do nothing, (2) treat, (3) test first, then treat if positive and don't treat if negative. The test is a good test

and has a .90 sensitivity and a .90 specificity for the disease in question.

Note the mortality that results from each option. Treatment reduces the mortality rate from 25% to 20%, which is only slightly worthwhile, whereas if you test first and then treat only if positive, the mortality rate is reduced to 11%—by more than half. You must bear in mind that treating a single patient with a 50% likelihood of having a disease is the same as treating 100 identical patients of whom 50 have the disease (D) and 50 do not (D̄). Also, note that option 2 risks killing a patient who does not even have the disease, whereas option 3 offers the double risk of not treating someone who has the disease, as well as killing someone who doesn't.

Based on trade-offs, ethics, and values, you and the patient are now able to decide which course to take. This chapter has presented some of the more important mathematical concepts that the problem solver must understand in order to interpret and evaluate patient information, make correct decisions regarding diagnosis and treatment, and deal with patients within the guidelines established by society, the medical profession, and managed care.

How to Use Tests

Paul Cutler

You have seen how the various types of information derived from the patient's data base may make a diagnosis more or less likely. Included in this data base are items from the history, the physical examination, and various diagnostic procedures that include tests from the laboratory, radiography department, and other ancillary diagnostic facilities.

Although the solution of most medical problems is to be found in the history and physical examination, it is frequently necessary to perform various tests in order to be more certain. A staggering array of information has become available with the mere puncture of a vein; with the ability to dissect every body fluid into picograms; with the skill to biopsy virtually any tissue; with the use of new imaging techniques that reflect the anatomy, physiology, and biochemistry of most organs; and with the wizardry to employ altered genes, electrons, positrons, magnets, and computers to track almost everything. The marriage of immunology and genetics at the biochemical altar has given birth to magic bullets, disease tracers, chemical factories, and yet more tests—all of which are as awesome as Star Wars.

Couple this diagnostic explosion with a new religion that deifies the measurement and looks upon simpler clinical methods with impiety. The result is an exponential increase in the ordering and performance of diagnostic tests and procedures, with only little knowledge of and little consideration for their necessity, cost, risk, benefit, and reliability. *It's easier, simpler, and more glamorous to order tests than to talk, examine, or think.*

There is an urgent need to overhaul some patterns for ordering diagnostic tests. Medical students must learn to follow new, more effective, and more efficient trends before they fall into the same bad habits that are often passed on

from one generation of house officers to the next. The fact that too many tests are ordered is undeniable. The fact that many tests are unnecessary, not helpful, and often misleading is well established, and the fact that the shocking rise of health care cost is in large part related to tests and procedures is a statistical reality.

Our challenge is to do whatever is possible to improve this situation without affecting quality care—to orchestrate the requisition of procedures for the patient's benefit rather than his or her detriment. To do this, *you must know* how your laboratory and procedure departments operate, why tests are ordered, how to order tests, how to interpret single and multiple test results, how much these tests cost, and how to decrease testing and avoid diagnostic overkill.

REASONS FOR TESTING

The fundamental reason for doing tests in conjunction with or following the history and physical examination is to help find out what is wrong with the patient. But in truth there are many other reasons. Some say that tests are done simply for the purposes of *discovery, confirmation,* or *exclusion*. To be more complete, we can list the following reasons for testing:

1. Diagnosis
2. Prognosis
3. Screening
4. Monitoring
5. Determination of baseline data
6. Decisions

Diagnosis is most important; a test or procedure helps to detect, confirm, document, or exclude a disease. Once a disease is suspected, further tests aim to increase or decrease the diagnostic certainty of one diagnosis to the exclusion of others.

Prognosis can be predicted, for example, by noting the degree of test abnormality. The higher the transaminase level in hepatitis, the higher the amylase level in pancreatitis, and the higher the creatine kinase MB isomer level in acute myocardial infarction, the more serious the disease and usually the worse the prognosis.

Screening is more complex, although in general, screening tests are done to exclude diseases in seemingly healthy persons. You screen for many diseases at the same time by ordering entire profiles or batteries of tests to be done by automated techniques—*multiphasic screening*. In so doing, you aim to exclude the presence of liver, bone, kidney, and parathyroid diseases, as well as electrolyte, lipid, and diabetic disorders. On the other hand, *targeting screening* is the ordering of a single test on a single person or an entire population, aiming to discover or exclude a specific disease—for example, the prostate-specific antigen, or mammography.

The use of tests for *monitoring* has many facets. You may wish to measure progression or regression of a disease, response to treatment, or drug levels of medication being used. A rising creatinine level indicates progressive worsening of kidney function. A falling cholesterol may indicate that dietary or drug treatment is effective. The blood level of an antiarrhythmic drug may not be high enough to achieve the desired effect.

Tests obtained for *baseline data* determination are akin to screening in that they tell you what is *not* wrong with the patient and establish patterns of normality. But they also permit you to detect problems that may crop up later during the course of a primary disease or as a result of treatment. It is important to note that the patient has a normal creatinine level before giving a possibly nephrotoxic drug and then noting its elevation.

A decision on treatment may depend on the result of a test; whether or not to use anticoagulants can hinge on a ventilation-perfusion scan; whether to continue or withhold digoxin treatment may depend on a blood digoxin level.

Not included in the list, but also important, is the fact that tests are ordered for patient and doctor reassurance and for defensive medicolegal reasons.

ON BEING IN ORDER

The sequence in which tests are ordered depends on many factors. If the situation is critical, the test with the highest yield is done, even though there may be some risk. But if there is time, perhaps lower yield, less risky procedures can be done first. If a massive myocardial infarction is impending, angiography might be the initial test. But if the situation is less fragile, an electrocardiogram (ECG) and cardiac muscle enzymes study come first, then perhaps a treadmill test, and a thallium scan thereafter.

Ordinarily, the order of testing is: (1) from cheap to costly, (2) from less to more risky, and (3) from simple to more complex. Within the constraints of time, risk, and cost, try to do the test or procedure with the most efficiency as soon as possible; that is, use the procedure with the highest sensitivity, specificity, and predictive values.

Ideally, all of the preceding objectives should be observed in deciding which tests to request first and the sequence in which they should be ordered. But this is not always practical. One or more objectives may be sacrificed for speed, convenience, accuracy, parsimony, a waiting list for procedures, time needed to await the results, and the condition of the patient. Sometimes it may be best to get the costly test done first; it may solve the problem quickly and save money in the long run.

KNOW YOUR LABORATORY

The discussions in this chapter do not relate only to what is commonly called "the lab." Included in the laboratory are the subdivisions of hematology, immunopathology, microbiology, histopathology, chemistry, and so forth. In addition, reference to "tests" includes all of those procedures done by radiologists, cardiologists, gastroenterologists, and pulmonary disease specialists. So what is said in this chapter regarding a simple blood chemical test also applies to computed tomographic (CT) scans, ultrasound studies, arteriography, programmed cardiac electrical stimulation, endoscopic procedures, and pulmonary function tests as well.

Familiarity Breeds Respect

One of the first things the beginning clinical person must do is visit the laboratory. Learn the tests that are available, how they are requested, what preparation is needed, the costs, the turnaround time, and the operating characteristics. The same should be done in the radiology and cardiology departments. Become familiar with all diagnostic procedures, their operating characteristics, their risks and complications, and who does them. Tactfully find out about the reliability of the results and the capability of the performer. You are now well on the way toward understanding what help you can expect from paraclinical sources.

Learn the Menus

Just as you would in a fine restaurant, carefully inspect the various offerings in each department. Become acquainted with the hematology, chemistry, endocrinology, cytology, microbiology, and immunopathology menus. Which tests are done in each subdivision? Learn what the chemistry profiles include in your hospital or laboratory. You may be offered 6, 18, 20, or 24 tests by the sequential multiple analyzer (SMA).

There is much to be gleaned as you inspect the request forms for each division. On the hematology form, the tests are listed, normal values are stated, and special procedures and entire profiles are grouped. Should you have a patient with a coagulopathy, one check mark generates a battery of 4, 6, 10, or even 15 tests.

A look at the endocrinology menu gives similar information. Here the tests are grouped for each endocrine gland. All four thyroid tests can be requested if you suspect a thyroid problem. Under the adrenals, there are 11 tests; if a problem is suspected here, you may order all of the tests; better yet, order à la carte—only what you want.

Profiles, batteries, and panels of tests are available with a simple check mark. You may order one or more, depending on the area you wish to investigate. A *coronary risk profile* includes the serum cholesterol level, high- and low-density lipoprotein levels, the cholesterol–high-density lipoprotein ratio, and triglyceride levels.

If the problem suggests arthritis of some sort, an arthritis profile will produce the rheumatoid factor titer, C-reactive protein, erythrocyte sedimentation rate, uric acid, and antinuclear antibody.

Additional available grouped studies include comprehensive viral agglutination titers, heavy metal screens, hypnotic profiles, prenatal profiles, and so forth.

Other facts must be learned. Which tests are available on an emergency basis? Which are not available on weekends? Which are done only once weekly, and on which day? Which tests must be sent to a distant laboratory because your hospital doesn't do them? Which drugs does a toxic drug screen include? How long does it take for a test result to be available? A blood count? A blood culture? Indeed, any test! You will be surprised by the huge amount of information on the urinalysis request form.

Ask your laboratory for the small pamphlet or instruction booklet that lists all tests alphabetically, tells you how much blood is needed for each test, what color-cap tube is used, and the cost of each test. Know what each test you order costs, and *calculate the expenses* every time you write some orders.

If you are not already impressed, peruse the CT scan, ultrasound, radiographic consultation, and cardiac study request forms. There you see not only what studies are offered, but you also get a good review of the possible uses for each procedure. The various nuclear scans are listed, but you don't know their operating characteristics; nor are the charges usually printed.

The multiple uses of ultrasound are impressive; the sensitivity and specificity for each use are not included, because rarely are they known. Costs are not stated, either. The same can be said for computed tomographic scans, digital subtraction angiography, magnetic resonance imaging, ultrasound, endoscopies, and the multitude of specialized cardiologic studies.

The foregoing is not meant to be anti-intellectual, but is rather a plea for prudence, deliberation, and consideration before ordering tests and diagnostic procedures. If the need and benefit far exceed the cost and risk, the test should be done. If the data derived are of questionable value, some risk, and high cost, *don't order the test*.

The number of tests ordered seems to be roughly proportional to the number of tests available. And the ultimate decisions that have such profound effect on the cost of health care depend on the physician or house officer who checks off the items on the menu.

What are the Costs?

The problem solver should know the monetary cost of every test or procedure he or she may order. And because the problem solver will initiate treatment that is dependent on the diagnosis, he or she should also know the cost of drugs and the treatment or treatments, if options exist.

The costs may be shocking, and it may be wise to consider carefully whether the additional set of electrolyte levels, the third chest radiograph, or the daily ECG is really necessary. You should be aware of who pays the bill. No matter who pays—the patient, the government, or the health maintenance organization—you should order tests only after profound regard for their costs, necessity, and possible benefits. When the clinical picture and the ultrasound study have already established a diagnosis with 99% certainty, it may not be wise to also order a CT, especially if medical management won't change, no matter what. Remember, too, that under managed care plans, the person who ultimately may have to pay for that extra and perhaps unnecessary procedure could be the patient—or you.

What Are the Risks?

Before requesting a diagnostic procedure, the ordering physician must consider the risks as well as the costs and benefits. Other than the trauma of venipuncture, the possible damage to veins that may be needed later, and the contribution to iatrogenic anemia, there are no risks attached to doing blood tests.

Certainly, there are no risks involved in obtaining urine for urinalysis or culturing body fluids, unless the urine is obtained by catheter, the sputum by transtracheal needle, and the spinal fluid by lumbar puncture. Scans and ultrasound are generally harmless. However, if a computed tomographic scan is dye-enhanced, renal damage may result, especially if there is diabetes mellitus or pre-existing renal disease. As for the more invasive procedures involving introduction of tubes and needles into tissues, arteries, and veins for pictures or biopsies, there are definite although poorly quantified risks.

Twenty-five procedures were studied in 434 published reports. Complications and risks were listed for lumbar puncture, Swan-Ganz catheter placement, bone marrow aspiration, thyroid as-

piration biopsy, transbronchial biopsy, kidney biopsy, stress ECG, and so forth. Not only were the complications staggering, but wide variations from place to place were noted in all instances.

WHAT NORMAL IS

There are many different definitions of "normal" that vary from "average" to "mean" to "usual." A test result that may be either positive or negative (dichotomous) is usually "normal" if negative, and "abnormal" if positive. But a test that measures a biologic distribution of variables is "normal" when the result falls within a predetermined range of values, which are called "referent values" or "cutoff points." They represent the range of normal values as determined by the performance of large numbers of measurements in healthy young people. The mean value is then determined, and the upper and lower limits of normal are set by calculating two standard deviations above and below the mean. Therefore, by mathematical edict, only 95% of normal persons will have normal values; 2.5% will be below normal, and 2.5% will be above normal. This latter 5% will be falsely abnormal (Fig. 8.1).

If the referent values for blood urea nitrogen are 10 to 20 mg/dL, a value of 200 mg/dL is def-

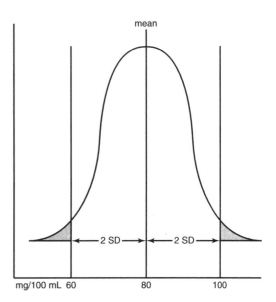

▶ **Figure 8.1.** Distribution of fasting serum glucose levels in a normal population. Shaded areas represent those persons who have abnormal test results (false positives).

initely abnormal. So is 40 mg/dL. But what about 25 mg/dL? Could this be a false positive? And how far above the referent interval must the result be to indicate the presence of disease? This becomes a very important issue, especially in the consideration of other tests, like those for transaminases (transferases) or alkaline phosphatase levels. How much above normal must the test result be before an intensive chain of studies is set into motion to determine the cause of the alleged abnormality?

The clinician who is seeking a "decision level" wants to know at which point above or below the referent values a test result becomes definitely abnormal and indicates the presence of disease. You must understand the effect of increasing the "degree of abnormality" of a test with nondichotomous results. How abnormal must a test result be before you become concerned? Common sense tells you to ignore a slightly abnormal result if the implied diagnosis is clinically highly unlikely but to regard it seriously if the implied diagnosis is clinically likely. Of course, you must be concerned if the result is markedly abnormal, even if unexpected.

At each increment of abnormality, the test has different operating characteristics, resulting in different true-positive and false-positive rates. Thus, the more abnormal the test result, the more likely it is to be truly positive and the less likely it is to be falsely positive.

The cutoff point between "worry—don't worry" will vary with the seriousness of the disease under consideration, the $P(D)$ before the test is done, the otherwise general health and age of the patient, the aggressiveness of the physician, and the decision level with which he or she can feel comfortable.

Sometimes, it may be difficult to interpret a laboratory test properly. The referent values may vary with age, gender, race, populations, time of day, method of test performance, and other interrelated factors. For example, the limits of normal hematocrit values differ for men and women. The upper normal limit of the serum creatinine level increases with age.

The Perfect Test

In order for a test to be perfect, it must be: (1) accurate, (2) precise, (3) discriminating, (4) pain free, (5) risk free, (6) inexpensive, and (7) useful.

The accuracy of a test refers to its ability to give *correct* results and hit the bull's-eye on retesting. Precision refers to reproducibility of results on replicate measurements, even though the results are not necessarily accurate. Ideally, a test should be both accurate and precise, although the two don't necessarily go hand in hand. For a test to be discriminating, it must be able to distinguish between health and disease. There should be a minimum number of false-negative and false-positive results. The other attributes of a perfect test need no further explanation. Obviously, there is no such thing as a perfect test!

Actually, tests that measure continuous variables, such as serum uric acid levels, white blood cell counts, and PR intervals do not clearly distinguish between health and disease.

Watch for Errors

Because many human beings and machines are involved in doing tests and procedures, it is only natural to expect a certain percentage of errors. Never forget that the more that tests are ordered, the more "red herrings" and errors may be introduced into the data base, and the more physicians may be misled. Mistakes are made at all levels—before the laboratory, in the laboratory, and after the laboratory.

Prelaboratory errors include improper preparation of the patient (e.g., diet, fasting state); the *taking of drugs* that interfere with accurate test performance; mislabeling of tubes; and obtaining poor specimens. Urine collected for culture may not be sterile, and sputum collected for culture may really be only saliva.

Intralaboratory errors are said to occur at a frequency of 3.65 per 100 tests. These include misplacing of specimens, errors in recording and filing, illegible reports, and poor referent values and referent intervals. And even if the referent values are well selected, by their very construction, there will be an additional 5% of false-positive results. If six unrelated tests are done, you can expect at least one test result to be falsely positive or abnormal in 26.5% of normal healthy individuals (1 minus $.95^6$ = 1 minus .735 = .265). If 12 independent tests are done, at least one test result will be abnormal in 46% of normal persons (1 minus $.95^{12}$ = 1 minus .54 = .46). Whether these abnormal results represent false positives and what to do about them will be discussed later in this chapter.

Once the results leave the laboratory, they may be placed on the wrong chart, or they may be incorrectly accessed by the computer. If a test result does not jibe with the clinical picture, always compare the name and the patient identification number in the report with the name and number on the chart.

The final error may be made by the physician who does not interpret results correctly because he or she either does not know or does not look. *There is no excuse for ordering a test and then ignoring or overlooking the result, which are actions that are commonly done.*

WHICH TESTS TO ORDER

The actual process of ordering tests may be simple or complex. In the section on Data Collection in Chapter 2, much was said about this subject, but because this is such an important issue in the light of today's efforts to contain costs, some concepts will be repeated and expanded here.

Admission Studies

For hospitalized patients, you usually order a complete blood count (CBC), urinalysis, SMA-20, chest radiograph, and electrocardiogram. This pattern is established by hospital policy, physician habit, and house officer perseveration. It may change from year to year, from hospital to hospital, from medical to surgical patient, from inpatient to outpatient, and according to the patient's age. Regulatory agencies, including third-party payers and hospital quality assurance and utilization programs, mandate changes from time to time.

For example, the elimination of the CBC and its replacement by the white blood cell count and hematocrit have cut costs without altering quality of care. Routine ECGs are not recommended for patients under 35. The need for chest radiographs and chemistry profiles must sometimes be documented on the chart. More and more tests require notations explaining their need. Attempts are being made to eliminate "standing orders" and preprinted uniform order sheets emanating from the attending physician's

office. Duplication of tests just done on an outpatient basis should be avoided. Reimbursement for some tests is denied if they are not truly indicated. These are all steps in the right direction.

Problem-Oriented Tests

Beyond the admission studies, subsequent tests should be geared to the identified diagnostic contenders. If jaundice is the principal problem, you can begin with a direct and indirect bilirubin level, alkaline phosphatase level, and hepatic cell enzymes levels (whichever transferase you prefer). But on the basis of clinical evidence, there is already an established likelihood of either obstruction or hepatic cell disease. The test results will decrease or increase an existing probability. Thus, when clinical judgment is used in ordering laboratory tests, the patient suspected of having a disease is placed in a new population with a higher $P(D)$, and the test therefore has a greater positive predictive value.

Should anemia be the problem, the clinical setting and study of the red blood cells help you decide whether to look for chronic blood loss from the gastrointestinal tract, a macrocytic anemia, altered bone marrow production, and so forth. At this point, you can order all tests for anemia in robot fashion or intelligently select those that are appropriate for the most likely diagnosis. For example, for weight loss, anorexia, indigestion, and microcytic anemia, order stool studies for occult blood, serum iron and iron-binding capacity, and gastrointestinal tract visualization. If the history, examination, and red blood cells suggest macrocytosis, determination of folate and vitamin B_{12} levels are indicated. In other circumstances, bone marrow aspiration, reticulocyte count, glucose-6-phosphate dehydrogenase levels, transferrin level, and so forth might be indicated. And this reasoning goes on and on for each clinical likelihood. *If the initial batch of tests does not confirm the prime clinical impression, tests may be ordered for the second likelihood.*

The other strategy, which is subject to some criticism even though it perhaps has timesaving benefits, is to order tests for all leading likelihoods at once and wait for all results to return. But it would seem wasteful and distasteful to aspirate the bone marrow for what is almost certainly an anemia caused by chronic blood loss.

Similarly, it would be premature, inappropriate, and fruitless to order a biopsy, CT scan, or endoscopic retrograde cholangiopancreatography if the clinical picture and initial few tests indicate that hepatitis almost certainly exists.

The Value of Special Tests

With the passage of time, certain tests become obsolete, some are proved valueless, and others assume greater value. You should be aware of such changes as they appear in the medical literature. For example, a Gram's stain of the stool is 43.5% sensitive and 99.4% specific for *Campylobacter* enteritis. This microbe has become an important cause of infectious diarrhea and needs unique antibiotic therapy. The very high specificity makes a positive stained smear essentially diagnostic. A negative smear is reasonably dependable at $P(D)$s between 5 and 20%. Treatment can be intelligently directed by this simple test that requires basic staining techniques.

For years, clinicians have pondered the best way to detect acute myocardial necrosis. The standard procedure had been to obtain the serum glutamic-oxaloacetic transaminase–creatine kinase–lactate dehydrogenase (SGOT–CK–LDH) triad on 3 consecutive days. More recently, studies have demonstrated that the parallel and series testing of the CK, its MB isomer, and LDH isoenzymes every 8 hours for 24 hours is preferable. The CK rises, and its MB fraction goes above its normal 5% portion; this rise is slightly preceded by an LDH "flip," whereby the LDH-1 fraction becomes greater than the LDH-2 fraction. Together, these two changes are essentially 100% specific for myocardial infarction—perhaps *the perfect test*. Remember, however, that new investigations may make even such excellent protocols obsolete. Indeed, many centers no longer study the LDH for this purpose.

The carcinoembryonic antigen has a sensitivity of .72 and a specificity of .80 for colorectal cancer. As a screening test, it would be worthless because of the high number of false positives. But in a patient whose $P(D)$ is already elevated by the clinical picture—for example, $P(D) = .50$-a positive test result raises the probability to .78; a negative test result reduces the likelihood to .26. So this test has value, although limited.

An acid-fast stain for tubercle bacilli has always been regarded as having questionable reliability. But studies that used a positive culture as a gold standard have revealed that a carefully and properly performed smear is highly specific (approaching .999) and moderately sensitive (.39).

Well-done studies of this type help us decide whether to use a test. And having used the test, we shoud know how to interpret the results. Data of this sort are needed for all tests and procedures. Most tests used today have never received critical evaluation at the medical decision level, and their predictive values remain unclear.

Acquired Immunodeficiency Syndrome (AIDS) Tests

The diagnosis of human immunodeficiency virus (HIV) infection depends on the demonstration of antibodies to the virus or on the direct detection of the viral DNA or one of its components in the blood. If AIDS is suspected, and permission for testing has been obtained, the *enzyme-linked immunosorbent assay* (ELISA) is the test to use. It is more than 99.5% sensitive, and although not optimal for specificity, it serves as an excellent screen. If the test is positive or indeterminate, a *Western blot* test is done next. The Western blot is highly specific but not sensitive enough to use for screening purposes. If the Western blot is positive, too, then HIV infection is present with absolute certainty. If the Western blot is negative, then the ELISA test was falsely positive.

Measurement of the number of CD4-positive T-lymphocytes per cubic millimeter of blood is a reliable indicator of the progress and stage of HIV disease. Other tests, such as DNA PCR (polymerase chain reaction), p24 antigen capture assay, viral density measurement, and direct cultivation of HIV from the plasma are mostly for research purposes and are just beginning to reach widespread clinical usefulness.

A Very Special Test

Take the important issue of whether serious coronary artery disease does exist as measured by the treadmill test. Few matters are more serious than the decision on whether a patient's chest pain means nothing or may lead to surgery or death. Because a "positive" test often leads inevitably to surgery, whereas a "negative" test results in medical treatment or nothing. Sensitivity and specificity must be carefully predetermined, and the consequences of false negatives and false positives must be weighed.

Before performing this test, the test protocol must be carefully designed. This includes the method of performance and the establishment of the criteria for positivity. The latter can be determined by a discriminant function analysis score that takes into account not only the slope and degree of ST-segment depression (or elevation) at the peak of exercise, but also the heart rate, the heart rate-pressure product, the presence and duration of symptoms, ECG abnormalities, arrhythmias, and so forth. Usually, only ST-segment abnormalities at a heart rate of 85% of the predicted maximum are the principal criteria for abnormality.

The sensitivity of this test hovers between .55 and .75 for severe coronary disease, and false negatives can occur with single vessel disease, with less stringent criteria for positivity, because of indefinable abnormalities in coronary anatomy, and for unknown reasons. The specificity is high but not high enough to exclude numerous false positives that can result from hyperventilation, mitral valve prolapse, and abnormal left ventricular depolarization and repolarization (e.g., left ventricular hypertrophy, digitalis therapy, or Wolff-Parkinson-White syndrome).

In order to quantify the predictive value of a positive or negative test result, an estimate of disease probability—$P(D)$—must be made. This clinical estimate depends on the presence and type of chest pain, gender, age, family history, blood glucose and cholesterol levels, and associated symptoms.

These are the multiple considerations required to make this test or *any test* worthwhile. Included are test performance, criteria for abnormality, efficient operating characteristics, and a reasonable approximation of disease probability before doing the test.

REASONS FOR OVERUSE

There are many. First is the greater availability and variety of tests resulting from technologic advances. Next, more and more, diseases are diagnosed, and their treatment is being monitored by laboratory tests. The ability to monitor drug levels and to do toxicologic studies has also increased laboratory use. For medicolegal reasons, too, tests are often unnecessarily done. Someone in the emergency department who has had an automobile accident may have a radiographic study performed wherever there is an ache or pain in order to rule out fractures. This is one example of the widespread practice of defensive medicine brought on in part by a litigious society.

Younger physicians tend to rely more on laboratory tests and procedures. Residents and interns may order large numbers of tests out of curiosity, in the interest of one-upmanship, according to established behavior, or because of the need to "be complete." Too often, the "chief" is more apt to criticize the house officer for a possibly helpful test that *wasn't* ordered than for an unnecessary test that *was* ordered. Omission is a greater sin than commission, so every conceivably related study is requested. These same house officers are then replaced by new ones who tend to *follow the leader.* Tests are especially overdone in teaching hospitals.

The lack of physician education in the proper use of tests, their operating characteristics, and their predictive values may be another root cause of misuse. Also, students are inadequately educated in most medical schools; courses in laboratory medicine have for the most part been eliminated from the curriculum.

The fact that most patients do not directly pay their own bills gives the physician an implied freedom to order tests. Another unfortunate situation is that diagnostic procedures are done by different departments in different specialties, each of which may be biased in favor of its own procedure. The patient may have three procedures done when one would suffice. Or the test done first may not have been the wisest choice, but it was done because its performer was more convincing. Not to be ignored is the realization that most procedures generate income, and that, in a few instances, dishonesty rather than bias may be the governing factor.

A final cause for the overuse of tests is the frequent need to follow up a false-positive result. The more procedures and tests that are done, the more false positives occur, and the more the need to track them down with yet more tests.

Unfortunately, false-positive results may even lead to harmful interventions, such as biopsies and exploratory surgery.

Unexpected Test Results

An inevitable outcome of multiple tests and *unsolicited data* is an unexpectedly positive test result. This presents the physician with problems and decisions. Is the result a false or true positive? Does another problem exist? What additional studies need be done?

First, you must realize that a slightly abnormal test result may merely represent the 2.5% on either end of the reference interval. A hemoglobin level of 11.5 g/dL, a lactate dehydrogenase level 10% above the upper limit of normal, or indeed any test result that is just outside the "normal range" may trigger a long search for nonexistent disease. Needless probes of this sort are common.

Next, the degree of abnormality must be considered. Nobody gets excited about a white blood cell count of 4500 or 11,000, but what if it's 1500 or 28,000? An alkaline phosphatase level slightly above normal might merely raise an eyebrow, but if it's three times normal, you worry and then search. A blood glucose level of 58 mg/dL or 116 mg/dL would be disregarded, but 40 mg/dL or 160 mg/dL would not. Both the true and false varieties of "chem profile disease" are common.

Given an unexpected abnormal test result, it may be ignored or acted upon. The basic approach for the action option would be: (1) repeat the test; (2) if normal, forget about it; (3) if still abnormal, consider the role of any drug the patient may be taking; (4) if still unexplained, consider a differential diagnosis for the abnormality; and (5) if a work-up is deemed appropriate after carefully weighing all aspects of the situation, track it down.

There are literally dozens of drugs that can cause each chemical aberration. And there are dozens of diseases that can do so too. You can easily develop or research a protocol to track down any abnormality. At times, the job will be easier if a group of abnormalities is uncovered that points to one organ or one disease. A distinctly increased alkaline phosphatase level requires an isoenzyme study, some type of liver scan, and a bone survey;

in this setting, a γ-glutamyltransferase level determination may help separate liver from bone disease. Hypercalcemia demands a detailed study for hyperparathyroidism or malignancy.

The investigation of every case of unexpected hypercalcemia opens Pandora's box. The public cost is over $100 million per year. A detailed voyage of discovery is indicated, which results in either surgery or inoperable cancer. Recent studies have shown that the removal of asymptomatic, unexpectedly discovered parathyroid adenomas may not be indicated in the long run. The question of surgery—now, later, or never—has not yet been resolved.

Then there's the patient with abdominal or back pain whose CT scan produces yet another quandary about adrenal lumps and bumps. These apparent abnormalities may be benign functionless adrenal tumors completely unrelated to the prime problem. But they *trigger prolonged odysseys* that often end in shipwrecks rather than in safe harbors.

Whether the worship of unsolicited laboratory data can result in more trouble than benefit is a matter to be decided on the basis of all the evidence in each individual case.

WHO DOES THE SHOPPING?

The Need for Change

Nobody denies that tests and procedures help in the management of patients. On the other hand, nobody denies that tests are overused, misused, and that they may create as well as solve problems. Furthermore, nobody denies the need to restructure the pattern for ordering tests. Can this necessary change best be accomplished by education, supervision, example, coaxing, incentive, or edict?

Those who write the orders in the chart are in large measure responsible for the control of hospital costs. The attending physician must set a good example by ordering only necessary and useful diagnostic and therapeutic measures, and must practice as he or she preaches and teaches.

Special Patterns

The most important test-ordering pattern to be established is that there be *no* pattern. As far as is humanly possible, the ordering of batteries should be abolished, and only those tests that are specifically indicated should be selected. It might be preferable to provide a blank order sheet rather than long printed lists. The former requires thought; the latter needs only mindless check marks.

A *separate catalog of tests* that lists everything in the paraclinical supermarket should always be available. But the catalog must be only a reference and not the sheet upon which tests are ordered. Everyone knows that those who shop in supermarkets buy more than they need because they are tempted by the vast array of goodies. Only the most budget-conscious shopper will purchase that which is absolutely needed. The same is true of the person who orders tests.

Nevertheless, the order writer must be aware of or know where to retrieve selected subsets of available studies if a particular diagnosis is suspected, or if there is a need to eliminate a possible diagnosis. This information either has already been taught, is becoming available in textbooks, or can be learned from material furnished by each diagnostic subunit. Note that standard textbooks usually merely list the tests that may be abnormal for a given disease without suggesting strategies.

If the problem is either jaundice, melena, hypochromic anemia, suspected hyperthyroidism, sore throat, chest pain, dyspnea on exertion, backache, and so forth, there are a limited number of *high-yield studies* to be done in each instance—after or during the extraction of data from the history and examination. The initial tests and any needed additional studies are usually well known. If not, you can read about them, discuss them with your peers, or consult appropriate experts. Section 2 of this book includes the diagnostic approach to many such common problems.

The patient suspected of having adrenal insufficiency needs only three or four well-selected tests, not a dozen, to cover all aspects of adrenal dysfunction. If panhypopituitarism is under serious consideration, only a handful of studies is needed to make sure; you need not do all tests for all endocrine abnormalities. Most thyroid problems need only two tests, not the complete four-test thyroid panel that is frequently requested. Although there are currently many serologic markers for viral hepatitis, they must be ordered in meaningful small groups depending on the clinical situation. Because of rapid advances in this field, the clinician may not know which tests to order first and which may possibly be needed later. Advice on current usage must be available.

STRATEGIES FOR TESTING

Whenever a patient tells you the chief complaint, you should immediately formulate and follow a protocol for getting more data. Usually, this format is self-designed, and each physician generates his or her own special protocol for each clinical problem seen. For common problems, the physician develops his or her own sequence. Less common problems may require some ingenuity or acquisition of additional knowledge from printed material or consultants.

Once the history and examination are completed and initial hypotheses are formed, further tests, studies, and procedures are often necessary. Generally, the physician has a preconceived problem-driven sequence for obtaining added information. Which tests first? Which later? All at once? Is one procedure enough? Are two better? Should all available tests and procedures be ordered? What if some are positive, and some are negative? All of these questions need careful consideration when tests are ordered.

In Series or Parallel

An important decision to be made is whether to order several studies at once or await the results of one test before ordering the next. Each strategy has its pros and cons. If you decide to order tests sequentially, you may find that as a result of the first test, the second may not be necessary. This would occur if the first study resulted in a positive or negative predictive value deemed sufficient for your purposes. The revised disease probability would have excluded or confirmed a diagnosis with enough certainty. However, if additional security or confidence is sought, a second study could be ordered. The predictive value resulting from the first study becomes the new $P(D)$ for calculating the performance and results of the second study.

The enigma of parallel testing (or, for that matter, series testing, as well) arises when one test is positive, and the other is negative. Sometimes patients are seen who have positive ultrasound study results and negative CT scan results, or vice versa. This causes confusion, and retests or additional tests must be done to add clarity. Always present is the disconcerting effect of "an equivocal test result." But, on the other hand, if test results are either all positive or all negative, greater confidence is established.

Which of Two to Do

If you should wish to do only one of a choice of many available tests, you may be faced with the question of doing the test with the greatest sensitivity or the test with the greatest specificity. Choose the one with the highest sensitivity if you cannot afford false-negative results. Choose the one with the highest specificity if you cannot afford false-positive results. The matter distills to a trade-off between the harm of missing a disease in a patient who has it, and the harm of diagnosing a disease in a patient who doesn't have it. To be considered are the seriousness and treatability of the disease, the chances of detecting the disease by additional tests, the psychologic and economic harm of a false diagnosis, the moral issues revolving around treating somebody for a disease he or she doesn't have, and so forth.

Specific Clinical Problems

Physicians have always had their favorite strategies for the diagnostic management of most problems. But as new procedures and tests become available, strategies have changed, are changing, and will continue to change. This will be especially true when the applications and properties of newer procedures become defined.

Consider a patient with blunt abdominal trauma in whom intra-abdominal bleeding is being considered. The choice lies between CT and peritoneal lavage. CT visualization is highly sensitive, can detect as little as 100 to 200 mL of blood in the peritoneal cavity, and can also note retroperitoneal trauma to the pancreas or duodenum. But it is costly and may not be immediately available. Needle lavage is simple, cheap, done in

the emergency department, and is essentially risk free. The presence of bile, amylase, or leukocytes may signal complications not yet suspected. But lavage may be overly sensitive and not quantitative; it is best for liver and spleen injury but is not good for retroperitoneal trauma. *The clinician must now make a choice.*

In another case, should the alkaline phosphatase level be surprisingly high, determination of isoenzymes should help pinpoint the organ source of the elevation—bone or liver. From there, you can either do bone radiographs (conventional or isotopic); search for a primary malignancy anywhere; or study the liver with added function tests, a CT scan or ultrasound study, and biopsy, if indicated. It is difficult to decide when to get off the *diagnostic treadmill* once you are on it. Multiple considerations enter the equation, and diagnosis cannot go on indefinitely. How important is it to track this isolated laboratory abnormality in the face of compounded risks and costs?

And in still another case, if acute pancreatitis is suspected, parallel serial measurements of serum amylase, serum lipase, and urine amylase are still very helpful. The amylase–creatinine clearance ratio may not be as good as was first thought. Chemical tests available in most 20-test profiles are good indicators; electrolytes, glucose, urea nitrogen, calcium, and bilirubin are included. Coagulation profiles are indicated on alternate days. Beyond the laboratory, ultrasound and CT aid in the diagnosis. Not all of these tests are necessary in each case, but the diagnosis can be substantiated, treatment can be directed, and the severity of disease can be gauged by some of the results.

For a patient who has suspected liver disease, there is an inexhaustible stimulus for diagnostic tests and procedures. But here the *concept of substrategies* should be introduced. Because there are separate batteries to measure hepatic viral infection, liver cell injury, cholestasis, metabolic derangement, and liver anatomy, you must select the test that fits the clinical problem. For hepatitis, only three or four antigen or antibody selections are enough. Liver cell injury is detected by the released enzymes (aspartate aminotransferase [AST], alanine aminotransferase [ALT], γ-glutamyltransferase [GGT], LDH). Cholestasis is measured by the levels of alkaline phosphatase, 5'-nucleotidase, and bile acids. To detect metabolic derangements resulting from liver disease, assay the total proteins, albumin, prothrombin, choline esterase, and so forth. The transition from acute to chronic liver disease is monitored by protein electrophoresis, immunoglobulins, and coagulation factors.

Anatomic delineation and histologic abnormalities of the liver can be detected by numerous more complex techniques that include scintigraphy, sonography, angiography, laparoscopy, biopsy, transhepatic cholangiography, and endoscopic retrograde cholangiography. Clearly, *not all tests are done for every liver problem*. The chosen substrategy depends on what information you need for the particular situation.

Printed Aids

Most strategies are well known and rapidly integrated into the physician's knowledge base. But there are excellent resources wherein organ panels and diagnostic strategies may be found. There you can research the protocols for acute renal failure, acute myocardial infarction, carcinoma of the prostate, hemolytic anemia, pulmonary embolism, and on and on. Then, decide on your own course of action, remembering that the exact niche for each new procedure has not yet been carved, and there is always room for disagreement.

Numerous new technologic procedures developed during the past three decades have substantially shortened and, for the most part, simplified the diagnostic process. These include:

- Fiberoptic endoscopy with extension into the distal bronchi, the pancreatic and biliary trees, and the entire colon;
- Biopsies of the lung, brain, heart, pancreas, liver, kidney, and prostate—some of which were formerly considered very risky, but now less so with imaging guidance;
- Tumor markers—immune-mediated or otherwise;
- Genomic patterns, whose applications seem infinite at this moment;
- Radioisotopic studies of many varieties, including measurement of blood flow and cardiac function, gallbladder function, organ imaging, abscess location, and proof of pulmonary emboli;
- Computed tomography (CT) of the head, chest, spine, abdomen, and pelvis;
- Ultrasound for cardiac anatomy, function, and disease; neck tumors; liver and gallbladder disease; pelvic tumors (ovary and prostate); and tubal pregnancies;
- Magnetic resonance imaging (MRI) for virtually the same purposes as computed tomography;
- Evoked brain potentials to measure specific neurologic and behavioral deficits; and
- Hosts of new and currently developing radiographic techniques such as magnetic resonance angiography, magnetic resonance spectroscopy, pulsed and continuous Doppler imaging, single photon emission computed tomography (SPECT), and others.

Serious consideration must be given to the impact of these techniques on the diagnostic process. In some instances, previous testing sequences have been made obsolete. For example, computed tomography and ultrasound studies of the kidney have almost relegated pyelography to the past. Ultrasound has virtually replaced the cholecystogram. The first step in the management of upper gastrointestinal bleeding is fiberoptic endoscopy, not contrast radiography. In many cases, magnetic resonance angiography has replaced cerebral arteriography.

COMPLEX CONSIDERATIONS

Some generalizations must be understood about recently adopted procedures. As new techniques appear on the horizon, old ones may fade into obsolescence. But new procedures must first be evaluated for reliability, and their operating characteristics must be established. Cost-benefit-risk factors need to be appreciated. The precise and proper position of each procedure in the array of diagnostic weapons will change from time to time. New applications for each procedure will appear in the literature, and each new one must pass stringent inspections. And as always for any new test, the pendulum will swing back and forth several times before the test's proper niche is found.

It is important to remember that in this decade of diagnostic revolutions, the situation concerning the various aspects of new technologic procedures is in a hyperdynamic state of flux. *Yesterday's discovery can become today's dictum and tomorrow's relic.* What is considered correct diagnostic traffic flow may be detoured, rerouted, bypassed, short-cutted, or even firmly established as a major highway.

In selecting your diagnostic protocol in each case, always consider the skill of the performer of the procedure, the concept of imperfect information, and the availability of technology at your work site.

There can be no question that many formerly used diagnostic plans have been radically altered by new imaging techniques. In most cases, the trend has been in the direction of using an expensive procedure that reaches the bottom line of a diagnostic problem while bypassing less efficient, time-consuming techniques. Generally, this *reduces costs* by decreasing the number of hospital days needed. But recall that false-positive results may require repeat studies and additional studies that increase heathcare costs.

To this moment, debates about optimal diagnostic protocols still exist over a wide range of medical and surgical problems. Consider a patient with cholestatic jaundice whose ultrasound study shows dilated intrahepatic ducts. The subsequent procedure of choice in most medical centers is a percutaneous transhepatic cholangiogram; in other centers, the endoscopic retrograde cholangiogram is preferred. Some centers will do both.

For other hepatic problems, the CT scan is preferred by some, ultrasound by others, isotopic scans still by a few; all three procedures are used when indecision exists. Each technical expert may tell you why his or her procedure is the one of choice. Unless you know better, the decision is a difficult one. Eventually, huge properly compiled data banks for each diagnostic study may be of help.

In hospitals where CT, MRI, ultrasound, and nuclear medicine sections have separate staffs, budgets, and scheduling arrangements, those who perform these procedures may become advocates and may compete for patients.

Given the same diagnostic problem, it can be seen why and how different doctors and different hospitals may pursue varied procedural sequences.

With some notable exceptions, CT, MRI, and ultrasound give similar information, and one study tends to reinforce the other. In many instances, the superiority of one technique over the other is still to be firmly established.

Although combinations of CT, MRI, nuclear imaging, angiography, and ultrasound should do much to elevate diagnostic likelihoods in cases where certainty is required, such combinations may not be in the best interests of patients, hospitals, health maintenance organizations, and all of their budgets.

ULTRASOUND

Images obtained from the reflection of high-frequency sound waves have proved their tremendous usefulness over the past two decades. Echos are now successfully used in diagnostic problems from head to foot. The technique is inexpensive, non-invasive, harmless, without radiation exposure, relatively simple to perform, and can be done at the bedside. It is available in all hospitals, emergency departments, and even some private offices.

The reliability of ultrasound examinations is especially dependent upon the expertise of the technician, the experience of the interpreter, and the quality of the equipment. This modality is being used more and more each year, and seems to be replacing some more expensive diagnostic methods. It is expected that this trend may continue. The ultrasound-emitting probe can be directed to various organs across the body skin surface, from the esophagus, or through the vagina or rectum.

The *M-mode method* is used primarily in heart disease (echocardiography). It is so named because it detects and measures motion of the ventricular wall. A single stationary ultrasound beam documents the activity of a linear needlelike projection of underlying tissue. Sound is reflected from each interface of tissues having different acoustical impedances, and the time between sending and receiving the signal is converted into distance between the reflecting surface and the transducer. A rolling drum synchronized with a simultaneous electrocardiogram (ECG) records continuous motion along the probe line in real time. Therefore, this mode's chief value lies in its precise delineation of motion and thickness of underlying cardiac tissue during the cardiac cycle (Fig. 9.1).

Two-dimensional (2-D) ultrasound uses a sound beam that sweeps rapidly across the chest, abdomen, or pelvis and generates a cross-sectional image in the plane traversed. Dynamic imaging at 30 or more frames per second can observe motion and 2-D detailed anatomy in *real time*.

The uses for such techniques are legion. Ultra-

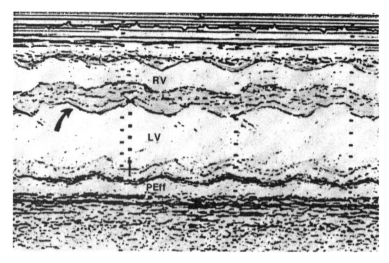

▶ **Figure 9.1.** M-mode echocardiogram demonstrates right ventricle (*RV*), left ventricle (*LV*), interventricular septum (*arrow*), and a pericardial effusion (*PEff*).

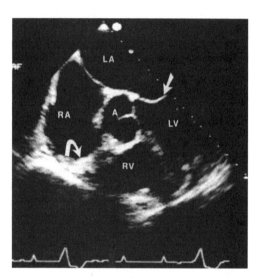

▶ **Figure 9.2.** Transesophageal two-dimensional echocardiogram. All four chambers of the heart and its valves can be identified. *A* is aorta. *Curved arrow* points to tricuspid valve. *Straight arrow* points to mitral valve.

sound is the procedure par excellence for demonstrating gallbladder stones, dilatation of hepatic bile ducts in obstructive jaundice, ascites, and subphrenic abscesses. It is especially good in cardiac diagnosis where motion is a factor, and anatomic and functional abnormalities can be detected. For example, some clinicians consider this diagnostic modality to be 100% sensitive for subphrenic abscess, 95% sensitive for demonstrating the dilated intrahepatic ducts of obstructive cholestatic jaun-

dice, and 95% sensitive for gallbladder stones. In these instances, it is highly specific, too.

In cardiovascular diagnosis, 2-D and M-mode ultrasound techniques are very helpful in confirming ventricular wall contraction abnormalities, valve defects, congenital ailments, pericardial effusions, aneurysms, mural thrombi, myxomas, mitral prolapse, and vegetations on valves (Fig 9.2).

Always an enigma in the past, cancers, inflammations, and pseudocysts of the pancreas are rendered more diagnosable by ultrasound. Retroperitoneal nodes and masses can be detected, and lymphoma staging may be done, too. The liver, spleen, and kidneys can be measured for size; and stones, tumors, metastases, cysts, and congenital abnormalities may be detectable in these organs. Differentiation can be made between cyst and tumor of the thyroid, kidney, or ovary. Pelvic masses can be outlined and sometimes diagnosed. In obstetrics, where radiation or isotopes are taboo, the expected date of delivery, placenta previa, and fetal gender and fetal abnormalities can be noted.

In the past 5 years, ultrasound has been particularly helpful in the detection of heart-valve vegetations by transesophageal probe, for the detection of ovarian cancer by transvaginal probe, and for the detection of prostatic cancer by transrectal probe.

Color Doppler

This very commonly used ultrasound study integrates the anatomic information provided by 2-

D with color-coded flow patterns within the heart, thus creating a graphic image of the direction, speed, and turbulence of blood flow through the various heart chambers, across the valves, and into the great blood vessels.

The Doppler principle is the process whereby moving objects reflect and alter the pitch of sound waves. The pitch of the reflected wave depends on the velocity of the reflecting tissue, in this case columns of blood, and whether the reflecting tissue is moving toward or away from the transducer.

Thus, Doppler color-coded flow imaging is particularly useful in measuring cardiac output, detecting and measuring valvular stenoses and insufficiencies, calculating valve size, delineating vascular obstructions such as carotid artery stenosis, and gauging pressure gradients. There are uses outside the heart, too—for example, in the measurement of the degree of obstruction and residual venous flow in a thrombosed deep leg vein.

COMPUTED TOMOGRAPHY

Since its introduction in 1972, CT has revolutionized the science of diagnosis perhaps more than any other procedure. It has proved to be most versatile and is widely accepted and used. X-ray signals from a body-encircling source are collected and computer-synthesized into a cross-sectional image of a body slice. Different tissues and different pathologic processes in the same tissue will display varying shades of gray. These variations may be enhanced by the intravenous injection of iodinated radiographic contrast material that not only increases density differentials between types of tissue, but also dynamically visualizes vascular structures. In this way, the sensitivity and specificity of the procedure are increased; the contrast not only helps in the detection of lesions, but aids in their differentiation and analysis.

CT is superior to conventional radiography in that the gray scale is more widely spread; thus, the radiographic densities of various types of juxtaposed soft tissue, air, and fat can be more clearly discerned, defined, and interpreted. The ability to visualize accurate 2-D transverse total cross-sections rather than traditional flat pseudo-3-D films is a decided plus (Fig. 9.3).

This modality has *outstanding* merit in the following diagnostic situations: brain disorders where distinctions must be made between trauma, types of strokes, hemorrhages, and tumors; adrenal tumors suspected by the clinical picture (but beware the incidence of benign nonfunctioning adrenal adenomas); possible herniated intervertebral discs or spinal stenosis, where intrathecal dye studies are often no longer needed; mediastinal masses where aneurysms, nodes, larger vessels, and tiny thymomas can be differentiated; lung lesions whose malignant or benign nature may often be determined; abdominal suppuration, when suspected; retroperitoneal tumors, nodes, or metastases; and the detection, staging, and resectability of malignant disease.

What a formidable accomplishment! Not only does CT do these positive things, but by so doing it often decreases or eliminates the need for more invasive tests, such as laparotomy, angiography, lymphangiography, biopsy, myelography, or endoscopic retrograde cholangiopancreatography (ERCP). The patient who is unconscious following head trauma can be spared invasive and risky cerebral arteriography; the scan can detect and discern intracerebral, subdural, epidural, and subarachnoid hemorrhage, as well as edema or contusion. Even though the procedure is expensive, it may result in shortened hospital stays and reduced costs, elimination of surgery or additional procedures, and improved patient care.

Other highly beneficial uses for CT scans include the detection of serious trauma to the liver, spleen, or kidney; the confirmation of dissecting aneurysms; the diagnosis and characterization of unusual or difficult-to-detect fractures of the vertebrae or pelvis; the distinction between cyst and tumor when a mass lesion is noted on renal pyelography; the identification of cancer and acute inflammation of the pancreas; and the fathoming of other abdominal masses.

But a word of caution must be added. CT scans must not be used to supply repetitive and redundant information. When scans are used strictly for screening vague problems, such as nonspecific abdominal pain, fever, or weight loss, very little significant information is obtained. But if the study is *goal-directed* with a more specific problem in mind, the positive yield is much higher. Not all fevers, coughs,

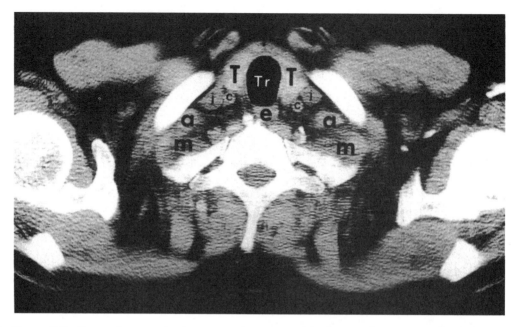

▶ **Figure 9.3.** Computed tomography demonstrates the anatomy of the thoracic inlet in exquisite detail. This procedure does equally well in other horizontal and sagittal body planes.

headaches, indigestion, or back pains need CT scans!

MAGNETIC RESONANCE IMAGING

This technique offers images that reflect not only anatomy but also biochemistry. Energy is released by certain elements in body sites that have been subjected to giant circumcorporeal magnetic fields and then bombarded with short bursts of radiofrequency waves. These energy signals from stimulated atomic nuclei, such as hydrogen and phosphorus, can be computer-imaged. This gives *structural and biochemical information* about tissue, thus tending to fingerprint some disease processes by performing "body chemical analyses" in the liver, brain, spinal cord, and neoplastic tissue.

Some of the known beneficial applications of this noninvasive diagnostic procedure are the detection of areas of cerebral edema, the delineation of the spinal cord, the discrimination of white from gray matter, the differentiation between liver disorders, the distinction between benign and malignant pathology, the diagnosis

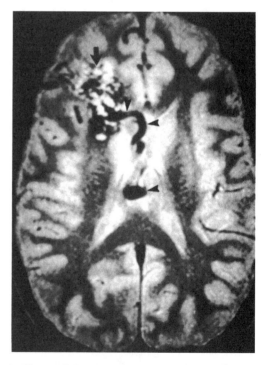

▶ **Figure 9.4.** Magnetic resonance imaging demonstrates a right frontal arteriovenous malformation (*arrow*) in a patient who has headaches. *Arrowheads* point to a large draining vein.

of bone and joint diseases, and the early detection of neoplasms. There is essentially no radiation exposure, and the injection of a contrast agent serves to enhance the clarity of images (Fig. 9.4).

Indeed, MRI appears to be useful in virtually the same array of disorders as is CT, and some clinicians predict that MRI will eventually replace CT. Magnetic resonance angiography (MRA), a recent modification of MRI, can now produce images of cerebral, cervical, renal, and peripheral arterial circulations in exceptional detail, but this procedure is not yet suitable for the coronary circulation. Magnetic resonance imaging cannot be used in patients who weigh more than 300 pounds, patients with pacemakers, and uncooperative patients.

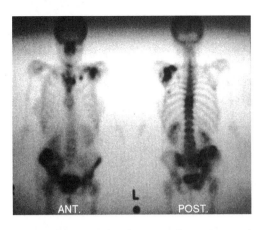

▶ **Figure 9.5.** Nuclear bone scan demonstrates multiple bone metastases from breast carcinoma.

NUCLEAR IMAGING

This is a procedure whereby chemicals tagged with radioactive isotopes are administered intravenously. Radioactivity is then measured over the special site to which the chemical is selectively attracted. Such scintigraphic techniques have been successfully used for four decades. The number of chemicals and dyes has multiplied, and all sorts of practical applications are now in use.

For example, the size and shape of the liver and spleen can be precisely delineated; tumors, cysts, and deformities can be detected; and even histopathologic abnormalities can be suggested. The ventilation-perfusion scan is highly sensitive for pulmonary emboli. Cerebral blood flow can be measured with serial scans. Multiple gated acquisition (MuGA) scans measure ventricular ejection fractions as a determinant of cardiac function. Ischemic areas can be detected in the heart, lung, brain, or kidney. Post-exercise thallium heart scans are highly sensitive for coronary artery insufficiency and myocardial ischemia.

Other popular uses include total body bone scans for inflammation or metastases, technetium-labeled compounds to diagnose or rule out acute cholecystitis; radio-iodinated fibrinogen to locate acute thrombosis anywhere; tagged erythrocytes to study their survival and sequestration, and to pinpoint the site of gastrointestinal bleeding; tagged leukocytes to locate occult abscesses; and on and on (Fig. 9.5).

BIOPSIES

Biopsy is another procedure that is being done with increasing frequency. Brain, heart, liver, kidney, spleen, thyroid, and pancreas are all accessible to the probing biopsy needle. Aspiration biopsy and cytologic study of thyroid nodules have replaced more formal biopsy procedures, eliminated nuclear scans, bypassed ultrasound, and avoided many instances of surgery.

Transthoracic and transbronchial lung biopsies are done almost with impunity under simple fluoroscopic guidance. Cervical mediastinoscopy for carinal node biopsy helps to determine the operability of lung cancers.

Perhaps the greatest encouragement for the biopsy of formerly inaccessible or dangerous sites is given by CT and ultrasound. With the precision and accuracy of guided missiles, real-time ultrasound or rapid sequence CT scanning can quickly direct a probing biopsy needle to a tiny 1-cm target or a drainage catheter to an occult abscess. This is an expensive, skill-requiring procedure, but it can bypass other less fruitful attempts at diagnosis and can save time and money in the long run.

DIGITAL SUBTRACTION ANGIOGRAPHY

This computerized system for visualizing arterial trees by the intravenous injection of a contrast material may eliminate the need for and risk of some intra-arterial contrast injections. Formerly, contrast materials reaching the arteries after intravenous injection were so dilute that they gave unsatisfactory images; the vessels could not be distinguished from the background soft-tissue densities. But the computer stores the digitized preinjection image and subtracts it from the postinjection image, leaving only the dye in the arteries to be seen.

This filmless system, which is stored and displayed by computer, dramatically increases the signal-noise ratio and *permits clear visualization of*

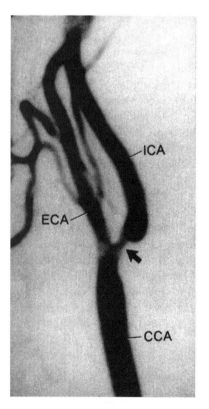

▶ **Figure 9.6.** Digital subtraction angiography demonstrates 60% reduction in diameter of internal carotid artery at its origin.

arteries. It demonstrates flow and perfusion defects.

So far, its greatest use has been to visualize carotid artery stenosis. It is reported that pulmonary artery occlusions by tiny emboli are detected with 100% sensitivity and rare false positivity. Renal circulation, coronary artery pathways, cerebral artery circuits, and other visceral and peripheral vessels may become clearly delineated by this almost harmless, slightly invasive procedure. The values of such visualizations are boundless (Fig. 9.6).

POSITRON EMISSION TOMOGRAPHY

This is another real-time imaging device used primarily in brain disorders. Tracer amounts of biochemically important substrates are labeled with very short half-life, positron-emitting radionuclides. The in vivo distribution of these tracers is measured by special scanning devices.

Thus, you can measure cerebral blood flow, oxygen consumption, glucose metabolism, and protein synthesis, depending on the chemical substrate used. Regional brain physiology and biochemistry can be observed, and areas of metabolic derangement can be pinpointed. With this device, implications for the diagnosis of stroke, schizophrenia, epilepsy, and multiple sclerosis become evident.

For example, the abnormal biochemistry in the plaques that occur in multiple sclerosis and the glucose metabolic defect that is found in an epileptogenic focus can be detected when other diagnostic methods are nonproductive. It has been noted that schizophrenics do not metabolize glucose equally in all areas of the brain. Cardiac, pulmonary, and abdominal disorders are still on the research agenda for this procedure.

This diagnostic and research tool is necessarily *limited to large institutions* for two reasons. First, the cost of the hardware alone is several million dollars. Second, because very short half-life radioisotopes are needed, they must be manufactured on site and cannot be transported elsewhere. It follows that only medical centers with cyclotrons or linear accelerators can perform positron emission tomography scans.

THE RADIOLOGIST'S NEW ROLE

Insofar as new diagnostic techniques are concerned, the great majority involve the radiology department, under whose aegis all types of imaging are done. The radiologist's role in the medical universe is undergoing evolution. In many cases he or she still deals with shadows and reads the films requested by the attending physician. But more and more, the radiologist is serving as a consultant. Being informed of the clinical situation, he or she may suggest the procedure or order of procedures best suited for each case.

A conference between the clinician and the radiologist is often very productive. In hospitals where such consultations are mandatory before CT scans are done, the number of procedures decreases, and the number of true-positive results increases.

ARE WE BETTER OFF?

Are the patient and clinician in a more advantageous position because of the newer diagnostic techniques? This question has three possible answers—yes, no, and maybe. Confusion, complications, and costs escalate. The accuracy of resulting diagnostic and therapeutic decisions may be enhanced or sometimes diminished in any individual case. Always present is the grim specter of imperfect information, because false-negative and false-positive results exist for some complex as well as simple tests. The skill of the performer of the procedure is a variable that must be considered.

Then, too, the clinician is often confounded by conflicting or indeterminate results that are "suggestive of" or "compatible with." In fact, uncertain tests or reports that neither exclude nor confirm a diagnosis only provoke the physician to order yet another test. And rapidly advancing technologies often leave him or her befuddled as to the appropriate test for a given problem; so one, two, three, or all tests may be ordered, with the hope that a uniformity of results will be obtained. When the results are not in accord, the physician is understandably stumped.

For the Opposition

The following case study demonstrates the pitfalls, snares, and entanglements that can result from reliance on new procedures.

A 55-year-old man has experienced malaise, jaundice, dark urine, and light stools for the past 10 months. He has had no weight loss, and his liver is slightly enlarged.

In the 1970s and 1980s, such a patient would have received a few liver function tests, possibly a liver biopsy, a gastrointestinal radiograph series, a barium enema to exclude a neoplasm, and then surgical exploration for obvious obstructive jaundice. Cancer, stone, or sclerosing cholangitis were the preoperative possibilities.

In the 1990s, *the same patient* undergoes additional multiple diagnostic procedures before a decision to operate is made. The carcinoembryonic antigen is strongly positive. Ultrasound shows subtly dilated intrahepatic ducts and a thickened gallbladder wall. But the CT scan reveals no dilated intrahepatic ducts and no gallbladder wall thickening. Percutaneous transhepatic cholangiography (PTC) shows constrictions of the hepatic ducts at their confluence. A liver biopsy is "consistent with obstructive jaundice." Endoscopic retrograde cholangiopancreatography shows normal distal ducts but gives no information about trouble higher up. Repeat PTC confirms strictures in the proximal hepatic ducts but also suggests a mass in the porta hepatis. The mass is confirmed by transfemoral selective arteriography.

Surgery is performed. Sclerosing cholangitis of the upper biliary ducts is found, and the mass is not there. So the preoperative impressions, decision to operate, and operative findings were the same in the 1970s, 1980s, and 1990s.

But for the 1990s, the CT scan and ultrasound were at odds. The carcinoembryonic antigen was falsely positive. ERCP was not helpful. The liver biopsy showed what was easily predictable. And the mass seen by PTC and arteriography was not present. In short, these additional complex procedures were confusing, added little helpful information, were redundant, were mostly not needed, and altered no decisions. They did, however, expose the patient to repeated dangers and to 47 rem of radiation (the equivalent of six barium enemas), and added many thousands of dollars to the bill (see Case 46, Chapter 16).

On the Flip Side

On the other side of the coin, there's no denying that the intelligent, appropriate use of new "hi-tech" tests can greatly benefit the patient. Diagnoses are often made more easily, more quickly, more correctly, and more cheaply; surgery may be simplified, or exploration may be avoided. Not only will more diagnoses be made, but disease processes will be better categorized and understood.

Consider, for example, the patient with *obstructive jaundice* just discussed. Assume that the initial study, ultrasound, had clearly shown dilated intrahepatic ducts and stones in the gallbladder. Assume further that the second study, a PTC, had shown a stone obstructing the common bile duct. No further studies would have been needed, and the therapeutic decision path would have been clear. Had the second test been an ERCP, the same necessary information might have been garnered.

Consider also a patient in whom *you suspect a pulmonary embolus.* Before starting expensive, lengthy, and risky anticoagulant treatment, you want to be more certain of the diagnosis, because the patient also has chronic liver disease and mild hypertension. The chest radiograph and ECG are both normal. There are many tests and procedures to choose from: arterial blood gases, ventilation-perfusion scan, pulmonary arteriography, and digital subtraction angiography.

Some clinical groups routinely perform pulmonary arteriography in such situations. After all, it is essentially a gold standard procedure and invades only the right side of the heart. However, the most universally used test is the ventilation-perfusion radionuclide scan. It is barely invasive, relatively inexpensive, universally available, and has moderately high sensitivity and specificity. Therefore, put your eggs in that basket. But if therapeutic surgical intervention is contemplated and 100% certainty is needed, arteriography should be done.

As a corollary, should you need to know if *iliofemoral venous thrombosis* is the source of the embolism, you can do a venogram, a plethysmogram, Doppler studies, or a radio-iodinated fibrinogen scan. The choice is not clear-cut and will vary from patient to patient.

A 60-year-old man with weight loss, anorexia, glucose intolerance, and no family history of diabetes mellitus is suspected of having *carcinoma of the pancreas.* Conventional radiography has been fruitless. You must now decide whether to order a CT scan, MRI, ultrasound, radionuclide scan, duodenal drainage cytology, ERCP, selective arteriography, serum markers, or a guided needle biopsy. Each test has its approximate operating characteristics, risk, cost, and availability.

So you consult your friendly unbiased radiologist, who will help you decide. One or two tests should suffice. Perhaps the best sequence is either ultrasound or CT scan followed by ERCP. The sensitivity and specificity of either combination are both in the 95% range. If one neoplastic area is delineated, a guided needle biopsy may raise the diagnostic probability to 100%. Then there will be no room for further doubt!

The next decision concerns a 64-year-old man with *transient ischemic attacks* and a right carotid artery bruit. Before suggesting surgery, you would like to perform the gold standard test for carotid stenosis—arteriography. But this procedure carries a 1% risk of causing a stroke. So you consider less invasive although perhaps not quite so accurate studies, such as ultrasound or digital subtraction angiography. If the results of one test are positive, and the results of the second are negative, you must now order a "tie-breaker." Even with its attendant risk, arteriography and perhaps better yet, magnetic resonance angiography, might be the best choice if surgery is anticipated. So do it first, because it will probably be all that you need.

In some instances, we can unequivocally state the best procedure for a prospective diagnosis. The "best test" for gallbladder stones is ultrasound; for acute cholecystitis, the best test is a radionuclide scan with techmetium-labeled iminodiacetic acid; for carotid stenosis, it is arteriography; for pulmonary emboli, it's the ventilation-perfusion scan; for suspected intracranial bleeding, do a CT scan; and for a herniated disc, it's the MRI. But for many other problems, the best choice is a toss-up or a slight edge for one procedure here and now but for another procedure there and later.

Into the Problem Solver's Mind

Paul Cutler

Through the medium of three interesting cases, this chapter brings you into the mind of the problem solver as he or she takes the history from the patient. The parenthetical sentences and paragraphs inserted in the course of the interview tell you what the doctor is thinking, why he or she asks certain questions, and how he or she evaluates the answers.

Before each physical examination, in the light of the history that has been obtained, the physician tells you the parts of the examination in which there is the most interest. Appropriate tests are then performed, and diagnostic closure is obtained.

CASE 1

Hoarseness in a 58-Year-Old Man

Doctor: Hello, Jim. What brings you here?

Patient: It's this voice of mine. I've been hoarse for the past 3 or 4 weeks, ever since we went to the Eagles-Rams game.

Doctor: Yes, I do notice that. Tell me more about it.

Patient: Well, you remember we both did yell a lot, especially when the Eagles held at the goal line, so at first I blamed my hoarseness on that. But it hasn't gotten any better. In fact, it's worse. I tried inhaling steam and stuff like that, but no help. This isn't so good for a salesman.

(Chronic persistent hoarseness—sounds like a possibly serious problem needing a thorough look. Jim still smokes a lot. Never did take my advice on that. If cheering at the game were the culprit, the hoarseness should have cleared in a few days. Besides, I made as much noise as he did, and my voice is OK.)

Doctor: Any other symptoms?

Patient: Like what?

Doctor: Like cough.

Patient: You know, I've had this annoying cough for years. That's why you told me to stop smoking. But I just can't stop. It's no worse than usual, but I do cough up a little grayish phlegm, which I never used to do.

(There are a number of companion symptoms that may be seen with hoarseness, depending on the cause and where the problem is located. These include cough, expectoration, hemoptysis, wheeze, stridor, stuffy nose, and postnasal drip.)

Doctor: Ever cough up any blood?

Patient: No, and I really look carefully for that.

(I'm sure Jim has chronic bronchitis, but I hope it's no more than that. Anyway, that couldn't account for hoarseness. I remember that his chest radiograph was normal 2 years ago. Could lung cancer have developed since then? Of course. And because probably less than 10% of persons who have lung cancer have hemoptysis, its absence doesn't help.

A vocal cord can be either diseased or paralyzed. Disease of the cord may result from chronic strain, as in singers and cheerleaders; from polyps, "granular laryngitis"; sinusitis with postnasal drip; tuberculosis; and cancer. Paralysis of a cord may result from an aortic aneurysm, a superior mediastinal mass, carcinoma near the apex of the lung, and carcinoma of the thyroid, all of which may impinge upon the recurrent laryngeal nerve, most notably on the left side. Further questions will aim to establish one hypothesis and exclude others.)

Doctor: Have you had a head cold recently? Perhaps a stuffy nose or a postnasal drip?

Patient: No.

(So much for sinusitis and a recent respiratory tract infection.)

Doctor: Jim, have you been doing an unusual amount of talking, singing, or hollering?

Patient: No, not really. You know, we salesmen make our living by talking. But with my voice, I never sing. Helen wouldn't stand for yelling, either.

(Continuous vocal cord strain seems unlikely.)

Doctor: Any trouble with breathing? Do you have any harsh noises or wheezes when you breathe?

Patient: No, I don't get short of breath, if that's what you mean. And my breathing sounds normal to me. Haven't had a wheeze since that bad chest cold you treated me for 5 years ago.

(A paralyzed vocal cord may be fixed either in the lateral or medial position; this may sometimes result in a high-pitched crowing sound when the patient breathes or, usually, in hoarseness.)

Doctor: What about pains in the chest?

Patient: None other than the usual tightness when I walk fast.

Doctor: Oh, yes! Has your angina gotten any worse?

Patient: No, it's about the same. If I monitor my activities carefully, I only rarely get chest pain.

Doctor: Any pains in the shoulders or arms?

Patient: No, just my usual bursitis in the right shoulder when I try my hand at tennis.

(Sounds like stable angina—no cause for immediate concern and certainly not related to his hoarseness. And he doesn't have the shoulder and arm pain seen in some lung cancers that impinge on the C-8, T-1, T-2 nerve roots. Pulmonary tuberculosis is always possible; it causes hoarseness if there is a highly active lung lesion producing sputum that yields positive test results for acid-fast bacilli. This seems most unlikely in view of Jim's outward good health. Anyway, I'll check with a chest radiograph.)

Doctor: OK, Jim, I'll come back to more questions later, but let's get to the physical examination now.

(My examination in this case will focus upon the eyes, the neck, the fingers, and the chest. If the patient has paralysis of a recurrent laryngeal nerve, he may also have involvement of the superior cervical sympathetic trunk, which is very close. In that event, he may have a homolateral Horner's syndrome—ptosis, miosis, enophthalmos, and anhidrosis.

If the superior vena cava is partially obstructed by an intrathoracic tumor, the veins of the patient's head, neck, and arms may be distended. If a pulmonary carcinoma exists, he may have cer-

vical lymphadenopathy or clubbed fingers. Thyroid carcinoma should easily be discovered by feeling the thyroid gland. The examination of the lungs may disclose telltale signs, such as tracheal deviation or dullness at the apex. But above all, examination of the larynx should furnish the key clue. One of the vocal cords will be either visibly diseased or paralyzed.)

Physical Examination: The patient has normal vital signs and a normal head and neck. Horner's signs are not present; there are no abnormal cervical lymph nodes; the thyroid gland is not enlarged; neck veins are not distended; and the trachea is in the midline.

The fingers are not clubbed, and the distal ends of long bones are not tender (hypertrophic pulmonary osteoarthropathy). Examination of the heart and lungs is within normal limits except for a fourth heart sound. The rest of the physical examination is also normal.

Mirror laryngoscopy reveals normal-looking vocal cords. The left cord does not move to the midline when the patient says "E-E-E-E." The right cord moves well (Fig. 10.1). Chest radiograph demonstrates an ill-defined, vague density in the left apex.

With almost 100% certainty, Jim has carcinoma of the lung that has enveloped the left recurrent laryngeal nerve where it arches under the aorta. So far, there is no evidence of cancer spread elsewhere. The absence of clubbing, nodes, and hemoptysis is not surprising, because these features have relatively low sensitivity for this disease.

Because the chest radiograph was inconclusive, a magnetic resonance image was obtained. It revealed a mass that was infiltrating the mediastinum and was contiguous with the aorta (Fig.

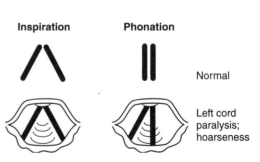

▶ **Figure 10.1.** Paralysis of the left vocal cord.

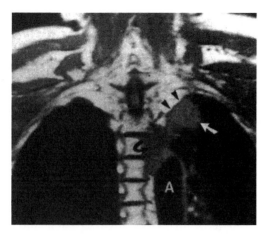

▶ **Figure 10.2.** Magnetic resonance image shows left superior sulcus tumor (Pancoast's) infiltrating the mediastinum.

10.2) Before therapy is initiated, a biopsy will be performed, and the cell type will be determined.

C A S E   2

Fever and Malaise in a 28-Year-Old Woman

Patient: I haven't felt well for a few weeks; I just have no pep and poop out in the late afternoon.

Doctor: Tell me more.

Patient: Well, it seems to have begun gradually. At first, I thought the kids were getting the best of me—so much to do at home after a day's work. But it's more than that. I just feel rotten. My temperature's been up, too. I started to check it some 8 or 10 days ago because I felt warm. It was over 100 on a number of occasions.

(Hmm!—young, seemingly healthy woman with fever and malaise for several weeks. Sounds like a low-grade infection somewhere—probably more than just a transient viral infection. She looks a little pale, too. I need more information.)

Doctor: Has this ever happened before?

Patient: No.

Doctor: Is it getting worse, or is it about the same?

Patient: I believe I'm feeling worse each day. Yesterday I put in a half-day's work. Today I could barely make it to your office.

(A chronic, progressive, unremitting illness. Malignancy doesn't seem likely at this age, ex-

cept perhaps for an occult lymphoma. I'll concentrate mainly on infections like tuberculosis and infective endocarditis, as well as systemic lupus erythematosus and sarcoidosis. These five illnesses are probably the most common ones that start like this.)

Doctor: Do you have any other symptoms?

Patient: Isn't that enough?

Doctor: Yes, I guess it is, but in order to find out what might be wrong, I must inquire about other symptoms. For example, do you have chills or night sweats?

Patient: No.

Doctor: What about cough and expectoration of phlegm?

Patient: Neither one.

Doctor: Has anyone at home or at work been sick?

Patient: No, I think. One or two of my fellow nurses were out with the flu last week, but that's all. My husband and two children are both well, thank God!

(Doesn't sound like she has gotten a respiratory tract infection from somebody else. The absence of cough, expectoration, and night sweats is a strong point against pulmonary tuberculosis, at least tuberculosis that is advanced enough to cause fever and malaise. Because most persons with sarcoidosis have respiratory tract symptoms, their absence is also a strong point against this disease.)

Doctor: Tell me about your work and your home life.

Patient: I'm a nurse at the Metropolitan Hospital where I do general duty nursing. As you know, we're very careful about precautions against infections. Both I and my husband work. He's a pharmacy store manager. Between the two of us, we earn enough money to live modestly and raise our two kids. It's not easy these days, you know. I'm grateful we have pretty good health insurance. I do the day shift, so we have all our dinners at home. After work each afternoon, I pick up the kids at the day care center, then shop and cook dinner. And it's to bed by 10 PM. I get up at 5 AM.

Doctor: Sounds like a not-too-easy life. How have your appetite and weight been?

Patient: My appetite is definitely off. I'm not sure, but I may have lost a few pounds.

(These are both nonspecific indicators that could go along with most illnesses. I'll have to get more specific.)

Doctor: Do you have itching of the skin?

Patient: No.

(Pruritus may be seen early with certain lymphomas like Hodgkin's disease.)

Doctor: What about your joints? Any aches, pains, or swellings of the joints—fingers, wrists, knees, ankles?

Patient: No.

(Arthralgias and even arthritis are common in systemic lupus erythematosus, as well as in sarcoid; their absence weighs against lupus and sarcoid, but certainly doesn't rule these diseases out.)

Doctor: Have you been having sharp pains anywhere in the chest, especially worse on breathing?

Patient: No.

(Inflammation of serosal cavities—pleura and pericardium—are not infrequently seen in lupus. Absence of this symptom is not a strong indicator, because pleuritis is not highly sensitive for this disease. If present, it would make me lean a bit toward lupus. But lest I forget, pleuritis occurs in tuberculosis, too. There's nothing else to suggest a lymphoma; for that disease, the physical examination will help. Now, for some questions that may point to endocarditis—acute or subacute.)

Doctor: Have you been told or do you know that you have a heart murmur?

Patient: When I was younger, the school nurse said I had a heart murmur. But my family doctor said it was innocent. In more recent years, some doctors noticed it, but most didn't.

(Hmmm. May be either nothing or unrelated. At any rate, I'll ask further.)

Doctor: Did you ever have acute rheumatic fever?

Patient: No.

(Only 50% of persons who have rheumatic valve disease report a history of having had acute rheumatic fever. So a negative history is not conclusive. The answer will be found in the physical examination.)

Doctor: Have you had any recent dental work?

Patient: Not real work. But I do have my teeth scaled every other month for gum problems. The last time was about 6 weeks ago. I'm due again in 2 weeks.

(Oh-oh! That's a red light. Recent dental work plus a heart murmur may equal infective endocarditis from mouth organisms and transient

bacteremia. The dental work may consist of extraction, gum surgery, or even a vigorous cleaning of teeth.)

Doctor: Did you take an antibiotic before having dental work done?

Patient: No. I was never told to.

(Sounds like we're on the right track. The physical examination should substantiate the impression of infective endocarditis, probably caused by *Streptococcus viridans*. I'll examine particularly for signs of anemia, embolic phenomena, heart murmur, and splenomegaly, each of which may be present or absent in this disease. If all are present, the diagnosis will be reasonably certain. If none is present, the diagnosis will be most unlikely.

I must also look for enlarged lymph nodes in the neck, axilla, and groin, because these signs, in combination with a large spleen, may indicate that the patient has a lymphoma rather than endocarditis.)

Physical Examination: The patient's vital signs are normal, except for a temperature of 100.5°F and a pulse rate of 106 bpm. Aside from several 1-cm lymph nodes in each axilla, there are no nodes palpable elsewhere. The conjunctiva and palms are pale. Several 3-mm petechiae are noted, one in the left conjunctiva, one in the right retina, and two on the fingertips. There are no Osler's nodes, Janeway spots, or subungual splinter hemorrhages. The head and neck are otherwise normal. There is a grade 2/6 soft late-systolic crescendo murmur heard over the mitral valve area. It is preceded by a short but noticeable click.

(These cardiac findings are typical for mitral valve prolapse. The location and size of the palpable lymph nodes suggest that they are benign.)

The rest of the physical examination is normal. In particular, the spleen and liver are not enlarged, and there is no clubbing of the fingers and toes.

(The diagnosis of infective endocarditis seems certain on the basis of the history and physical examination. The transient bacteremia that often results from oral operative procedures may settle on previously damaged or otherwise abnormal heart valves, such as exist in this patient. Other than for the identification of the causative organism, the laboratory will give little added information.)

The blood count showed 3 million red blood cells (RBCs) per cubic millimeter; 10 g of hemoglobin per 100 mL; and 10,500 white blood cells per cubic millimeter, with a normal differ-

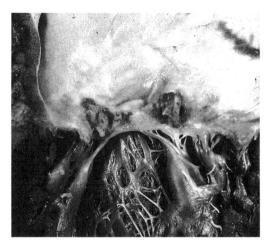

▶ **Figure 10.3.** Mitral valve showing vegetations of bacterial endocarditis.

ential. The urinalysis was normal, except for 10 to 20 RBCs per high-powered field. Three consecutive blood cultures drawn from different sites over a 4-hour period of time all showed positive results for *Streptococcus viridans.*

(Most cases of endocarditis will manifest microscopic hematuria which, together with petechiae, are evidence of microembolization from valve vegetations (Fig. 10.3.)

Transthoracic or transesophageal ultrasound study for the presence of mitral valve vegetations was not deemed necessary.

Appropriate antibiotic treatment was begun.

C A S E   3

Jaundice in a 68-Year-Old Man

Doctor: Haven't seen you for a year. Why did you come to see us today, Mr. Brown?

Patient: Doctor, I noticed my eyeballs were yellow while shaving yesterday. At first I thought it was a reflection from the sun, but on looking carefully, I could see that the whites of my eyes were yellow.

Doctor: Yes, I can see that. Have you had any other problems?

Patient: Not really.

(He's definitely jaundiced—sclera and skin— and he has no other complaints, so it would seem to be painless jaundice. If so, I'm thinking of either obstruction of the bile duct by a tumor such as that

of the bile ducts, pancreas, or ampulla of Vater, or an intrahepatic lesion like cirrhosis, infectious hepatitis, or metastatic carcinoma. In any event, this appears to be a serious problem. First, I would like to know if the bile duct is obstructed, for if so, there will be no bilirubin entering the gut.)

Doctor: Have you noticed any changes in the usual color of your urine or stool?

Patient: Yes, now that you mention it. For the past week or two, my urine has been almost as dark as Coca-Cola. On the other hand, my stool has been an unusual light tan color, especially yesterday and today.

(He has obstructive jaundice; there's little or no bilirubin entering the gut, and large amounts of bilirubin are spilling over into the urine as the serum bilirubin rises.)

Doctor: Does your skin itch?

Patient: Yes, it does. Look at my scratch marks. I thought it might be the new underwear I just bought.

(Pruritus is common with obstructive jaundice—it may result from an increase in bile salts in the blood.)

Doctor: Have you been having any sort of pain anywhere in the abdomen?

Patient: No, not at all, lately. You remember I had an episode of severe pain up here under my right ribs about 3 years ago. You did some tests and found gallstones. You recommended surgery, but I didn't want an operation because of my heart condition. So here I am, 3 years later. I never had that pain again.

Doctor: Yes, of course I remember. It's here in your chart. Which reminds me, how is your heart doing?

Patient: No problems there, either. Since I had my heart attack 7 years ago, I haven't had any chest pains. No shortness of breath either.

(Hmmm! Gallstones. Could there be a stone in the common bile duct obstructing the flow of bile? Not likely—he's had no recurrent right upper quadrant pains. A stone in the duct doesn't remain silent for long. However, gallstones may encourage the development of cancer of the gallbladder, or sometimes the stones are seen in association with acute pancreatitis. But again, no pain, so pancreatitis too is out of the picture. His heart problem is no doubt unrelated. Seems to be doing well there—no angina or congestive heart failure. It's time to search for symptoms that might be related to the general debility seen with many cancers, as well as symptoms that might be related to specifically located cancers.)

Doctor: Have you lost weight, and how have your appetite and general strength been?

Patient: I feel good, other than what you see. My appetite is as good as ever. I haven't lost any weight, and I still play a mean game of tennis—singles.

(Sounds generally OK. I'll get more specific.)

Doctor: Do you have indigestion, nausea, or vomiting?

Patient: No.

(Infectious hepatitis can cause transient obstructive jaundice when it peaks. Swollen hepatocytes crowd the bile canaliculi. But if so, I would expect the patient to have nausea, vomiting, and right upper quadrant pain or discomfort. That possibility seems most unlikely, but I'll be sure to check for liver size and tenderness.)

Doctor: How have your bowels been?

Patient: Regular.

Doctor: Do you ever notice black or bloody stools?

Patient: No.

Doctor: Do you look?

Patient: Yes.

Doctor: Have you had any recent injections or blood transfusions?

Patient: No.

Doctor: Are you taking any medications?

Patient: No.

Doctor: Have you traveled out of the country lately?

Patient: No.

Doctor: Have you eaten raw seafood?

Patient: No.

(So much for infectious and drug-related hepatitis.)

Doctor: Do you have a cough? Do you cough up phlegm or blood?

Patient: None of those.

Doctor: Do you still smoke?

Patient: No, I quit after my heart attack 7 years ago.

Doctor: Do you have any difficulty in passing urine? For example, how many times per night must you go to the bathroom?

Patient: No problem there. I get up once a night, but that's been for years. My stream is good.

(There are no symptoms pointing to the common malignancies seen in men—stomach, colon, lung, and prostate—but the absence of symptoms certainly does not rule any of them out. Each could be present and have extensive metastases to the liver, yet be asymptomatic.

I know that Mr. Brown was once a heavy drinker. He said that he gave it up a few years before my last examination a year ago. When I checked him then he had no stigmata of cirrhosis, but I'll check for them when I examine him again.)

Doctor: How much alcohol are you drinking?

Patient: Just one or two Scotches daily.

(Well that's not a lot, provided he speaks the truth. Cirrhosis could indeed have a presentation of jaundice only, but it would not tend to be obstructive in nature. Some bile should be entering the gut. Besides, if that were the case, there should be abnormalities on the physical examination. I'll check that.)

Doctor: I note in your chart that we found a trace of glucose in your urine a year ago. The blood glucose was normal then. Did you follow up on this possible problem when you moved to California?

Patient: No, I was too busy.

Doctor: Do or did any members of your family have diabetes?

Patient: No. Nobody. I did check on that.

(This is worrisome—the recent onset of possible non-genetic diabetes in an older man, especially with painless jaundice—suggests the possibility of pancreatic cancer.)

Doctor: Mr. Brown, I'm going to examine you now. There will be more questions later. First, though, please go to the bathroom and give me a urine sample. You will find containers there.

(In doing the physical examination, I will focus on the liver and abdomen. I want to know if the liver is enlarged, nodular, and/or tender, and if there are any of the various stigmata of cirrhosis. I will examine the abdomen most carefully for the presence of a mass. On the rectal examination, I will look for cancer of the rectum or prostate, check the color of the stool, and test for occult blood.)

Physical Examination: The skin, cornea, oral mucosa, tongue, and palms are deep yellow. The liver is 10 cm on percussion in the right midclavicular line and non-tender, and the edge is not palpable. There are no abdominal masses, tenderness, or guarding. Peristalsis is normal in all quadrants. There is no pallor. Stigmata of chronic liver disease such as spider angiomata, palmar erythema, and distended abdominal veins are not present. Rectal examination reveals no masses; the prostate is slightly and diffusely enlarged and without nodules, and the sample of stool removed is the color of clay and negative for occult blood. The rest of the examination is normal.

The urine sample is brownish tan and, upon shaking, the foam is golden yellow.

(Cirrhosis and hepatitis are out of the picture. Carcinoma outside of the biliary tract is rendered unlikely, although still possible. I must focus on cancer of the bile ducts, gallbladder, ampulla, and pancreas. The history of glycosuria centers most of my concern on the pancreas, especially because the common bile duct traverses the head of the pancreas.)

Pertinent laboratory values are presented in Table 10.1. The laboratory tells you what you already knew or suspected. There is no liver cell damage. There is obstructive jaundice, as evidenced by the high bilirubin level, high alkaline phosphatase level, and normal transaminase level. There is no evidence for obstruction of pancreatic ducts.

The absence of urine urobilinogen confirms the presence of complete obstruction of the common bile duct. If there is no bilirubin entering the gut, there is no conversion of bilirubin to urobilinogen by intestinal bacteria. Therefore,

Table 10.1. Pertinent Laboratory Values for the Patient in Case 3

TEST	RESULT	INTERPRETATION
Serum fasting glucose	132 mg/dL	above normal
Serum transaminase	80 IU/L	normal
Serum alkaline phosphatase	240 IU/L	three times normal
Serum amylase	60 IU/L	normal
Serum bilirubin	8.5 mg/dL	very high

Urine: 4+ bilirubin, negative for urobilinogen.

urobilinogen is not reabsorbed through the portal vein, and none spills over into the urine (see Table 16.6, Case 47).

It now becomes necessary to pinpoint the precise location of the obstruction. An ultrasound study of the liver may confirm that there are no discrete tumors within the liver, but what is more important, the ultrasound may indicate the presence of dilated bile ducts. If the bile ducts are dilated, which they almost certainly will be, percutaneous transhepatic cholangiography (PTC) or endoscopic retrograde cholangiopancreatography (ERCP) will locate the obstruction.

Ultrasound study of the liver showed normal parenchymal architecture and dilated hepatic ducts and common bile duct (Fig. 10.4). No intrahepatic masses were seen. A mass was suspected in

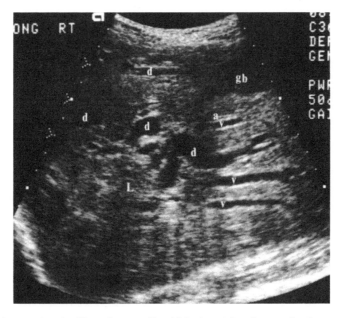

▶ **Figure 10.4.** Ultrasound study of liver showing dilated bile ducts (d); color Doppler distinguishes ducts from arteries and veins by the velocity of fluids within these vessels.

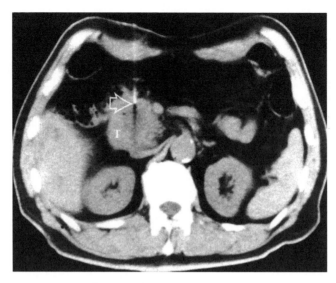

▶ **Figure 10.5.** Percutaneous computed tomographic-guided biopsy of pancreatic adenocarcinoma; tip of needle is in the head of pancreas. *T* is a tumor.

the head of the pancreas. PTC demonstrated the previously noted dilated ducts and an area of complete obstruction in the region of the head of the pancreas. Computed tomography (CT) confirmed a mass in the head of the pancreas. A CT-guided biopsy of the mass disclosed adenocarcinoma of the pancreas (Fig. 10.5). An abdominal surgeon was consulted.

AFTERWORD

None of the preceding three cases was simple or easy to solve with just a few questions. But 2 minutes of conversation should have been enough to establish a list of leading diagnostic contenders, rank them in the order of likelihood, and establish one or two possibilities as being most likely.

In each case, there were distracting bits of information that mandated the consideration of other hypotheses. Most other cases are usually more easily solved. For example, if the patient with hoarseness also had a chronic cough, weight loss, and hemoptysis, lung cancer would have been the prime suspect from the outset. And if, on the other hand, this patient had been a 24-year-old homeless person with a chronic cough, ex-

pectoration, weight loss, fever, and night sweats, pulmonary and laryngeal tuberculosis, as well as the acquired immunodeficiency syndrome, would have been likely contenders.

The second patient, a young woman who had been experiencing several weeks of malaise and fever, could have had any one of many different diseases. Such presenting constitutional symptoms are not specific for any organ or any type of malady. However, if there were an associated history of aches and pains in various joints, as well as a recent episode of "pleurisy," and the examination did not reveal a heart murmur or evidences of microemboli, lupus erythematosus would have been the prime suspect.

The patient in case 3 was jaundiced. Had there also been a history of weeks of anorexia, nausea, weight loss, and indigestion, stomach cancer with liver metastases might have been the hypothesis of choice. But on the other hand, if the jaundice had been associated with several days of nausea, vomiting, fever, and right upper quadrant discomfort, consideration would have been given to infectious hepatitis or acute cholecystitis.

Thus, as additional historical information is compounded with the chief complaint, the flow of data acquisition and resolution goes this way or that.

From Patient to Paper

Paul Cutler

What follows is a dialogue between a patient and a physician. Note the conversational quality of the interview. Also, especially notice the use of open-ended questions and see who does most of the talking. Observe that the physician follows no rigid format, yet misses very little, tracks positive clues, goes off on tangents, and then returns to the departure point. If it seems that too many questions are sometimes asked at one time, you are correct. This is done here for the purpose of editorial brevity, but should not be done when taking a history. On occasion, *a parenthesized paragraph* is inserted during the colloquy; this text denotes the physician's interim thoughts and impressions.

At the conclusion of the interview, the physical examination is presented. Try to formulate a problem list based on the history and physical examination alone. Subsequently, you will note the author's version of how this case should be written up. If any information was not obtained in the original interview, this can be ascertained by inspecting the written version. Then, go back to the patient and fill in the gaps.

The initial problem list, assessment, plan for each problem, test results, and a final problem list follow the written history and physical examination.

PATIENT INTERVIEW

Doctor: Good morning, Mrs. Smith. I haven't seen you in several years. How are you?

Patient: Well, not so good, doctor.

Doctor: What's troubling you?

Patient: Lots of things, but mainly I can't eat.

Doctor: Oh?

(That could mean any one of lots of things—I need much more information.)

Doctor: Tell me more about that!

Patient: It's been going on for 3 or 4 months. First I thought it was just my nerves. You see, I've been depressed about my daughter who just got divorced; and my son isn't making such a good living. But the appetite doesn't get better. In fact, it's gotten worse. It's such an effort to eat.

Doctor: Have you lost weight?

Patient: Oh, yes, my clothes don't seem to fit anymore. My usual weight is 165 pounds, but I'm down to 146. All my life I've been overweight, and now it's finally coming off.

Doctor: You don't want it to?

Patient: Yes, but not this way.

Doctor: How do you feel otherwise?

Patient: Not really good. I tire easily and have to take a nap each afternoon. You know me, doctor, I usually keep busy from morning to night. But I've been feeling too weak; in fact, I stopped my volunteer work at the hospital. And that's not like me.

(Anorexia, weight loss, and weakness. That's an ominous triad. I'm thinking in terms of either depression or a major debilitating physical illness such as cancer or a chronic infectious process. In addition to delving more deeply into her psychologic state, I will search each body system for symptoms that might indicate malignancy there.)

Doctor: I know, Mrs. Smith. How old are you now?

Patient: Fifty-eight, and I've always been so well!

Doctor: Well, not really. You remember, I've treated you for several problems. And then when you lived in California, you saw a doctor a few times.

Patient: Oh, yes, I forgot about my blood pressure and blood sugar.

Doctor: Where do these two situations stand right now?

Patient: Well, the blood sugar seems to be under good control with the two pills I take each day. As for the blood pressure, it doesn't bother me, so I don't bother it!

Doctor: If you remember, I started you on both medications about 10 years ago. What happened?

Patient: The doctor in California checked me and told me to continue with the blood sugar pills. He said the blood pressure was normal, so I stopped the pills for that.

Doctor: Do you have severe thirst or frequent urination?

Patient: No, I checked my blood sugars often, and they're normal.

(Sounds like her diabetes is reasonably well controlled. If her current symptoms resulted from uncontrolled diabetes, she would have polyuria and polydipsia. I'm not sure where her hypertension stands. I must not forget to review her systems, but because we're into the diabetic issue now, I'll ask for symptoms that might indicate diabetic complications.)

Doctor: What about chest pains, trouble with your vision, leg pains and cramps, burning sensations in the feet?

Patient: None of those, either. I wear glasses, but see well. The eye doctor gave me new glasses a year ago and told me my eyes were perfect.

(There are no symptoms to indicate coronary disease, peripheral vascular disease, neuropathy, or retinopathy. I'll check later for physical signs of these complications.)

Doctor: Any headaches, dizziness, nosebleeds, shortness of breath, swollen legs, or palpitations?

Patient: Never.

(There are no symptoms to indicate left ventricular failure from longstanding or severe hypertension, nor are there any symptoms supposedly associated with severe hypertension.)

Doctor: Tell me what you do each day.

Patient: I'm up at 7 AM and get my husband off to work with breakfast and a packed lunch. Eating out is so expensive these days. I pass the morning straightening up the apartment, have a bite of lunch, and then have a nap. Can you imagine that! By 4 PM, I begin supper. Bill gets home at 5 PM, and he's real hungry. After dinner, he helps me with the dishes, and we spend the evening watching TV. Then to bed by 11 PM.

Doctor: Any other activities?

Patient: Well, it's church on Sunday. I wouldn't miss it. Our minister gives such good sermons. Occasionally, we visit friends, but I've cut down on that. I really get too tired, and I'm embarrassed by not being able to eat. No more dancing, either, and I did so want to learn the Macarena. Oh well, my knitting will have to do.

Doctor: Tell me about where you've lived, your education, and your family.

Patient: I've lived in Pennsylvania all my life, except for the past 7 years in California. We left and returned when my husband changed his place of employment. He works so hard; I'm worried for him, too. Being a construction manager isn't easy, but he's managed to make a good living for all of us these past 35 years. I dropped out of college to marry him—it was wartime, you know. My education stopped, but I do manage to keep reading. I read lots about everything. Between reading, knitting, watching TV, the house, and the kids—that takes care of my time. I told you my children are a great concern to me. I have three. One son is 33 and can't seem to find himself or get a job. My daughter is 31, has two children, and just got a divorce. The 22-year-old fancies himself as a musician, plays in local bands on Saturdays, but otherwise just hangs around the house.

(Although Mrs. Smith has some situations in her life that might conceivably cause a reactive depression, I get the feeling that she is a well-adjusted person, that her principal problem is not psychiatric, and that in all likelihood a serious organic problem exists.)

Doctor: What about your parents, and your sisters or brothers?

Patient: My father died suddenly when I was young. I'm told he had diabetes. Mom died at 80 of cancer—stomach, I think. I have three younger sisters and one brother. They're all well so far. Oh, yes, one sister has high blood pressure, and my brother has a touch of sugar.

Doctor: Well, I see things aren't completely pleasant for you. Do you take any medications, and what about tea, coffee, alcohol, and cigarettes?

Patient: I've never smoked, drink coffee or tea several times a day, have a cocktail or two with my husband on weekends, and take no medications other than my diabetes pills. Oh, yes, I do take an occasional aspirin for knee pains, and a teaspoon of paregoric for loose bowels.

Doctor: Paregoric?

Patient: Just for the past few weeks. My bowels have been a little loose from time to time, so I've taken 1 or 2 teaspoons a day. It always worked for the children.

Doctor: What are your bowel movements like?

Patient: Usually, I have one bowel movement a day. The past few weeks, on certain days, I have two or three. They're slightly loose, and occasionally watery.

Doctor: What color are they?

Patient: I don't notice.

Doctor: Is diarrhea unusual for you?

Patient: Oh, yes. If anything, I tend to be on the constipated side. I think the diarrhea is from my nerves, too. Nerves can do anything, can't they?

Doctor: Well, uh, I guess so. Any trouble swallowing?

Patient: No.

Doctor: Any indigestion, heartburn, gas, belching, abdominal pain, or jaundice?

Patient: None of those. I do seem to fill up easily when I eat, but I guess that's my bad appetite.

(Oh, oh! Easy satiety suggests stomach cancer, although the 3 weeks of diarrhea hint at colon cancer. Either disease could explain the problem, especially if metastatic cancer exists. I should have asked about gastrointestinal symptoms right off, but I got to it through the drug and medication route. I'll check the other systems now.)

Doctor: Do you have any other symptoms?

Patient: No, not really.

Doctor: What about difficulty, pain, or frequency of urination?

Patient: No.

Doctor: When did your menstrual periods stop?

Patient: They began at 12 and stopped at 50. I've had no periods since then—but—I do notice a few drops of blood after intercourse.

Doctor: Tell me about that.

Patient: It's only been for the past 6 or 8 months. There's just a little bleeding after my husband and I have sex. It lasts a day or two. I guess my membranes are thin.

Doctor: No vaginal discharge or pain?

Patient: No.

Doctor: What about your chest? Do you have a cough, or do you bring up phlegm or blood? Any shortness of breath?

Patient: No.

(Post-menopausal vaginal bleeding is a red flag. She seemed hesitant to tell me about it. I'll check that on the physical examination. The ab-

sence of cough and hemoptysis and the history of no smoking are strong points against lung cancer, at least lung cancer that is so advanced as to cause this patient's presenting symptoms.)

Doctor: Any trouble with your eyes, ears, nose, or mouth?

Patient: No.

Doctor: Let me be more specific. Do you have spots before your eyes, difficulty with vision, inflammation or pain in the eyes, double vision, or tearing?

Patient: No. But I do wear glasses.

Doctor: Is your hearing good? Do you get earaches, ringing in the ears, or discharge from the ears?

Patient: No.

Doctor: How about your mouth and throat? Are your teeth OK?

Patient: They're all gone—had them extracted 5 years ago. They were all bad, anyway. I wear dentures.

Doctor: Any trouble with your lips, mouth, tongue, or voice?

Patient: No, except for a little hoarseness if I talk to my husband too much. He's almost deaf, you know.

Doctor: Do you have any pain or stiffness in your joints?

Patient: My knees are stiff when I get up in the morning. I've had that for several years. It seems to get better when I'm up and about. Come to think of it, they're a little aching and stiff after I've watched TV for a few hours, too.

(Sounds like she may have osteoarthritis of the knees. I'll check this on the physical examination too.)

Doctor: What about your breasts? Any pain, swelling, lumps, or discharge from the nipples?

Patient: No. I used to have swollen lumpy breasts before my menstrual periods, but that doesn't happen anymore.

Doctor: Is your sex life satisfactory?

Patient: I'd say "yes." We don't do it as much as we used to, but we still enjoy it. Guess we're both getting old. Do you think it causes my bleeding?

Doctor: We'll have to see. Refresh me on your past health. Any serious illnesses, operations, or accidents?

Patient: No illnesses we haven't discussed. No accidents, either, thank God! But you do remember my gallbladder was removed 20 years ago for stones.

Doctor: Oh, uh, yes. A few more questions, and then we can begin our examination. Have you ever had allergies, wheezing, or hives?

Patient: No.

Doctor: How about headaches and dizziness?

Patient: I already answered that one.

Doctor: Any trouble with your skin, hair, or nails?

Patient: My hair seems to have gotten thinner in the past 10 years, but they tell me that's natural.

Doctor: What about chills and fever?

Patient: Never.

Doctor: You've always considered yourself to be in good health, haven't you?

Patient: Yes, until recently.

Doctor: Are you very concerned about your health?

Patient: Not really. You've got to get sick sometime!

Doctor: Well, let's do your physical examination now. Come with me.

(Let's see, now. I plan to do an orderly, complete physical examination, because there seem to be a number of problems here. But I will focus particularly on those areas related to the history-driven hypotheses I've already formed. Insofar as malignant disease is concerned, I will examine for pallor, pathologic lymph nodes, breast lump, abdominal mass, liver size, rectal mass, and stool for occult blood. A pelvic examination and Pap smear are vital. As for yet asymptomatic complications of diabetes, I will check the fundi and arterial pulsations and sensation in the lower extremities. For the effects of hypertension, I will check the blood pressure in both arms, the fundi, the carotid arteries for bruits, and the heart for size and abnormal heart sounds.)

The physical examination shows a well-developed, fairly well-nourished woman appearing to be her stated age, comfortably sitting in a chair and in no distress. Height, 62 inches; weight, 144 lb; temperature, 36.5° C, blood pressure, 188/110 in both arms; and respirations, 16 per minute. On inspection, she appears pale and shows some evidence of weight loss in that her skin folds are loose. No jaundice, rashes, abnormal pigmentation, venous distention, or deformities are present.

The hair is gray and slightly thinned. Her conjunctiva, tongue, and nailbeds are pale, and the palmar creases are not pink. She is edentulous, wears dentures, and has a deviated nasal septum. There are no other abnormalities noted around the head, face, eyes, ears, nose, mouth, and throat, except for the fundi that show a few tiny round punctate hemorrhages and arteriolar narrowing and tortuosity. The thyroid gland is not palpable, and the trachea is in the midline. No abnormal lymph nodes are felt in the neck or anywhere in the body. There are no carotid bruits.

The lungs are normal on examination; the diaphragm moves well and equally on both sides. The cardiac apex beat is 11 cm from the midsternal line in the fifth left intercostal space and occupies an area with a diameter of 3 to 4 cm; it feels forceful. An S_4 is heard over the apex. Otherwise, there is nothing of note. The breasts show no abnormalities in the sitting and reclining positions. There is no tenderness, rigidity, or mass palpable in the abdomen. The liver is 12 cm on percussion from top to bottom in the right midclavicular line, but this is imprecise because of the breasts; the liver's edge is not palpable. A right upper quadrant scar is noted.

Rectal examination is normal. The feces are brown and test +2 for occult blood. Speculum examination of the cervix reveals a 1-cm-wide bleeding friable area at 6 o'clock. A Pap smear is taken. Pelvic bimanual examination shows the uterus to be normal in size and position and freely movable. The adnexa are not palpable. Peripheral pulses are normal. No varicose veins are present. Both knees are slightly swollen, and Heberden's nodes are noted on the hands. Orthopedic and neurologic examinations are normal.

WRITTEN RECORD: AUTHOR'S VERSION

Mrs. Smith is a 58-year-old housewife whose history is reliable and accurate and whose chief complaint is "I can't eat" for the past 3 or 4 months.

History of Present Illness

For the past 3 to 4 months, the patient has had anorexia and 19 lb of weight loss. She also tires easily and, unlike her busy routine, has been obliged to stop volunteer hospital work and take a nap each afternoon. She thinks this may well be related to her nerves because she has been depressed about her divorced daughter and two jobless, aimless sons.

Past Medical History

She has had diabetes and hypertension for 10 years. For the diabetes, she takes glyburide twice daily, frequent checks of her blood show normal glucose levels, and she has no severe thirst or polyuria. She started medication for hypertension 10 years ago, but was subsequently told her blood pressure was normal, so she decided to stop the medication. She has no symptoms attributable to hypertension or its complications, such as headache, dizziness, visual disturbance, dyspnea on exertion, swollen legs, or palpitations. She takes an occasional aspirin for headache and paregoric for loose bowels. The gallbladder was removed 20 years ago.

Patient Profile

Mrs. Smith is an intelligent, somewhat anxious woman who seems to show no more than a normal concern for her symptoms and possible illnesses. Her diabetes and hypertension hardly seem to matter. She does think a lot of her trouble is due to nerves, but isn't sure. She is a sturdy, considerate, kind woman who cares for her husband and seems well adjusted, adaptable, and in control. One gets the feeling that her problems are organic. She has lived in Pennsylvania all of her life except for the past 7 years, during which time she had been in California; the move was because of her husband's change in job site. He is a construction foreman who has always provided well and is now getting old and deaf.

Mrs. Smith dropped out of college to get married during wartime, and although her formal education stopped, she has kept busy reading, doing charity work, and watching TV. She knits; likes to dance, although she fatigues too much for that now; attends church regularly; and seems to have good psychosocial and sexual relationships with her husband. She gets to bed by 11 PM, is up at 7 AM, makes breakfast and lunch for her husband, naps in the afternoon, makes dinner, and she and her husband clean up to-

gether. She does not smoke, drinks two to three cups of coffee or tea daily, and has one or two cocktails with her husband on weekends.

Family History

Her father died suddenly when he was young, and he had diabetes. Her mother died at 80 of cancer, possibly of the stomach. She has three younger sisters and one brother; one sister has hypertension, and her brother has diabetes.

Systems Review

- *General*. There have been no chills or fever, and the patient considers herself in good health until recently.
- *Head*. There are no headaches or dizziness.
- *Skin, hair, nails*. There has been thinning of the hair for 10 years, but the nails and skin show no abnormalities.
- *Eyes, ears, nose, throat*. She wears eyeglasses and has no spots before the eyes, visual difficulty, inflammation or eye pain, double vision, or tearing. She has good hearing and no tinnitus or aural discharge. She has no teeth and wears dentures. There are no symptoms referable to the lips, mouth, tongue, or voice. She gets a little hoarse sometimes but attributes this to her husband's deafness.
- *Pulmonary*. The patient has no cough or expectoration.
- *Cardiovascular*. Covered under the past medical history.
- *Breast*. No pain, lumps, swelling, or discharge.
- *Allergy*. The patient has had no allergies, wheezing, or hives.
- *Gastrointestinal*. Although she is usually constipated, she has had diarrhea for the past 3 weeks. This consists of two to three bowel movements a day, which are slightly loose and occasionally watery. She doesn't observe whether the stool is black or bloody. There is no dysphagia, indigestion, heartburn, gas, belching, abdominal pain, or jaundice. She does seem to have early satiety.
- *Genitourinary*. There has been no pain, frequency, or difficulty with urination. Her menses began at age 12 and ended at age 50. For the past 6 to 8 months, there has been postcoital

bleeding lasting a day or two each time, but no vaginal discharge or pain.

- *Musculoskeletal.* The knees are stiff and aching on getting up in the morning and after sitting a while.

The physical examination has been detailed in the protocol. In summary, however, the physical examination shows a 58-year-old white woman who looks drawn and pale. The blood pressure is 188/110, and she demonstrates pallor, particularly in the palmar creases, weight loss, no teeth, a deviated nasal septum, diabetic and grade 1 hypertensive changes in the fundi, an enlarged heart with a diffuse, forceful apical beat, an S_4, 2+ occult blood in the stool, a cervical lesion, swollen knees, and Heberden's nodes.

Problem List

1. Weakness, weight loss, anorexia, anemia
2. Easy satiety
3. Diarrhea
4. Hypertension
5. Left ventricular hypertrophy
6. Diabetes
7. Anxiety and depression
8. Cervical lesion
9. Hypertrophic osteoarthritis
10. No teeth
11. Postcholecystectomy

ASSESSMENT OF PROBLEM LIST (AND PLAN) Problem 1 consists of weakness, weight loss, anorexia, and anemia. This is the most urgent problem in this case and is the cause for the patient's presentation to the physician. The first three symptoms could be compatible with a large variety of organic problems as well as depression. However, the presence of anemia makes one think more in terms of an organic lesion. These four clues direct your attention to a malignancy, especially in a patient of this age. But the possibility of uremia, tuberculosis, or a hematologic disorder must be considered. Studies to be done would include a complete blood count to assess the degree and type of anemia, repeat stool examinations for occult blood to confirm the original finding, a chest radiograph, sigmoidoscopy, barium enema or colonoscopy,

and a gastrointestinal series. A gastrointestinal malignancy must be strongly considered in a woman of this age who has this type of presentation.

As for problems 2 and 3, these suggest that the site of her disease process is in the gastrointestinal tract and could relate to either carcinoma of the stomach or carcinoma of the colon.

Hypertension (problem 4) is noted by her history, blood pressure reading, and changes in the fundi. It needs treatment. Left ventricular hypertrophy (problem 5) is listed as a separate problem, although it is merely an extension of problem 4. It is evidenced by the enlargement of the heart, the strong apical impulse, and the fourth heart sound. The patient does not appear to be in left ventricular failure.

Her sixth problem, diabetes, seems to be under good control, as shown by the history, lack of symptoms, and test results that she obtains. However, further evaluation necessitates repeated blood glucose determinations.

The anxiety and depression (problem 7) exist for obvious reasons, and these must be dealt with at some future date.

Problem 8, a cervical lesion, is probably a serious one. Postmenopausal bleeding must always be considered with gravity. The lesion that was noted could be malignant, but at this point we can only call it a cervical lesion and may label it as carcinoma of the cervix only when and if a Pap smear or biopsy is conclusive.

Problem 9 is based on the history of joint stiffness plus the findings of swelling of the joints and Heberden's nodes.

STUDIES
- Urinalysis is normal except for 3+ albuminuria.
- Complete blood count shows 3 million red blood cells per mm^3, 6 g Hb/100 mL, white blood cells and platelet normal, and hypochromic microcytic red blood cells.
- Successive stools are +2, +3, negative, +3 for occult blood.
- Eighteen-test blood chemistry profile is normal, except for 136 mg of glucose/dL. The sodium, potassium, chloride, bicarbonate, urea nitrogen, protein, albumin, calcium, phosphorus, cholesterol, uric acid, creatinine, total bilirubin, alkaline phosphatase, creatine phosphokinase, lactate dehydrogenase, and glutamic-oxaloacetic transaminase are all normal.

- Chest radiograph is normal, except for mild-to-moderate left ventricular enlargement.
- Pap smear of cervical lesion shows clumps of *cancer cells* (grade 5).
- Electrocardiogram (ECG) shows mild left ventricular hypertrophy and strain.
- Proctosigmoidoscopy is normal.
- Barium enema reveals a *polypoid irregular lesion of the cecum.*
- Colonoscopic biopsy diagnoses adenocarcinoma.
- Upper gastrointestinal radiographic series is normal.

FINAL PROBLEM LIST Problems 1, 2, and 3 can now be combined into one problem—adenocarcinoma of the cecum. Problem 8 can be elevated to a diagnostic resolution—carcinoma of the cervix. A new problem has been detected, and it must be given a new number: 12. albuminuria. This may be a separate problem related to kidney disease of undisclosed origin, or it may result from diabetic nephropathy.

REASSESSMENT The ECG and chest radiograph confirm the previous impressions. It should be noted that Mrs. Smith's anemia is caused by the cecal carcinoma and not by cancer of the cervix.

The amount of blood loss from the cervical lesion would be minimal in this instance. However, large quantities of blood can be lost in the stool over a long period of time and not be apparent to the patient. Even though the patient has an enlarged heart, she does not have basal rales or any other evidence of heart failure.

Until recently such a patient would undergo immediate intestinal surgery, followed perhaps a bit later by treatment for the cervical cancer. But newer technology enables a search for metastases, which, if present, might preclude unnecessary and noncurative surgery. You might order computed tomographic scans of the lung and liver, and a radionuclide bone scan in order to rule out metastases before deciding on surgery. Others would not search so intensively.

EPILOGUE

The preceding sections of this chapter dealt with data acquisition, data synthesis, and data analysis. These are the processes a physician uses with each patient he or she sees. Fortunately, most cases are much simpler than Mrs. Smith's. But, in any event, these are some of the skills a student must acquire and master.

Problem Solving in Action

INTRODUCTION

This section consists of 86 carefully selected cases that exemplify the many common ways in which patients present to their physicians. The cases are solved by using various problem-solving techniques described in Section 1.

Individual cases are presented in a "think along with me" style whereby chunks of data and chunks of corresponding logic are alternately interspersed. This method was chosen because it simulates what goes on in the clinician's mind as he or she gathers each new bit of information, and, furthermore, because it is easier to understand serialized reasoning than to benefit from a lengthy discussion that follows a complete case presentation.

The reader can block out the intermittent logic and compare his or her own data interpretation with that of the author. And by the iterative process of following the data-logic sequence portrayed in each case, and then identifying the strategies used, you can begin to solve problems in much the same way.

The 86 cases are divided into 11 chapters, each chapter representing a module of disease such as hematology, endocrinology, cardiology, etc. Each module includes cases that represent the common ways in which patients within that subset present to the physician. For example, 90% of patients with heart disease complain of either chest pain, shortness of breath, syncope or palpitations; and they present to the physician in only seven or eight finite ways. In this regard, the primary care physician needs to know mainly about coronary disease, heart failure, hypertension, aortic and mitral valve disease, and a few common arrhythmias. The rest can be researched or referred for consultation. Other modules are similarly constituted.

It is not uncommon for a single mode of patient presentation to require a consideration of diseases in many modules for its resolution. For example, in the patient whose abdomen is swollen, the problem solver needs to know about heart, liver, kidney, and malignant diseases.

HOW MUCH TO LEARN

While a Renaissance man could know all of medicine, astronomy, and architecture, and a physician of 50 years ago could know all there was to know about medicine, these former feats are no longer possible. The memorization of a 2000-page textbook may well be an exercise in futility and the student of today should therefore learn about common presentations, common diseases, problem-solving techniques, and where to get more information. Since most problems are simply and easily solved, only a few need more detailed information, which can usually be gleaned on the job.

ORGANIZATION

Each chapter starts with an introduction that presents an overview of the problems and patient presentations within that module, and includes that system's symptoms and physical signs, new testing methods, and the problem-solving techniques that may be especially useful.

Virtually every case consists of a patient presentation, a detailed data-logic sequence, and a diagnosis, followed by questions and answers, the editor's comments, and suggested readings.

A question and answer section follows most of the logic sessions. This is designed not only to test comprehension of the concepts in the case discussions, but also to enlarge the information base and teach additional material. (Try to supply your own answers before reading those of the author.)

Most case discussions are followed by a "Comment" in which the particular problem-solving methods, decision points, and pathways of logic used in that case are noted. The reader may try his or her hand at identifying the techniques used in each case before reading the editor's commentary.

At the conclusion of the first case study in each chapter, there is a list of subjects that should be learned or reviewed in order to acquire the knowledge base sufficient for this case in all of its ramifications (problem-based learning). But for other cases, the reader should devise his or her own list of related materials to be reviewed in standard textbooks. If more information is needed for a case presentation on teaching rounds or for more detailed study, several recent review articles on the subject should be selected from your favorite information database.

In addition, a "Suggested Readings" list follows every logic session. Each list is designed to furnish references that elaborate on the didactic information discussed in the case study. Almost all recommended readings are from publications in the 1990s, many as recent as 1996. Textbook readings are intentionally not included because they are readily available and simply accessed.

ONE LAST WORD OF CAUTION!

The reader should not get the impression that all problems are solved as neatly and smoothly as those described here. Some sick hospitalized patients defy accurate diagnosis for long periods of time in spite of and even because of diagnostic measures. These patients are usually polypathic, replete with complications, and often made more undiagnosable by iatrogenic problems. The solution may come only with an autopsy—or perhaps not even then. *(P.C.)*

Hematologic Problems

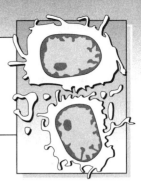

Although the examination of the stained blood smear is usually the keystone to problem solving in the patient who has a blood disease, the history, physical examination, and a profusion of other laboratory tests play an important role too. Many aspects of the patient profile and family history are especially significant, because the key clue may be found in the patient's occupation, race, habits, medications, nutrition, environment, or the presence of a similar illness in his/her family.

Exposure to bone marrow toxins in the environment or at work is probably more common than realized; this may include food additives, paint solvents, and insecticides. House painting used to carry the risk of lead poisoning, which is also seen in battery workers; and bone marrow depression caused by benzene-like solvents is well known. High blood lead levels and lead intoxication in ghetto children result at least in part from eating old varieties of lead-containing paint that peel from the walls. Cases of aplastic anemia for which a cause is never found may follow undetected exposures to as yet unrecognized bone marrow depressants.

As for race, Mediterranean anemia in persons from the Eastern basin, sickle cell anemia in blacks, and pernicious anemia (PA) in Scandinavians are well-recognized relationships. Family history may offer the key clue; hemoglobinopathies, congenital hemolytic jaundice, hereditary telangiectasia, and familial polyposis may each account for anemia as well as a host of other related clinical manifestations. The patient who tells you that his/her siblings or parents are also anemic may have one of these inherited diseases.

A careful history of drug ingestion is critical. The list of drugs that can cause depression of one or all three cellular components of the bone marrow could fill many pages. But the ones to be regarded with particular concern are the anticonvulsants, gold, sulfonamides, propylthiouracil,

phenothiazines, penicillins, and quinidine; they are all in common use. Peculiar eating habits should alert you to the possibility of iron deficiency anemia; the craving for large quantities of ice, clay, or starch (a condition referred to as pica), once thought to be the cause of this form of anemia, is now considered to be its result.

Last, diet may also play an important part in deciding on the cause of an anemia. Taking a nutritional history that seeks iron, vitamin B_{12}, or folic acid deficiency due to inadequate intake demands that the history taker know the foods wherein those elements are found. Iron is present in spinach, beef, eggs, chicken, and liver; vitamin B_{12} is found in glandular organs, muscle, eggs, cheese, and milk; folic acid is contained in green vegetables ("foliage") and organs like liver and kidney.

The presenting pictures of patients who have blood diseases are multiple, but only a handful are commonly seen. First, there is the patient who has no symptoms but is found to have anemia, polycythemia, or a white blood cell count abnormality during a routine examination or during the course of an unrelated illness. Next, perhaps the most common symptomatic presentation is that of anemia—weakness and easy fatigability—a picture that can be caused by many diseases and pathophysiologic mechanisms.

Acute and chronic anemias have different presentations, and it is important to realize that most anemias are apt to be manifestations of some underlying disease, such as carcinoma of the colon or duodenal ulcer. "Anemia" is a clinical finding, not a diagnosis, and is not commonly a disease in and of itself.

Then, there is the common complaint of "I bruise easily," which needs careful evaluation. A sizable percentage of women have this symptom; it usually turns out to be of no consequence. But spontaneous bruising, with a history of prolonged or late bleeding after tooth extractions or after minor injuries, may indicate a significant coagulopathy. In this instance, a good history is usually more reliable than many laboratory tests.

Other less common presentations must be mentioned. The patient notes enlarged lymph nodes or a left upper quadrant mass that may be an enlarged spleen. Bone pain from myeloma, leukemia, or lymphoma may bring other patients to your office. In some instances, chronic leg ulcers, postural syncope, a sore tongue, neurologic symptoms, dark urine, persistent cough, or dysphagia may each be the initial complaint.

But be especially careful of the patient who has latent coronary disease, mild peripheral vascular disease, nascent chronic obstructive pulmonary disease, subclinical cerebral ischemia, or incipient heart failure, whose symptoms of angina, claudication, dyspnea, or lightheadedness may surface because of a gradually developing anemia. His or her complaint may be referable to the underlying chronic disease, not to the anemia or to the disease causing the anemia.

The subset of the physical examination concerned with blood diseases includes evidence of pallor; jaundice; smooth and/or red tongue; large lymph nodes; splenomegaly; hemorrhages or vascular abnormalities in the fundi, skin, and mucous membranes; tender bones; manifestations of high cardiac output; and neurologic evidence of posterior and lateral column disease.

The following are some common clusters and their usual causes. Anemia, bone pains, and uremia often signify multiple myeloma; anemia and jaundice suggest hemolytic anemia or metastatic cancer; anemia and weight loss often result from malignancy; anemia and bruises suggest myelodysplasia or leukemia, lymphoma, hemolytic anemia with thrombocytopenia, or aplastic anemia; anemia plus gallstones hints at a chronic hemolytic anemia; and anemia, jaundice, and severe abdominal pain suggest a hemolytic crisis.

New technology has made it possible to determine the size and nature of histopathologic abnormalities that may exist in the liver and spleen. This can be helpful in hematologic diagnosis.

Controversy persists concerning the staging of lymphomas. Some experts still resort to exploratory laparotomy, although most are now content with scanning techniques and lymphangiography. With the better understanding of lymphocyte populations, the nosology of lymphomas is undergoing repeated revision.

Classic blood studies have not changed appreciably in the past decade. Exceptions are the *serum ferritin concentration* that is used to reflect total body iron stores accurately, and the *mean corpuscular volume* (MCV) that is now thought to be the most significant index for classifying anemias. The red blood cell (RBC) distribution width (RDW) is very helpful in evaluating microcytic anemias. The MCV, the RDW, and the *reticulocyte index* (or even better, the absolute reticulocyte count by flow cytometry) are the three important determinants in the algorithmic pursuit of an anemia's cause.

Anemias that have been caused by new technology and new fads must be mentioned. The mechanical damage of red blood cells by aortic and mitral prosthetic heart valves can result in hemolytic anemia. Some joggers and marathon runners have also been found to develop a mechanical hemolytic state. And hosts of new anticancer, anti-psychotic, and anti-thrombotic drugs have caused a profusion of blood diseases. These diseases include those resulting from depression of one or more bone marrow elements and also some that result from the induction of autoimmune disorders.

It is particularly noteworthy that, during the past decade, there has come about a better understanding of the impact of molecular biology on the diagnosis and treatment of hematologic disorders. This revolves in great measure around the use of recombinant DNA technology and the ability to identify DNA sequences and specific genetic defects in various disorders such as sickle cell anemia, β-thalassemia, and others. *(PC, RML)*

WEAKNESS AND JOINT PAINS

David A. Sears

Data A 46-year-old woman comes to your office complaining of increasing fatigability and a "tired and weak" feeling for the past 3 or 4 months. She has had rheumatoid arthritis (RA) for 8 years, and her joint symptoms have been controlled by regular use of aspirin and non-steroidal anti-inflammatory drugs (NSAIDs).

Logic Symptoms of weakness and fatigue are so common and nonspecific that, taken alone, they provide little guidance. More details are needed. Is the patient tired immediately on arising in the morning, or does fatigue increase throughout the day? Fatigue on arising is often psychoneurotic in origin, whereas fatigue coming on after some work or activity tends to be organic. Have her activities actually changed as a result of the symptoms? For example, does she still clean house, work at her job, and pursue her hobbies? One must ask questions to distinguish between weakness, shortness of breath, and fatigue, which are different symptoms with different implications, but which may be used interchangeably by patients describing how they feel. In the present patient, with a known chronic disease of fluctuating severity, you need information about the activity of her RA.

Data The patient says that she has had no severe pain, tenderness, redness, swelling, or heat in her joints for 2 years while taking regular doses of anti-inflammatory drugs. She has some mild morning stiffness in her metacarpophalangeal and proximal interphalangeal joints as well as occasional soreness in the wrists, elbows, and knees. In answer to your step-by-step questions about her level of daily function, she indicates that she has continued to carry on most of her activities as a housewife and mother but with less energy than in the past. She finds that she must stop and rest during her household chores, and by the end of the day she is exhausted. What limits her is more fatigue than true weakness or shortness of breath.

You are unable to detect any significant changes in her environmental or living situation. Her husband and two children, ages 17 and 13, are in good health, and she describes no tension in her relationships with them or others. She denies crying spells or feeling "blue" and has had no anorexia, weight loss, or insomnia.

Logic At this point, you have no positive indications of emotional causes for her symptoms and no evidence of increased activity of her arthritis, although these cannot yet be ruled out as causes of her symptoms. You simply need more information and proceed to complete your data base.

Data History reveals no additional pertinent information. Results of systems review are negative, except for the following. For several years she has noted some mild postprandial nausea and eructations after eating fried or greasy foods, and therefore avoids them. Six months ago, she had a 1-hour episode of dull right upper quadrant pain. In addition, she sometimes experiences mid-epigastric and substernal burning pain that is

relieved by an antacid. She denies other abdominal pain, vomiting, jaundice, and black or tarry stools. There has been occasional urinary frequency and nocturia once or twice a night. For the past year, her menstrual periods have been irregular. They have occurred at shorter or longer intervals than previously, and many have been prolonged, with heavier than normal flow. She has had occasional hot flushes and assumed that she might be entering the menopause. Family history reveals that she is of Italian extraction and that one sister was mildly anemic and was told she had Mediterranean anemia.

On physical examination, the patient is a slightly obese white woman whose vital signs are: pulse, 76, regular; blood pressure (BP), 115/70; respirations, 14/min; temperature, 37°C. Slight pallor of the skin, tongue, and palms is noted. Results of examination of other skin areas, head and neck, heart and lungs, and pelvis and rectum are normal. There is no stool in the rectum for guaiac testing. No lymph nodes are palpable. The abdomen is mildly obese, but there is no tenderness, palpable mass, or organomegaly. Slight swelling of the proximal interphalangeal joints gives her fingers a fusiform appearance, and there is some thenar and hypothenar atrophy, but not ulnar deviation or subluxation. The wrists and knees too are slightly swollen, but there is no restriction of joint motion. Neurologic examination is normal, peripheral pulses are normal and equal, and there is no ankle edema.

Logic You decide to obtain routine laboratory studies to complete your data base: blood count, urinalysis, chest radiograph, and also an erythrocyte sedimentation (ESR) rate as a nonspecific test of activity for rheumatoid disease. You also schedule an ultrasonographic examination of the abdomen because of fatty food intolerance, the episode of abdominal pain, and your suspicion of gallbladder disease. The cause of her presenting symptoms is not at all apparent thus far, although the information available is leading you toward an organic cause.

Data Laboratory results are: hematocrit, 28%; hemoglobin (Hgb), 8.4 g/dL; MCV, 70 fL; white blood cell (WBC) count, 11,200/mm^3 with 2% bands, 76% segmented neutrophils, 18% lymphocytes, and 4% monocytes; and platelet count, 420,000/mm^3. The urinalysis shows specific gravity 1.016, pH 5, glucose and protein negative; microscopic examination of the spun sediment reveals 6 to 8 WBCs per high-powered field (HPF), and no RBCs or casts. The ESR (Westergren method) is 62 mm/h.

The chest radiographic finding is normal. The abdominal sonogram shows that the gallbladder has a thickened wall and contains two stones. When the anemia is recognized, you examine the blood smear and order a reticulocyte count. The blood smear is shown in Figure 12.1. The reticulocyte count is 2.2%.

Logic Your suspicion of gallbladder disease is confirmed, and this may explain at least some of the gastrointestinal (GI) symptoms. The ESR is moderately elevated, but you are unsure if this is due to her RA, which by history and physical examination seems inactive. The urinary symptoms, low-grade pyuria, and slight blood leukocytosis warrant a search for urinary tract infection, and you order a urine culture.

The anemia is one of underproduction of red blood cells, as indicated by the calculated reticulocyte index of less than 1 ($2.2 \times 28/45 \times 1/1.85$). The 28/45 fraction corrects for the degree of anemia and the fact that the reticulocyte count is expressed as a percentage. The 1.85

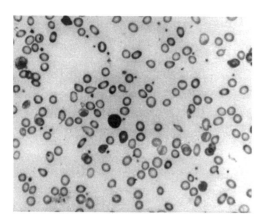

▶ **Figure 12.1.** Blood smear. A normal small lymphocyte is shown in the photomicrograph. Normal-sized red blood cells have a diameter close to that of a small lymphocyte. Note that most red blood cells here are significantly smaller. Also, the area of central pallor in the red blood cells is larger than normal. (As a rule of thumb, the central pallor occupies approximately one third of the diameter of the cell.) Thus, this blood smear shows microcytic, hypochromic red blood cells. There are mild abnormalities of red blood cell shape as well, with some thin ("pencil") cells and teardrop cells.

value represents the number of days needed for a circulating reticulocyte to mature into an RBC because of early release of reticulocytes from the bone marrow in the anemic patient. These adjustments to the reticulocyte count result in a reticulocyte index that measures bone marrow production of red blood cells.

When this index is regarded along with the RBC morphology determined from red blood cell indices and your personal examination of the blood smear, the anemia can be classified as that of abnormal cytoplasmic maturation (defective hemoglobinization). This immediately suggests a problem in iron metabolism, and your differential diagnosis would include true iron deficiency, the anemia of chronic disease, sideroblastic anemia, thalassemia minor, and lead poisoning. Let us consider each of these.

Iron Deficiency Anemia. With rare exceptions, this condition is due to blood loss. Menstruating women are often in a precarious state of iron balance, and this patient has a history of heavy menses. The GI tract is the other common site of blood loss and must be considered even when another etiology may be present, as occurs in this patient. In addition, this woman takes aspirin and other NSAIDs and could very well have hemorrhagic gastritis as a result. Examination of stools for occult blood and measurement of the serum iron, total iron-binding capacity, and ferritin are in order. The association of unusual appetites (pica) with iron deficiency is sufficiently common to warrant some additional specific questions.

Anemia of Chronic Disease. This is very common, perhaps the most frequent cause of anemia in hospitalized patients. The patient has a disease (RA) that is often associated with this type of anemia.

Sideroblastic Anemia. This disorder may occur as a hereditary or idiopathic acquired disorder or secondary to other diseases (such as RA). Because sideroblastic anemia is a disease of excessive iron loading, the serum iron will distinguish it from the previously mentioned disorders.

Thalassemia Minor. Although worldwide in distribution, this disorder is particularly common in individuals of Mediterranean ancestry. Your patient is of Italian extraction, and there is a history of the disorder in the family. The blood smear does not show target cells or basophilic stippling to suggest thalassemia minor, but with this history, hemoglobin electrophoresis for the determination of hemoglobins A$_2$ and F is warranted.

Lead Poisoning. The patient has no history of exposure. The blood smear shows no basophilic stippling. This diagnosis seems unlikely and need not be pursued further.

The combination of gallstones and anemia makes you briefly consider a hemolytic type of anemia. But this becomes most unlikely when you consider the facts that the reticulocyte index is less than 1 and the anemia has many features suggesting iron deficiency.

Data Additional history indicates that the patient does not eat clay or starch, but she likes to chew on ice cubes; for the past 5 to 6 months she has consumed the contents of one or two refrigerator trays of ice daily. Further laboratory data are as follows: urine culture results negative; serum iron, 29 μg/dL; hemoglobin F, 1.5% (normal <2%); and hemoglobin A$_2$ 3.0% (normal <4.0%). The patient fails to bring in stool specimens as requested. The serum ferritin value is not yet reported.

Logic Sideroblastic anemia is excluded by the low serum iron level, and β-thalassemia minor is excluded by the normal levels of A$_2$ and F hemoglobin; α-thalassemia minor is not ruled out but would not explain the low serum iron level. True iron deficiency is strongly suspected on the basis of the low serum iron level and normal binding capacity, which combine to give an abnormally low calculated saturation of 10%. The history of pagophagia (ice pica) is also suggestive of iron deficiency. However, the patient has a chronic inflammatory disease (RA) often associated with anemia of chronic disease, and that form of anemia cannot be absolutely differentiated from iron deficiency by the data thus far available. Determination of tissue iron stores will distinguish iron deficiency from the anemia of chronic disease, because storage iron is absent in the former and present in the latter. Iron stores may be assessed directly by an iron stain of aspirated bone marrow. Iron stores may be assessed indirectly by measurement of the serum ferritin level. They are usually normal or elevated in the anemia of chronic disease and low in true iron deficiency.

Data The serum ferritin level is 6 ng/mL. See Table 12.1 for interpretation of serum ferritin levels.

Logic The diagnosis of iron deficiency is established, and therapy with oral ferrous sulfate can

TABLE 12.1. Serum Ferritin Level Interpretation^a

SERUM FERRITIN (NG/ML)	PROBABLE DIAGNOSIS
< 20	Iron deficiency
20–50	Iron deficiency + anemia of chronic disease
> 50	Anemia of chronic disease

^{a}This table provides approximate guidelines for the interpretation of the serum ferritin level in the patient with a subnormal serum iron value. It indicates that the serum ferritin value may be in the normal range in iron deficiency if the anemia of chronic disease coexists with the iron deficiency. However, iron deficiency is very rare if the serum ferritin level exceeds 50 ng/mL.

begin. However, occult GI bleeding has not been excluded. It must be sought even though there are other explanations for the patient's iron deficiency (menorrhagia and possible gastritis due to NSAID use).

Data The patient brings in samples from three stools, and two are found to test positive for occult blood. Results of sigmoidoscopy and an upper GI radiograph series are negative, but the barium enema shows a definite filling defect in the cecum. The patient is taken to surgery, and a carcinoma of the cecum is resected (Fig. 12.2).

Logic Statistical probability would suggest that this patient's iron deficiency was due to her menorrhagia or to drug-induced gastritis, and the cecal carcinoma was an unexpected finding.

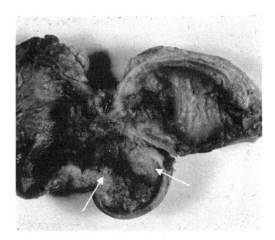

▶ **Figure 12.2.** Resected carcinoma of cecum. The lesion is polypoid and ulcerative, causes chronic blood loss, but does not obstruct unless it is strategically positioned at the ileocecal valve.

However, this patient illustrates the importance of ruling out the serious diagnosis of GI malignancy in a patient with iron deficiency. The elevated ESR and mild leukocytosis were probably due to the tumor.

Carcinoma of the cecum has a notoriously silent onset, often with only intermittent bleeding and iron deficiency anemia, as in this patient. It causes obstruction less commonly than do tumors of the descending or sigmoid colon. It is uncertain whether her presenting complaint of easy fatigue can be attributed directly to her moderate degree of anemia, because many persons tolerate this degree of anemia with no symptoms. Her future course will settle the issue.

Several loose ends remain to be tied up. You might question why the surgeon did not remove the diseased gallbladder at the same time. His judgment was against doing two major procedures, although many might disagree. This matter may need management in the future. Results of the urine culture were negative, but in view of her previous history of frequency, this test should be repeated if symptoms recur.

Because several possible causes for iron deficiency anemia were not ruled out in this patient, we have only assumed that carcinoma of the colon was the cause. It may not be so. Should the anemia recur, endoscopy for gastritis may have to be done. Furthermore, the alleged early menopause with increased menstrual blood loss is worrisome. Usually, menses are diminished. This, too, could be a source of continuing blood loss, and needs observation and possible endometrial biopsy to make sure that an endometrial carcinoma is not present.

Questions

1. If the evaluation of this patient had led to a diagnosis of anemia of chronic disease due to active RA rather than iron deficiency, the correct therapy would have been:
   (a) parenteral rather than oral iron.
   (b) transfusion.
   (c) more vigorous treatment of the arthritis.
   (d) a multivitamin preparation containing iron, pyridoxine, and folic acid.
2. Aspirin may predispose to GI blood loss for each of the following reasons except:
   (a) a direct effect on gastric mucosa.
   (b) inhibition of prostaglandin synthesis.
   (c) interference with platelet function.
   (d) production of thrombocytopenia.
3. Assume your patient's barium enema had not disclosed a carcinoma of the cecum. Your next step would have been to:
   (a) treat with oral iron and observe.
   (b) do fiberoptic gastroscopy.
   (c) start steroid therapy for arthritis.
   (d) do an endometrial biopsy.
4. Who of the following is/are particularly prone to have iron deficiency?
   (a) A 9-month-old baby girl fed only cow's milk
   (b) An adolescent female
   (c) A man with a prosthetic aortic valve that has become partially loosened, leading to hemodynamic abnormalities and traumatic hemolysis of red blood cells
   (d) A man with multiple telangiectases on his face, lips, oral mucosa, and hands

Answers

1. **(c) is correct.** With control of the underlying disease (RA), the anemia will correct itself. A major mechanism responsible for the anemia of chronic disease is inability to mobilize reticuloendothelial iron for red blood cell production. Thus, iron therapy, either by mouth or by injection, is not effective. Transfusion would not be warranted for this patient and would be of transient, if any, benefit for her symptoms. Use of "shotgun" hematinics is never appropriate. Specific diagnosis is the key to therapy for anemia.
2. **(d) is correct.** Aspirin does not produce thrombocytopenia. It does cause gastritis by direct mucosal injury and perhaps by decreasing the mucosa-protecting effect of prostaglandins. Even small doses inhibit the platelet release reaction and, therefore, platelet aggregation and primary hemostasis.
3. **(b) is correct.** In the presence of iron deficiency anemia and occult blood in the stool, your next step would be to consider and rule out hemorrhagic aspirin gastritis, or some other bleeding lesion in the stomach or duodenum. Its finding would necessitate a change in therapy. **(d)** might be a reasonable answer at this stage, but blood in the stool makes **(b)** more appropriate. Treatment with iron may be in order, but a cause of the GI bleeding must be discovered, if possible. The arthritis seems quiescent and well controlled,

so steroids would be a poor choice, especially if there is already demonstrated GI bleeding from an unknown source.

4. **All are correct.** Unsupplemented cow's milk is a poor source of iron, and rapidly growing infants have a large requirement. The adolescent female has the combined increased iron requirements imposed by rapid growth and menstruation (and may have a deficient diet as well). Chronic intravascular hemolysis may lead to iron deficiency due to loss of iron as hemosiderin and ferritin in the urine. In hereditary hemorrhagic telangiectasia (Osler-Rendu-Weber disease), the telangiectases are often in the GI tract, too, and may bleed recurrently.

COMMENT This case study emphasizes the importance of finding the precise cause of anemia before beginning treatment. Furthermore, the study is notable for the number of problem-solving techniques used by the author.

First, he found a key clue—anemia; the other clues, fatigue and weakness, were too nonspecific to use as a departure point. This was a difficult problem because there were many distracting possibilities, each of which could have caused the anemia, but did not. These included RA, aspirin ingestion, indigestion and abdominal pain from a possibly bleeding upper GI lesion, irregular menses, and Mediterranean anemia. Instead, because of unexplained occult blood in the stools and the high incidence of cancer in this age group, the author pressed on to find carcinoma of the colon. This was the probable cause of the anemia, but we are left with another possibility yet to be reckoned with—abnormal vaginal bleeding.

Although cholelithiasis is present and is already causing symptoms, it has nothing to do with iron-deficiency anemia. This condition will have to be addressed shortly.

Having established the presence of a problem in iron metabolism, a list of possibilities was constructed, several likely hypotheses were chosen, all but one were excluded, and that one was eventually proved. (*P.C.*)

PROBLEM-BASED LEARNING To get the most out of this seemingly complicated presentation, much reading must be done. There are many facets to this patient's illness about which the reader may need to be reinformed. A thorough study of this case should cover:

- Classification of all anemias by both the RBC indices and the reticulocyte index
- Ability to calculate reticulocyte indices and RBC indices given the necessary data
- Symptoms and signs of various common anemias
- Understanding of the relationship between RA and anemia, and how to determine the activity of arthritis
- Relationship between aspirin ingestion and anemia
- Comprehension of the clinical picture of gallbladder disease
- Knowledge of the clinical features of thalassemia, anemia of chronic disorders, and sideroblastic anemia
- Kinetics of iron deficiency anemia and its relationship to chronic blood loss
- Detection of and work-up for chronic GI blood loss
- Clinical features of carcinoma of the colon
- Familiarity with the laboratory aspects of an anemia study, with special attention to occult blood in the stool, reticulocyte index, RBC indices, and the serum iron, total iron-binding capacity, and ferritin

It should be clear that a complete study and comprehension of just this one case entails the mastery of a large body of information that goes beyond hematology into the GI tract, the genitourinary tract, and the diseases of joints. Ten or 20 cases like this and you know a lot of medicine.

Suggested Readings

Massey AC. Microcytic anemia: Differential diagnosis and management of iron deficiency anemia Med Clin North Am 1992;76:549–566.

Moore DF Jr, Sears DA. Pica, iron deficiency, and the medical history. Am J Med 1994;97:390–393.

Rockey DC, Cello JP. Evaluation of the gastrointestinal tract in patients with iron-deficiency anemia. New Engl J Med 1993;329:1691–1695.

Sears DA. Anemia of chronic disease. Med Clin North Am 1992;76:567–579.

CASE **2**

MILD ASYMPTOMATIC ANEMIA

Allan J. Erslev

Data   A 45-year-old engineer working for a New Jersey computer company was expecting a second child and wanted to increase his life insurance. He was told to get health clearance and was seen by his family physician. He felt well, had no complaints, and his physical examination was entirely normal. However, routine blood counts revealed a mild-to-moderate anemia with a hemoglobin concentration of 9.6 g/dL. Red blood cell indices were within normal limits, as were the white blood cell count, differential count, and platelet count.

Logic   When the laboratory results were received, the physician immediately recognized that he had a difficult diagnostic problem to solve. If the patient had been a 45-year-old woman, the anemia would probably have been an iron deficiency anemia due to menstrual blood loss. The normal daily intake of iron is approximately 15 mg, of which 1 to 2 mg are absorbed. The daily loss is approximately the same, but menstruation adds approximately 30 mg of iron lost every month, making the balance between intake and loss of iron in a young woman somewhat precarious. Actually it makes a mild anemia the most common affliction of mankind—or rather, of womankind.

However, the patient was a middle-aged man with no history of chronic blood loss, such as black or bloody stools, bloody urine, or frequent nosebleeds. For a brief moment, the physician wished for a microscope to look at the blood smear, but then realized that the anemia was quite mild and the red blood cell indices were normal, indicating that the examination of a blood smear would not have been very rewarding.

On the other hand, severe iron deficiency anemias that result from chronic blood loss are manifested by lower than normal RBC indices and blood smears that show decreased size and color of RBCs. In severe anemias caused by folic acid or vitamin B_{12} deficiency, the RBC indices are higher than normal, and the blood smear shows increased size and color of the RBCs (Fig. 12.3).

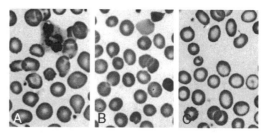

▶ **Figure 12.3.** Note preponderance of large, well-stained RBCs and a multilobed polymorphonuclear leukocyte in **A.** The cells in **B** are normal in size and stain, whereas the cells in **C** are small and have large areas of central pallor. **A.** Macrocytic, normochromic red blood cells, as seen in vitamin B_{12} or folic acid deficiency. **B.** Normal. **C.** Hypochromic, microcytic red blood cells, as seen in iron deficiency anemias.

Although the physician had done a rectal examination and examined and tested a stool specimen for blood, more than one specimen needed to be examined. The physician also needed a much more thorough history and physical examination than the one carried out during the first routine visit.

The patient was not black or Asian, which ruled out sickle cell trait or hemoglobin E disease, both conditions associated with mild asymptomatic anemia. However, the physician had not inquired as to the parents' European origin, and if the parents had emigrated from the Eastern Mediterranean basin, thalassemia trait was a definite possibility. The patient obviously needed to come back for a more thorough history as to past chronic illnesses, especially autoimmune diseases, and as to hospitalizations and old blood counts. It was also important to know if he had been exposed to potential bone marrow toxins in his work as an engineer or during private hobbies. Had he taken any over-the-counter medications, especially aspirin? It would also be of interest to find out if he had been drafted in the Vietnam war and if not, why not.

Data   At his repeat visit, the physician found the man to be in excellent health, never hospitalized, and with no recollection of having had his blood examined before. His high draft number had exempted him from serving in Vietnam. He had had no exposure to potential bone marrow toxins such as paint solvents, insecticides, antimetabolites, and some antibiotics, and had no significant exposure to aspirin, NSAIDs, or other medications that might cause gastric bleeding or depress erythropoiesis. His family origin was English and German, and there was no family history of blood diseases. Both parents were alive and well, as were two siblings. Except for slight pallor, the physical examination was again completely normal. A number of blood tests were drawn, and the patient was sent home with five Hemoccult tests to be used for examinations of successive stools for blood.

Logic The blood tests obtained were designed to discover if the anemia was due to increased destruction of red blood cells or decreased production. The most important and most easily obtained test was the reticulocyte count. Although this count usually is expressed in percent, it should be expressed in total number of reticulocytes per mm^3. Transforming it into a reticulocyte count may no longer be appropriate, because the printout from the electronic counters always gives the total red blood cell count, making it easy to calculate total reticulocyte numbers. In patients with increased red blood cell destruction, the reticulocyte count is usually increased, showing a compensatory response, although it is decreased in anemia due to decreased red blood cell production.

Unfortunately, a mild anemia is not apt to change the reticulocyte count significantly, a feature that is shared with almost all of the blood tests used to diagnose an anemia. It is actually much easier to diagnose a severe anemia than a mild one.

Among the other tests obtained, the results of the Coombs' test, bilirubin, lactate dehydrogenase, and haptoglobin would tend to be abnormal if the rate of red blood cell destruction were increased. Tests likely to show a decreased rate of red blood cell production are vitamin B_{12} and folic acid levels and iron, iron binding capacity, and ferritin. The likelihood that the patient had a mild megaloblastic anemia due to folic acid deficiency was very low because of his lack of history of alcoholism. However, megaloblastic anemia may occur in patients who have gastric atrophy and malabsorption of vitamin B_{12}; because this disorder can be easily cured, it should always be included in the differential diagnosis of anemia.

A hemoglobin analysis was also requested to rule out the unlikely possibility of β-thalassemia or an abnormal hemoglobin. The physician planned to await the results of all these tests before he asked for a bone marrow aspiration and biopsy. Such an examination, when combined with iron stains and chromosomal analysis, could rule out other possibilities, such as refractory anemias, preleukemias, bone marrow replacement, or bone marrow hypoplasia.

Data With the exception of the iron studies, all blood count and blood test results were within normal limits. The urine examination was also normal. All stool samples were negative for occult blood. However, the serum iron was 20 μg/dL; iron binding capacity, 400 μg/dL; and ferritin, 20 ng/mL.

Logic The course of action was now clear and the physician felt that a bone marrow analysis was not necessary, at least not right away. The patient had a mild iron deficiency anemia; the high iron binding capacity and low ferritin level ruled out the anemia of chronic disease, which is also associated with a low serum iron level. Because iron deficiency always or almost always indicates blood loss, a search for the site of the blood loss had to be initiated.

The possibilities that the iron loss was caused by poor iron intake or inadequate iron absorption were too remote to be considered. Iron is present in most foods, especially in meat, spinach, eggs, chicken, and liver, and unless the patient has serious malabsorption due to destruction or removal of the gastric, duodenal, or ileal mucosa, iron absorption is normal.

Iron deficiency in a man is primarily due to gastrointestinal blood loss, and in rare cases due to urinary blood loss. The latter takes place in patients with chronic hemolytic anemia, especially paroxysmal nocturnal hemoglobinuria, in which there is depletion of haptoglobin, a compound that usually prevents hemoglobin from being filtered through the kidney. Consequently, one would expect to find urinary losses of hemoglobin only in severe hemolytic anemia, a condition that had already been ruled out. Bleeding from urinary stones or bladder lesions could be quite asymptomatic; however, the normal urine examination pretty well ruled out this possibility. That left gastrointestinal bleeding either from a colonic tumor or polyp, a duodenal ulcer, or a small varix. The bleeding obviously would have had to be sporadic because five consecutive stool specimens were all negative for occult blood.

Data The patient was referred to a gastroenterologist who performed a thorough colonoscopy followed by endoscopy of the esophagus, stomach, and duodenum. No lesions were found anywhere.

Logic Although the results of all studies were negative, the physician did not give iron as a diagnostic trial because it was fairly certain that the patient would respond to the iron, that the hemoglobin would return to normal, and that a potential future problem would be temporarily concealed. Therefore, the physician referred him to a hematologist for bone marrow examination and a second opinion.

Data The hematologist was also certain that the patient had experienced blood loss, and asked if the patient ever had donated blood at the Red Cross. The patient proudly informed him that he was a two-gallon blood donor and regularly gave blood four times a year.

Logic Blood contains approximately 1 mg of iron in 1 mL of packed red blood cells and each donation of 450 mL of blood, with a hematocrit of approximately 44%, represents a loss of 200 mL of packed red blood cells, or 200 mg of iron. If he had given blood every 3 months, this represented a loss of approximately 2 mg a day, far in excess of the normal daily intake. Consequently, he had slowly depleted his tissue iron stores that normally consist of 2 to 5 g of iron. Because the bone marrow is a preferred organ for iron utilization, red blood cell production and hemoglobin synthesis as measured before each blood donation had been normal until now. Now there was only a limited amount of tissue iron available as shown by the low ferritin level, and consequently the red blood cell production had decreased.

Data Based on this logic, the patient was started on ferrous sulfate tablets 300 mg three times a day, and when seen a month later, his hemoglobin level had returned to normal. He was urged to continue his most admirable hobby as a blood donor, but to take regularly one ferrous sulfate tablet a day.

Logic Such a tablet contains 67 mg of metallic on, and because 5 to 10% is absorbed, it should him a safe reserve and, in addition, over the n rebuild his iron stores to normal.

Questions

1. In which of the following clinical situations are you apt to find an iron-deficiency type of anemia demonstrating hypochromia and microcytosis?
   (a) Glossitis, dysphagia, spoon-shaped nails in a 65-year-old woman
   (b) Chronic indigestion and stools 2+ for occult blood in a 48-year-old executive
   (c) Easy fatigability in a 38-year-old multigravida patient with irregular vaginal bleeding
   (d) Difficulty with balance and walking in a pale 70-year-old woman
   (e) Right upper quadrant pains, anemia, and jaundice in a 20-year-old black man

2. A hemoglobin concentration of 10 g/dL may be normal in which one of the following subsets?
   (a) Teenagers
   (b) Pregnant women
   (c) Persons older than 85 years
   (d) Newborn babies

3. Your 65-year-old male patient is weak and pale. The rest of the history is non-contributory, and the physical examination is otherwise normal. Laboratory test results show 7g/dL Hgb, 4 million RBC/mm^3, and hematocrit 30%. Which of the following tests should be done, and in what order?
   (a) Folic acid and vitamin B$_{12}$ blood levels
   (b) Upper gastrointestinal series
   (c) Sternal bone marrow aspiration
   (d) Stool examination for occult blood
   (e) Serum iron, iron binding capacity
   (f) Colonoscopy
   (g) CT of abdomen
   (h) Reticulocyte count

Answers

1. **(a), (b), and (c) are all correct.** They might represent the Plummer-Vinson syndrome, duodenal ulcer or gastric cancer, and menometrorrhagia. (d) points to the macrocytic anemia of pernicious anemia, and (e) suggests the normochromic normocytic anemia of hemolysis, possibly due to sickle cell anemia with associated gallstones.

2. **(b) is correct.** Pregnancy is associated with increased plasma volume that causes a dilution of a normal red blood cell mass. Consequently, a mild dilutional anemia is common and physiologic in the second and third trimester. In all other age groups, a hemoglobin concentration of 10 g/dL warrants further investigation.

> 3. This is a severe iron-deficiency anemia. The calculated MCH is 20, and the MCV is 70—hypochromia and microcytosis. Tests (d), (e), (f), and (b) may be done, and in that order. (c) offers nothing additional. (a) helps in macrocytic anemias. (h) is helpful in normocytic and hemolytic anemias. CT offers limited information and is costly, but may be used to search and scan if all other test results are negative.

COMMENT As the author states, mild anemias are more difficult to diagnose than severe ones. In the former circumstance, the blood smear, red blood cell indices, and reticulocyte count are not very helpful. But in the case of severe anemia, they help direct further inquiry into one or another subset of hematologic disorders.

First, it was determined that iron deficiency existed. Because chronic blood loss in the male most often results from gastrointestinal bleeding, the GI tract was thoroughly studied—nothing found.

This case study presents a perfect example of the value of a good and thorough history. One appropriate question during the first interview would have solved the problem. There would have been no need for detailed hematologic and radiographic studies. *(P.C.)*

Suggested Readings

Finch C. Regulation of iron balance in humans. Blood 1994;84:1697.

Massey A. Microcytic anemia: differential diagnosis and management of iron-deficiency anemia. Med Clin North Am 1992;76:549.

Rockey DC, Cello JP. Evaluation of the gastrointestinal tract in patients with iron-deficiency anemia. N Engl J Med 1993;329:169.

BLEEDING GUMS AND BRUISING

Shirley P. Levine

Data A 23-year-old woman comes to the emergency department complaining of bruises over her body and bleeding gums for the preceding 36 hours.

Logic The combination of bruising and oral mucosal bleeding suggests a widespread coagulopathy rather than a local process such as trauma or gingival disease.

Data The patient has never had easy bruisability, epistaxis, gum bleeding, or bleeding into the joints. Menarche was at age 13, and menses have been normal. The last menstrual period was 16 days before admission and was normal in amount and duration. The patient had several dental extractions at age 17 and oozed slightly for 6 to 12 hours thereafter. There has not been excessive bleeding with minor trauma. She has not had surgery or pregnancies. Family history indicates no bleeding disorders.

Logic These negative clues strongly suggest an acquired bleeding abnormality. It is important to establish any prior bleeding history and to evaluate carefully the hemostatic response to previous trauma or surgical procedures. You may be worried about her bleeding following dental extraction, but this was only slightly prolonged. Oozing lasting longer than 24 hours, or fresh bleeding occurring after a few days would definitely arouse suspicion of abnormal hemostasis. Therefore the recent onset of bruising and mucosal bleeding, the absence of post-extraction bleeding, and the negative family history exclude hereditary disorders such as hemophilia A, hemophilia B (Christmas disease), and von Willebrand's disease (vWD).

Acquired coagulation defects can result from disease processes affecting any one or several of the major divisions of the coagulation system: (1) vascular endothelium, (2) platelets, and (3) plasma clotting factors. Now, you seek to determine which basic defect or combination of defects is operative in this case.

1. Abnormalities of blood vessels, capillaries, and their endothelium are seen in allergic vasculitis, thrombotic thrombocytopenic purpura (TTP), scurvy, long-term steroid use, and meningococcemia.
2. Platelet abnormalities consist of insufficient numbers (thrombocytopenia—less than 20,000/mm^3) or deficient function (thrombocytopathy). Low platelet counts can result from insufficient production, excessive destruction, or splenic pooling. Platelet malfunction, if acquired, can result from use of drugs such as aspirin, nonsteroidal anti-inflammatory drugs, and some antibiotics, as well as from uremia.
3. Abnormalities of plasma clotting factors can

result from vitamin K deficiency (malnutrition or malabsorption), liver disease, warfarin sodium overdosage, and inhibition of activity or decreased quantity of any of the Roman-numeraled plasma factors.

Data On physical examination the patient is a well-developed young woman without pallor or jaundice. Vital signs are normal. Ophthalmoscopic examination is unremarkable. There is oozing of the gingivae, with several small hemorrhagic bullae on the buccal mucosa. There is an ecchymosis and oozing in the right antecubital area secondary to a venipuncture, and there are several ecchymoses and multiple petechiae on both lower extremities. There is no palpable adenopathy or splenomegaly. The results of the remainder of the physical examination are normal. **Logic** Purpuric bleeding (ecchymoses and petechiae) is characteristic of abnormalities of the platelets or blood vessels. Ecchymoses can occur in apparently healthy individuals, often without trauma, and account for a lifelong history of "easy bruisability." They are especially common as isolated small ecchymoses on the hips and thighs of some women ("devil's pinches"). Ecchymoses and petechiae on the extremities can also be seen with the previously-named vascular abnormalities.

Acquired defects of platelet function rarely cause a profound coagulopathy, and in such cases the visible manifestations are of insidious onset and are associated with other symptoms and manifestations of the underlying disease processes, such as dysproteinemia and uremia. Hemorrhagic bullae are nearly specific for thrombocytopenic bleeding.

The facts that the liver is not enlarged, there are no stigmata of chronic liver disease, and the spleen and lymph nodes are not palpable—all tend to rule out liver disease and lymphoproliferative disorders as the cause for the coagulopathy. **Data** The physician in the triage area had immediately ordered a blood count, prothrombin time (PT), and partial thromboplastin time (PTT). Results were as follows: PT, 13.2/12.0 sec control; PTT, 31.0/32.0 sec control; hematocrit, 38%; hemoglobin, 12.5 g/dL; white blood cell count, 6700/mm³; differential, normal; **platelet count, 8000/mm³**. Results of the SMA-20 were pending. Review of the peripheral smear confirmed

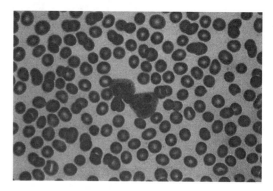

▶ **Figure 12.4.** Note two normal white blood cells, normal red blood cells, and the striking absence of platelets.

the thrombocytopenia, revealing several large platelets (megathrombocytes). Red blood cells and white blood cells appeared normal (Fig. 12.4). **Logic** Review of the peripheral smear ruled out artifactual thrombocytopenia secondary to platelet clumping; however, the presence of ecchymoses and petechiae already made this an unacceptable diagnosis.

The normal PT and PTT make a combined clotting factor/platelet disorder unlikely. Liver disease can cause a prolongation of the PT or PT/PTT due to decreased production of clotting factors and thrombocytopenia due to hypersplenism. However, the thrombocytopenia of hypersplenism is almost never this severe. Acute disseminated intravascular coagulation (DIC) is the other common cause of multifactorial bleeding and would also cause a prolongation of the PT and PTT as well as thrombocytopenia—all due to consumption.

Because this patient clearly has severe thrombocytopenia as the cause of her problem, the possible pathophysiologic processes at this point include:

1. Decreased platelet production due to ineffective thrombopoiesis, bone marrow injury, or bone marrow infiltration
2. Increased peripheral platelet destruction, utilization, or pooling
   a) Autoimmune thrombocytopenic purpura (AITP), which is either idiopathic or secondary to certain immunologic diseases, viral infections, a few specific drugs, and conditions in which the spleen is enlarged. Human immunodeficiency virus (HIV)-AITP is very common, and thrombocy-

topenia is frequently the presenting problem in patients who do not know they are HIV-positive.

b) Peripheral platelet consumption due to thrombotic microangiopathy (TTP, chronic DIC, or hemolytic uremic syndrome [HUS]).

Ineffective thrombopoiesis due to vitamin B_{12} and folate deficiency can be eliminated because there is no anemia or neutropenia. You can see thrombocytopenia as the presenting manifestation of malignant diseases that infiltrate the bone marrow, but again, this level of thrombocytopenia would be most unusual without a concomitant decrease in hematocrit or white blood cell count.

It is also unlikely that this patient has a thrombotic microangiopathy because there is no anemia nor are there fragmented red blood cells in the peripheral blood smear.

Chronic DIC, which may occur in patients who have cancer, can have a presentation of thrombocytopenia and evidence of fibrinolysis (elevated D-dimer and fibrin split products [FSP]), but there is no change in PT or PTT because synthesis of the clotting factors can keep pace with consumption. However, schistocytes would usually be present in the blood smear.

Peripheral destruction of platelets remains likely. The next step is to perform a bone marrow aspiration in order to determine megakaryocyte number and morphology. If they are absent or dysplastic, the problem resides with poor production. If they are present in good numbers, the culprit is excessive destruction.

Data On further questioning, the patient states that she has not been exposed to chemicals and has only an occasional social drink. She has taken a variety of pills from the local health food store but believes that they contain only vitamins. She smokes 10 to 20 cigarettes per day.

A bone marrow aspiration and biopsy were performed and demonstrated normal cellularity, and an increased number of megakaryocytes, with normal morphology, normal myeloid and erythroid maturation, and no abnormal cells.

Logic The increased number of megakaryocytes in the bone marrow indicates that the thrombocytopenia is secondary to excessive platelet destruction and not to underproduction. Even before the bone marrow examination, decreased

production of platelets was rendered far less likely, because the patient took no drugs such as estrogen, heparin, gold compounds, and ethanol, all of which could sometimes cause underproduction.

You may still want to obtain FSP or D-dimer to rule out chronic DIC. Also, TTP should be briefly considered. The peak incidence of TTP is from 10 to 40 years of age, and women are more commonly affected than men. It is characterized by microangiopathic hemolytic anemia, thrombocytopenia, fluctuating neurologic signs, fever, and mild renal insufficiency with microscopic hematuria. Microangiopathic hemolytic anemia is invariably present at the time of diagnosis; however, you should still review the results of her lactate dehydrogenase (LDH) and total bilirubin and order a reticulocyte count to be certain. Without prompt initiation of plasmapheresis or plasma infusion, TTP is an invariably fatal disease.

It is most likely that the patient has antibody-mediated AITP. This can be seen as a complication of drugs, collagen vascular diseases, lymphoproliferative disorders, and viral infections, especially human immunodeficiency virus (HIV). She is in the age range for both SLE and Hodgkin's disease, so these diagnoses should be briefly considered, especially because the development of AITP may predate other manifestations of these diseases.

Data More information—the patient did admit to occasional joint pains but denied swelling or erythema of the involved joints. She was thought to have viral pericarditis at age 21, but has had no further episodes of chest pain. She has no rashes, alopecia, or arthritis. You check the results of her SMA-20, which are normal, and her urinalysis, which shows only 2 to 3 WBCs per HPF. You should order an antinuclear antibody (ANA) and discuss with the patient whether an HIV test is appropriate.

Logic This patient had a classic presentation of acute AITP. You may have immediately suspected this diagnosis, but because of the number of other disease processes that can produce thrombocytopenia, you had to take a very complete history, perform a complete physical examination, and examine the blood smear, especially for schistocytes to rule out TTP.

It would be helpful if there were platelet antibody tests that were both sufficiently sensitive and specific for platelet autoantibodies. There is a new generation of tests ("antigen capture assays") that are able to detect platelet autoantibodies and determine their specificity. These assays, when available, will allow a positive diagnosis of AITP instead of this being a diagnosis by exclusion.

If the patient has negative results from the ANA and HIV test, she will be presumed to have idiopathic autoimmune thrombocytopenic purpura, even though SLE or lymphoma may still be found at a future date.

More than 90% of children with AITP have spontaneous remissions, but remission is rare enough in adults to warrant prompt steroid therapy. If there is no response to steroids, splenectomy may be indicated. Intravenous immunoglobulin (Ig) infusions provide only temporary responses in adults and should be reserved for acute thrombocytopenic bleeding.

Questions

1. If this patient's chief presenting complaint was mucosal bleeding and a lifelong history of bruisability and heavy menses, which of the following diagnoses would be most likely based on this history?
   (a) von Willebrand's disease
   (b) Hemophilia A
   (c) Protein C deficiency
   (d) Factor XII deficiency

2. If this patient had presented with mucosal bleeding, a lifelong history of bruisability and heavy menses, and a prolonged PTT with a normal platelet count and PT, which of the following tests would you order next?
   (a) Bleeding time, factor VIII activity
   (b) Bleeding time, factor VIII activity, von Willebrand's factor (vWF) activity, and vWF antigen
   (c) Lupus anticoagulant (LA) assay
   (d) Fibrinogen level

3. If you were trying to differentiate coagulopathies on the basis of bleeding characteristics, which of the following abnormalities would make you favor a deficiency of clotting factors?
   (a) Petechiae
   (b) Hemarthroses
   (c) Multiple superficial ecchymoses
   (d) Significant bleeding from superficial cuts

4. Which of the following drugs has not been implicated as a cause of AITP?
   (a) Heparin
   (b) Cimetidine
   (c) Danazol
   (d) Quinine

5. Which of the following statements about HIV-AITP is not true?
   (a) Commonly occurs when the CD4 count is only modestly decreased (i.e., 400)
   (b) Is always accompanied by palpable splenomegaly
   (c) Frequently responds to treatment with AZT
   (d) Is associated with platelet autoantibodies

Answers

1. **(a) is correct.** von Willebrand's disease is an autosomal dominant coagulopathy characterized by both a deficiency in factor VIII and abnormal platelet function. In contrast to hemophilia A, mucous membrane bleeding—including epistaxis and menometrorrhagia—is common, and spontaneous soft-tissue and joint bleeds are uncommon. Hemophilia is also sex-linked and therefore uncommon in women. Protein C is an inhibitor of activated factors V and VIII, and when it is deficient, there is an increased incidence of clotting, not bleeding. Factor XII deficiency is characterized by a prolonged PTT on laboratory testing, but no clinical bleeding.

2. **(b) is correct.** This patient needs to be evaluated for von Willebrand's disease, and the next phase of laboratory testing would usually include these four tests. If vWD were diagnosed, multimer studies would permit you to distinguish among classic vWD and its variants. The lupus anticoagulant is characterized by a prolonged PTT, but only rare clinical bleeding. It is almost always characterized by hypercoagulability and can be suspected if there is no correction of the PTT when patient plasma is mixed with normal plasma ("mixing test"). A fibrinogen deficiency would produce an increase in the PT and PTT because of the position of fibrinogen in the final common pathway of plasma coagulation.

3. **(b) is correct.** Petechiae, ecchymoses, and bleeding from superficial cuts are all characteristics of abnormal primary hemostasis (blood vessel and platelet phase). Hemarthroses are the most common bleeding manifestation of severe hemophilia, a deficiency of either factor VIII or factor IX.

4. **(c) is correct.** Heparin, cimetidine, and quinine are all associated with autoimmune thrombocytopenia. It has been recently demonstrated that heparin-induced thrombocytopenia results from binding of immune complexes of heparin-platelet factor 4 and antibody to the platelet surface. The other two drugs appear to be associated with the development of platelet autoantibodies. Danazol is not associated with thrombocytopenia and has been used successfully as salvage therapy for pa-

tients who have severe refractory immune thrombocytopenia.

5. **(b) is correct.** HIV-AITP is frequently one of the earliest complications of the HIV infection. Patients are seen in the early phase of their infection with isolated thrombocytopenia, which can respond both to AZT and the conventional modalities used to treat other forms of immune thrombocytopenia. Platelet autoantibodies have been implicated in the pathophysiology. A palpable spleen would make the etiology for the thrombocytopenia more uncertain because both hypersplenism and immune thrombocytopenia have normal bone marrow examinations, with normal to increased numbers of megakaryocytes.

COMMENT This case exquisitely demonstrates some of the prime problem-solving methods used by the clinician. The problem-solver's pattern of data collection and data evaluation develops along a path that uses five separate decision points:

1. Is the bleeding problem local or diffuse?
2. If diffuse, is the defect congenital or acquired?
3. If acquired, is the condition caused by defects in capillaries, platelets, or clotting factors?
4. If there is deficiency of platelets, is it due to inadequate production or excessive destruction?
5. If caused by excessive destruction, what are the various causes—TTP, DIC, or AITP?

A divide-and-conquer strategy was employed at each decision point, with the liberal use of positive and pertinent negative clues as the case logic developed. The final diagnosis was reached more by a process of eliminating all contenders save one, which was already the most likely diagnosis by virtue of the gender, age, and otherwise well-being of the patient, in addition to the fact that AITP is statistically the most common cause of acquired coagulopathies. *(P.C.)*

Suggested Readings

George JN, El-Harake MA, Raskob GE. Chronic idiopathic thrombocytopenic purpura. N Engl J Med 1994;331:1207–1211.

Harrington WJ, Minnich V, Hollingsworth JW, et al. Demonstration of a thrombocytopenic factor in the blood of patients with thrombocytopenic purpura.

J Lab Clin Med 1951;38:1–10. [This is the classic paper on immune thrombocytopenia. The authors themselves were the non-thrombocytopenic recipients who were transfused, which makes this one of the unique experimental papers in medical literature.]

McMillan R. Clinical role of antiplatelet antibody assays. Sem Thromb Hemostas 1995;21:37–44.

Rutherford CJ, Frenkel EP. Thrombocytopenia: Issues in diagnosis and therapy. Med Clin North Am 1994;78:555–575.

Thompson CE, Damon LE, Ries CA, Linker CA. Thrombotic microangiopathies in the 1980s: Clinical features, response to treatment, and the impact of the human immunodeficiency virus epidemic. Blood 1992;80:1890–1895.

CASE 4

LETHARGY AND CONFUSION

David A. Sears

Data A 78-year-old woman of Italian ancestry is brought to the emergency room by her family because of increasing lethargy and mental confusion. She can provide little medical history, but her daughter reports a gradual decline in her mother's previous good health during the past 3 to 6 months. During this period she spent much of her time sitting in a chair or napping and evidenced occasional memory lapses, which the family attributed to old age. An episode of urinary incontinence led them to bring her to the hospital.

Logic These are nonspecific chronic symptoms that suggest deterioration of cerebral function. In a woman her age you consider various dementias and a host of other causes, such as anemia, uremia, diabetes, cancer, liver disease, cardiac or respiratory disease, and depression.

Data Further history from the daughter reveals that the patient has stumbled and fallen two or three times when she has arisen at night to go to the bathroom, but not at other times. Her appetite has been poor, her eating habits erratic, and she has lost 10 pounds. She has always abstained from alcohol and tobacco and takes no medications. There is no history of renal disease, and she has had no polydipsia or polyuria. There have been no significant changes in her living situation. No additional history is immediately available.

Logic The weight loss is worrisome, and you consider the possibility of malignant disease. Falling at night suggests that she depends on her vision to maintain balance. You suspect a defect in one of the other systems that control balance—that is, cerebellar function, proprioception, and the vestibular apparatus. In any case, this history suggests that you will want to check certain portions of the neurologic examination carefully. The absence of past renal disease speaks against uremia but does not rule it out. Diabetes causing the clinical pattern of weight loss and confusion is unlikely in the absence of severe thirst and frequent urination. The absence of alcohol intake tends to make liver disease less likely.

Data On physical examination the patient is a slightly confused, elderly, gray-haired woman. Vital signs are normal, and the pulse and blood pressure are not significantly altered when she changes from a supine to a sitting posture. Her skin is generally pale and palmar creases are white. You think that the skin and sclerae may be slightly icteric, but you are not sure. The breath is not uremic, fruity, or musty. She has a large ecchymosis on the right thigh from a recent fall.

Logic These few simple observations serve to focus your thinking. The normal vital signs speak against cerebral anoxia due primarily to a cardiac or pulmonary cause. The pallor suggests anemia, and the stability of her blood pressure and pulse with changes in posture weighs against hypovolemia. Thus, if she has anemia, it is most likely chronic. The questionable icterus will be important in considering the cause of anemia if present and, of course, raises the possibility of liver disease. In evaluating her ecchymosis, try to decide if it is excessive for the amount of trauma. If it is, you think of thrombocytopenia or a coagulation factor deficiency. Normal odor of the breath weighs against uremia, diabetic ketoacidosis, and hepatic failure.

Data The remainder of the physical examination reveals normal retinae. The tongue is red and devoid of papillae. There is no palpable lymphadenopathy or thyromegaly. The lungs are normal. Examination of the heart reveals a strong apical impulse 2 cm to the left of the mid-clavicular line in the fifth intercostal space. Heart sounds are normal, and the rhythm is regular, but a grade 2/6 non-radiating systolic ejection murmur is heard at the base of the heart. The ab-

domen is soft and nontender with normal bowel sounds and no palpable masses. The liver edge is felt 2 cm below the right costal margin in the mid-clavicular line; its vertical height by percussion at this point is 8 cm. The tip of the spleen is felt at the left costal margin in deep inspiration. Rectal examination is normal, and the finger specimen of stool is negative for occult blood.

Neurologic examination shows intact cranial nerves, normal reflexes, and no pathological reflexes. She is oriented to place and person but not to time, has impaired recent memory, and performs serial sevens poorly. Light touch and pinprick are normally perceived, but vibratory sensation is lost from the iliac crests down; position sense is abnormal in both big toes. The Romberg test result is positive with the eyes shut. Stereognosis, rapidly alternating movements, and finger-to-nose test are normal, and there is no nystagmus.

Logic You continue to suspect anemia in this patient, and the finding of a palpable spleen is important. It indicates an enlarged spleen, and the enlargement must be explained. On the other hand, although her liver is palpable, it is not enlarged. The vertical height is thought by some to be crucial in deciding about liver size. The absence of lymphadenopathy indicates that her splenomegaly is not part of a general process affecting lymphoid organs. Diseases like malignant lymphomas may effect the spleen alone but more commonly involve lymph nodes as well.

Examination of the stool specimen for occult blood is an important part of the evaluation of the anemic patient. Although one negative test result does not rule out gastrointestinal blood loss as a cause of anemia, it makes it less likely. Your neurologic examination indicates cerebral dysfunction and posterior column disease, but there is no evidence of disease of the lateral columns, cerebellum, or vestibular apparatus. The cluster of anemia, posterior column disease, and atrophic glossitis in an elderly person suggests the diagnosis of pernicious anemia.

Data A tube of blood is sent to the laboratory for blood counts, and the printout of the automated determinations reads as follows: hematocrit, 20%; hemoglobin, 6.4 g/dL; red blood cell count, 1.6 million/mm^3; mean corpuscular volume, 125 fL; mean corpuscular hemoglobin, 40 pg; mean corpuscular hemoglobin concentration, 32%;

white blood cell count, 4100/mm³; differential white blood cell count, 48%; segmented neutrophils, 44% lymphocytes, 5% monocytes, and 3% eosinophils; and platelet count, 82,000/mm³. Results of urinalysis and "chem 7" (electrolytes, glucose, blood urea nitrogen [BUN], and creatinine) are normal.

Logic Your suspicion of anemia has been confirmed, and attention should now be directed at defining it by mechanism and morphology. For the former, a reticulocyte count will be most useful and should be ordered immediately. For the latter, consider the red blood cell indices and examine the blood smear. The high mean corpuscular volume indicates macrocytosis. The mean corpuscular hemoglobin concentration shows normal cellular hemoglobin concentration. Both are mean values and do not tell you anything about the degree of variation in cell size and shape. Because of the patient's questionable icterus, you order the serum bilirubin and liver function tests. An electrocardiogram (ECG) and chest radiograph are also done.

Data The additional data are as follows: reticulocyte count, 4.2%; total serum bilirubin, 2.8 mg/dL , 0.3 mg/dL conjugated; serum glutamic-oxaloacetic transaminase, 17 mIU/mL; serum glutamic-pyruvic transaminase, 24 mIU/mL; lactate dehydrogenase, 975 mIU/mL (normal <220); and alkaline phosphatase, 78 mIU/mL (normal <125). The ECG is normal, and the chest radiograph shows minimal cardiomegaly. The blood smear is shown in Figure 12.5.

Logic When the reticulocyte count is corrected for the patient's anemia and for the consequent early release and prolonged circulation of reticulocytes, you arrive at a reticulocyte index of 1.0. Thus, red blood cell production has not increased in response to the severe anemia. Impaired red blood cell production and the abnormalities noted on the blood smear strongly suggest megaloblastic anemia. The term megaloblastic refers to morphologic features of precursor cells in the bone marrow, and examination of the bone marrow is an appropriate next step.

Data The bone marrow shows marked megaloblastic changes in nucleated red blood cells and white blood cell precursors.

Logic The patient has now been proved to have megaloblastic anemia. The ineffective erythropoiesis (death of red blood cell precursors before leaving the marrow) associated with megaloblas-

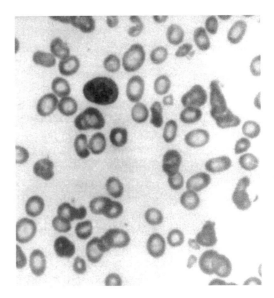

▶ **Figure 12.5.** The red blood cells are generally normochromic. They vary a great deal in size (marked anisocytosis), with a predominance of macrocytes but also microcytes. Note that many of the large red blood cells are oval in shape (oval macrocytes). The red blood cells vary in shape as well (moderate poikilocytosis), particularly the small fragmented cells. A single segmented neutrophil is seen whose nucleus is hypersegmented (over 5 lobes), and platelets are diminished.

tic anemia explains the patient's unconjugated hyperbilirubinemia (due to hemoglobin catabolism) and the very high lactate dehydrogenase level (released from destroyed red blood cell precursors). The mild leukopenia and thrombocytopenia are also characteristic of megaloblastic anemia, and splenomegaly is commonly present. The heart murmur and slight cardiomegaly may be due to the severe anemia per se.

Except for rare circumstances, megaloblastic anemia is due to vitamin B_{12} or folic acid deficiency. These two causes cannot be distinguished by blood counts or morphology of blood or marrow, but the clinical setting in which they occur is different and provides clues as to which vitamin is lacking. Vitamin B_{12} deficiency is almost never due to dietary lack. It results from impaired absorption of B_{12} caused by atrophic gastritis with failure of intrinsic factor secretion (pernicious anemia) or malabsorption due to intestinal diseases or surgery. Folic acid deficiency, on the other hand, is usually related to inadequate diet and less often to underabsorption. Alcoholic patients are often folate deficient. Lack of vitamin B_{12} may produce a variety of neurologic abnormalities, although lack of folic acid rarely or never does.

Data Further history from the patient and her daughter reveals that although she has been eating poorly, she does have some meat every day and usually eats a green salad at lunch. The stools were described as loose on occasion but not light-colored, foamy, frothy, greasy, or unusually foul smelling.

Logic The clinical picture strongly suggests classical pernicious anemia. There is no evidence of dietary folic acid deficiency or malabsorption. She has atrophic glossitis, which commonly accompanies the atrophic gastritis of PA, and posterior column disease is one of the common neurologic abnormalities associated with PA. Her cerebral dysfunction may also be a direct result of vitamin B_{12} deficiency ("megaloblastic madness") and may account for the weight loss that occurs in only 5% of PA patients. The classical triad of weakness, sore tongue, and paresthesias is present in only a minority of patients. Because PA necessitates lifelong therapy with parenteral vitamin B_{12}, confirmation of the diagnosis is important. A serum vitamin B_{12} assay is ordered.

Data The serum vitamin B_{12} level is reported to be <100 pg/mL (normal> 200).

Logic This unequivocally low serum vitamin B_{12} level confirms vitamin B_{12} deficiency as the etiology of the megaloblastic anemia. The clinical picture suggests that the deficiency is probably due to classical PA. Certain other tests will add additional confirmatory evidence if such is deemed necessary:

- Gastric analysis after pentagastrin stimulation. Absolute achlorhydria accompanies failure of intrinsic factor secretion in atrophic gastritis. This is a quick and simple test that will add weight to the diagnosis of PA.
- Schilling test for vitamin B_{12} absorption. This is a theoretically elegant test, or series of tests, which has, however, practical drawbacks in some cases.
- Testing for serum anti-intrinsic factor antibodies. This test is fairly sensitive and quite specific for PA.

Data Fasting gastric analysis shows achlorhydria after pentagastrin administration. The diagnosis of PA is made, and the patient is begun on vitamin B_{12} injections.

Questions

1. Megaloblastic anemia due to folic acid deficiency may be associated with each of the following except:
   (a) pregnancy.
   (b) gastric carcinoma.
   (c) phenytoin therapy.
   (d) severe hemolytic disease.
2. Vitamin B_{12} deficiency may result from each of the following except:
   (a) subtotal gastrectomy.
   (b) fish tapeworm (*Diphyllobothrium latum*) infestation.
   (c) strict vegetarianism for 3 months.
   (d) intestinal "blind loop" syndromes.
3. If this patient had had a resection of her terminal ileum 5 years earlier for regional ileitis, the most likely cause of her megaloblastic anemia would have been:
   (a) vitamin B_{12} deficiency.
   (b) folic acid deficiency.
   (c) vitamin B_{12} and folic acid deficiencies.
   (d) iron deficiency.
4. Which of the following is/are associated with pernicious anemia?
   (a) Antibodies to gastric parietal cells
   (b) Antibodies to intrinsic factor
   (c) Antithyroid antibodies
   (d) All of the aforementioned
5. Which of the following abnormalities will be reversed by vitamin B_{12} therapy in this patient?
   (a) Anemia, leukopenia, and thrombocytopenia
   (b) Neurologic abnormalities
   (c) Achlorhydria
   (d) All of the aforementioned

Answers

1. **(b) is correct.** Gastric carcinoma occurs with increased frequency in patients with PA, not in those with folate deficiency. Demands on folic acid stores are increased by fetal requirements in pregnancy and by increased cell turnover as occurs with active hemolysis, so folate deficiency may occur in each of these states. Anticonvulsant drugs, particularly phenytoin, may produce folate deficiency through still uncertain mechanisms.
2. **(c) is correct.** Individuals who avoid not only meat but also eggs and milk ("vegans") may develop dietary vitamin B_{12} deficiency, but much longer periods of time (years) would be required because of the large stores of vitamin B_{12} in the liver. Even though subtotal gastrectomy leaves some intrinsic factor-producing cells, there is a significant incidence of vitamin B_{12} deficiency after re-

moval of most of the stomach. The intestinal fish tapeworm may compete with its host for ingested vitamin B_{12} and prevent absorption of the vitamin. Although this rarely occurs outside of Finland, there are recent reports of fish tapeworm infestation in the vicinity of the Great Lakes. Changes in the bacterial flora of the small bowel due to stasis or altered circulation of intestinal contents (as may occur in "blind loops") can produce vitamin B_{12} deficiency by a similar mechanism in which overgrowing bacteria compete with the host for available vitamin B_{12}.

3. **(a) is correct.** Vitamin B_{12} (linked to intrinsic factor) is bound by receptors and absorbed in the terminal ileum. Because of body vitamin B_{12} stores, deficiency may not appear until several years after absorption of food vitamin B_{12} stops. Folic acid is absorbed in the proximal small bowel. Iron deficiency does not produce megaloblastic anemia.

4. **(d) is correct.** Although it is not clear what pathogenic role the antibodies against parietal cells and intrinsic factor play in PA, they are found in a high percentage of patients. Antibodies against intrinsic factor are fairly specific for PA, although anti-parietal cell antibodies are found in other groups of patients as well. Hypothyroid patients may share some of the autoimmune manifestations of patients who have PA, and the two diseases coexist with a frequency that is greater than chance would dictate.

5. **(a) is correct, and (b) may be correct.** The hematologic abnormalities are completely corrected by vitamin B_{12} therapy. The neurologic abnormalities of vitamin B_{12} deficiency may be irreversible, partially reversible, or completely reversible over long treatment periods. It is important to remember that neurologic manifestations in vitamin B_{12} deficiency are extremely variable. They may be the presenting complaint in a patient with little or no anemia, or they may be entirely absent. The achlorhydria will persist because it is part of the basic pathologic defect of PA—atrophic gastritis.

COMMENT At first, the nonspecificity of symptoms causes you to consider a wide variety of possibilities. As more data are gathered, many diagnoses are ruled out. A cluster of anemia, mental changes, posterior column disease, and atrophic glossitis is found, suggesting PA. But anemia becomes the key clue. A few well-chosen studies establish the presence of a megaloblastic anemia; further data and logic result in a diagnosis of PA rather than folate deficiency.

The presence of weight loss and anorexia is a distracter because these are uncommon in PA. Common clues, such as fever, sore tongue, and paresthesias, are lacking, showing that not all classical findings need be present. Palpable splenomegaly is present in fewer than half the patients. Mild neurologic signs may occur in as many as 30% of these patients, although this used to be more common when the disease was diagnosed later.

Probability theory is especially applicable here. The odds are that an elderly woman with megaloblastic anemia who eats adequately, does not drink alcohol, and does not have malabsorption has PA rather than folic acid deficiency. Treatment was initiated on the basis of a strongly presumptive diagnosis, and then confirmed by the serum vitamin B_{12} level. *(P.C.)*

Suggested Readings

Carmel R. Subtle and atypical cobalamin deficiency states. Am J Hematol 1990;34:108–114.

Pruthi RK, Tefferi A. Pernicious anemia revisited. Mayo Clin Proc 1994;69:144–150.

Stabler SP, Allen RH, Savage DG, Lindenbaum J. Clinical spectrum and diagnosis of cobalamin deficiency. Blood 1990;76:871–881.

Tefferi A, Pruthi RK. The biochemical basis of cobalamin deficiency. Mayo Clin Proc 1994; 69:181–186.

CASE 5

A FAMILY AFFAIR

Frank Beardell and Sandor S. Shapiro

Data A dentist refers a 17-year-old female high school student to you because she has recurrent bleeding gums and a history of easy bruising and occasional nosebleeds.

Logic It is sometimes difficult to decide if either of these symptoms, occurring singly, is definitely pathologic, because many persons complain of one or the other, yet have no disease. The precise point at which bruises resulting from moderate trauma are normal and where bruises from slight trauma become abnormal is a judgment call. Many patients, especially older women, say that they "bruise easily."

Bleeding gums may result from too vigorous tooth brushing, so it might be helpful to know the circumstances in which bleeding, as well as bruising, occur. Because the patient was seen by a dentist, it must be assumed that she has no gum disease that was causing her to bleed.

Nosebleeds can be caused by trauma, nose-picking, and intranasal inflammation or tumor.

Last, while having three symptoms, each of which might possibly be the result of a different circumstance, their concurrence is far more likely to be the result of a single disease.

Hemorrhagic disorders to be considered as possible causes of the symptoms in this case include:

- Diseases of small *blood vessels* and capillaries
- *Platelet* disorders due either to *insufficient numbers* or to *malfunction*
- Diseases associated with deficiency of one or more *clotting factors*

A detailed personal and family history is in order.

Data The patient notes a lifelong history of easy bruising after minor trauma and intermittent bleeding from her gums after brushing, even after light brushing. Nosebleeds occur occasionally, sometimes from the right nostril, and at other times from the left. She claims not to pick her nose. There is no history of hemarthroses, gastrointestinal bleeding, hematuria, or intracranial bleeding. Her mother gives her own history of easy bruising since infancy, with multiple, often unexplainable, bruises on the arms and legs.

Both mother and daughter report normal menses. On further questioning, it is learned that their periods generally last 7 to 9 days, with the use of up to 10 pads per day. Neither the mother nor the daughter ever had surgery, and the mother does not recall any bleeding problem at her daughter's birth.

Logic The fact that both mother and daughter have similar histories from early childhood suggests strongly that an *inherited* disorder of coagulation exists. The importance of obtaining specific details of the menstrual history is illustrated in that although both mother and daughter report normal menses, their menstrual bleeding is clearly excessive.

The two most common hereditary hemorrhagic diseases are von Willebrand's disease (vWD) and hemophilia A. Defective platelet function—vWD—is the commonest hereditary coagulopathy. A deficiency of factor VIII—hemophilia A—is the second most common hereditary coagulopathy.

A factor weighing against hemophilia A in this case is the fact that the patient is female. Hemophilia is an X-linked recessive disorder that is only rarely seen in women. Furthermore, the pattern of bleeding—gums, skin bruising, nosebleeds—is more suggestive of a defect involving platelet function (vWD) than a primary defect in the coagulation mechanism (hemophilia A).

vWD is transmitted in an autosomal dominant hereditary pattern and has approximately twice the prevalence of hemophilia A. von Willebrand's factor is an unusually large, multimeric plasma glycoprotein that serves both as a carrier for factor VIII and as a *mediator of initial platelet adhesion* to the blood vessel wall at the site of vessel injury (Fig. 12.6). Thus, patients with low levels of vWF, and a consequently prolonged bleeding time, commonly also have low levels of factor VIII. The synthesis of vWF is a multistep process resulting in the formation of high molecular weight multimers. As a result, a number of variants of vWD can arise in which functionally defective vWF rather than its total absence may be the problem. Analysis for the presence or absence of these multimers forms the basis for the diagnosis of the various subtypes of vWD.

Platelets have multiple roles in achieving hemostasis. They act mechanically to seal defects in the vascular endothelium, they provide a surface upon which the coagulation cascade can be activated, and they promote clot retraction by interaction with strands of fibrin. For platelets to function, they must not only be adequate in number, but they must have available ample amounts of functional vWF. Healthy blood contains 200,000 to 300,000 platelets per mm^3, and serious bleeding because of platelet deficiency is rarely seen until the platelet count falls below 10,000 to 20,000/mm^3. When platelets are inadequate in number and/or function, the bleeding time is prolonged. If the bleeding time is prolonged and platelet numbers are normal, abnormal platelet function is likely.

At this point, most evidence points to the presence of a hereditary disease associated with abnormalities in platelet-vessel wall interaction, such as due to insufficient vWF or to disorders of platelet receptors. Abnormalities in the blood vessels themselves, such as in vascular and collagen disor-

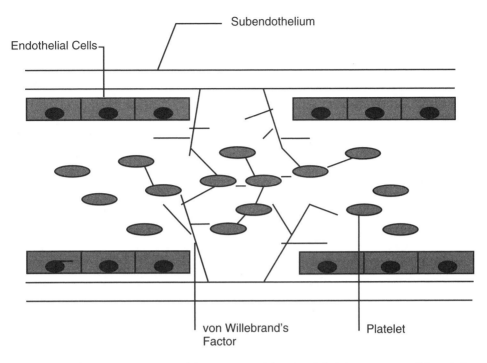

Endothelial Cells

Subendothelium

von Willebrand's Factor

Platelet

▶ **Figure 12.6.** Schematic representation of the interaction of the subendothelial matrix, von Willebrand's factor, and the platelet after tissue injury, which results in exposure of the matrix to the blood proteins.

ders, are weak diagnostic contenders. And until the platelet count is done and found to be normal, diseases such as autoimmune thrombocytopenic purpura (AITP), thrombotic thrombocytopenic purpura (TTP), disseminated intravascular coagulation (DIC), and thrombocytopenic conditions due to primary bone marrow failure (such as in leukemia and aplastic anemia) are still diagnostic possibilities—even though they are all acquired diseases of relatively recent onset.

Data Physical examination reveals a pleasant, well-developed young female who is pale. The vital signs are normal and she is afebrile. Fundoscopic examination shows no evidence of retinal hemorrhage and the sclerae appear normal. There is blood oozing from a single site of the gingival mucosa. Multiple small ecchymotic areas are seen on the extremities at various stages of resolution. A large tender ecchymotic area overlies the left antecubital fossa at the site of a previous venipuncture. The abdomen is normal and there is no lymphadenopathy. No petechial rash is noted. The patient's skin is of normal tone and

no joint laxity or hyperextensibility is found. The remainder of the physical examination is normal.

Logic Examination confirms the bruises and bleeding gums. The absence of splenomegaly and enlarged lymph nodes argues against disorders such as leukemia or lymphoma. The lack of joint laxity and of hyper extensibility and the normal skin turgor tend to rule out disorders of collagen formation such as the Ehlers-Danlos syndrome. Her otherwise general good health plus the absence of commonly associated clues are against the diagnoses of systemic lupus, vasculitis, TTP, and DIC. Factors weighing against AITP is the absence of the very commonly present petechial rash, plus the fact that the patient's symptoms have been present for her lifetime.

Data Laboratory tests follow: hemoglobin, 10.5 g/dL; hematocrit, 31.5%; MCV, 80; WBC, 8800/mm³; and a normal differential. The automated *platelet count* is 250,000/mm³. The PTT is 44.5 sec (control 30.0), and the PT is 12.5 sec (control 11), INR 1.1. The template bleeding time is

>15 minutes. The RBCs appear microcytic and hypochromic. No schistocytes, helmet cells, or platelet clumping seen.

Logic The most prominent abnormalities are the mild microcytic anemia and the prolonged PTT and bleeding time. The normal number of platelets signifies that the defect of platelet function is probably caused by a critical deficiency of normally functioning vWF.

The anemia is of the iron-deficiency type and probably is a result of her menorrhagia.

Platelet clumping seen on peripheral smear has a variety of causes and is itself a cause of spurious decreases in the platelet count—not an issue in this case because the platelet count was normal and platelet clumping was not seen on the peripheral smear.

TTP is a fulminant disorder that is characterized by a pentad of clinical signs and symptoms: fever; thrombocytopenia; renal failure; fluctuating levels of consciousness and transitory focal neurologic defects; and a hemolytic anemia whose hallmarks are schistocytes and otherwise deformed RBC's seen in the blood smear. These features are not present in this case.

DIC is usually associated with catastrophic illnesses such as metastatic cancer, massive trauma, burns, and sepsis. Small thrombi occur throughout the microvasculature. Consumption of platelets and several coagulation factors takes place, particularly fibrinogen and factor V, resulting in a prolongation of the PT and PTT. This, together with the effects of the body's effort to dissolve the clots by activating fibrinolysis, results in bleeding, as well as in deformed RBC's in the blood smear and increased levels of fibrin split products (FSP) in the blood.

Data The plasma factor VIII level is 12% (normal, 50–100%). The fibrinogen level is 212 mg/dL. There is no increase in FSP and all other coagulation factors are normal. Mixing studies using half patient and half normal plasma show complete correction of the PTT. Renal function is normal, and the urinalysis indicates no RBCs.

Logic Normal renal function and urinalysis and the absence of evidence of fibrinolysis are further assurances that this patient does not have a consumptive coagulopathy such as TTP and DIC.

Complete normalization of the PTT in mixing studies is diagnostic of a factor deficiency, in this case factor VIII. This factor circulates in the

blood bound to vWF; when vWF is deficient, so, frequently, is factor VIII. Factor VIII is crucial to normal hemostasis but is not involved in platelet function.

The Bernard-Soulier syndrome (BSS) is a rare autosomal recessive bleeding disorder caused by a derangement of the platelet receptor complex known as the glycoprotein Ib-IX-V complex, resulting in compromised interaction between platelets and the vWF in the blood vessel subendothelium. BSS patients have normal factor VIII levels, so it can be ruled out in this case.

Data The patient's vWF function, measured as ristocetin cofactor activity, was 10%; her vWF concentration, measured immunologically, was 15%. A sample of plasma was electrophoresed on an agarose gel in the presence of sodium dodecyl sulfate, and vWF multimers were visualized with a radioiodinated anti-vWF antibody. There was a moderate decrease in all molecular weight multimers.

Logic Although a variety of molecular defects may result in vWD, the underlying abnormalities may be divided into three groups:

1. Type 1 vWD exhibits a partial quantitative deficiency of vWF.
2. Type 2 vWD exhibits qualitative variants of vWF.
3. Type 3 vWD exhibits virtually complete deficiency of vWF.

A diagnosis of type 1 von Willebrand's disease was made, and a detailed discussion ensued with the patient and her mother about treatment and the prevention of future bleeding problems.

Therapy for patients with vWD aims to raise the plasma vWF and factor VIII to hemostatically effective levels, especially before surgery. Various forms of treatment include cryoprecipitate, factor VIII concentrates, and intranasal desmopressin.

COMMENT The first branching point in the problem-solving algorithm in this case depended on a determination of whether the bleeding disorder was inherited or acquired. Because there are basically only two major hereditary diseases to consider—hemophilia A and von Willebrand's disease—one was easily eliminated from consideration by virtue of the patient's gender and the type of bleeding seen. Nevertheless, the problem solver felt it important to consider and then exclude the various acquired coagulopathies. Whereas a detailed analysis of the findings (or absence of findings) in the history, physical examination, and laboratory studies helped to eliminate most diagnostic possibilities, the vWF determination and the platelet count were crucial clues in pinpointing the correct diagnosis. (P.C.)

Suggested Readings

Lethagen S, Harris AS, Nilsson IM. Intranasal desmopressin (DDAVP) by spray in mild hemophilia A and von Willebrand's disease type 1. Blut 1990;60: 187–191.

Miller JL. von Willebrand's disease. Hematol/Oncol Clin North Am 1990;4:107–128.

Sadler JE, Gralnick HR. A new classification system for von Willebrand's disease. Blood 1994;84:676–679.

COUGH, FEVER, THEN FATIGUE

David A. Sears

Data A 24-year-old black man is admitted to the hospital because of increasing fatigue following a respiratory tract infection. He felt well until 5 days ago when he developed nasal stuffiness, a sore throat, and a dry cough. Three days later his cough became productive of thick yellow sputum, his temperature rose to 39.4°C, and he began to note sharp pain in the left posterior thorax with deep inspiration. His physician made a clinical diagnosis of pneumonia and prescribed azithromycin and three to four aspirin tablets daily for fever. Cough and fever abated, but he felt progressively weaker and was therefore hospitalized.

Logic Thus far, the history sounds most compatible with a viral upper respiratory tract infection followed by the development of pneumonia. However, the latter diagnosis must be confirmed, and the etiology must be established. Increasing weakness raises the possibility of a complication of the respiratory tract infection.

Data History reveals that the patient had been healthy all his life. He had been told that he had "yellow jaundice" as a newborn but that he had not required transfusion or other specific therapy. The results of systems review are entirely

negative, except for the fact that he has noted his urine to be dark brown for the past 1 or 2 days. Family history is negative or unobtainable. His parents are dead, and his only sibling, a sister, is in good health.

Logic The history of jaundice as a newborn is difficult to evaluate. Alloimmune hemolytic disease of the newborn or prematurity would be the most likely causes. The recent history of dark urine is important. Because urine in the febrile, dehydrated patient is concentrated and often appears darker than usual, it is important to ascertain its color by careful questioning and direct observation. Among the causes of dark urine are ingested foods or drugs (beets, phenolphthalein), bilirubin, red blood cells, hemoglobin, myoglobin, porphyrins, and melanin. The cause in this patient is not yet apparent.

Data On physical examination he appears acutely ill. Nail beds and mucous membranes are not cyanotic but appear slightly pale. His pulse is 95/min, BP 120/70 without postural changes, respirations 18/min, and temperature 37.3°C. The sclerae are slightly icteric and the pharynx is slightly reddened without exudate. Respiratory movements of the thorax are asymmetrical with splinting on the left. There is dullness to percussion, breath sounds are bronchovesicular, and many fine to medium moist rales are heard over the left lung posteriorly. The heart is not enlarged to percussion, and the apex beat is normally located, but the precordium is active with a forceful left ventricular impulse. The heart sounds are normal, and there is a grade 1/6 systolic ejection murmur heard best along the left sternal border. The abdomen is soft and nontender, and the liver and spleen are not palpable. The remainder of the examination—including the rectum, nervous system, and extremities—is normal.

Logic The physical examination is consistent with the expected pneumonia and does not give evidence of complications, such as pleural effusion, empyema, pericarditis, endocarditis, or meningitis. Scleral icterus may rarely occur in pneumonia due to lysis of red blood cells in the pneumonic lesion, but it is much more likely to reflect a complication like focal hepatic necrosis, underlying liver disease, or hemolysis. Taken together with the dark urine in this patient, you may consider liver disease with bilirubinuria or hemolysis with hemoglobinuria. Laboratory studies are important at this point.

Data Results are as follows: hematocrit, 25%; reticulocytes, 15%; and white blood cell count, 14,500/mm³ with 81% segmented neutrophils, 12% bands, 2% metamyelocytes, and 5% lymphocytes. The blood smear is shown in Figure 12.7. A quick screening test for the presence of sickle hemoglobin yields a positive result. The urine is clear and mahogany brown in color; specific gravity 1.025; pH 5.0; protein 1+; glucose, ketones, and bilirubin test negative; and blood tests positive. The spun sediment contains amorphous debris but no cells or casts. Stool tests guaiac negative. Sputum is thick and yellow; Gram's stain reveals occasional white blood cells and a few gram-positive diplococci. It is cultured. Chest radiograph: a homogeneous density involves much of the left lower lung field; no pleural fluid is seen; the heart is of normal size and configuration. The levels of blood urea nitrogen, glucose, electrolytes, serum glutamic-oxaloacetic transaminase, serum glutamic-pyruvic transaminase, and alkaline phosphatase are normal. Total serum bilirubin is 5.2 mg/dL, and conjugated bilirubin is 0.5 mg/dL. The serum has a red-yellow color.

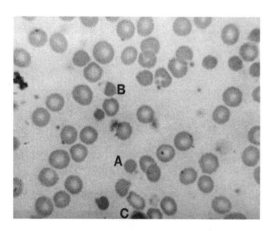

▶ **Figure 12.7.** Blood smear. The red blood cells are normochromic. There is moderate variation in size, with small cells (mostly microspherocytes), and large cells, many of which are polychromatophilic—probably reticulocytes. Note the microspherocytes (A) and one "blister" cell (B). The non-hemoglobinized portion of the latter is probably occupied by oxidatively denatured hemoglobin (Heinz bodies) that do not stain with Wright's stain. Part of a nucleated red blood cell (C) is seen at the edge of the smear.

Logic A good deal of light has been shed on the patient's problems. The reticulocyte index of 4.5 ($15 \times 25/45 \times 1/1.85$) indicates accelerated bone marrow production of red blood cells. Therefore the mechanism of the anemia is either acute blood loss or hemolysis, and the clinical picture clearly indicates the latter. The blood smear suggests red blood cell fragmentation but does not indicate a specific cause for the hemolytic process. The mild leukocytosis and granulocyte immaturity are compatible with acute hemolysis and/or the patient's pneumonia. The dark color of the urine is due to heme pigment, as shown by the positive dipstick test result for blood, which could be due to red blood cells, free hemoglobin, or myoglobin. However, red blood cells were not seen in the sediment, and the urine specific gravity was not low enough to suggest osmotic lysis of red blood cells. The myoglobin molecule is only one fourth the size of hemoglobin and is rapidly cleared from the plasma by filtration in the kidney.

Therefore, in the absence of renal failure, myoglobin does not accumulate in the plasma and produce visible pigment. We can conclude that the urinary pigment is hemoglobin (or more likely methemoglobin, its oxidized form, which is brown in color) and that hemoglobin is also responsible for the reddish color of the plasma. Thus, the patient has intravascular hemolysis with hemoglobinemia and hemoglobinuria. The unconjugated hyperbilirubinemia is also due to his hemolysis.

Data The tentative diagnosis of partially treated, probably pneumococcal, pneumonia is made, and parenteral ceftriaxone started. Attention is turned to further evaluation of his hemolytic anemia.

Logic The differential diagnosis includes both congenital and acquired disorders and can be fairly lengthy at this point. Among the more common ailments to be considered are the following:

Congenital
- Sickle cell disease or other hemoglobinopathy: The history of good health and the absence of sickled forms on the blood smear make homozygous sickle cell disease unlikely. The history and absence of target cells make doubly heterozygous states like hemoglobin SC dis-

ease and sickle cell-β-thalassemia unlikely as well. Sickle cell trait is most likely. Hemoglobin electrophoresis should be ordered for further evaluation of the hemoglobinopathy.

- Red blood cell glucose-6-phosphate dehydrogenase (G-6-PD) deficiency: This is a good possibility. A special stain of the patient's red blood cells for Heinz bodies may be helpful as well as a G-6-PD assay on his red blood cells.
- Hereditary spherocytosis: The absence of family history, lack of splenomegaly, and acute nature of the hemolysis weigh against this diagnosis.

Acquired
- Drug-related immune hemolysis: Only azithromycin was administered before the hemolysis, and this drug is not known to cause immune hemolysis.
- Idiopathic autoimmune hemolytic anemia: This cannot be excluded, and a direct Coombs' test should be done.
- Cold agglutinin hemolysis due to *Mycoplasma pneumoniae* infection. Although the patient's pneumonia is not characteristic of *Mycoplasma* infection, its cause is not yet established, so this possibility should be considered. A Coombs' test for complement on the red blood cell surface, serum cold agglutinin titer, and complement fixation test for *M. pneumoniae* should be obtained.

Data Additional studies are done as follows: hemoglobin electrophoresis shows 58% A, 2% A_2, and 40% S hemoglobin. Methyl violet staining reveals Heinz bodies in a few of the patient's red blood cells. A screening test for red cell G-6-PD gives equivocal results, and an assay shows 5.8 IU of G-6-PD per gram of hemoglobin (normal 5.6 to 12). The direct Coombs' test result is negative for both γ-globulin and complement on the red blood cell. The serum cold agglutinin titer is 1:4. The complement fixation test for *Mycoplasma* will not be available for several days. Serum hemoglobin level is 35 mg/dL (normal <5), and methemalbumin is present. Haptoglobin is absent.

Logic The elevated serum heme pigment, methemalbuminemia, and absent haptoglobin merely confirm the intravascular hemolysis, which has already been appreciated by other simpler observations. The negative Coombs' test virtually excludes immune hemolysis, and the normal serum cold agglutinin titer rules out hemolysis secondary to *M. pneumoniae* infections. The hemoglobin electrophoresis and sickle preparation allow the diagnosis of sickle cell trait to be made with certainty. This abnormality has no apparent relationship to the patient's hemolysis or pneumonia.

The finding of Heinz bodies in the patient's red blood cells is a crucial observation. Heinz bodies represent membrane-bound hemoglobin, denatured and precipitated due to oxidative damage. Increased susceptibility to this oxidative change can result from an inherited defect in the reductive mechanisms of the red cell (by far the most common of which is G-6-PD deficiency) or from an inherited unstable hemoglobin. The presence of these rigid intracellular precipitates predisposes the red blood cell to fragmentation injury or destruction in the splenic microcirculation. Because G-6-PD deficiency occurs in approximately 10% of black men in the United States, this is by far the most likely diagnosis in the present patient. The low normal enzyme level by assay does not exclude this diagnosis. The enzyme level is higher in younger red blood cells, and a deficient individual with a marked reticulocytosis (i.e., a young population of red blood cells) may have a level in the normal range. This also explains why the hemolysis may be self-limited and the anemia begins to correct itself even while the affected individual continues to be exposed to the triggering drug or illness. The oxidative challenge that precipitates hemolysis in a patient with G-6-PD deficiency is often caused by a drug but may result from an acute illness, as in this patient. Neither azithromycin nor aspirin, in the doses taken by this patient, precipitates hemolysis in the G-6-PD deficiency common to black men in this country (Table 12.2).

Data The patient's sputum culture results are negative, probably due to the prior antibiotic therapy. Serologic testing of acute and convalescent sera shows no evidence of *Mycoplasma* infection. He responds to ceftriaxone therapy, with clearing of the pneumonia that is assumed to have been pneumococcal. Hemolysis ceases, and the hematocrit slowly returns to normal. A G-6-PD assay on his red blood cells months later shows a level approximately 10% of normal. The neonatal jaundice may have been due to his G-6-PD deficiency, with hemolysis precipitated by an acute illness or oxidative drug (such as vitamin K).

TABLE 12.2. Drugs and Illnesses Precipitating Hemolysis in African-Americans with G-6-PD Deficiency[a]

Nitrofurantoin and other nitrofurans
Nalidixic acid
Methylene blue
Phenazopyridine hydrochloride
Primaquine
Various sulfonamides
Naphthalene (moth balls)
Certain infections such as pneumonia and hepatitis
Diabetic ketoacidosis (?)

[a]This common type of glucose-6-phosphate dehydrogenase (G-6-PD) deficiency (G-6-PD A) is relatively mild. Among whites G-6-PD Mediterranean is a common variant and is associated with more severe deficiency of the enzyme and thus a longer list of drugs that may cause hemolysis.

Questions

1. The patient's sister:
   (a) cannot have inherited the gene for G-6-PD deficiency.
   (b) may have inherited the gene for G-6-PD deficiency from her father.
   (c) has a 50% chance of carrying the gene for G-6-PD deficiency and, if affected, may be susceptible to hemolysis induced by oxidant drugs.
2. Although hemoglobin was demonstrated in this patient's urine, his pigmenturia could have been due to:
   (a) hemosiderinuria.
   (b) urobilinogenuria.
   (c) bilirubinuria.
   (d) none of the aforementioned.
3. Sickle cell trait is characterized by:
   (a) the absence of clinical illness, normal blood counts, and normal blood smear.
   (b) rare episodes of pain in the extremities due to the hemoglobinopathy.
   (c) normal hematocrit, slightly elevated reticulocyte counts, and slightly shortened red blood cell survival.
   (d) hemolytic episodes during severe exertion.
4. A positive direct Coombs' test result may be seen in each of the following except:
   (a) hemolysis due to a cold agglutinin appearing after *M. pneumoniae* infection.
   (b) an Rh-negative (D−) woman who has borne an Rh-positive (D+) baby.
   (c) a patient receiving large doses of penicillin who develops hemolysis due to anti-penicillin antibodies.
   (d) a patient with systemic lupus erythematosus who develops hemolytic anemia.
5. Hereditary spherocytosis is characterized by each of the following except:
   (a) splenomegaly.
   (b) red blood cells on the blood smear with reduced diameter and absent central pallor.
   (c) return to normality of red blood cell shape following splenectomy.
   (d) red blood cells with increased osmotic fragility.

Answers

1. **(c) is correct.** G-6-PD deficiency is transmitted as an X-linked recessive trait. Therefore, the patient inherited it from his mother, a presumed heterozygote, and his sister would have a 50% chance of being a heterozygote as well. Although female heterozygotes on the average have higher enzyme levels than the male hemizygotes because of their second (normal) X chromosome, the Lyon hypothesis of random inactivation of the X chromosome predicts that some female heterozygotes will have very low enzyme levels. Furthermore, clinical experience has shown that heterozygous women may have hemolytic episodes, and the diagnosis must be considered in women as well as in men.
2. **(d) is correct.** The patient could have hemosiderin in his urine due to uptake of filtered hemoglobin by tubular cells and conversion of the iron to this insoluble storage compound. Usually more prolonged hemolysis is required to produce detectable urinary hemosiderin, which is identified by staining the sediment with Prussian blue. However, hemosiderin does not discolor the urine. Urobilinogen, arising from bacterial degradation of bilirubin in the gut, is increased in the urine in hemolysis, but it also does not discolor the urine. Bilirubin may produce a yellow to brown color in the urine, but only conjugated (direct-reacting) bilirubin is excreted by the kidney. This patient's increased bilirubin was unconjugated (indirect) and would not appear in the urine.
3. **(a) is correct.** Painful crises do not occur in sickle cell trait as implied in answer **(b).** Red blood cell survival is normal, and hemolysis is not precipitated by exertion, illness, or other common stresses.
4. **(b) is correct.** Such a woman might have a positive *indirect* Coombs' test result due to anti-D antibodies in her serum but would not have a positive *direct* Coombs' test result (i.e., antibodies on her D-negative red blood

cells). A positive direct Coombs' test result occurs in cold agglutinin hemolysis, usually because of the presence of complement on the red blood cell surface that has been fixed there by the cold-reactive IgM antibody. Penicillin-related immune hemolysis occurs when penicillin, present in high concentration, binds to the red blood cell surface and reacts there with anti-penicillin immunoglobulin G (IgG) antibodies. The red cell is damaged even though the antibody is not directed against red blood cell antigens. If penicillin is present, a positive direct Coombs' test result may be seen. Obviously, the Coombs' test will not yield positive results if administration of penicillin has been stopped, and the drug is cleared from the circulation. Autoimmune hemolytic anemia may complicate systemic lupus erythematosus, and the anti-red blood cell autoantibody is detected by the direct Coombs' test.

5. **(c) is correct.** Although splenectomy virtually cures the hemolytic process so that red blood cell life span returns to near normal, the inherited abnormality of red blood cell shape persists. Mild splenomegaly is characteristic of hereditary spherocytosis. Spherocytes in hereditary spherocytosis are microspherocytes and appear on the blood smear as described in (b). Because of their decreased surface area-volume ratio, hereditary spherocytes have a limited ability to swell in hypotonic solution and therefore characteristically have increased osmotic fragility.

COMMENTS It was evident in this case that the patient had another disease process coincident with or caused by the pneumonia. Any one of several key clues could have led to the correct diagnosis using a branching process. You could start with either dark urine, anemia, or icterus. An analysis of the urine would have pointed directly to hemoglobinuria. Myoglobinuria is ruled out by special tests or by the absence of pigment in the serum. Had you begun with anemia, the high reticulocyte index in the absence of obvious hemorrhage would lead to the same conclusion. Bilirubin fractionation would have indicated hemolysis had you started with jaundice as the key clue.

From that point, it was simply a matter of pinpointing the cause for the hemolysis. This too was easily accomplished by a branching process. The results of the Coombs' test, *Mycoplasma* complement fixation, hemoglobin electrophoresis, and G-6-PD measurement led in one direc-

tion or another. In essence, the author followed a self-constructed flowchart. *(P.C.)*

Suggested Readings

Beutler E. G6PD deficiency. Blood 1994;84:3613–3636.

Burka ER, Weaver Z III, Marks PA. Clinical spectrum of hemolytic anemia associated with G-6-PD deficiency. Ann Intern Med 1996;64:817–825.

Tabbara IA. Hemolytic anemias. Diagnosis and management. Med Clin North Am 1992:76:649–668.

NECK LUMPS

Paul Cutler

Data A 17-year-old female sought medical attention because she noticed lumps in the left side of her neck. She had been in excellent health until 2 years ago when she had similar neck lumps. That illness was associated with fever, sore throat, and malaise from which she recovered in 2 weeks. On the basis of examination and blood tests, a physician had diagnosed infectious mononucleosis (IM). At the present time, the patient has none of the symptoms that were associated with her previous neck lumps.

Logic The earlier illness sounds like IM and you make a note to contact the previous physician and confirm that impression; you expect that she had atypical lymphocytes and a positive heterophil antibody test result. Even so, the current lumps are not likely to be recurrent IM and probably represent something new.

A problem of this sort could be solved by the traditional complete history, physical examination, and laboratory tests. But who could proceed without first feeling the lumps, verifying what they are, seeing if there are others, and asking parallel questions?

First, what are the lumps? Are they lymph nodes, tumors, cysts, or congenital remnants? Localized lymph node swelling can be caused by viral diseases, upper respiratory tract infections, recent immunizations, tooth abscesses, cat-scratch disease, metastatic cancer, lymphoma, tuberculosis, or an infection anywhere that is draining into regional lymph nodes.

Generalized lymphadenopathy, on the other

hand, suggests lymphoma, leukemia, sarcoidosis, systemic lupus erythematosus (SLE), brucellosis, IM, syphilis, lipoidosis, Graves' disease, the use of hydantoins for epilepsy, and HIV disease.

Data There is a 3 × 3-cm firm, nontender, freely movable nodule in the left neck just above the sternoclavicular joint, and several smaller nodes to the left along the clavicle. At the same time you examine the rest of the head and neck and check the vital signs. All else is normal. There is no fever, no icterus, the thyroid gland is normal, the trachea is not deviated, and there are no signs of hyperthyroidism. The nodule does not move upward on swallowing.

Logic You are clearly dealing with large pathologic nodes. An inflamed branchial cleft cyst or aberrant thyroid can be dismissed. Absence of tenderness weighs against acute inflammation or rapid growth. A rubbery consistency, mobility, and the discreteness of nodes suggest Hodgkin's disease. Later on, Hodgkin's and tuberculous glands become matted together. Metastatic cancer is unlikely at her age.

The next important points to determine are whether the lymphadenopathy is local or generalized and whether the spleen (the largest of lymphoid organs) is enlarged.

Data A firm nontender 2- × 2-cm node is felt high in the left axilla. The chest, heart, breasts, and lungs are normal, although there seems to be some increase in splenic dullness in the midaxillary line. This finding is confirmed by a spleen that is palpable 2 cm below the left costal margin on deep inspiration. The liver has a 10-cm vertical span by percussion. No other lymph nodes are palpable. Indirect nasopharyngoscopy and indirect laryngoscopy show these areas to be normal and free of tumor. The results of the rest of the examination, including the rectopelvic and neurologic portions, is entirely normal.

Logic The association of large lymph nodes in two areas (supraclavicular and axillary) with enlargement of the spleen raises the serious question of lymphoma in your mind. But other diseases associated with generalized lymphadenopathy are all still possible. A palpable spleen is already twice normal size.

Lipoidosis has been noted at a very young age. Metastatic cancer is unlikely in a 17-year-old. Primary sites have not been found, although at this age melanoma must be carefully sought and

ruled out. There is no rash or arthritis to go with SLE. Anemia, bruises, and petechiae are not present—points that weigh against leukemia. A few questions are indicated to detect constitutional symptoms or symptoms related to specific diseases that could cause adenopathy. These questions were all asked while doing the examination.

Data She has no cat, has never drunk unpasteurized cow's or goat's milk, denies any recent illness, did receive immunizations for a trip to Europe 8 months ago, has had no weakness, anorexia, weight loss, fever, chills, night sweats, or pruritus, never had arthritis, and takes no medication. She recalls taking some sort of medicine with each acute illness as a child because she had suffered a convulsion in infancy, but she has not taken any in recent years. There is no history of frequent recurrent infections. She has never been sexually active and does not use drugs.

Logic Hydantoin anticonvulsants are associated with lymphoid hyperplasia, pseudolymphoma, and lymphoma, but their administration so long ago makes the relationship most unlikely. Animal-related diseases such as cat-transmitted viruses, tuberculosis, and brucellosis are ruled out, and her immunizations are too remote. The absence of clinically detectable anemia, visible coagulopathy, and recurrent infections tells you that even though we may still be dealing with a lymphoma or leukemia, the bone marrow is not being replaced.

Last, you have virtually excluded some diseases associated with generalized lymphadenopathy such as SLE, secondary syphilis, sarcoidosis, and AIDS, because there are no manifestations or associated clinical features of these diseases present.

At this point, serious consideration must be given to the possibility that a malignant lymphoma exists in this patient. Such lymphomas are of two types: (1) *Hodgkin's disease,* and (2) *non-Hodgkin's* lymphoma. Besides differences in histology, there are a number of distinguishing clinical features.

Patients who have *Hodgkin's disease* usually are initially seen by the physician in one of three ways: (1) nodes in the neck; (2) asymptomatic mediastinal widening seen on routine chest radiograph; and (3) B symptoms (systemic)," which consist of fever, night sweats, and significant weight loss (10% body weight in 6 months). Pruritus was once considered a member of this group, but is no longer. B symptoms were not present in this patient, but because only 30% of patients with Hodgkin's disease have B symptoms, this diagnosis is not excluded. These symptoms are uncommon in non-Hodgkin's lymphoma, and if present, they occur late in the course of the disease.

The clinical features that tend to differentiate Hodgkin's disease from non-Hodgkin's lymphomas are noted in Table 12.3. But it must be pointed out that the non-Hodgkin's lymphomas include a large number of subtypes, such as those that are related to renal transplantation, AIDS, human T-cell lymphotropic virus (HTLV-1), Epstein-Barr virus, and Burkitt's lymphoma.

Although a biopsy must ultimately be done, laboratory studies are indicated at this time. If lymphoma is present, the cell type and precise architecture are required to determine prognosis and treatment.

Data Thyroxine (T_4) test result is normal. Blood studies show hemoglobin, 11.0 g/dL; hematocrit, 33%; red blood cell count, 4.5 million per mm³; mean corpuscular volume, 73 μm³; mean corpuscular hemoglobin, 24 pg; white blood cell count, 6,200/mm³; differential, normal; and platelet count, 186,000/mm³. The smear shows red blood cell hypochromia.

Chest radiograph demonstrates a normal posteroanterior view, but encroachment on the retrosternal clear space is noted on the lateral view. Liver function tests are normal, but the alkaline phosphatase level is slightly increased (10% above normal). The Venereal Disease Research Laboratory test result is negative. Protein electrophoresis, serum calcium, and antinuclear antibody test results are normal or negative.

Logic The patient has a mild hypochromic microcytic anemia by indices and smear. This was not detected clinically. In a 17-year-old, the most common cause is iron lack due to heavy menses. Platelets are slightly low, but you realize that platelets have a tendency to pool in a large spleen. Leukemia is virtually ruled out.

The normal posteroanterior chest radiograph, serum calcium, and proteins are strong evidence against sarcoidosis. SLE can now be eliminated by the absence of commonly associated clinical features. But the suggestion of involvement of the anterior mediastinum as reflected in the retrosternal mass makes lymphoma an increasingly likely diagnosis in a patient with three other lymphatic sites involved. Remember that the thymus and substernal thyroid are in this location too.

The elevation of alkaline phosphatase is slight and may be inconsequential, although it raises the question of liver or bone involvement. More studies are needed to prepare for surgical biopsy of the large node.

Data Results of urinalysis, blood urea nitrogen, creatinine, prothrombin time, and partial thromboplastin time are all normal. Computed tomography of the chest confirms the presence of anterior mediastinal adenopathy.

Logic You call the surgeon to examine the node with you so that there is no confusion as to which

TABLE 12.3. **Distinguishing Clinical Features Between Hodgkin's Disease and Non-Hodgkin's Lymphomas**[a]

| Feature | LYMPHOMA | |
	Hodgkin's	Non-Hodgkin's
Cell origin	Not determined	B cell 90%; T cell 10%
Genetic translocation	Not determined	Common
Reed-Sternberg cell	Always present	Rare
B symptoms	Common	Rare
Localized disease	Common	Uncommon
Special sites		
Mediastinum	Common	Uncommon
Abdominal nodes	Uncommon	Common
Bone marrow, bones, skin	Uncommon	Common

[a]Involvement of cervical nodes, liver, and spleen is common to both disorders.

one is to be removed. You want the largest supra-clavicular node to be sampled. Then you call the pathologist to do a touch preparation of the lymph node by pressing the cut surface immediately to a microscope slide and making multiple impressions. The tissue will be fixed and sectioned.

Data These studies are all done following removal of the node. The following day you and the pathologist review the tissue. The touch preparation, stained by Wright's stain, shows normal lymphocytes and not much else. The fixed tissue shows bands of collagen, a nodular pattern, and rare classical Reed-Sternberg cells.

Logic The pathologist calls this typical nodular sclerosing Hodgkin's disease. There are four histologic types of Hodgkin's disease:

1. Lymphocyte predominant
2. Nodular sclerosis
3. Mixed cellularity
4. Lymphocyte depleted

Nodular sclerosis, as exists in this patient, is the most common type, and it consists of lymphoid nodules interspersed with collagen bands. The Reed-Sternberg (R-S) cell is a giant multinucleated cell with eosinophilic nucleoli; it is present in each of the four types, and the diagnosis of Hodgkin's disease can be made only if these cells are found. Although the malignant cell lineage cannot be traced to B or T cells, nor can a genetic translocation be identified as in non-Hodgkin's lymphoma, it is interesting to note that the genome for the Epstein-Barr virus can be found within the R-S cell (Fig. 12.8).

Because the prognosis and the selection of appropriate treatment depend in large measure on the extent of disease, it is important to determine the various sites that have been involved. Are the anemia and slight thrombocytopenia a reflection of bone marrow involvement? Is the elevated alkaline phosphatase level a result of liver involvement? Is the enlarged spleen due to Hodgkin's disease? Could there be lymph node involvement below the diaphragm? Further studies are indicated.

Data A bone marrow biopsy shows no evidence of Hodgkin's disease, but the metarubricytes are small and show delayed hemoglobinization. An iron stain shows no stainable iron. A percutaneous liver biopsy shows normal liver. The patient undergoes a lymphogram, whose results are negative.

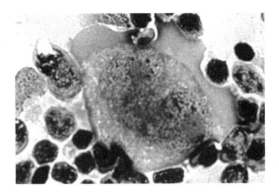

▶ **Figure 12.8.** Reed-Sternberg cell and adjacent lymphocytes (highly magnified).

Logic Computed tomography is useful to detect enlarged lymph nodes at any site in the abdomen. Lymphography, however, is particularly useful in staging Hodgkin's disease. It visualizes the retroperitoneal nodes, most commonly involved in Hodgkin's disease, and it can detect lymph nodes that are not only enlarged, but of abnormal structure. In addition, it is useful in directing the surgeon to the diseased nodes, the removal of which can be confirmed by a scout film of the abdomen in the operating room. Finally, if abnormal nodes are visualized, their response to therapy can be followed by periodic scout films of the abdomen to visualize changes in the conformation and size of the retained contrast material.

We now have a patient who has four lymphatic areas involved, including the supraclavicular, axillary, and mediastinal nodes and the spleen. She has a clinical stage (CS) III$_S$A, meaning that she has disease above and below the diaphragm (III), that she has clinical involvement of the spleen (s), and that she has no systemic symptoms (A). We know that in patients who have splenic enlargement in Hodgkin's disease, approximately one third do not have Hodgkin's disease in the spleen when it is removed and examined. Similarly, if the spleen is normal in size, one third have Hodgkin's disease as revealed by pathologic examination. Furthermore, the lymphogram does not visualize upper abdominal, splenic, porta hepatic, or mesenteric nodes. Finally, splenic involvement with Hodgkin's disease enhances the likelihood of liver involvement, despite a negative percutaneous biopsy result. You would like the patient to have as little therapy as possible because of the risk of complications and a second malignancy. You ask the surgeon to do a staging laparotomy.

Data The patient is taken to the operating room and, through a midline incision, the liver undergoes biopsy, the spleen is removed, and multiple lymph nodes undergo biopsy. She is returned to her room without event. The pathologist slices the spleen in 2-mm-thick slices and finds no gross Hodgkin's disease. All abdominal tissue shows no abnormalities. The spleen shows follicular hyperplasia.

Logic You know that the enlarged spleen is not due to Hodgkin's disease. She has disease above the diaphragm only (stage II) and has no symptoms (A). There are three sites above the diaphragm involved, so the notation would be (II_3). We thus have a patient with CS III_SA who, after further tissue was obtained, was found to have a different, less extensive pathologic stage (PS), IIA. The convention is to use a subscript to note all additional tissue for which a biopsy is performed, such as liver $(_H)$, spleen $(_S)$, nodes $(_N)$, and bone marrow $(_M)$; and a $(+)$ or $(-)$ to indicate whether Hodgkin's disease was found on biopsy. Thus, the complete clinical and pathologic staging notation for this patient would be: CS III_SA PS $II_3A_{M-S-H-N+}$.

It should be emphasized that staging laparotomy is indicated *only* when it is likely that the outcome would influence the choice of therapy. The splenomegaly suggested the presence of upper abdominal disease, which may have changed the patient's therapy from radiotherapy alone to combined radiotherapy and chemotherapy.

A doctor-patient conference concerning treatment options can now take place.

Questions

1. Lumps in the left groin bring a healthy 28-year-old man to your office. On examination, the lumps are firm, nontender, pathologic lymph nodes. Furthermore, he has a 1-inch scar on his left foot where a "small tumor" was removed 6 months ago in a nearby town. Severe "athlete's foot" is also present. The first and most helpful action to do is:
   (a) biopsy a node.
   (b) special test on urine.
   (c) liver scan.
   (d) get pathologic report on "small tumor."
2. In reference to Hodgkin's disease, which *one* of the following statements is true:
   (a) Mediastinal, splenic, mesenteric, or para-aortic nodes may be involved.
   (b) Mediastinal node involvement suggests intra-abdominal node disease.
   (c) The bone marrow is involved in 20% of patients who have Hodgkin's disease.
   (d) Anemia may result from bone marrow involvement, hypersplenism, or hemolysis.
3. Hodgkin's disease can have many different presentations. Which of the following presentations is/are possible?
   (a) Episodic fever and sweats
   (b) Superior vena cava obstruction
   (c) Generalized pruritus
   (d) Hilar adenopathy on routine radiograph
4. You see a 40-year-old man who complains of fevers, night sweats, and considerable weight loss. On examination, there are enlarged nodes on both sides of the neck and in both axillae, the spleen is palpable, and the liver has a vertical diameter of 15 cm. Chest radiograph and bone marrow aspiration are normal. High-resolution CT scan of the abdomen and pelvis confirms the enlarged liver and spleen, but there are no enlarged nodes. Lymph node biopsy reveals typical findings of mixed cellularity Hodgkin's disease. Derive the clinical and pathologic stages in this patient.
5. While shaving, a 60-year-old man notices a lump in his neck. It is firm, nontender, and the size of a walnut. There are no other symptoms, and his examination is otherwise not remarkable. The lump is just anterior to the midpoint of the right sternomastoid muscle. Which of the following items of information may be helpful, and in what order?
   (a) Nasopharyngoscopy
   (b) Chest radiograph
   (c) Thyroid function tests
   (d) History of cigarette smoking
   (e) Biopsy
   (f) CT or MRI of the neck
   (g) Upper gastrointestinal radiographs

Answers

1. **(d) is correct.** Melanoma sounds likely, and a simple telephone call may solve the problem. The urine can be tested for melanin, but the result is not commonly positive. A liver scan may disclose large hepatic metastases—common in melanoma. A node biopsy will give a positive diagnosis. Fungal infections can cause large nodes from repeated

episodes of cellulitis. All the answers are correct, but (d) is simple, easily done, and may be most productive.

2. **(d) is correct.** The anemia may have one or more of several causes. Mesenteric node involvement is uncommon in Hodgkin's disease. It is common in non-Hodgkin's lymphoma and should raise suspicion about the histologic classification of the original lymph node biopsy if discovered at staging laparotomy. The other nodes mentioned are commonly involved. Abdominal node involvement is suggested by the presence of nodes in the supraclavicular and axillary areas, not in the mediastinum. This relates to the anatomic proximity of the celiac nodes and thoracic duct. Only 5% of patients with Hodgkin's disease have bone marrow involvement, in contrast to patients with non-Hodgkin's lymphoma, in whom the incidence is 40 to 50% for the nodular forms.

3. **All are correct.** Each symptom can be the initial manifestation or presentation. Large nodes high in the mediastinum can obstruct the vena cava and cause distention of veins and swelling of the neck, arms, and face. Itching is common in younger women. The fever is called Pel-Ebstein fever.

4. $CS\ IV_{4N,\ H,\ S}\ B$
   $PS\ IV_6\ B_{M-\ S?\ H?\ N+}$

Clinical staging

IV indicates diffuse disease, above and below the diaphragm, including liver involvement. Four nodal sites as well as the spleen appear diseased. B symptoms are present.

Pathologic staging

Six sites are involved, although the bone marrow is not involved; spleen and liver are probably also involved, although this will require tissue verification.

Recent additions to the staging nomenclature (Cotswolds seminar) include X for bulky disease and E for disease in extranodal contiguous sites such as bone, lung, pericardium.

5. **(d)-(b)-(a)-(g)-(f)-(e).** The preferred order may vary. (c) is of no value because the mass is not thyroid-related. The other items may all be helpful. Until proved otherwise, in this age group metastasis from a malignancy of the upper aerodigestive tract is the number one contender. Studies may stop if the endpoint is reached early.

COMMENT Pursuit of a diagnosis here is ideally suited to an algorithmic approach whereby a decision path or flowchart is used. Numerous questions and tests can be avoided and diagnostic possibilities quickly eliminated, depending on the direction taken at key branching points.

The following decisions must be made:

• Are the lumps caused by enlarged lymph nodes?
• Are they local or disseminated?
• Is the spleen palpable?
• Is there evidence of bone marrow involvement and constitutional symptoms, and are there clues for other diseases causing lymphadenopathy? "Yes" or "no" answers direct you to a terminal branch of the diagnostic tree.

Age and gender enter the picture. Most patients with enlarged glands will have malignancy, infection, or connective tissue disease; the likelihood of each will vary with age and gender.

Likelihoods were listed and excluded one by one. At the same time, a pattern for lymphoma was gradually woven and proven with the decisive clue—a biopsy. A previous episode of swollen glands (IM) and the former taking of medication for convulsions were misleading clues. The specificity, sensitivity, and importance of liver and spleen size were carefully considered. And last, the need for a team approach by three physicians was demonstrated. *(P.C.)*

Suggested Readings

Levine AM. Acquired immunodeficiency syndrome-related lymphoma. Blood 1992;80:8.

Pangalis GA, Vassila Kopoulos TP, Boussiotis VA, et al. Clinical approach to lymphadenopathy. Semin Oncol 1993;20:570.

Urba WT, Longo DL. Hodgkin's disease. N Engl J Med 1992;326:678.

Williams SF, Golomb HM. Non-Hodgkin's lymphoma. Semin Oncol 1990;17:1.

CASE 8

ELEVATED HEMATOCRIT

Roger M. Lyons

Data A 55-year-old male oil rig worker was admitted to the hospital for an elective herniorrhaphy. The preoperative work-up revealed a hematocrit (Hct) of 56, and surgery was delayed.

Logic In considering a patient with an elevated Hct, you must first distinguish between a transient and a persistent increase in Hct above the upper limit of normal (52% for a man and 47% for a woman). Even with the limited information given previously, it is clear that the patient is not severely ill, as is usually the case in patients who are dehydrated with a transient increase in Hct (e.g., diarrhea, diabetic ketoacidosis, heat prostration, and severe burns).

Data Six months before this admission he was told that he had "too much blood," and a review of his records revealed elevated Hct levels recorded on two separate occasions during the previous year.

Logic In view of this information, both a transient elevation in Hct and a laboratory error can be excluded. The following is a pathophysiologic classification of patients who have persistently elevated Hct levels:

- Polycythemia rubra vera (P. vera)
- Polycythemia secondary to physiologically appropriate excessive erythropoietin production associated with hypoxia: for example, pulmonary disease, high altitude, cyanotic heart disease, hemoglobinopathy with high oxygen affinity, and carboxyhemoglobinemia
- Polycythemia secondary to physiologically inappropriate production of erythropoietin by a tumor or renal cyst or excessive administration of recombinant erythropoietin
- Relative (spurious) polycythemia

Relative polycythemia is separated from P. vera and the secondary polycythemias by the fact that the elevated Hct in relative polycythemias does not indicate a true increase in body red blood cell mass. The plasma volume is decreased, so that the red blood cell count is only relatively increased. It is important to note that the relative or spurious polycythemia is the most common cause of an elevated Hct in the general population in this country.

Normally the red blood cell mass is hormonally controlled by a negative feedback loop. A persistent fall in arterial oxygen saturation results in the production of erythropoietin, a glycoprotein that is made almost entirely by the peritubular cells of the renal interstitium in adult humans. Erythropoietin acts on the red blood cell precursors in the bone marrow, resulting in an increase in red blood cell production, red blood cell mass, and oxygen-carrying capacity of the blood. If the

red blood cell mass increases to abnormally high levels, the viscosity of the blood increases, resulting in decreased blood flow and paradoxical tissue hypoxia, particularly in the central nervous system. This sequence is physiologically appropriate for chronic hypoxia.

On the other hand, certain tumors can elaborate an erythropoietin-like substance. This is not physiologically appropriate and can be caused by seemingly unrelated tumors like cerebellar hemangioblastoma, renal carcinoma or cyst, hepatoma, and unusual uterine tumors.

P. vera is not associated with increased erythropoietin levels. In this case an abnormal clone of red blood cell precursors appears to be exquisitely sensitive to stimulation by erythropoietin, and red blood cell production continues despite a very low level of erythropoietin.

With the information available, none of these possibilities can be excluded. If the patient were a woman rather than a man, relative polycythemia would be unlikely because that condition rarely occurs in women. The patient's age is not helpful, because the average onset of P. vera is 60 years and that of relative polycythemia is 52 years.

Data On further questioning the patient admitted to a 30 pack-year cigarette history. He had a chronic morning cough productive of small amounts of brown sputum, but he had no shortness of breath. He had been a heavy drinker but had not had any alcohol intake for more than 5 years. Recently he spent a 2-week vacation in Mexico but had not been at high altitude. He gave no family history of blood problems, but there was a significant family history of hypertension. He had previously been diagnosed as having mild hypertension but had not taken the medication prescribed. There was no history of renal disease. There was no bleeding, thromboembolism, weight loss, or night sweats. He did have mild pruritus with dry skin.

Logic The history of smoking suggests the possibility of carboxyhemoglobinemia as the result of carbon monoxide in cigarette smoke. Carbon monoxide binds to hemoglobin and prevents the latter from binding oxygen and also increases the oxygen affinity of hemoglobin; the half-life cycle of the carbon monoxide-hemoglobin complex is approximately 4 hours. Tissue hypoxia may result, and this stimulates erythropoietin production with a resultant increase in the Hct. Approximately 45% of smokers have been noted to have an elevated carboxyhemoglobin level and 3% have an elevated Hct.

The absence of a family history of blood problems suggests that a hemoglobinopathy is unlikely, but this possibility cannot be completely ruled out. Time spent at high altitude can be ruled out as a cause for the increased Hct. Hypoxia due to low atmospheric pressure causes an almost immediate increase in erythropoietin concentration, with resultant reticulocytosis at 3 to 5 days, and then a slow increase in the Hct. Many months may pass before the Hct reaches a new stable level. The rise in the Hct is roughly proportional to the altitude.

Data The initial part of the physical examination revealed a moderately obese man in no acute distress. His vital signs were normal, with the exception of a blood pressure of 140/95. On inspection, he had a ruddy complexion but was not cyanotic.

Logic The general appearance and absence of weight loss suggest that he does not have a widespread malignancy. However, both localized hypernephromas and hepatomas have been associated with ectopic erythropoietin production, and the incidence of hepatoma is increased in patients with alcoholic liver disease. These are rare and thus unlikely, but are not ruled out. The patient's ruddy complexion is consistent with his elevated Hct, hyperviscosity, and resultant inadequate oxygenation of circulating hemoglobin. One must be careful not to overinterpret the complexion, because persons who spend much of their time outdoors, as this man does, frequently have ruddy complexions.

Data Further examination revealed dilatation of his conjunctival blood vessels and retinal veins. His heart and lungs were normal. The liver was not tender but was palpable 3 cm below the right costal margin with a total vertical span of 15 cm. The tip of the spleen was clearly palpable 1 cm below the left costal margin on deep inspiration. No other abdominal masses could be felt. He did not have calf tenderness, pedal edema, or adenopathy. Neurologic examination, including gait and coordination, was completely normal. Stool guaiac test result was negative.

Logic The dilatation of conjunctival and retinal vessels suggests an increased blood volume and hyperviscosity of the blood as is seen in poly-

cythemia, but which may also be seen in association with the hyperviscosity of paraproteinemia, or occasionally in patients who have CO_2 retention. The lack of significant cardiac or pulmonary abnormalities suggests that cyanotic heart disease or severe pulmonary disease is unlikely.

The abdominal examination in a patient who has an elevated Hct is of critical importance. Hepatomegaly in this man is consistent with his drinking history, but the lack of gynecomastia, spider hemangiomas, palmar erythema, and testicular atrophy suggests that he does not have extensive alcohol-induced hepatic damage. Splenomegaly could be present on the basis of hepatic cirrhosis and portal hypertension but, as just indicated, he probably does not have severe liver disease. Hepatomegaly is present in 30 to 50%, and splenomegaly is present in 75% of patients who have P. vera. Splenomegaly is a major point in the differential diagnosis of an elevated Hct because it is not likely to be present in either secondary or relative polycythemia. The normal neurologic examination is strong evidence for the absence of a cerebellar hemangioblastoma, a third type of tumor that has been associated with ectopic erythropoietin production.

Data The Hct was 55 and 56% on two separate occasions, along with an MCV of 76 and RDW of 17. The white blood cell count was 14,000/mm³ with a normal differential, and the platelet count was 550,000/mm³. The blood smear did not show rouleaux formation, and the red blood cell morphology suggested mild micro-ovalocytic hypochromic changes. An 18-test chemistry profile was normal except for a uric acid of 9.5 mg/dL and an LDH of 235 U/L. Prothrombin time and partial thromboplastin time were normal, as was a serum protein electrophoresis.

Logic An elevated white blood cell and platelet count are strongly suggestive of P. vera. This is one of the myeloproliferative disorders that are presumed to be manifestations of disease of the hematopoietic stem cell. In these disorders (P. vera, chronic granulocytic leukemia, essential thrombocytosis, myelofibrosis), erythrocytic, granulocytic, monocytic, and megakaryocytic cell lines proliferate en masse (to a variable degree in each disorder) rather than individually. However, a moderately elevated WBC count is commonly seen in smokers.

The hypochromic micro-ovalocytic red blood

cells with a low MCV and elevated RDW suggest iron deficiency that almost universally accompanies P. vera (bone marrow iron stores are absent in 95% of patients with P. vera). This is usually due to a combination of increased gastrointestinal blood loss and increased utilization of iron to enlarge the red blood cell mass. An elevated RBC count with a low MCV is the hallmark of erythrocytosis with iron deficiency and is occasionally seen in thalassemia. There is a defect in hemostasis in P. vera on two bases. First, local vessel dilatation from hyperviscosity and tissue anoxia results in a defect in the vascular phase of hemostasis with an inability of the vessels to contract normally when injured. Second, platelet function is frequently defective. The incidence of peptic ulcer disease is increased in P. vera (15% of patients), most likely because of the increased basophil count and blood histamine levels that have been observed in this disease; this results in increased gastric acid production.

At this point, despite the strong suggestion that the patient might have P. vera, the diagnosis has not been definitely established, and therapy would be inappropriate. The Hct is only a relative number reflecting the ratio of red blood cell mass to plasma volume. Thus a decrease in plasma volume in association with a normal red blood cell mass (as in relative polycythemia) might be present. It is not until the Hct is more than 60% that one can be assured that the red blood cell mass is increased. We have not ruled out the possibility of hypoxia (i.e., physiologically appropriate secondary polycythemia) as the cause of this man's problem.

Frequently patients with chronic hypoxic pulmonary disease will have a normal Hct despite a persistently decreased arterial oxygen saturation. All causes of anemia should be considered in a patient with a normal Hct who is hypoxic and should be polycythemic. Chronic infection as seen in many patients with bronchitis or bronchiectasis could result in the observed Hct. In addition, many patients with chronic pulmonary disease have an increased plasma volume and an increase in red blood cell mass appropriate for their hypoxia. The resultant Hct would be normal.

Data Arterial blood was drawn, and the PO_2 was 85 mm Hg, with a saturation of 96%. The ^{51}Cr red blood cell mass was 40 mL/kg (normal is <36 mL/kg for a man), and the plasma volume measured as the ^{125}I albumin space was normal. A leukocyte alkaline phosphatase score was 130 U/L (normal is 20 to 100 U/L), and the vitamin B_{12} level was 1100 pg/mL (normal is 200 to 900). Serum iron was 30 $\mu g/dL$, and the total iron-binding capacity was 400 $\mu g/dL$, with a low saturation of 7.5%. Serum ferritin was 10 ng/mL.

Logic The diagnosis of polycythemia rubra vera is established on the basis of an elevated red cell mass, and polycythemia due to hypoxia is excluded on the basis of the normal arterial oxygen saturation (i.e., >92%). In association with splenomegaly, these findings are adequate criteria for the diagnosis of P. vera. If splenomegaly were absent, two of the following (all present in this patient) would have been necessary to confirm a diagnosis of P. vera:

- Thrombocytosi > 400,000/mm^3
- Leukocytosis > 12,000/mm^3 in the absence of fever or infection
- Leukocyte alkaline phosphatase score > 100 U/L in the absence of fever or infection
- Vitamin B_{12} > 900 pg/mL or unbound vitamin B_{12} binding capacity of > 2200 pg/mL

The increased vitamin B_{12} binding capacity and vitamin B_{12} level are seen in only 10% of patients with P. vera and likely should be removed from the diagnostic criteria. The etiology of the increased leukocyte alkaline phosphatase is unknown.

If adequate criteria to diagnose P. vera were not present, the other major causes of secondary polycythemia would have been evaluated as follows:

- Renal or hepatic cyst or tumor—CT of the abdomen is the study of choice to evaluate liver and kidneys and has the advantage of providing information about splenic size.
- Carboxyhemoglobinemia—carboxyhemoglobin level.
- Hemoglobinopathy with increased oxygen-binding affinity—$P_{50}O_2$; a decrease in $P_{50}O_2$ (the oxygen tension at half-maximal saturation of hemoglobin with O_2) indicates an abnormal hemoglobin with increased oxygen binding.

To evaluate the presence of excessive erythropoietin production, reliable measurements of erythropoietin can be commercially obtained. This measurement is occasionally needed to separate different types of erythrocytosis. Growth of erythroid colonies in bone marrow tissue cultures in the absence of exogenous erythropoietin is presumptive evidence for a myeloproliferative disorder. A diagnosis of relative polycythemia (normal red blood cell mass and decreased plasma volume) does not necessarily indicate a benign prognosis because these patients have an increased incidence of hypertension and thromboembolic disease with a shorter life span than the general population.

Data The patient had 1 U of blood removed per week until his Hct was below 45%; it was maintained at this level by phlebotomy for 4 months. At that time, he was readmitted to the hospital and underwent herniorrhaphy without complications.

Logic Hemorrhage and thrombosis are common complications in a surgical patient with uncontrolled P. vera. The complication rate for bleeding and thromboembolism is immediately lowered by phlebotomy to a Hct of < 45%, but the hemorrhage rate does not return to baseline until the patient has been under adequate control for approximately 4 months. The increased rate of thromboembolism does not return to baseline until the Hct has been controlled for 3 to 4 years.

Data The patient was followed up on a regular basis, and his Hct was maintained at less than 45% by phlebotomy. The elevated uric acid was controlled with allopurinol. However, his platelet count continued to rise until it was persistently greater than 1.5 million per mm^3. He began to complain of easy bruisability and distressing pruritus, especially after bathing. The pruritus did not respond well to antihistamines, antiserotonins, H$_2$ blockers, cholestyramine, or lowering his platelet count to less than 1 million per mm^3 with hydroxyurea. His pruritus decreased in severity after interferon was initiated at 3 million units subcutaneously three times per week. He had the onset of painful cyanotic fingertips (erythromelalgia), but this responded promptly to daily aspirin administration.

Logic P. vera is associated with increased cellular production and turnover giving rise to hyperuricemia, hepatomegaly, and splenomegaly. The

etiology of the pruritus is unclear, but it is associated with the increased cellular turnover.

Occasionally, as the fibrosis progresses it may transform into another myeloproliferative disorder. Post-polycythemic myeloid metaplasia and myelofibrosis (PPMM) develops in 10 to 20% of patients with P. vera. The increased risk of developing acute leukemia is influenced by the type of treatment given; this complication occurs in 0.8% of patients treated with phlebotomy alone or short pulses of busulfan; in 11% of those receiving chlorambucil; and in 8% of patients treated with radioactive phosphorus. A possibly increased leukemia risk with hydroxyurea is controversial. The risk is much higher in patients who develop PPMM. Despite complications, the prognosis with good care for patients diagnosed with P. vera is excellent; median survival is 9 to 16 years.

COMMENT This problem is readily solved by a flowchart approach (Fig. 12.9). We are dealing with one key clue that has a limited number of causes and specific tests to prove each one. The use of two tests (red blood cell mass and oxygen saturation) determines which branch of the diagnostic tree to follow. Additional clues guide you further (depending on their positivity or negativity) until a solution is reached.

In general, patients with P. vera need not have studies beyond the arterial oxygen saturation, and the diagnosis is then confirmed by the total clinical picture. But 10% of patients with P. vera will have an arterial oxygen saturation between 88 and 92%. Here the diagnosis is made if other criteria are present, and diseases causing a low PO$_2$ are excluded.

You must cope with other bits of imperfect information too. Because most patients with hemoglobinopathy or carboxyhemoglobinemia may have normal oxygen saturation, you should test for those conditions whenever polycythemia exists in the appropriate clinical setting. The *dotted line* in Figure 12.9 indicates the paradox involving the latter two hemoglobin disorders; although the measured arterial oxygen saturation is usually normal, functional tissue hypoxia is present, and the polycythemia is erythropoietin-produced. *(P.C.)*

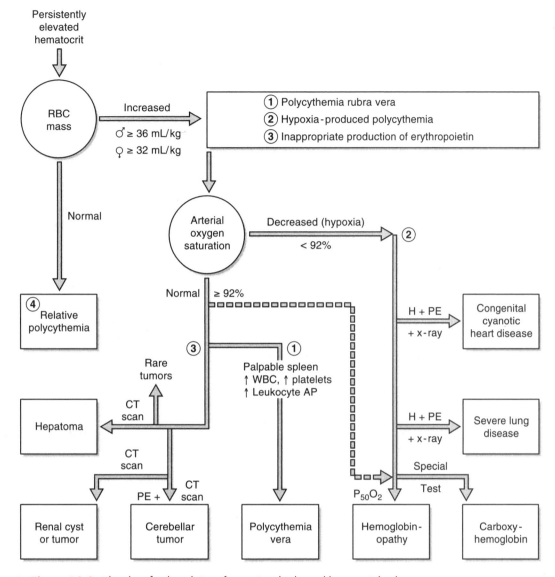

Persistently
elevated
hematocrit

RBC
mass

Increased

♂ ≥ 36 mL/kg
♀ ≥ 32 mL/kg

① Polycythemia rubra vera
② Hypoxia-produced polycythemia
③ Inappropriate production of erythropoietin

Normal

Arterial
oxygen
saturation

Decreased (hypoxia)
< 92%

②

④ Relative
polycythemia

Normal ≥ 92%

H + PE
+ x-ray

Congenital
cyanotic
heart disease

③

Rare
tumors

① Palpable spleen
↑ WBC, ↑ platelets
↑ Leukocyte AP

CT
scan

Hepatoma

H + PE
+ x-ray

Severe lung
disease

CT
scan

CT
scan

Special

PE +   CT
scan

$P_{50}O_2$ Test

Renal cyst
or tumor

Cerebellar
tumor

Polycythemia
vera

Hemoglobin-
opathy

Carboxy-
hemoglobin

▶ **Figure 12.9.** Flowchart for the solution of a persistently elevated hematocrit level.

Suggested Readings

Belgrami S, Greenberg R. Polycythemia rubra vera. Semin Oncol 1995;22:307.

Berlin NI (ed). Polycythemia. Semin Hematol 1975; 12:4;1976;13:1.

Kaplan ME, et al. Polycythemia vera: An update. Semin Hematol 1986;23:167.

Landau SA. Polycythemia vera and other polycythemic states. Clin Lab Med 1990;10:857.

Murphy S. Polycythemia vera. DM 1992;158.

CASE 9

BACKACHE, WEAKNESS, NOSEBLEEDS

Sherri S. Durica and James N. George

Data Recurrent nose bleeds and low back pain bring a 60-year-old woman to your office. She noticed intermittent brief nosebleeds for approximately 6 weeks. Three days ago one episode of bleeding lasted through the entire day. Epistaxis is a new problem for her. She has had middle and lower back pain for the past 3 months but denies any trauma before the onset. She did, however, experience a sudden worsening of the lower back pain a few weeks ago while attempting to lift a basket of laundry. The pain largely subsided with rest and local heat. The patient has also noticed a large bruise and hematoma of her left thigh that followed minimal trauma. In addition, she recently became aware of a patchy rash on her lower legs.

The patient has been a healthy, active woman all her life with no previous hospitalizations. However, for the past 4 months she felt progressively more fatigued, and during the past 2 months she was unable to do her housework. She denies fever, dyspnea, orthopnea, and chest pain. She has had a recent problem with constipation and anorexia and admits to a 10-lb weight loss to 110 pounds during the last 3 to 5 weeks.

Logic Symptoms of excessive bleeding are not specific. Epistaxis can result from many underlying causes: vascular abnormalities such as telangiectases, increased blood pressure, or a hemostatic abnormality. The recent onset of this problem indicates that it is an acquired, not a congenital, abnormality, and makes a vascular problem unlikely. Her other symptoms suggest the possibility of a chronic, progressive disease. Weakness, backache, anorexia, and constipation are all common and nonspecific symptoms, but the combination is ominous. The history that the fatigue was severe enough to change her life-style (inability to do housework) makes this a clinically important problem.

Data Examination reveals a temperature of 37 °C; pulse 90, blood pressure, 130/70; and respirations, 18/min. She appears chronically ill but is alert and well-oriented. The conjunctivae, oral mucous membranes, and tympanic membranes are pale. There is a moderate amount of dried blood in both nares. Results of examination of the chest are normal. There is an area of tenderness over the lower thoracic spine and another area of tenderness over the midlumbar spine. Heart sounds are normal; no friction rub, murmurs, or gallop rhythm sounds are heard. There are no breast masses, lymphadenopathy or hepatosplenomegaly. Examination of the extremities reveals the left thigh bruise and hematoma as

well as a faint petechial rash in the pretibial and ankle areas bilaterally. The reults of the neurologic examination are normal.

Logic The physical examination rules out hypertension as a predisposing cause for the epistaxis. The left thigh hematoma and petechiae suggest a hemostatic defect, which may be due both to abnormal coagulation (the hematoma) and platelet defect (the petechiae). The localized areas of tenderness over the thoracic and lumbar vertebrae are a serious concern. Although this could be caused by benign osteoporosis with vertebral compression fractures, such discrete and localized painful areas raise the question of a malignant disease. The exacerbation of low back pain with lifting suggests the possibility of a recent compression fracture.

Data Initial laboratory in the office were: hematocrit, 27%; reticulocyte count, 3%; white blood cell count, 3000/mm^3 with a normal differential; and a platelet count of 27,000/mm^3. The blood smear confirmed a reduced platelet count and revealed normal red blood cell morphology but significant rouleaux formation; white blood cell and platelet morphology were normal. One nucleated red blood cell was noted. Urinalysis: clear, yellow, specific gravity 1.010, no glucose or protein (by Clinistix), and no cells or bacteria in the sediment. Chest radiograph showed a lytic lesion in the left clavicle, diffuse osteopenia, and compression fractures of several thoracic vertebra. Lateral spine films revealed compression fractures of T-11 and T-12 (Fig. 12.10).

Because the patient is not currently bleeding, you elect to continue her evaluation on an outpatient basis. You give her some analgesics for her back pain and a container for a 24-hour urine collection.

Logic These initial findings indicate the presence of a disease that may account for the 4 months of chronic progressive symptoms. The anemia is due to bone marrow failure, because the reticulocyte count corrected for the degree of anemia (reticulocyte index) is only 0.9. Also the added presence of thrombocytopenia and leukopenia (pancytopenia) indicates bone marrow failure.

The other major and alarming abnormality is the presence of vertebral compression fractures and an osteolytic lesion of the clavicle. These bone changes are most likely due to a widespread malignant disease, and the associated hematopoietic ab-

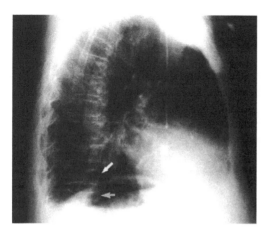

▶ **Figure 12.10.** Diffuse osteopenia and compression fractures of T-11 and T-12 in a patient who has multiple myeloma.

normalities suggest bone marrow replacement. Metastatic carcinoma may cause this, and now the normal breast examination assumes new importance. Leukemias and lymphomas do not usually cause osteolytic lesions. At this age, multiple myeloma, a malignant proliferation of plasma cells, is probably the most common cause of widespread osteolytic lesions with bone marrow failure.

Now the back pain may be explained. The anemia, which probably developed gradually, may be less responsible for the fatigue than is the underlying chronic disease. The platelet count, estimated from the blood smear to be less than 50,000/mm³, may account for the nosebleeds and petechial rash but would be less likely to cause the large thigh hematoma. The constipation and anorexia remain unexplained. Because of these abnormalities, blood chemistry measurements and routine coagulation studies are ordered.

Data The laboratory reports shows further abnormalities: ESR, 120 mm/h; creatinine, 4.2 mg/dL; total protein, 9.3 g/dL; serum albumin, 2.7 g/dL; calcium, 11.2 mg/dL; lactate dehydrogenase, 250 U/L (normal, 90 to 190 U/L); partial thromboplastin time, 43 seconds (normal, 21–36 sec); prothrombin time, 13 seconds (normal, 9.5–12.5 sec); and thrombin time, 18 seconds (normal, 9–14 sec). It is noted that the clot in the tube collected for serum failed to retract. You see the patient in clinic the next day to give her the laboratory results and discuss further diagnostic work-up.

Logic At this time multiple myeloma is the presumptive diagnosis for many reasons:

- Very high serum globulin could be the myeloma paraprotein.
- Increased globulin in myeloma typically causes marked rouleaux formation of red blood cells in the peripheral blood smear and an extremely high ESR. Occasionally, Ig paraproteins of the non-IgM type can cause plasma hyperviscosity and increased blood volume. A physical sign of this phenomenon is engorgement of the retinal veins and sometimes even "sausage linking" of the veins due to intense rouleaux formation and sluggish circulation.
- Paraproteins can interfere with blood coagulation, most commonly by inhibiting fibrin polymerization. This abnormality is most apparent in the prolonged thrombin time and poor clot retraction.
- Myeloma can be associated with the renal failure indicated in this patient by the high creatinine level. This is usually related to renal excretion of the immunoglobulin light chains (Bence-Jones protein) resulting from unbalanced immunoglobulin synthesis. The absence of proteinuria on the routine initial urinalysis is due to the insensitivity of the routine Clinistix test to immunoglobulin light chains.
- The osteolytic bone lesions are characteristic of multiple myeloma, although occasionally patients will have a presentation of diffuse osteopenia.
- The bone lesions may result in hypercalcemia, which could account for the patient's constipation and anorexia. Also, the hypercalcemia itself can cause renal damage.
- Anemia due to decreased red blood cell production is characteristic of myeloma, and granulocytopenia and thrombocytopenia are also common. To confirm the diagnosis of multiple myeloma, more studies were done.

Data Further characterization of the hyperglobulinemia is obtained by routine serum protein electrophoresis with immunofixation, and quantitative serum immunoglobulin levels. The 24-hour urine specimen that the patient collected is tested for total protein and protein electrophoresis with immunofixation.

These studies demonstrate a tall narrow "spike"

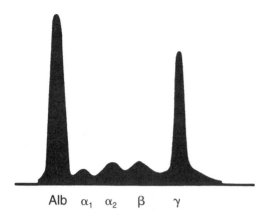

▶ **Figure 12.11.** Serum protein electrophoresis that demonstrates a paraprotein spike in the gamma (γ) region.

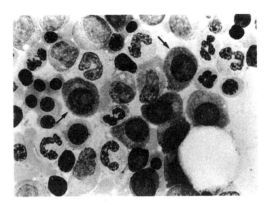

▶ **Figure 12.12.** Bone marrow aspirate showing many immature plasma cells (arrows).

of protein in the γ-globulin region of the protein electrophoresis (Fig. 12.11). Immunofixation defines this paraprotein as an IgG immunoglobulin with only κ light chains. The homogeneity of the light chains suggests a monoclonal origin of the paraprotein. Quantitative analysis of the immunoglobulins demonstrates: IgG, 5300 mg/dL; IgA, 47 mg/dL; and IgM, 23 mg/dL. The analysis of the 24-hour urine demonstrates 1.4g of protein that migrates in the globulin region and was identified as κ immunoglobulin light chains.

Additional radiographs demonstrate multiple osteolytic lesions of the skull as well as a large lytic lesion near the neck of the right femur. A bone marrow aspiration and biopsy are performed. Cellularity appears normal, but megakaryocytes are decreased. On the low-power examination a marked increase in plasma cells, readily identifiable by their deep blue cytoplasm, is immediately apparent. Both erythropoiesis and myelopoiesis appear morphologically normal under oil immersion, but the percentage of plasma cells is increased to 37% (normal, less than 5%). Many of the plasma cells are large, with immature-appearing nuclei (Fig. 12.12).

Logic These explain the patient's chronic symptoms and provide an explanation for her presenting symptom of epistaxis; the picture is classic for multiple myeloma. The occurrence of an IgG paraprotein is most common, because myeloma proteins occur with the same relative frequency as the concentration of immunoglobulins in normal serum (i.e., IgG >

IgA > IgM >> IgD >> IgE). Similarly, κ light chains are more common both in normal IgG immunoglobulins and IgG myeloma paraproteins. A decreased concentration of the other major serum immunoglobulins, IgA and IgM, is common in myeloma. Also, it is presumed that the patient is deficient in normal functioning IgG. The urine paraprotein is merely the excreted excess κ light chains synthesized by the neoplastic plasma cells but not assembled into a complete IgG molecule. The urine dipstick (Clinistix) is insensitive to these immunoglobulins and will yield negative test results in a patient who has a documented urinary paraprotein.

These immunoglobulin abnormalities are the hallmark of multiple myeloma, and it is extremely difficult to make this diagnosis without such an abnormality. Seventy-five percent of patients will have a globulin spike on serum protein electrophoresis, and one third of these patients plus almost all of the remainder will have a paraprotein in the urine. Approximately one fourth of patients with multiple myeloma will have no serum paraprotein spike revealed on standard electrophoresis. These patients synthesize only the immunoglobulin light chain that is rapidly cleared from the plasma and appears in the urine. Their clinical disease is the same as that of other patients with multiple myeloma.

The bone marrow aspirate is typical of multiple myeloma. But as the name of the disease implies, there may be nonuniform distribution of malignant plasma cells. Therefore, different results may be obtained by bone marrow aspiration from different sites.

Benign monoclonal serum immunoglobulin paraproteins occur with increasing frequency with advancing age. This situation is distinguished from multiple myeloma by the absence of urinary paraproteins, skeletal lesions, and bone marrow replacement by plasma cells.

Waldenström's macroglobulinemia is an IgM paraproteinemia that resembles but is clinically distinct from multiple myeloma. Its major presenting clinical problem is hyperviscosity. The malignant cell resembles a lymphocyte more than a plasma cell, but liver, spleen, and lymph nodes may be enlarged, renal damage is uncommon, and osteolytic lesions are rare.

Questions

1. Which one of the following statements about a serum monoclonal immunoglobulin is false?
   (a) It appears as a narrow peak in the β- or γ-globulin region of the serum protein electrophoresis.
   (b) It may appear in otherwise normal persons.
   (c) It contains only one heavy chain type.
   (d) It contains both κ and λ light chains.
2. Which one of the following is least likely to be found in a patient with newly diagnosed multiple myeloma?
   (a) Splenomegaly
   (b) Hypercalcemia
   (c) Renal insufficiency
   (d) Abnormal plasma coagulation studies
3. Which one of the following statements is false?
   Urinary immunoglobulin light chain excretion (Bence-Jones proteinuria):
   (a) is related to renal failure in multiple myeloma and is therefore a poor prognostic sign.
   (b) may be the only manifestation of a paraprotein in multiple myeloma.
   (c) consists of immunoglobulin κ or λ light chain peptides.
   (d) is ruled out by a standard Clinistix negative test result for proteinuria.
4. A "broad-based" polyclonal increase in γ-globulin may occur in all of the following diseases except:
   (a) multiple myeloma.
   (b) tuberculosis.
   (c) osteomyelitis.
   (d) decubitus ulcers.

Answers

1. **(d) is the false statement.** The definition of a monoclonal paraprotein is that it is homogeneous by all criteria, consisting of only a single chain and light chain type. The homogeneity of a monoclonal immunoglobulin is also the explanation for statements (a) and (c) being true. Monoclonal immunoglobulins of low concentration, not associated with any clinical signs of multiple myeloma, occur with increasing frequency with increasing age. Estimates of the incidence have been as high as 1% of the normal population in their sixth decade, increasing to 5% in their ninth decade.
2. **(a) is correct.** Whereas plasma cells are derived from B lymphocytes, the tumors of malignant cells occur almost exclusively in the bone marrow, and lymphadenopathy and splenomegaly are not seen. Hypercalcemia is a common sequela of bone destruction, and renal insufficiency is a common sequela of urinary immunoglobulin light chain excretion. Abnormal plasma coagulation is usually related to interference with fibrin polymerization by the myeloma paraprotein.
3. **(d) is the false statement.** The standard clinical laboratory urine test by Clinistix is sensitive only to albumin, not immunoglobulin peptides. Other standard clinical tests of proteinuria, such as drop-testing with 20% sulfosalicylic acid, will detect immunoglobulin light chains. The classic method of detecting immunoglobulin light chains is their precipitation at 56°C and their solubility when the temperature is increased to 100°C. This distinguishes them from albumin, because albumin is soluble at 56°C but precipitates as the temperature approaches 100°C. Immunoglobulin light chains are filtered by the renal glomerulus but are toxic to renal tubules, and are therefore associated with the development of renal failure and a poor prognosis in patients who have myeloma.
4. **(a) is correct.** The development of the abnormal monoclonal paraprotein in myeloma is associated with a decreased concentration of normal immunoglobulins. Therefore, the β-and γ-globulin regions of the protein electrophoresis adjacent to the narrow paraprotein spike are usually flat. A broad-based hyperglobulinemia is typical of a normal polyclonal antibody response to a severe chronic infectious or inflammatory disease, such as tuberculosis, osteomyelitis, or decubitus ulcers.

COMMENT Multiple myeloma has clinical manifestations in many organ systems; therefore, the presenting symptoms may vary. In this patient, the distressing problem of persistent epistaxis caused her to seek medical help. A downhill course, back pains, and renal failure can be seen in other diseases too (metastatic cancer, lymphoma, coincidental renal disease). But nosebleeds, anemia, and lytic bone lesions weighted the evidence heavily for myeloma, especially in a 60-year-old woman. Protein studies and bone marrow examination made the diagnosis certain. Cause and effect were thoroughly explored in relating the pathophysiology to the clinical picture. The sensitivity and specificity of monoclonal spikes, bone marrow aspirate abnormalities, and lytic bone lesions were included in the logic.

A good physician noting anemia, bone pain, renal failure, and a previous downhill course would immediately study the serum and urine proteins, bone marrow, and skull and vertebral films. The problem would be solved in 24 to 48 hours. *(P.C.)*

Suggested Readings

Barlogie B, Hoover R, Epstein J. Multiple myeloma—Recent developments in molecular and cellular biology. Curr Top Microbiol Immunol 1995;194:37–41.

Bergsagel D. The incidence and epidemiology of plasma cell neoplasms. Stem Cells 1995;13(suppl)(2):1–9.

Hussein M. Multiple myeloma: An overview of diagnosis and management. Cleve Clin J Med 1994;61(4):285–298.

Kyle RA. Diagnostic criteria of multiple myeloma. Hematol Oncol Clin North Am 1992;6(2)347–358.

CASE 10

JAUNDICE, WEAKNESS, PALLOR

Sherri S. Durica and James N. George

Data A 19-year-old man came to your office because of increasing weakness and fatigue. He had been very healthy and active all his life until 4 months ago when his family physician diagnosed hepatitis. At that time, he had anorexia, nausea, vomiting, and jaundice, preceded by several days of fever and chills. There had been no known exposure to needles and no known contact with a source of infectious hepatitis. He was in bed at home with this illness and his doctor had treated him with prochlorperazine for his nausea and vomiting. After 3 weeks of bed rest he was not jaundiced, but he continued with prochlorperazine almost daily for nausea and anorexia. He never regained enough strength to return to his job as a truck mechanic, and in the past few weeks had become even more tired and lost approximately 15 pounds. Finally, he had subjective fevers for the past 2 days but had not taken his temperature.

On physical examination, the patient was a very muscular young man who did not appear chronically ill. Vital signs: blood pressure, 110/70; pulse, 100; respirations, 12/min; and temperature, 38.8 °C. Pallor was evident in the skin and mucous membranes. The skin and sclerae were not icteric. There were no petechiae, purpura, or rashes. The lungs were clear. Cardiac examination revealed a grade II/VI early systolic ejection murmur, but no gallops or friction rubs were heard. The liver was palpable at the right costal margin, but not enlarged or tender to percussion. When the patient lay on his right side, the spleen was palpable 3 cm below the left costal margin on inspiration. There was no lymphadenopathy.

Logic At this time there was not enough to make a diagnosis. The history was consistent with the previous doctor's diagnosis of hepatitis. Because of the general principle of relating all symptoms to one diagnosis, if possible, it was reasonable to suspect that the illness was a continuing activity of his hepatitis. The liver was not enlarged or tender, but it was possible that hepatitis had progressed to cirrhosis. Splenomegaly could be due to cirrhosis with resulting portal hypertension, but there were no other physical signs of portal hypertension or cirrhosis such as ascites, distended periumbilical veins, spider angiomata, and so forth. It did seem certain that a serious illness was present. Routine blood counts and urinalysis were performed in the office.

Data Laboratory were as follows: hematocrit, 12%; white blood cell count, 300/mm³; and platelet count, 63,000/mm³. Examination of the blood smear demonstrated normochromic red blood cells with moderate anisocytosis and poikilocytosis. Red blood cell volume appeared normal. All white blood cells seen were small, mature lymphocytes. Platelets were moderately decreased, averaging three per oil field. Urinalysis was normal.

Logic These abnormalities clearly demonstrated that the illness had been present for some weeks or months, because the patient was able to tolerate the severe anemia. The presence of fever with such severe leukopenia is common and is generally due to infection with gram-negative or gram-positive bacteria, or viral or fungal organisms. These clearly explained the presenting symptoms, but finding the cause of the abnormal blood counts became urgent.

- Aplastic anemia, consistent with this degree of pancytopenia, may occur following hepatitis. To confirm this, a bone marrow aspiration and biopsy are required. It is significant that the patient had no exposure to certain drugs or organic chemicals that may have caused aplastic anemia. Many drugs have a reported association, but chloramphenicol, phenylbutazone, hydantoins, sulfonamides, gold, and benzene appear to carry a greater risk of bone marrow toxicity than other agents. Although splenomegaly is not present in aplastic anemia, the spleen may be enlarged if chronic liver disease is also present.
- Phenothiazines, such as prochlorperazine, are common causes of leukopenia, but they do not cause anemia, thrombocytopenia, and splenomegaly.
- Megaloblastic disease due to a deficiency of vitamin B_{12} or folic acid can cause severe pancytopenia, and occasionally splenomegaly. Although pernicious anemia (vitamin B_{12} deficiency) is unusual at this age, the long period of anorexia may have led to folic acid deficiency. However, there is nothing to suggest this from examination of the peripheral blood smear; the absence of oval macrocytes, striking poikilocytosis, and neutrophils would be unusual. The spleen may be palpable in 20% of patients who have pernicious anemia.
- Severe granulocytopenia and splenomegaly can also occur on an autoimmune basis. Felty's syndrome is a well-recognized cluster of granulocytopenia, splenomegaly, and rheumatoid arthritis; thrombocytopenia may also occur. But arthritis is not present in this case. And although chronic autoimmune or chronic inflammatory disease may also cause mild-to-moderate anemia, the degree of anemia in this case is inconsistent with such diseases.

- Acute leukemia must be suspected as a cause of extremely severe anemia and leukopenia, especially when accompanied by splenomegaly. Although approximately one fourth of patients with acute leukemia initially have leukopenia, it is unusual not to find myeloblasts or lymphoblasts when the peripheral blood smear is searched. Patients with acute leukemia who have a low neutrophil count are at risk of infection with a variety of organisms and must be treated with empiric antibiotic therapy if they are febrile. Chronic myelocytic leukemia and chronic lymphocytic leukemia are always associated with leukocytosis and are not a consideration.

Data Because of these severe abnormalities, the patient was admitted to the hospital. Serum chemistries were obtained and reported as normal, with the exception of an elevated LDH level of 515 U/L (normal, 90 to 190 U/L) and a uric acid level of 11.5 mg/dL (normal, 2.5 to 7.2 mg/dL). An attempt to aspirate bone marrow from the iliac crest was unsuccessful, but a core biopsy was obtained. Transfusion with 3 U of red blood cells was given. Blood cultures were drawn and broad-spectrum antibiotics begun. The next morning, the patient was afebrile and the cardiac murmur was gone.

Logic The fact that a skilled physician cannot aspirate bone marrow is very significant. Three possibilities exist: (1) the bone marrow is severely aplastic with only fat present, (2) the bone marrow is packed with leukemic or tumor cells in association with fibrosis, or (3) the bone marrow is entirely replaced by dense reticulin and collagen fibrosis. The inability to aspirate bone marrow, together with the history and physical examination, allow the following diagnostic considerations:

- Aplastic anemia is consistent with the inability to aspirate bone marrow but does not explain the splenomegaly.
- Leukopenia due to phenothiazine toxicity should not cause total bone marrow aplasia or fibrosis, and the bone marrow should be easily aspirated.
- Megaloblastic disease is associated with a very cellular bone marrow that is easily aspirated.
- Autoimmune neutropenia is also associated

with a cellular bone marrow that is easily aspirated.

- Acute leukemia may have a presentation of a densely infiltrated bone marrow that cannot be aspirated.
- Myelofibrosis with myeloid metaplasia of the spleen is consistent with inability to aspirate bone marrow and also consistent with the history and physical examination. But it rarely occurs in young persons; 60 is the average age of onset.

Therefore, acute leukemia was thought to be the most likely diagnosis, and is was probable that the previous hepatitis was *entirely coincidental*. Although there is a well-documented association between viral hepatitis and aplastic anemia, no such association had been demonstrated of acute leukemia of either lymphoblastic or myeloblastic origin, because approximately half of patients who are initially seen with these diseases have no palpable lymphadenopathy.

Transfusion was indicated not just because of the severe anemia but also because there was no apparent quickly reversible cause of the anemia. If, for example, severely megaloblastic hematopoiesis had been found by bone marrow aspiration, then rapid recovery would be expected after appropriate treatment with the deficient vitamin (B_{12} or folic acid), making immediate transfusion unnecessary even for this severe degree of anemia. Fever in a neutropenic patient must be treated empirically with broad-spectrum antibiotics in order to avoid fulminant bacterial sepsis. The presence of a heart murmur in a febrile patient should raise the possibility of endocarditis. The appropriate initial steps are the drawing of blood cultures and initiation of empiric antibiotic therapy. The observation that the murmur disappeared with correction of the anemia suggests, however, that this was most likely a flow murmur due to hyperdynamic heart action.

The observation of elevated serum LDH and uric acid levels could be related to a disease such as acute leukemia with accelerated cell turnover and release of nucleic acid urate precursors. This strengthens the suspicion of acute leukemia versus aplastic anemia.

Data Wright's-Giemsa stains of the touch imprints of the biopsy, available immediately, provided a definite diagnosis 2 days before the per-

manent histologic sections of the bone marrow could be available. The imprints demonstrated a nearly solid sheet of uniform mononuclear cells with multiple nucleoli, fine nuclear chromatin, and scant cytoplasm. These cells were primitive blast cells, precursors of either lymphocytes or granulocytes. No other normal bone marrow cells were seen—no megakaryocytes, no erythroid precursor cells, and no intermediate granulocyte precursors (Fig. 12.13).

Logic The accumulation of immature cells that are unable to differentiate but continue to divide and eventually replace normal hematopoietic tissue establishes the diagnosis of acute leukemia. The previous hepatitis was entirely coincidental. The conventional Wright's-Giemsa stain may not definitely distinguish lymphoblasts from myeloblasts (the latter being the precursor cell of granulocytes and monocytes), and this distinction is important for therapy and prognosis. Special studies were performed later that day.

Data Careful examination of the bone marrow biopsy imprint revealed no Auer rods in the cytoplasm of the blast cells and no development of granules to suggest promyelocytes. Either of these findings would be diagnostic of acute myeloblastic leukemia. A peroxidase reaction, to demonstrate cytoplasmic granules with peroxidase activity that are not apparent in the Wright's stain, was negative. This result made the diagnosis of acute myeloblastic leukemia unlikely. A periodic acid-Schiff's reaction to detect cytoplasmic glycogen granules demonstrated large blocks of periodic acid-

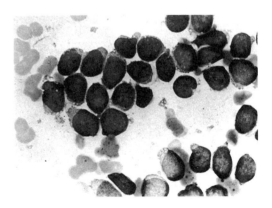

▶ **Figure 12.13.** Touch imprint of bone marrow biopsy showing solid sheets of primitive blast cells.

Schiff-positive material in some of the blasts, thus identifying these cells as lymphoblasts and diagnosing the disease as acute lymphoblastic leukemia. The definitive diagnosis was made within a day of the patient's presentation to the office, the nature of the illness was discussed with the patient and his family, and therapy was begun. A lumbar puncture was done before initiation of therapy; no leukemic cells were found on cytologic examination.

The patient underwent induction therapy with an aggressive regimen using a combination of daunorubicin, vincristine, prednisone, and L-asparaginase. He achieved remission after the initial induction cycle and underwent central nervous system prophylaxis with intrathecal methotrexate. Consolidation therapy with multiagent chemotherapy was given, followed by 30 months of maintenance therapy with oral methotrexate and 6-mercaptopurine. The patient did well for 1 year after completion of maintenance therapy, at which time he was noted to have a white blood cell count of 43,000/mm³ with 5% circulating blasts. Bone marrow biopsy confirmed a relapse. He underwent re-induction therapy, followed by allogeneic bone marrow transplantation. Now 2 years later, he is doing well, is married, and continues to work as a truck mechanic.

Logic The treatment of acute lymphocytic leukemia typically includes an induction phase in which several chemotherapeutic agents including vincristine and prednisone are administered. With this aggressive type of therapy, the majority (more than 80%) of patients will achieve hematologic remission. Treatment of the central nervous system is important because it is relatively inaccessible to intravenous chemotherapy and may serve as a "sanctuary" site for early relapse (the testes also serve as a sanctuary site, but isolated testicular relapse is unusual). Consolidation or intensification therapy is given after remission is achieved; chemotherapeutic agents are generally similar to those used in the induction phase. Maintenance therapy is given for several months to help decrease the relapse rate. Patients who relapse with acute lymphoblastic leukemia may undergo another induction phase and allogeneic bone marrow transplantation is considered in those who have a suitable bone marrow donor.

Questions

1. A 34-year-old asymptomatic man is discovered to have an enlarged spleen at the time of his routine physical examination. His hematocrit is 42%, and his white blood cell count is 42,000/mm³. Examination of the peripheral blood smear demonstrates normal red blood cell morphology and normal numbers of platelets. The white blood cell differential is: segmented neutrophils, 36%; band neutrophils, 12%; metamyelocytes, 10%; myelocytes, 14%; promyelocytes, 4%; myeloblasts, 3%; basophils, 5%; eosinophils, 4%; lymphocytes, 8%; and monocytes, 4%. A special stain of the peripheral blood demonstrates absent leukocyte alkaline phosphatase. You immediately suspect:
   (a) acute myelocytic leukemia.
   (b) chronic myelocytic leukemia.
   (c) polycythemia vera.
   (d) neutrophilic leukemoid reaction.
2. Which of the following statements about acute lymphocytic leukemia is correct?
   (a) Usually occurs in the elderly
   (b) A complete remission (normal peripheral blood and bone marrow) is commonly (more than 85% of patients) achieved with chemotherapy
   (c) Always has a presentation of a high white blood cell count
   (d) Commonly has a presentation as the terminal phase of chronic lymphocytic leukemia.
3. Which of the following abnormalities causes the greatest risk of death in a patient who has acute leukemia?
   (a) Thrombocytopenia
   (b) Granulocytopenia
   (c) Hyperuricemia
   (d) Leukocytosis
4. A 62-year-old man notes a mass in the left side of his abdomen. On examination, the mass moves with respiration and feels like a spleen. Enlarged lymph nodes are found in the neck, axillae, both groins, and epitrochlear areas. The patient's tonsils are markedly enlarged. He does not appear anemic. The diagnosis is most readily and dependably made by:
   (a) lymph node biopsy.
   (b) antinuclear antibody determination.
   (c) complete blood count (CBC).
   (d) computed tomographic scan of the liver and spleen.

Answers

1. **(b) is correct.** In contrast to acute leukemia, chronic myelocytic leukemia always has a presentation of a high white blood cell count. The peripheral white blood cell

differential is approximately the same as in normal bone marrow, which suggests a defect in bone marrow release. The histochemical stain demonstrating absent alkaline phosphatase activity in the neutrophils is an empiric but important observation that helps to distinguish this disease from a normal reactive leukocytosis. But the clinical setting and persistence of leukocytosis in chronic myelocytic leukemia make the distinction more definite. The normal-appearing granulocyte maturation seen on the peripheral blood smear rules out acute leukemia, a disease in which the primitive cells (blasts) are unable to differentiate and mature. Polycythemia vera is a disease closely related to chronic myelocytic leukemia, but diagnostic criteria include an increased red blood cell mass (not present when the hematocrit is 42%).

2. **(b) is correct.** As shown by many studies, the peak age incidence for acute leukemia is less than 10 years. Approximately half of patients are initially seen with normal or low total white blood cell counts. Acute lymphocytic leukemia is an entirely different disease from chronic lymphocytic leukemia, and there is not a transition between these diseases. Chronic lymphocytic leukemia affects older adults. In chronic lymphocytic leukemia, B lymphocytes cannot differentiate into immunologically competent cells and accumulate in the circulation.

3. **(b) is correct.** Granulocytopenia cannot be corrected by transfusion, and the risk of fatal infection is great. Extreme leukocytosis due to blasts is also a threat because these large and rigid cells have difficulty passing through the microcirculation. Clinical studies have suggested that a blast concentration in the peripheral blood of greater than 100,000/mm³ is commonly associated with leukothrombi and infarction of the lung and brain. Appropriate chemotherapy can reduce this leukocytosis within 24 to 48 hours. Hyperuricemia can cause acute renal failure but should be well controlled by maintaining a good output of alkaline urine and treatment with allopurinol (a xanthine oxidase inhibitor). Thrombocytopenia can be effectively managed by platelet transfusions. Clinically important bleeding rarely occurs unless the platelet count is <10,000/mm³ and unless fever and infection are also present.

4. **(c) is correct.** This is a typical presentation for chronic lymphocytic leukemia. The blood count will likely show a marked leukocytosis, which is sometimes dramatic (e.g., >100,000 white blood cells per mm³, 95% mature lymphocytes), but there may be no anemia, thrombocytopenia, or systemic symptoms. Lymph node biopsy is not necessary if chronic lymphocytic leukemia is apparent on the peripheral blood smear. Choices (b) and (d) offer nothing useful.

Suggested Readings

Devine SM, Larson RA. Acute leukemia in adults: Recent developments in diagnosis and treatment. Ca: Cancer J Clin 1994;44(6):326–352

Preti HA, Kantarjin HM. Acute lymphocytic leukemia in adults: An update. Texas Med 1994;90(1):52–59.

Preti A, Kantarjin HM. Management of adult acute lymphocytic leukemia: Present issues and key challenges. J Clin Oncol 12(6):1312–1322.

CASE 11

LEG PAIN

Barbara A. Konkle

Data A 39-year-old sales executive comes to your office complaining of leg pain. She noticed persistent pain in the back of her right leg after an aerobics class that she attended 2 days previously. Because she did not remember any injury during the exercise, she thought the pain might be the result of missing classes while on a recent business trip. Ibuprofen every 6 hours and applied heat gave no relief. She has been in excellent health all of her life.

Logic At this point it seems most likely that the pain is musculoskeletal in origin. However, it would be unusual to have a major injury such as a plantaris tendon tear without a major memorable event during the exercise. Also, mild musculoskeletal injuries should respond, at least in part, to anti–inflammatory medication. Another possibility would be lumbar vertebral disc disease with radiculopathy giving referred pain to the leg.

Data The pain is located over the entire right calf, is more in the nature of a dull ache, seems fairly constant, is not worse when she walks or stands, bothers her even at rest or in bed, and is not accompanied by numbness or pins-and-needles sensations. She has noticed no swelling or redness.

Logic The nature of the pain, its constancy, unilateral nature, not worsening with activity or motion, and the absence of paresthesias point away from a musculoskeletal injury or nerve root impingement.

Data You ask more about her recent business trip. She tells you the trip was to South America. She was gone for 5 days and had time for nothing other than business. She had flown to Buenos Aires, gone directly to her hotel and, except for dinner out, had remained at the hotel where the business sessions were held. Because of the tight schedule, the meetings had lasted up to 16 hours per day, and she had been under a lot of pressure. There was no pain then nor during the return trip. On specific questioning, she had not been having any chest pain, shortness of breath, palpitations, or syncopal feelings.

Logic With the history of prolonged relative immobilization, you now consider the possibility of deep vein thrombosis, although you do not yet eliminate musculoskeletal and neurologic causes. If thrombosis exists, there are as yet no symptoms to suggest embolization.

Data Two younger sisters are in good health and there is no history of venous thrombosis in her or in her family members. She has been pregnant twice, had two normal spontaneous vaginal deliveries without problems, and is not pregnant at present. She has never taken oral contraceptives.

Logic There is no family history to suggest a hereditary disposition to hypercoagulability. Oral contraceptives are known pre-disposers to clot formation, but she does not take them.

Data On physical examination, the vital signs were within normal limits and she had no adenopathy. The lungs were clear to percussion and auscultation and the breasts were without masses or discharge. The cardiac examination displayed a normal apex beat and normal S_1 and S_2 without murmurs or extra heart sounds. The abdomen was soft without organomegaly; there were no masses felt. Results of pelvic and rectal examinations were normal, and there was no pain on percussion along the spine.

Upon examination of her legs, there was distinct tenderness to palpation behind the right knee and posterior thigh, and no discrete masses were felt. Measurements of the thighs 10cm above the upper border of the patella showed that the right thigh was 3 cm greater in circumference than the left. The right calf measured 1cm greater than the left calf at 10 cm below the patella. The pain in her right leg increased slightly with extension of the knee, but the pain was not increased when the leg was flexed at the hip with the knee extended (straight leg raise). Homan's sign was absent. The leg was not warm or discolored, there was no swelling of the ankles, and the neurologic examination, including all reflexes, was normal.

Logic The physical examination suggests that the pain and swelling result from a unilateral local process. There is no evidence for a pelvic tumor or lymph node disease that might compress and obstruct lymphatic flow. Illnesses such as congestive heart failure or conditions that are associated with decreased serum albumin, such as cirrhosis or the nephrotic syndrome, may result in lower extremity swelling, but in those cases the swelling would be bilateral, greater distal than proximal, and not associated with pain or tenderness. Local swelling would not occur with referred pain due to vertebral disc disease.

Also, the straight leg raise would elicit pain with lesions of the fifth lumbar or first sacral root, the two most commonly involved roots. Lesions of the first sacral root would decrease or abolish the ankle deep tendon reflex.

Pain in the calf plus swelling of the extremity point strongly to the presence of deep vein thrombosis, but objective studies have shown that this initial clinical diagnosis is correct less than half the time. The gold-standard test for the detection of a deep vein thrombosis has been ascending venography. This involves the injection of contrast dye into the veins of the foot. It can detect both distal thrombi located in the calf and more proximal thrombi in the thigh. But this test is time-consuming, may be technically difficult, and may be painful to the patient.

Ultrasonography supplemented by Doppler flow imaging to measure venous blood flow has been shown to have high sensitivity and specificity, especially for proximal thrombi, and is well tolerated by patients. Its operating characteristics are not as good in calf vein thrombosis, but detection there is not so critical because there is less risk from pulmonary embolism.

Data The patient underwent ultrasonography and Doppler flow studies and was found to have an occlusive thrombus in the right popliteal vein (Fig. 12.14). No other thromboses were noted. The CBC, PT, and PTT were normal. A chemistry profile showed normal renal function, and normal calcium, uric acid, albumin, and LDH levels.

Logic Immediate anticoagulation is indicated. Patients with proximal thrombi (above the knee) have a 4 to 6% chance of having a pulmonary embolus. There are so far no symptoms or signs of an embolus, and further studies to rule this out are not indicated at this time.

You must now decide whether the patient

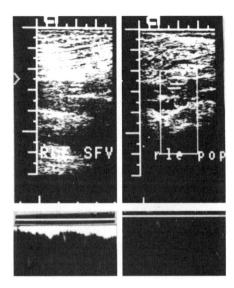

▶ **Figure 12.14.** Doppler flow studies of right lower extremity. Flow is present in the femoral vein (bottom left), but not in the popliteal vein (bottom right). The femoral vein is compressible; the popliteal vein is not.

needs further evaluation of the thrombosis. She did have prolonged immobilization as a risk factor, but was this sufficient reason? In assessing an adult who has venous thrombosis, it is important to exclude an acquired disorder for which the thrombosis may be an indicator.

Foremost on this list is malignancy, especially of the lung, breast, and uterus; this may be associated with a markedly increased risk of thrombosis. Your careful examination, her age and good health, and normal counts and chemistries make this unlikely. Oral contraceptives predispose to thrombi, too, but as previously noted, this patient takes none.

Myeloproliferative diseases, particularly essential thrombocythemia and polycythemia vera, may be associated with thrombosis. These may be arterial or venous and may present at unusual sites such as in mesenteric or hepatic veins. Her normal CBC makes these unlikely.

The lupus anticoagulant syndrome is also associated with an increased risk of arterial and venous thrombosis, as well as with mid-trimester abortions. Paradoxically, the LA is associated with clotting and, less frequently, bleeding syndromes. It may be seen with an increased PT or PTT due to interference of the anticoagulant with the phospholipid component of the test. In conjunction with thrombocytopenia, or with an acquired deficiency of factor II (prothrombin), bleeding may occur. This syndrome's presentation may include a normal PT and PTT, which would require further testing to establish the diagnosis.

The question of whether to do further testing in this 39-year-old woman does not have a clear-cut answer. It is unlikely that further findings would alter your initial management and length of warfarin sodium therapy. Even with inherited or acquired hypercoagulable states, the risk of long-term anticoagulation usually outweighs the benefits until someone has more than one thrombotic event. Many of the results of studies used in the diagnosis of acquired or inherited hypercoagulable states are affected by an acute thrombosis and/or anticoagulation. They are on the whole very expensive and, if abnormal in the setting of acute thrombosis, may need to be repeated anyway. These should be done at initial presentation only in patients in whom long term anticoagulation seems warranted. This would include patients with a history of prior thrombosis or a strong family history of thrombosis.

Data The patient is admitted to the hospital for heparin therapy, followed by oral anticoagulation therapy with warfarin sodium, which is to be maintained for 3 months.

Logic You advise the patient that she is at risk of thrombosis in the same leg in the future. She will need to guard against prolonged immobilization and should be prophylaxed with heparin or an alternative therapy for any major surgical procedure. Because her job requires long international flights that may put her at risk for recurrent thrombosis, you decide to do further tests to rule out an acquired lupus anticoagulant and inherited protein C, protein S, or antithrombin III *deficiency*. Protein C, protein S, and antithrombin III are *inhibitors* of the coagulation cascade. Their sites of action are depicted in Figure 12.15. You know that these tests have at least a 90% chance of being within normal limits in this patient.

Data Results of lupus anticoagulant and anticardiolipin antibody tests are negative. Protein C, protein S, and antithrombin III levels are within normal limits. A test for activated protein C resistance (APC) is abnormal.

Logic Until recently, known inherited deficiencies or abnormalities of clotting factors were only infrequently known to be causes of thrombosis.

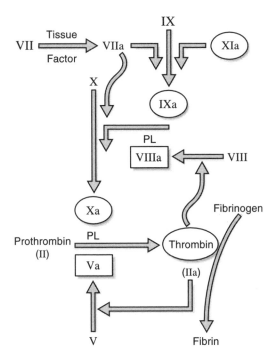

▶ **Figure 12.15.** A schematic representation of the coagulation cascade. Factors inhibited by activated protein C in the presence of activated protein S are enclosed by a rectangle. Factors inhibited by antithrombin III are enclosed by an oval. PL = phospholipid.

studied for APC resistance. If they test positive, they too should avoid risk factors. And if available, you may wish to confirm that she has factor V mutation by molecular diagnostic studies (Table 12.4).

TABLE 12.4. Disorders That Promote Thrombosis

Acquired Disorders
Congestive heart failure
Stasis and inactivity
Metastatic cancer
Myeloproliferative disorders
Oral contraceptives
Lupus anticoagulant
Trauma
Pregnancy
Inherited Disorders
Antithrombin deficiency
Protein C deficiency
Protein S deficiency
Activated protein C resistance
Dysfibrinogenemia

In 1991, researchers described an abnormality in a large number of patients with thrombosis that was associated with an abnormal response to the addition of APC to their plasma in a PTT reaction. In a normal individual this results in prolongation of the PTT, but in affected individuals the degree of prolongation is markedly reduced. APC inhibits the coagulation cascade by inactivating factor Va and VIIIa by cleaving these proteins. Protein S is a cofactor in this reaction. It was further determined that this resistance to APC was due to a mutation in the factor V gene at the site of APC-mediated cleavage. This mutation is present in 3 to 4% of the general population and appears to be a major risk factor for various thrombotic diseases.

This finding would not change the recommendations you made to the patient. However, you would need to be firm in your advice to avoid risk factors, to ambulate frequently on long trips, and to avoid hormonal therapy. You would advise her parents, siblings, and children to be

Questions

1. Six months after the initial thrombosis, the patient returns to your office. She is doing well, but complains of intermittent swelling of the left leg, especially after being on her feet all day. The swelling is gone when she gets up in the morning. There is no pain or tenderness. The most likely reason for the leg swelling is:
   (a) recurrent deep vein thrombosis.
   (b) post-phlebitic syndrome.
   (c) arterial thrombosis.
   (d) a pelvic mass.
2. At the time of initial presentation of the patient, the screening laboratory tests reveal a slightly prolonged PTT. The test is repeated using 1:1 mixing (½ patient plasma, ½ normal plasma), and the PTT remains slightly prolonged. The most likely reason for this abnormality is:
   (a) a deficiency of a coagulation factor tested in the PTT assay (XII, XI, IX, VIII, V, II).
   (b) an acquired inhibitor to a coagulation factor tested in the PTT assay.

(c) an acquired inhibitor that interferes with the phospholipid requirement of the PTT assay (lupus anticoagulant).

(d) vitamin K deficiency.

3. While in your office, the patient develops right-sided chest pain that she describes to you as sharp and worse with inspiration. You suspect she has had a pulmonary embolism originating from the leg thrombus. In this situation, the most common finding on physical examination is:

(a) an increased respiratory rate.

(b) a pleuritic rub on chest auscultation.

(c) an increased pulmonic component of the second heart sound.

(d) an increased heart rate (tachycardia).

Answers

1. **(b)** is correct. Patients with lower extremity thrombosis, especially those involving the more proximal veins, have a high risk of developing the post-phlebitic syndrome. This is due to distortion of the normal venous architecture by the clot. Symptoms range from mild dependent edema to chronic edema, pain, and venous stasis ulcers, and they can be decreased by having the patient wear specially designed support stockings. The incidence of post-phlebitic syndrome can be significantly reduced by using thrombolytic therapy with streptokinase, urokinase, or tissue plasminogen activator as the initial therapy. These agents result in clot dissolution, whereas heparin only prevents clot propagation. The use of these agents is associated with a higher incidence of bleeding complications, but should be considered for treating large proximal deep venous thromboses of the lower extremity.

2. **(c)** is correct. Understanding mixing studies is essential to understanding the evaluation of coagulation disorders. Factor activity in normal pooled plasma is defined as 1 U/mL. However, to obtain a normal PTT, one only needs 30 to 40% of normal values. Thus, if the PTT is prolonged due to a factor deficiency, including vitamin K deficiency, a 1:1 mix will result in normalization of the PTT, although if the prolongation is due to an inhibitor, the PTT will usually not correct. The patient's results suggest the presence of an inhibitor. Acquired inhibitors to coagulation factors are usually associated with a marked prolongation of the PTT and bleeding.

A mild prolongation of the PTT in a patient who has a history of thrombosis is more likely to be due to a lupus anticoagulant. Frequently in such patients the PTT will be normal, but tests that are more sensitive to the phospholipid component (dilute Russell's viper venom time or tissue thromboplastin inhibitor test) will be abnormal and will not correct with mixing.

3. **(d)** is correct. Although all of the findings listed can be seen in the setting of pulmonary embolism, sinus tachycardia is the single consistent finding. If pulmonary embolism is associated with infarction of the lung tissue, associated irritation of lung pleura can be detected by auscultation of a friction rub. However, infarction occurs in only 10% of episodes of pulmonary embolism. Acute pulmonary hypertension that may accompany a large pulmonary embolism may be associated with an increased pulmonic component of the second heart sound. However, greater than 50% of the pulmonary vascular bed needs to be compromised before signs of right heart strain and pulmonary hypertension are evident.

COMMENT First and foremost, this case demonstrates that thrombophlebitis usually has an underlying cause, whether it be so simple as trauma or so complex as an inherited deficiency of natural clot inhibitors. Second, this case takes you through the causes of leg pain, leg swelling, and a combination of the two, which points almost irrefutably to deep vein thrombosis. Third, the various acquired and hereditary causes of hypercoagulability are detailed. Last, the intelligent management of leg vein clots and their complications as well as their prevention are presented. Difficulties often arise in the understanding of clotting disorders, particularly in grasping the concept of a deficiency of clot inhibitors—a sometimes confusing double negative. (P.C.)

Suggested Readings

Dahlback B. Physiological anticoagulation. J Clin Invest 1994;94:923–927.

Hirsch J, Fuster V. AHA medical/scientific statement: Guide to anticoagulant therapy, Part 1: Heparin. Circulation 1994;89:1449–1468.

Hirsch J, Fuster V. AHA medical/scientific statement: Guide to anticoagulant therapy, Part 2: Oral anticoagulants. Circulation 1994;89:1449–1461.

Weinmann EE, Salzman EW: Deep-vein thrombosis. New Engl J Med 1994;331:1630–1641.

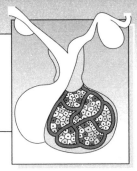

Only 40 years ago, endocrinology was still in its infancy, and diseases of the endocrine glands were poorly understood. Today the situation is much improved, thanks largely to the ability to measure blood hormone levels by radioimmunoassay and to new-generation imaging procedures.

Endocrine diseases were simple. There was either hyperfunction or hypofunction of the pituitary, adrenal, thyroid, gonad, or parathyroid glands. To a great degree this is still true. Hyperfunction is caused by tumor, hyperplasia, or stimulation; and hypofunction results from replacement, destruction, or atrophy. But we now recognize feedback mechanisms, many of which are the basis for testing a gland's function. The pituitary gland, once thought to be the king and supervisor of all endocrine glands, is now known to be subjugated by feedback mechanisms and to be governed by a power behind the throne—the hypothalamus.

Because there are so many different endocrine diseases, each with its own set of symptoms, physical signs, and diagnostic measures, very little overlap exists, and one endocrine disease cannot easily be confused with another. But they may be confused with diseases of other systems because of overlapping symptoms or clusters. You must remember too that, if the pituitary gland is diseased or destroyed, multiple endocrine hypofunction can exist. Furthermore, several simultaneously functioning adenomas may exist independently of the pituitary in the multiple endocrine neoplasia syndromes.

As for problem solving, pinpointing the diseased organ should be simple. There are many well-known clusters and key clues. For example, tachycardia, tremor, exophthalmos, and thyromegaly equal hyperthyroidism; no menses since childbirth points to Sheehan's syndrome; weakness, pigmentation, and hypotension suggest Addi-

son's disease. But remember that such diagnostic clusters are not infallible.

Clues that alert you to the possibility of an endocrine disease include hypertension, hyperglycemia, nervousness, amenorrhea, loss of libido, polyuria-polydipsia, altered growth pattern, changes in facies and body build, qualities of hair and skin, hair distribution, sweat pattern, and tolerance to heat or cold. Weakness and loss of vigor are common.

Pattern recognition is simple if you have the disease in mind. Hyperthyroidism, myxedema, acromegaly, and Cushing's disease can be spotted on the sidewalk or in mental institutions if you specifically look for them. Sometimes the manifestations are so prominent you notice the disease even if you are not seeking it. One look at the face, and you know the diagnosis.

This is an area where Sherlock Holmes would be at his best. Questions such as—"Do you change your dentures more frequently than you used to?"; "Have your hat and shoe sizes gotten larger?"; "Do you argue with your husband over whether the windows should be open or closed, or the air-conditioner on or off?"; and "May I see your former photograph?"—can furnish the single clue that solves the mystery.

However, despite all that has been said, endocrine disease is often overlooked. There are several reasons: (1) the physician is not thinking of it; (2) the early symptoms are often vague and nonspecific—for example, weakness, nervousness, anorexia; and (3) the onset is often subtle and not noticed by the patient. Thyroid disorders, in particular, are often overlooked in the elderly for these reasons.

Don't neglect the possibility of an endocrine disease if the patient's complaints seem neuropsychiatric in origin. Most endocrine abnormalities may have a presentation of symptoms suggesting either depression, confusion, anxiety, personality changes, organic brain syndrome, and so forth. Consider the clinical pictures of Addison's disease, Cushing's disease, hyperparathyroidism, hypoparathyroidism, hyperthyroidism, hypothyroidism, hypoglycemia, pheochromocytoma, and hypo- and hyperosmolar states. Note that each may have neuropsychiatric manifestations as a major or minor portion of the history.

New technology has given rise to quantum leaps in the diagnosis of endocrine diseases. For nodules of the thyroid gland, accurate cytologic diagnosis of aspirated specimens drawn in the physician's office has saved countless patients from unnecessary thyroidectomies. Ultrasound, magnetic resonance imaging (MRI), and high-resolution computed tomography (CT) of the endocrine glands have revolutionized our ability to detect endocrine tumors. However, with the more frequent use of these sensitive imaging techniques, even small tumors can be identified in the pituitary, parathyroid, and adrenal glands. Appearing in patients without signs of overt endocrine disease, these tumors can pose diagnostic challenges, but when small they are often benign and functionless.

Perhaps the most rapid strides in the study and diagnosis of endocrine disorders have been catalyzed by peptide radioimmunoassays. Measurable hormones include insulin, gastrin, secretin, prolactin, adrenocorticotropic hormone (ACTH), thyroid-stimulating hormone (TSH), luteinizing hormone (LH), follicle-stimulating hormone (FSH), human growth hormone (HGH), vasopressin (antidiuretic hormone [ADH]), and parathyroid hormone (PTH). These sensitive assays can reliably detect when a hormone is deficient as well as when it is excessive. In this way the TSH assay has become the single most useful screening test for hyperthyroid or hypothyroid disease—suppressed values in the former and increased values in the latter.

Here are a few words about the relative frequency of endocrine disorders. Almost universal is the menopause—not really a disease. Amenorrhea is often encountered too, but in the young adult woman it is likely to be due to pregnancy. Diabetes mellitus (DI) is actually the most common endocrinopathy; the average physician sees several to many cases each day. Thyroid diseases are not infrequent; approximately 10 to 20 new patients with hyperthyroidism and hypothyroidism may be seen yearly by a physician. Male hypogonadism resulting from pituitary insufficiency or from primary gonadal hypofunction is relatively common too; it manifests itself as incomplete sexual maturation or infertility. Hyperparathyroidism is not unusual; however, the diagnosis nowadays most often results from asymptomatic hypercalcemia discovered on routine testing. On the other hand, diseases of the adrenal and pituitary glands are uncommon and may at most be encountered only a few times per year. Other endocrine diseases are rarities. (*P.C./B.G.*)

CASE 12

A THYROID NODULE

Carlos Pestana

Data A 29-year-old white man undergoes a physical examination for the purpose of taking flying lessons. A nodule is found in his thyroid. The patient comes to you, his regular physician, for further advice.

Logic Here is an asymptomatic patient who has something discovered by someone else in a routine physical examination. Your first task is to confirm the presence of the physical finding.

Data With the patient suitably disrobed, standing in front of you in a good light, you can see no asymmetry or abnormality in his neck. He is a rather thin young man, and you can actually see his sternomastoid muscles, the pulsation of his carotids, and the prominence of his thyroid cartilage. You ask him to swallow, and as he does so, you suddenly see it: his larynx goes up, and a round lump approximately 2 cm in diameter comes up from behind the right sternoclavicular joint. It lifts the sternomastoid muscle and also bulges medial to it, just lateral to the trachea, then moves down again and out of view. You palpate the area, and there is no question in your mind. A 2 x 2-cm round, smooth, fleshy-feeling mass is present at the base of the neck, to the right of the midline. It moves up and down with swallowing, is not tender, and has no pulsations. You cannot feel the rest of the thyroid gland.

Logic You have answered your first question. In fact, you have answered two. He does have a lump in his thyroid as suggested by the location, and the fact that it moves up and down with swallowing; but you have also determined that this is a single nodule, as opposed to enlargement of the whole thyroid gland. Had his whole gland been enlarged, cancer would not be a likely consideration. Instead you would be concerned with the possibilities of Graves' disease, multi-nodular goiter, compensatory overgrowth because of hypofunction, or thyroiditis. An assessment of thyroid function and autoimmune inflammation would then be indicated. But with a distinct single nodule, the main concern is cancer. Thyroid function must be evaluated here too because a benign nodule can be thyrotoxic. Let us complete the history and physical examination before considering further tests.

Data There is no chief complaint or present illness, so the entire history is a review of systems; but we stress some questions that are particularly pertinent to his problem. He could have a toxic adenoma, and thus have symptoms of hyperthyroidism. Has he lost weight despite increased appetite? Any diarrhea? Does he have palpitations? Has he noticed intolerance to heat? Has anyone noticed that he is jumpy, fidgety, or on the move all the time? Any changes in emotional stability? The answers are all negative.

We are also concerned about cancer of the thyroid, but there are few symptoms specifically referable to this disease. These cancers are usually painless, silent, and unobtrusive until they become huge. We ask him about hoarseness, and he denies it. He has no difficulty swallowing. It would be nice to know (1) how long the mass has been there, and (2) how fast it has grown, but he did not even know of its existence until now. We ask a few specific questions regarding the past medical history and family history. Has he ever had radiation exposure to the head and neck area? This is a well-known carcinogenic event for the thyroid. Has anyone in his family had cancer of the thyroid? (One type, medullary carcinoma, often occurs in families.) The answers are no.

In the general physical examination we continue to stress the pertinent areas. His eyes look normal: no staring gaze, no lid lag, no exophthalmos. He can focus on a close object without one of his eyes wandering off. The skin, hair, and nails are normal; his pulse rate is 78 beats per minute and regular. We ask him to stick out his tongue; a 3- × 5-in card is placed over his outstretched hands—no tremors are detected. The neck is carefully examined for possible lymph node metastasis along the jugular chain, but none is found. The rest of the physical examination is unremarkable.

Logic It does not look as though he has a toxic adenoma; we are left with the question of cancer vs. a benign lump. Further studies of his thyroid function will help define the issue only in a roundabout way. Most thyroid cancers are not functional, and the ones that are—the medullary type—produce thyrocalcitonin, not thyroxin. But on the other hand, it is rare for cancer to occur in a hyperthyroid patient; and, more specifically, a hyperfunctioning nodule is almost never cancer. If we could show that he has a toxic adenoma, we could deal with that and stop worrying about cancer. Furthermore, if we get to the point of surgical exploration, we must be certain that unsuspected hyperthyroidism does not exist. It could be lethal to do an operation in a hyperthyroid patient without appropriate preparation. Let us get laboratory confirmation that he is euthyroid.

What shall we order? The most accurate assessment of thyroid function that would reveal hypothyroidism or hyperthyroidism would be a sensitive determination of TSH, at a cost of approximately $68.00. If our only concern is hyperthyroidism, we could be reasonably reassured with a free thyroxine (T_4) determination, at a cost of only $24.00. We order the latter.

Data His free T_4 is 1.2 μg/dL. Normal values in males range from 0.8 to 1.5.

Logic With negative clinical findings and a normal free T_4, we are confident that he is euthyroid. Now we have a euthyroid patient with a thyroid nodule. Is it cancer? Only your pathologist can tell you for sure.

In the case of papillary, medullary, or anaplastic cancers, the diagnosis can be made with just a sample of the tumor; that is, a biopsy. In fact, in most cases it can be made with even less—with cytology specimens obtained by fine needle aspiration.

Unfortunately, for the second most common cancer of the thyroid, follicular cancer, the whole tumor is needed. Capsular invasion, blood vessel invasion, and other architectural features are often the clues needed to distinguish benign from malignant.

So, should we schedule the patient for surgery? No, not yet. As it happens, the incidence of cancer in thyroid nodules is very low. Most thyroid nodules are benign. If we did thyroidectomies— a major operation—for all of them, a lot of unnecessary, expensive, and risky negative explorations would be done. This is a situation that calls for a *selective* approach.

We know of several factors that increase the likelihood of cancer: young age (older patients are more likely to have benign lumps), male gender, a single nodule as opposed to several nodules, a history of radiation exposure to the neck, a solid as opposed to a cystic mass, and a cold nodule as revealed by radioactive iodine scan. Some of these data we can get at minimal cost by just doing the history and physical—bearing in mind that physicians do not work without pay; their time is valuable too!

In this case we have already gathered several of those worrisome items: he is a young man with a single nodule. But that is not enough to go ahead with surgery. We need more. We are going to have to spend some serious money to make up our minds, but it behooves us to do it wisely, and in the most expeditious and economic way. A high-resolution sonogram will cost approximately $300 to $400, and a radioactive scan will cost another $400 to $500. Armed with the information provided by those two tests, and thus operating only on the patients that have solid, cold nodules, the yield of cancer is approximately 20%.

Sounds good enough. You would not want a lump left in your neck if you had a 20% chance that it was cancer. And thus for years and years, we did operate on that basis. While we were doing so, we were also humoring our pathologists who wanted to gain experience with another test, fine needle aspiration cytology (FNA). We allow them to perform this test in all our patients. Well, they got the experience!

Nowadays, if you have a reliable cytologist you can bypass the sonogram and the radioactive scan. For approximately $350 you can get the FNA, and if you make your surgical decision on that basis, the yield of cancers goes up to approximately 40%. Many unnecessary operations are thus avoided, while very few cancers are missed. We ask that our patient get an FNA of the thyroid nodule.

Data The fine needle aspiration is reported as "Indeterminate. Compatible with follicular neoplasm. Cannot rule out cancer."

Logic Have we wasted our $350? No, not really. In fact, the test has been quite helpful. In experienced hands (persons who do at least 50 of these per year), approximately 75% of thyroid nodules can be diagnosed with confidence as benign. None of those needs surgery, and very few of them will turn out to be actually malignant. The very rare cases of false negatives will become evident clinically in due time, and given the slow growth and relatively nonaggressive nature of most thyroid cancers, those patients will still do reasonably well. Another 5% or so of FNA diagnoses will be malignant, and we operate on those.

In approximately 20% of samples, the pathologist cannot tell. We then get the evasive "compatible with . . ." and the defensive "cannot rule out . . .," but in that subgroup of patients cancer is relatively frequent. The bulk of patients with benign lumps was already excluded. Surgery in the indeterminate cases will yield approximately 20% cancer; about as selective as the older and more costly route of sonogram plus radioactive scan. Some surgeons will do the additional tests in that subgroup, but many feel that surgery is justified without further ado.

In this case it certainly is: remember that he is a young man with a single nodule. Furthermore, when a pathologist writes down "cannot rule out cancer" you are trapped. *You* have to rule it out.

We schedule the patient for surgery. He is an otherwise healthy young man, so the preoperative work-up does not need to be extensive. Our hospital has a single absolute requirement on all presurgical patients: a hematocrit. Other absolute requirements do not apply to this patient: females of childbearing age must have a pregnancy test, patients older than age 40 require an electrocardiogram (ECG), and black patients must be tested for sickle cell disease. Based on medical indication, we could add white blood cell (WBC) count, electrolytes, blood urea nitrogen (BUN) and creatinine, blood glucose, chest radiograph, coagulation studies, and flexion and extension neck radiographs. We order the hematocrit, and add the chest radiograph. We are going to operate on the thyroid, where an abnormality has already been detected. Tracheal displacement or intrathoracic extension of the gland would be nasty surprises to find at the time of intubation and operation. Admittedly, these are not likely to be present given the physical findings, but a chest radiograph does not cost a fortune.

Data The chest radiograph is normal. The hematocrit is 45. A sample of blood is drawn and stored to be sent for thyrocalcitonin levels only if the tumor should prove to be a medullary cancer. This test is expensive and must be sent to a specialized center to be done. However, if medullary cancer is found, serial calcitonin levels may alert you to tumor recurrence.

A right subtotal thyroid lobectomy is done under general anesthesia. A frozen section diagnoses benign thyroid adenoma. Four days later, at the time when sutures are removed and the patient is ready to go home, the final pathologic diagnosis is still benign, but now somewhat embellished to read "macrofollicular colloid adenoma" (Fig. 13.1).

Logic The story has a happy ending. The pathologist confirms the clinical impression of a benign adenoma, and no further surgery is needed. Had it been a carcinoma, further pathologic classification would have been necessary because the operative management is different for each of the four types of thyroid cancer.

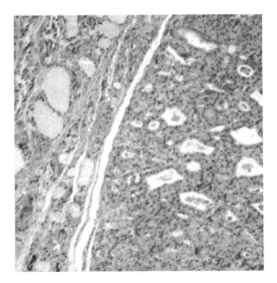

▶ **Figure 13.1.** Thyroid adenoma. Note normal thyroid tissue on left side, adenoma on the other.

Questions

1. A palpable mass in the neck is most likely to arise from the thyroid gland if:
   (a) it is located in the midline, at approximately the level of the hyoid bone, and moves up and down with swallowing.
   (b) it is located at the base of the neck, or a few centimeters from the midline, and moves up and down with swallowing.
   (c) it is located in the lateral aspect of the neck, in the vicinity of the sternomastoid muscle, and does not move with swallowing.
   (d) it has a history of repeated episodes of inflammation, drainage of pus, and reappearance of the mass.

2. Diffuse enlargement of the thyroid gland can be found in all of the following conditions except:
   (a) Graves' disease
   (b) Simple goiter
   (c) Hashimoto's thyroiditis
   (d) Papillary cancer

3. Which of the following thyroid nodules is most likely to be malignant?
   (a) A hot nodule in a middle-aged woman
   (b) A nodule that is slightly larger than several others in the same gland
   (c) A nodule known to have remained the same size for 2 years, which suddenly becomes tender and twice its size
   (d) A cold nodule in a young man

Answers

1. **(b) is correct.** More often than not, thyroid masses are off the midline because they arise from either lobe, but they could be at the midline if arising from the isthmus. Choice (a) describes the location of a thyroglossal duct cyst. Only rarely will a mass arising from an elongated pyramidal lobe be found in that location. Choice (c) suggests a mass originating from lymph nodes along the jugular chain—either inflammatory, primary neoplastic, or metastatic. Beware if a biopsy from that site is read as "normal thyroid." The thyroid gland is never at the lateral neck during embryologic formation and migration, and thus there is no such thing as "lateral aberrant thyroid." Such a case is sooner or later proved to be metastasis from a thyroid cancer. Choice (d) suggests a congenital cystic mass (thyroglossal duct cyst or branchial cleft cyst) with repeated infection.

2. **(d) is correct.** Cancers of the thyroid do not produce diffuse enlargement, except for a far-advanced anaplastic tumor that can reach a very large size. Papillary cancer would typically be a single palpable nodule, even though pathologically it is often multicentric and seldom large. In fact, at times there are palpable metastases in the neck nodes before the primary lesion can be detected. Diffuse thyroid enlargement occurs in (a), (b), and (c). Simple goiter is not so simple; it can result from diverse causes such as iodine deficiency or the taking of lithium.

3. **(d) is correct.** This answer gives the most suspicious combination of factors. Choices (a) and (b) are variations of the opposite situation: being female, capture of iodine, middle age, and multiplicity of nodules are all factors that lower your level of suspicion. Choice (c) describes a situation that is seen when bleeding occurs inside a thyroid nodule, most often an adenoma. Of course, bleeding can also occur in a carcinoma, and the fact that the nodule has been inactive for 2 years does not rule out cancer. Papillary and follicular carcinomas grow very slowly.

COMMENT To solve this problem, the author first used an anatomic approach. He confirmed the presence of the nodule and established its location in the thyroid gland. Rather than collect a complete data base, he immediately branched into a subset of data to determine if the nodule was malignant or causing hyperthyroidism. The latter was quickly ruled out by the absence of very commonly occurring signs and symptoms. For how could the patient be in a toxic state in the absence of symptoms, tremor, tachycardia, and eye signs? In choosing thyroid function studies, the author was selective and cost-conscious—ordering only what was necessary. Then he invoked Bayes' theorems in considering the likelihood of a thyroid nodule's being malignant and further evaluated these odds in terms of sex, age, and cytology.

Actually, a dendrogram with three decision points solved this problem:

1. Confirm anatomy
2. Assess thyroid function
3. Evaluate fine needle aspiration cytology

The rest of the information was helpful but not crucial. (*P.C.*)

PROBLEM-BASED LEARNING To get the most from this case study, learn all about the following:

- Thyroid nodules and their causes
- Thyroid enlargement
- Thyroid carcinoma, the pathologic types and their clinical pictures
- Substernal thyroid nodules
- How to examine the thyroid gland by palpation and auscultation
- Determination of thyroid function by the clinical picture and tests
- Relationship between radiation exposure and subsequent thyroid neoplasia
- Other endocrine adenomas associated with medullary thyroid cancer
- Latest information on needle aspiration cytology, ultrasound, and computed tomographic scans of the thyroid gland
- The role of radioactive iodine in thyroid studies
- Hashimoto's thyroiditis
- "Simple" goiter

Suggested Readings

Gharib H. Fine needle aspiration biopsy of thyroid nodules: Advantages, limitations and effect. Mayo Clin Proceed 1994;69:44–49.

Mazzaferri EL. Review article, current concepts: Management of a solitary thyroid nodule. New Engl J Med 1993;328(8):553–559.

Rifat SF, Ruffin MT. Management of thyroid nodules. Am Fam Phys 1994;50(4):785–790.

Woeber KA. Cost effective evaluation of the patient with a thyroid nodule. Surg Clin N Am 1995;75(3): 357–363.

C A S E 13

GLYCOSURIA

Carlos A. Moreno

Data Two-plus glycosuria is detected on routine urine dipstick in an 18-year-old female. Because her father died of diabetes and heart disease at age 42, her mother has taken her to a physician for a checkup at least once a year. The results of these checkups have all been negative, including one done 6 months ago.

Logic Concern for the daughter is understandable. You get the impression that testing may be excessive. At any rate, further tests must now be done. Although only one third of random positive urine sugar test measurements turn out to be caused by diabetes mellitus, the odds are greater with this background. Given the ready availability of portable glucometers, urine testing for diagnosis and management of diabetes mellitus is now rarely used.

Data Further history reveals that the patient has been very nervous and has lost weight during the past few months. Contrary to advice, she has been drinking lots of soft drinks because she likes them, although she says she has not been thirsty. She gets up twice a night to urinate because she has a "Coke and coffee" before going to bed. She has no dysuria. Despite weight loss, her appetite has been as good as ever. While her mother is out of the room, the patient confides that she has a boyfriend, is sexually active, and takes birth control pills. Sometimes during the day she gets very nervous and weak and finds that a soft drink makes her feel better.

Before going further, you have your nurse perform a finger-stick blood glucose determination and, while waiting for the results, continue with your thoughts. The time is 3 pm, 2 hours after the patient's substantial lunch.

Logic On the surface, this case seems simple. But the more data you gather, the more complicated the problem becomes. Diabetes is foremost in your mind because of the family history and one-plus glycosuria. Was the test done accurately? Probably so, but you will never know. You have found nothing so far.

The nervousness is puzzling. Although she may have enough to be nervous about; having a boyfriend and being sexually active, failure to follow carbohydrate restriction, an overly concerned mother, and the stresses of adolescence—all can foster severe anxiety. The weight loss is worrisome; diabetes could be the cause, but she does not seem to have the degree of glycosuria, polyuria, and polydipsia that would be expected if diabetes were causing the weight loss. She drinks sweetened beverages and urinates twice a night, but this is difficult to evaluate. It is not a straightforward history of extreme thirst and excessive urination.

Other factors test your logic. Hyperthyroidism can cause nervousness, weight loss, and even gly-

cosuria in the presence of a good appetite. It must be considered. Birth control pills diminish glucose tolerance and can cause glycosuria too. Nervousness and weak spells relieved by soft drinks suggest hypoglycemia. In early diabetes this can occur several hours after eating, but she cannot pinpoint the times of day; hypoglycemia would not occur if symptomatic diabetes were already present. Symptoms of this sort may be used as excuses by patients who wish to partake of sweets. Your thoughts are interrupted by the arrival of the result of the blood glucose test.

Data The blood glucose is 100 mg/dL.

Logic You press on for more data, remembering that the patient's mother had an overactive thyroid gland removed 20 years ago and that there is an increased coincidence of diabetes and hyperthyroidism.

Data There has been no excessive sweating, tremor, or heat intolerance. The pulse is 80; blood pressure (BP), 106/80; temperature 36.6°C; and respirations, 16. A quick focused physical examination shows no exophthalmos, lid lag, stare, or loss of convergence; the thyroid gland is not enlarged; the breasts are turgid and enlarged. This reminds you to ask if she has missed any menses. The answer is no. Because she is sexually active and takes oral contraceptives, you perform a pelvic examination; it reveals a nulliparous cervix with normal adnexa.

Logic There is no evidence of hyperthyroidism, hypoglycemia, diabetes mellitus, or pregnancy. Birth control pills could cause the breast changes and the glycosuria (if it were indeed present). The weight loss is still unexplainable, although according to your own scale she has lost only 6 lb in 6 months. All the other symptoms could be explained on nonorganic bases. A normal fasting glucose does not rule out impaired glucose tolerance. Not wishing to miss anything, such as tuberculosis, you order additional studies.

Data A chest radiograph shows no evidence of tuberculosis. The triiodothyronine (T_3) resin uptake and T_4 determinations are also in the normal range. After 3 days' preparation with a high carbohydrate intake, a 75-g oral glucose tolerance test is done. The results are 96, 160, 204, 145, and 100 mg/dL at fasting, and at 1/2, 1, 2, and 3 hours. A trace of glucose is noted in the third urine sample. Blood count and routine urinalysis are normal.

Logic This is a slightly abnormal glucose tolerance test and indicates impaired glucose tolerance. The 1- and 2-hour values are above normal, as is the trace of glycosuria. You bear in mind the fact that oral contraceptives can diminish glucose tolerance, but the family history weights your judgment. You also recall that oral contraceptives, pregnancy, and estrogen administration can elevate the T_4 level (by increasing the thyroid-binding globulin) and decrease the T_3 resin uptake—thus altering your thyroid function studies. Whereas this may have occurred in this case, the results are still within the normal range. Hyperthyroidism can be ruled out.

Data You explain to the mother and daughter that she has impaired glucose tolerance, prescribe a sensible 1800 calorie diet, advise restriction of extra carbohydrate, and ask the patient to return in 3 months. Privately, you tell the patient to stop birth control pills and explain why. You also give her some advice about boyfriends, soft drinks, and use of barrier contraception. One year later, the patient returns. She has not been living at home and has not watched her diet, although she did stop taking oral contraceptives. Her symptoms include nausea, weight gain, frequent urination, and intense thirst.

Logic It sounds like severe insulin-deficient juvenile diabetes is now upon us. The nausea and weight gain do not fit the picture.

Data Further questions elicit amenorrhea for 3 months, considerable morning nausea, bloated feeling, and swollen ankles in the evening. The results of a rapid pregnancy test are positive, and the uterus is enlarged to the size of a pregnancy of 3 1/2 months' duration. The blood glucose is 228 mg/dL, and the urine shows 4+ glycosuria. She is pregnant and has florid diabetes (Class B gestational diabetes).

Logic The nausea and weight gain go with her pregnancy. She manages to eat well after the nausea wears off, and much of the weight gain is salt and water retention. Hospitalization is indicated, because her diabetes will need considerable attention. This will allow control of her diabetes and permit a baseline evaluation of her vascular, renal, and obstetric status. It is also an ideal time to educate the patient about her diabetes and nutritional needs.

Data After 7 days in the hospital, the patient leaves much improved. Except for some persistent nausea, her symptoms are gone. She is on an 1800-calorie, 2-g sodium chloride, diabetic diet that allows for three meals daily and a bedtime snack. A split insulin regimen of 40 U of human neutral protamine Hagedorn (NPH) insulin and 20 U of regular human insulin before breakfast, and 20 U of NPH insulin and 10 U of regular insulin before dinner is required to keep her daily fasting blood glucose in the 60 to 90 mg/dL range and the urine free of glucose and ketones. The patient performs self blood glucose monitoring at home.

Logic Maternal and fetal welfare improve with tight diabetic control. Patients are taught to monitor their blood glucose at home, and good control is thus usually achievable.

Data She is followed closely through her pregnancy with only minor adjustments in insulin dose, goes into labor, and spontaneously delivers a healthy child at 38 weeks. After promising to adhere to a strict regimen, she moves back with her mother who takes care of the baby while the patient works during the day. Now she takes 25 U of NPH insulin in the morning and 5 U of regular insulin before lunch and dinner, and she is instructed to continue her home glucose self-monitoring.

Several weeks later, her employer informs her mother, who in turn informs you, that the patient is acting strangely from time to time. Her actions seem incoordinate, and she does not respond properly to questions. This is especially noticeable before quitting work for the day. A 4 pm blood glucose taken during an episode of strange behavior is 30 mg/dL. There is no evidence of perspiration, trembling, rapid pulse, or dilated pupils that you might expect in insulin-induced hypoglycemia. Oral sweets alleviate the disorder in several minutes. Insulin dosage is reduced to 20 U daily, and the patient is advised to have a 200-calorie carbohydrate snack daily at 3 pm. The behavior disorder does not return.

Logic Insulin requirements generally decrease postpartum and need adjustment. The hypoglycemia might have been anticipated. Many patients are able to remain off insulin after the immediate postpartum period.

Data You next see this woman 10 years later. She is 28 years old, has been living in another city, and has just returned. There have been several hospitalizations in the past 5 years, two for regulation of her diabetes. Several years ago she had pneumonia and was admitted to the hospital in a comatose state. Although meningitis and brain abscess were suspected, it turned out to be simply ketoacidotic coma. This information is obtained by telephoning the hospital record room.

Recently her diabetes has been under "good control," but her glycosylated hemoglobins have been running 9 to 11%. She takes insulin daily but does not monitor her glucose at home. An occasional fasting glucose is between 140 and 180 mg/dL, and the morning urine specimen usually tests negative for glucose. She complains of blurred vision in both eyes.

Logic Visual difficulty in a 28-year-old juvenile diabetic may represent diabetic retinopathy, cataracts, or ordinary presbyopia. Elevated glucose levels can cause blurry vision, but so can retinal detachment or progressive diabetic retinopathy. An examination should give the answer. You also wonder how good her diabetic control really is. Most authorities feel that good diabetic control will delay microvascular complications. She has missed her yearly ophthalmologic examination.

Data The fundi show numerous microaneurysms, small and large hemorrhages, neovascularization, and waxy exudates (Fig. 13.2). No cataracts are seen. An ophthalmologist finds that she needs glasses, but these only partially correct her visual problem. Fluorescein angiography confirms the presence of diabetic retinopathy, and panretinal argon laser or xenon arc light photocoagulation is recommended to prevent further deterioration.

Blood glucose taken at different times of the day is 150 mg/dL at 7 am, 260 mg/dL at 11 am, 340 mg/dL at 4 pm, and 382 mg/dL at 9 pm; urine glucoses are all 4+ except for 1+ in the morning. A urinalysis shows 3+ proteinuria and occasional fine granular casts in addition to the glucose. The hemoglobin A1c is 11%. The rest of the examination findings and laboratory tests are normal, except for weak pulsations in the arteries of both legs as well as decreased sensation in the lower extremities, and a creatinine level of 2.1 mg/dL. An angiotensin converting enzyme (ACE) inhibitor is added to her medication.

Logic The diabetes is poorly controlled. She now has proliferative diabetic retinopathy with early renal failure and a peripheral neuropathy. These three microvascular complications are usually seen together. It has been demonstrated that laser photocoagulation reduces the rate of visual

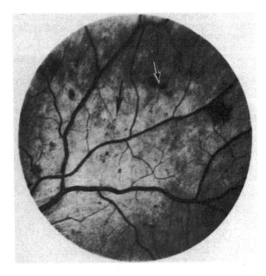

▶ **Figure 13.2.** Fundus of a diabetic patient showing hemorrhages and exudates as varying size.

loss. Also the elevation of glycosylated hemoglobin corroborates poor diabetic control for at least the previous 4 to 6 weeks. The incidence of nephropathy, retinopathy and neuropathy could have been reduced with intensive therapy. ACE inhibitors are added to prevent progression of renal disease in diabetes with albuminuria. ACE inhibitors have a greater benefit if used early when the patient has microalbuminuria.

Data The insulin dose is modified. She is to take 40 U of NPH insulin each morning and 20 U before supper. Diet and activities are again discussed and the nature of her problems is explained.

Only 2 months later, the patient revisits you. She has had recurrent bouts of high epigastric discomfort that are unrelated to meals and unrelieved by alkali. The first episode was prolonged and occurred 5 weeks ago. Antacids did not give relief. She feels better now, but comes to see you because she still fatigues easily.

Logic Although you consider peptic ulcer disease, gastroesophageal reflux disease, and cholelithiasis, your prime concern in a female patient with long-standing diabetes is silent myocardial infarction (MI). Diabetic gastroparesis is common and may be improved with cisapride.

Data An ECG shows an inferior wall myocardial infarction of undetermined age. ST segments are isoelectric, so you conclude that the MI is not

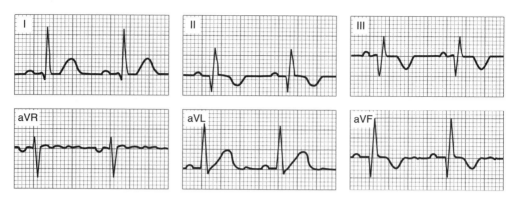

▶ **Figure 13.3.** Old inferior myocardial infarction. Q waves and inverted T waves in leads II, III, and aVF. ST segments are isoelectric. V leads are normal (not shown).

acute (Fig. 13.3). The ECG taken only 2 months ago was normal. You advise a month of restricted activity plus the same diabetic regimen. Just as she is about to leave your office, she mentions that her feet are numb, and her legs have been hurting during the past month. At first she says they hurt all the time, but closer questioning tells you her calves ache and get tired when she walks one or two blocks.

Logic Leg pains in a diabetic person can be caused by vascular insufficiency and by arthritis or varicose veins as in anybody. If caused by arterial occlusion, the pains come with walking and go away with rest (intermittent claudication). If neuropathy is the cause, the pain is more or less constant and is associated with other sensory changes and hyporeflexia. Arthritic pain is limited to the joints and is accompanied by stiffness. In severe varicose veins, the entire leg may become achy and tired when the patient is on her feet for a long time. Foot numbness is a common complication resulting from a peripheral neuropathy associated with decreased nerve conduction.

Data Quick examination show no joint swelling or deformity, no varicose veins, normal reflexes, and decreased normal sensory perception. No arterial pulses are felt in either leg from the femoral arteries down, and the legs are pale and cool.

Logic In addition to her other problems, she has another diabetic complication—arteriosclerosis obliterans of the lower extremities. The thought occurs to you that she may have had a saddle embolus from a mural thrombus. But remembering that her peripheral pulses were weak 2 months

ago, you favor progressive sclerosis as the cause. At any rate, the result is the same. The thought of aortofemoral bypass occurs to you, but in view of all her other problems you decide to wait and see what happens. Good foot care and prevention of infection is essential.

You wonder which of her many diabetic complications will eventually end her life. Diabetic complications can be lessened by tight control of blood glucose and by maintaining normal blood pressure, as well as by decreasing cardiovascular risk factors such as smoking, hyperlipidemia, and obesity. Perhaps the patient would have benefitted from a subcutaneous insulin pump. Newer therapies include pancreatic transplantation and new medications. Intensive education, the use of multiple daily injections of insulin and three to four times a day monitoring are the current standards of care. Nutritional evaluation and dietary management, as well as an exercise regimen, would have improved her care.

Data As she leaves your office, she makes an appointment—for herself and her young unmarried daughter . . . .

Questions

1. Your 58-year-old insulin-requiring diabetic patient develops nausea, vomiting, lethargy, and stupor. You last saw him well only 7 days ago. Except for signs of dehydration and deep breathing, all examination findings are normal. Which is the single most likely diagnosis?

(a) Nonketotic hyperosmolar coma
(b) Hypoglycemic coma
(c) Uremic coma
(d) Ketoacidotic coma
(e) Stroke
(f) Lactic acidosis

2. To solve the foregoing problem, what are the *three* crucial bits of information you seek?
(a) Glycosylated hemoglobin
(b) Serum electrolytes
(c) Blood gases
(d) CT scan of the abdomen
(e) Serum glucose level
(f) serum creatinine

3. A 65-year-old diabetic woman with long-standing type II diabetes develops pains in both legs. What are the fewest essential items needed to decide what may be wrong?
(a) Questions about the nature of the pain and what brings it on
(b) MRI of lumbosacral spine
(c) Palpation of lower extremity arterial pulsations
(d) Lower extremity venograms
(e) Neurologic examination for lower extremity reflexes and altered sensory perception
(f) Pelvic examination

Answers

1. Although all are theoretically possible, **(d)** is most likely. Deep breathing (Kussmaul's sign) indicates acidosis, making choices (a) and (b) unlikely. Choice (c) takes long to develop. Choice (e) should show neurologic abnormalities. Choice (f) may result from oral agents like phenformin.

2. **(b), (e), and (g) are correct.** The glucose level will be high (300 to 500 mg/dL?), the blood pH low (7.2), the bicarbonate level low (10 mEq/L), and the urinalysis will show 2 to 4+ ketones. Choice (a) will only tell you the degree of diabetic control for the previous 6 weeks. Electrolyte levels may be abnormal or normal. The creatinine level may be elevated from dehydration, and the CT is a waste of money.

3. **(a), (c), and (e)** When combined will determine with reasonable certainty whether the problem lies with vascular disease or neuropathy. If (c) and (e) are normal, and if (a) guides you away from these two diabetic complications, unrelated problems may be uncovered in the spine, the leg veins, or in the pelvis.

COMMENT The family history and subsequent development of diabetes mellitus influence our logic throughout this case study. First, we are confronted by the significance of newly discovered glycosuria and the errors that can be induced during testing. Altered glucose tolerance has three possible explanations here; pertinent negative and false-positive clues are considered as we think of diabetes, hyperthyroidism, and oral contraceptives. Distracters are present in the form of nervousness, weight loss, possible polyuria and polydipsia.

When true diabetes eventually comes, it is associated with pregnancy, so we have an overlap of symptoms associated with pregnancy that need sorting. As each diabetic complication develops, a new list of possible diagnoses appears, but the odds are that they all relate to diabetes—which they do. Each new problem presents a key clue and is easily solved with a few bits of information. The value of personally contacting a formerly used hospital for information is cited. Sequence of events and cause-and-effect are frequently used (poor control and complications, claudication following infarct, oral contraceptives and enlarged breasts).

Branching techniques are used for data gathering, sometimes to a fault. Interest in the infarct almost caused peripheral vascular disease and the peripheral neuropathy to be overlooked. Bayesian probability theories mold our thoughts as we consider causes for glycosuria, weight loss, leg pains, numbness of the feet, epigastric pains, diminished vision in diabetics, and the presence or absence of various diabetic complications in this patient or any diabetic patient. *(P.C.)*

Suggested Readings

American Diabetes Association. Clinical practice recommendations. Diabetes Care 1995;18(suppl)1:1–96.

Clark CM, Lee DA. Prevention and treatment of the complications of diabetes mellitus. New Engl J Med 1995;332:1210–1217.

The Diabetes and Complications Trial Research Grant. The effort of intensive treatment of diabetes on the development and progression of long-term complications in insulin-dependent diabetes mellitus. New Engl J Med 1993;329(14):977–986.

Hirsch IB. Surveillance for complications of diabetes. Postgrad Med 1996;99:147–172.

CASE 14

WEAKNESS, ANXIETY, SWEATING

David J. Kudzma

Data   Ever more frequent spells of generalized weakness, anxiety, sweating, tremulousness, and palpitations bring a 38-year-old woman to your office. She is unmarried, an executive in an advertising agency, and always felt well until 3 months ago when these spells began. They occur mainly in the late afternoon and while watching the late show.

Logic   Symptom clusters like these are common reasons for seeing a physician. Some of the features mentioned may be absent, additional ones may be present, or one or two of them may dominate the picture. Age, sex, and race notwithstanding, this general group of complaints would immediately suggest the following possibilities: (a) anxiety, (b) menopause, (c) hypoglycemia, (d) paroxysmal cardiac arrhythmia, (e) hyperthyroidism, (f) pheochromocytoma, or (g) serotonin-producing tumor. The first few conditions listed are common; the last two are rare. Some can be easily eliminated by a single question or observation.

Data   Between episodes she is well. She never had surgery, knows of no heart disease or murmur, and never had acute rheumatic fever. Menses are still normal, and she has no flushes. There are no gastrointestinal symptoms. Appetite is normal, and weight is stable. Although she feels palpitations during the spells, they do not seem persistent and have no clear-cut onset or finish. During a spell, she experiences no breathlessness, dry mouth, or numbness around the mouth and fingertips. She denies being nervous or tense but does relate that she has had to work especially hard to attain an executive position in such a "high-pressure, all male" profession.

Logic   These few questions immediately eliminate many possibilities. Anxiety with hyperventilation seems unlikely. The symptoms of hyperthyroidism are not episodic; furthermore, her appetite is normal, and she has not lost weight. Menopause can be excluded by her age and normal menses. Paroxysmal arrhythmias are unlikely in view of the description of palpitations and the absence of known heart disease. A serotonin-

producing carcinoid produces similar spells, but gastrointestinal symptoms are usually present too; in addition, this disease is rare. Four possibilities have been reasonably well eliminated. You are left with anxiety, hypoglycemia, and pheochromocytoma.

Examination of the patient during a spell would be infinitely helpful. Is the blood glucose level low? Is the blood pressure high? Although we may have to await an attack for final diagnosis, more information may provide an answer now.

Data   There are no other symptoms in the history or review of systems. Her mother and older sister have hypertension, and her father is an insulin-dependent diabetic. She has remained unmarried because she chose to do so; there were several marriage offers that she declined because they would have meant giving up her career. She smokes half a pack of cigarettes a day and drinks two cups of coffee. On social occasions she has one alcoholic drink.

Physical examination findings are completely normal, except for the blood pressure that is 160/96 in both arms and does not decline when she stands up. In particular, there are no abnormal eye signs, thyromegaly, heart murmurs, tachycardia, or tremor. Pelvic, rectal, and neurologic examination findings are normal. Forty-five seconds of hyperventilation makes her dizzy but fails to produce a typical spell. Electrocardiogram, chest radiograph, complete blood count, urinalysis, and 18-test chemistry profile results are normal also (including the blood glucose).

Logic   A little has been added. Hyperthyroidism is clearly excluded. So is organic heart disease. Rheumatic heart disease, a common cause of arrhythmias, is virtually ruled out by the absence of murmurs. Hypertension is often familial, although the possibility of pheochromocytoma still exists. Roughly one third of those with the latter disease have normotension between attacks, one third have hypertension with paroxysms superimposed, and one third have persistent hypertension without paroxysms. So this is still possible, even though the usual orthostatic changes are not present. The psychosocial status concerns us, although it may be of no consequence.

Three possibilities persist. *Pheochromocytoma* may be diagnosed by examination during an attack and by urine studies for epinephrine derivatives. *Anxiety with hyperventilation* remains a diagnosis to be made by exclusion and psychiatric evaluation, although this condition now seems most unlikely. If *hypoglycemia* is present, you are in a different universe and a host of other considerations enter the picture. Because both pheochromocytoma and hypoglycemia have symptoms resulting from hyperepinephrinemia, their distinction may be difficult. The former is rare; the latter is more common. Beware the frequent error of using hypoglycemia as a wastebasket diagnosis in individuals who are chronically fatigued, depressed, lethargic, "have no pep," and whose blood glucose levels are borderline low. You decide that she will need additional studies, beginning with a determination of the blood glucose level during a symptomatic episode. She is taught to self-monitor her blood glucose level and instructed to test during a spell.

Data At 3 PM 2 days later, your patient develops another of her episodes. An immediate blood glucose is 40 mg/dL. Symptoms are relieved by orange juice. Urinary vanillylmandelic acid, metanephrines, and 5 hydroxyindoleacetic acid determinations from a urine sample collected several hours after the episode are normal.

Logic Hypoglycemia is clearly diagnosed; pheochromocytoma and carcinoid are ruled out. Now a search for the cause of the hypoglycemia must begin. In general, there are three groups of hypoglycemias: *reactive, fasting,* and *factitious.*

Reactive hypoglycemia occurs as a reaction to a meal—often a high-carbohydrate meal. As such, it appears 2 to 4 hours after eating. If no meal is eaten, no attack occurs. Therefore, if episodes of hypoglycemia result from a missed meal or in the early morning hours after an overnight fast, they must have some other cause. From the initial history, it is clear that this patient's episodes are postcibal or reactive because they only occur several hours after a meal.

There are three types of reactive hypoglycemia—*functional, mild diabetic,* and *alimentary.* The first is the most common cause of hypoglycemic attacks in adults. It is often seen in tense, striving individuals with emotional disorders or maladjustments. The fasting blood glucose level is normal and remains so even after a 24- or 72-hour fast. It was once thought that excessive insulin response to a normal glucose load was the cause, but insulin assays have proved that

this is not the case; the mechanism remains unclear. Attacks are usually short and mild, last 15 to 30 minutes, are not accompanied by central nervous system manifestations, and clear spontaneously. A 5-hour oral glucose tolerance test (GTT) should precipitate an attack from 3 to 4 hours after the glucose load; the blood glucose at that time should be less than 40 to 50 mg/dL. Blood glucoses taken a few hours after meals often reveal similar levels.

In some instances, patients have what appear to be typical hypoglycemic episodes several hours after eating, yet clear-cut hypoglycemia cannot be synchronized with the attacks; here a rapidly falling blood glucose may be a factor. Complex psychosomatic elements may be operative too. Remember, too, that some normal persons may show low glucose levels during a GTT, but they may not have clinical hypoglycemic episodes.

Because of these variances, the GTT as a means of determining the cause of hypoglycemia has recently fallen into disrespect. Too many false negatives and false positives!

The second most common cause of hypoglycemia is early mild diabetes mellitus. Here large amounts of insulin are released, albeit late, and the glucose falls to low levels several hours after eating. The family history of diabetes suggests this possibility.

A third type of postcibal or reactive hypoglycemia is called alimentary hypoglycemia. This is caused by an excessive insulin response to rapid glucose absorption. It is most commonly seen in patients who have had gastroenterostomies or gastric resections whereby glucose enters the small intestine rapidly. Occasionally it is seen in the absence of surgery.

Data A 5-hour oral GTT is done. The results are 90, 140, 150, 94, 68, 36, and 68 mg/dL at zero, ½, 1, 2, 3, 4, and 5 hours after glucose ingestion. Between 3 and 4 hours after glucose ingestion she develops the cluster of symptoms that characterized each previous attack.

A detailed nutrition history is now taken. It should have been done earlier. Breakfast consists only of coffee. But for lunch she has a sandwich, a soft drink, and ice cream. Dinner includes meat and potatoes, bread, and a sweet dessert.

Logic The GTT result is characteristic of *functional hypoglycemia* in that she seems to overreact to a glucose load. Early diabetes is ruled out. The initial hyperglycemia that would be seen in alimentary hypoglycemia is not present. Her diet is a bit high in carbohydrate, especially in the meals preceding her attacks. No further studies need to be done, and treatment can be initiated. Her intake of sweets must be reduced and more frequent feedings given. Antihypertensive therapy is also begun.

On the other hand, if the patient had had attacks at 4 or 5 am or after a missed meal, especially in the presence of vigorous exercise, organic hyperinsulinism would have been a prime consideration. A beta-cell insulin-secreting adenoma is both serious and curable.

Also to consider, if the attacks occurred on fasting, are severe liver disease (where the liver is depleted of glycogen), glycogen storage disease (where the liver exhibits glucose greed), pituitary or adrenal insufficiency (where hormones that counteract the falling glucose level induced by insulin are lacking), severe inanition and wasting, and massive fibromas, sarcomas, or fibrosarcomas found in the chest, retroperitoneal space, or pelvis. The latter tumors cause hypoglycemia in an unclear manner. Insulin levels are normal, but these tumor cells may synthesize a polypeptide that is similar in action to insulin but not recognized immunologically as such.

An alcoholic debauch, especially in the presence of poor food intake, can cause hypoglycemia and even coma. It results from alcohol-induced impairment of hepatic gluconeogenesis.

Most of these disorders are easy to diagnose. Severe liver disease is quickly apparent on physical examination, alcoholic excess with malnutrition may be solved with a question, and glycogen storage disease in children is suspected by hepatosplenomegaly and proved by biopsy. Pituitary and adrenal diseases have numerous other clues, and large connective tissue tumors are usually palpable or noted on pelvic examination or chest radiograph.

Factitious factors cause another subset of hypoglycemias. Insulin overdose and oral hypoglycemics are obvious causes in diabetics, especially if a meal is missed or late. But non-diabetics, especially relatives of diabetics whose hypoglycemic drugs are available, have been known to self-inflict mysterious attacks for secondary gain. The history gives the key clue. But if suspicion and mystery persist, the presence of insulin autoantibodies and a plasma sulfonylurea determination may give proof despite denial.

Questions

1. Insulin-secreting adenomas must always be considered in patients with fasting hypoglycemic episodes. A 56-year-old otherwise healthy man has convulsive seizures associated with bizarre behavior on six different mornings during the past month. Each episode occurs at 4 or 5 am while he is still asleep, and is vividly described by his wife. Physical examination findings are normal. Fasting blood glucose is 60 mg/dL. You suspect an insulinoma and wish to prove it. The following reflections are all correct except one.
   (a) This disease is surgically curable, 90% of the tumors are benign, and some are associated with multiple endocrine neoplasia (MEN) type I in which adenomas occur in the pituitary and parathyroid glands as well as in the pancreatic islets.
   (b) The pattern of symptoms is repetitive in the same person, and central nervous system symptoms usually follow the less serious manifestations also seen in reactive hypoglycemias. Attacks are severe and persistent, usually requiring glucose for relief.
   (c) The fasting blood glucose level is often well below 60 mg/dL. If not, a 24-hour or even a 72-hour fast may be required to elicit severe hypoglycemia (less than 40 mg/dL). Because abnormal insulin-glucose homeostasis exists, the inappropriate elevation of plasma insulin concentration in the presence of hypoglycemia after an overnight or more prolonged fast remains the cornerstone of diagnosis (abnormal immunoreactive insulin-glucose ratio).
   (d) Whipple's triad consists of: (1) the clinical picture of episodic hypoglycemia, (2) proof of hypoglycemia by blood tests during an episode, and (3) relief of symptoms by the administration of glucose. The fact that the triad exists in this patient is proof that he has an insulinoma.

2. Non-pancreatic large tumors have in recent years been identified as causes of fasting hypoglycemia. Which one of the following statements is incorrect?
   (a) Tumors are usually of mesodermal origin, grow slowly, and attain huge size before causing symptoms.
   (b) Occasionally, carcinomas with metastases will also cause hypoglycemia; hepatomas are notable in this respect.
   (c) The immunoreactive insulin-glucose ratio will be abnormally high.

(d) A total body scan, computed axial tomography, chest radiograph, pelvic examination, and liver scan should be able to detect almost all large tumors associated with hypoglycemia.

3. The following four disorders may be associated with hypoglycemic episodes. In only one of these disorders, the fasting blood glucose level is normal, the blood glucose remains normal even after a 3-day fast, and its hypoglycemic episodes do not occur if a meal is missed or late. Which disorder does this description fit?

(a) Insulinoma
(b) Severe liver disease
(c) Adrenal insufficiency (Addison's disease)
(d) Functional hypoglycemia.

Answers

1. **(d) is correct** because it is partially incorrect. Whipple's triad is present in virtually all cases of hypoglycemia, regardless of the cause. All other statements—(a), (b) and (c)—are correct and matters of fact. To be reasonably certain that an insulinoma exists, Whipple's triad must be present *and* blood tests drawn during a symptomatic episode should reveal (1) inappropriately elevated insulin and C-peptide levels, and (2) the *absence of sulfonylureas*. Once proved biochemically, the tumor must be located; ultrasound of the pancreas is best. If MEN is suspected, MRI of the pituitary and serum calcium should be obtained.

2. **(c) is correct** because it is incorrect. The precise mechanism for hypoglycemia in these instances has not yet been resolved. It is not caused by high insulin production, and thus the immunoreactive insulin level is not elevated; in fact, it is often low. Excessive utilization of glucose by the tumor is one theory. Others place blame on the tumor's secretion of insulin-like substances that lower the glucose level but do not immunoreact like insulin. Bear in mind that endodermal malignancies sometimes cause hypoglycemia too. The diagnostic measures listed in (d) may all be useful in locating tumors that are not externally palpable.

3. **(d) is correct.** In functional hypoglycemia, episodes occur only in response to the stimulation of a meal—usually 3 or 4 hours later. No meal—no hypoglycemia! Not so for the other choices.

Comment The two major decision points in this case were: (1) are the episodes caused by hypoglycemia or hyperepinephrinemia? and (2) what is the cause of the hypoglycemia? In the development of clinical logic, a differential diagnosis was laid out, and all disorders save one were eliminated. Case 19 later on in this chapter deals with a patient who also had hypoglycemic episodes, but the logic branches into a different direction. It is interesting to note how two clinicians from disparate academic environments approach the same problem. *(P.C.)*

Suggested Readings

Cryer PE. Banting Lecture. Hypoglycemia; The limiting factor in the management of IDDM. Diabetes 1994;43(11):1378–1389.

Cryer PE, Fisher JN, Shamoon H. Hypoglycemia. Diabetes Care 1994;17(7):734–755.

Marks V. Recognition and differential diagnosis of spontaneous hypoglycemia. Clin Endocrinol (Oxford) 1992;37(4):309–316.

Prince MJ. Hypoglycemia of non-diabetic origin. Curr Ther Endocrinol Metab 1994;5:412–416.

Service FJ, O'Brien PC, Kao PC, et al. C-peptide suppression test: Effects of gender, age, and body mass index; implications for the diagnosis of insulinoma. J Clin Endocrinol Metab 1992;74(1):204–210.

CASE 15

OBESITY AND HIRSUTISM

Paul Cutler

Data In an attempt to make herself more attractive, a 38-year-old recently divorced woman seeks your advice because she is overweight and has excessive hair all over her body.

She has been in good health all her life. Although the patient has always been slightly overweight (height 64 in, weight 148 lb), in the past 3 years her weight gradually increased to 192 lb despite the fact that she eats "practically nothing." She is convinced there is something wrong with her glands and that her metabolism and hormones must be "out of balance." As further evidence for her opinion, she says she has been hairy ever since she can remember and would like to have this treated, too.

Logic This lady has two chief complaints—obesity and hirsutism. Your first thoughts revolve around whether these are part of one endocrine disease, or are they unrelated, and are we simply dealing with a "fat hairy woman?"

Although nutrition and "nutritional value" of the diet may have become an issue of unwarranted popular concern, the greatest dietary problem in the United States remains the excessive consumption of food. In more than 95% of cases, obesity is simply the result of eating too much. This usually stems from familial and cultural eating habits, psychologic factors, lack of exercise, or combinations of these three. Only the rare fat person has an endocrine disease. Of these, we must consider hypothyroidism, Cushing's syndrome, polycystic ovaries, hypothalamic disorders and tumors, and various causes of hypoglycemia, especially insulinoma. Furthermore, diabetes mellitus and obesity often coexist. So much for the causes of obesity!

Next you quickly run through the causes of hirsutism to see if there are conditions common to both lists: familial, idiopathic, ovarian (polycystic ovaries, stromal hyperthecosis, or virilizing tumors), adrenal (virilizing tumor, congenital hyperplasia, adenoma, carcinoma, or Cushing's syndrome), porphyria cutanea tarda, and medications (steroids, androgens, diphenylhydantoin, minoxidil, danazol, diazoxide, and oral contraceptives).

A number of endocrine overlaps are noted.

You recall that *ethnic hirsutism* in Mediterranean persons appears at puberty, worsens into the twenties, and is not associated with endocrine abnormalities. Furthermore, *idiopathic hirsutism,* the most common type, probably has some basis in androgen abnormality. In fact, 70 to 85% of women with idiopathic hirsutism have mild elevation of plasma testosterone (.8 to 2.0 ng/mL) if sophisticated measuring techniques are used. Those patients who have idiopathic hirsutism without frank virilization have abnormal secretion of various androgens from the adrenal gland or ovary; there are no detectable structural abnormalities.

If hirsutism of sudden onset is associated with menstrual disturbances and is accompanied by *virilism* (acne, frontal balding, enlarged clitoris, low-pitched voice, and increased muscle mass), then an endocrine disease caused by increased androgens must be strongly suspected and is usually clearly manifested. Virilization is most commonly secondary to an androgen-secreting adrenal or ovarian tumor. In these cases the testosterone level is greater than 2 ng/mL.

Harvey Cushing first described the clinical picture of bilateral adrenal hyperplasia caused by excess ACTH secretion from a pituitary basophil adenoma. The abundant ACTH secretion resulted in adrenal cortisol hypersecretion. This specific set of circumstances is known as "Cushing's disease."

All other clinical disorders that have the same clinical presentation and that are caused by the presence of excess cortisol, but in which a pituitary adenoma is *not* present, are known as "Cushing's syndrome." Hypercortisolism caused by a primary adrenal tumor or adrenal carcinoma is an example of Cushing's syndrome.

Notwithstanding the foregoing, by far the most common cause of Cushing's syndrome is the exogenous administration of steroids for the treatment of patients with asthma, rheumatoid arthritis, ulcerative colitis, renal transplantations, and some malignancies.

Also, be aware of "ectopic ACTH" syndromes in which ACTH-like substances are produced by bronchogenic carcinomas (mainly oat cell) and thymomas, and less often by malignancies of the breast, colon, ovaries, and elsewhere (Table 13.1).

The common substrate in all cases of Cushing's syndrome and Cushing's disease is the excessive secretion of cortisol by the adrenal cortex. If you exclude iatrogenic and ectopic causes, the pituitary gland is responsible for two thirds of cases and autonomous adrenal disease for the remaining third.

Various textbook sources do not clearly distinguish between the disease and the syndrome. Semantics aside, from the diagnosis and treatment standpoint, it is important to know only whether the primary pathologic process results from disease in the pituitary area, disease of the adrenal cortex, tumors elsewhere, or the exogenous administration of steroids.

It is necessary to understand the various hormonal relationships and feedback mechanisms operative in the hypothalamic-pituitary-adrenal axis. The hypothalamus, under the control of circadian rhythm, neurotransmitters, and physical and emotional stress, secretes corticotrophic releasing hormone (CRH), which stimulates the pituitary to secrete ACTH. In turn, the ACTH stimulates the adrenal cortex to form cortisol.

TABLE 13.1. Causes of Cushing's Syndrome

1. Excessive CRH production
   a. Hypothalamic disorder
   b. Ectopic CRH production—carcinoid, islet cell tumor, pheochromocytoma, thyroid medullary cancer

2. Pituitary adenoma (Cushing's disease)
   a. 90% micro
   b. 10% macro

3. Ectopic ACTH production—oat cell, breast, ovary, colon carcinomas

4. Adrenal gland—adenoma, carcinoma

5. Exogenous steroid administration

CRH = corticotropin-releasing hormone; ACTH = adrenocorticotropic hormone.

The plasma level of cortisol regulates the further secretion of CRH and ACTH by feedback to both the hypothalamus and the pituitary gland (Fig. 13.4). Ectopic ACTH-like substances stimulate the adrenal to form cortisol. Another group of tumors may in some instances secrete CRH-like peptides, which results in formation of more ACTH and cortisol. Included in this group are carcinoids, islet cell tumors, pheochromocytomas, and thyroid medullary carcinoma.

Data This patient's menarche was at age 13 and sexual development was normal. However, her menses have been irregular at times, dysmenorrhea has been a problem, and she has no children. Recently her menses had become more irregular, and she has not had a menstrual period for 4 months.

Excessive body hair has been present since age 15. She describes several black hairs on the upper lip and chin that require shaving, long black hairs on the forearms, and a few hairs around her nipples and abdomen. The amount of hair present seems to have increased steadily over the years, and she shaves her legs frequently.

She also complains of frequent headaches and occasional episodes of depression. Two years ago she almost fainted on several occasions and had to eat to keep from passing out. These episodes were accompanied by weakness and sweating. A physician obtained a blood glucose at that time; it was normal, and the episodes never recurred. A review of her current eating habits reveals that her "eating nothing" is grossly understated.

Both parents are of Mediterranean origin, and her father and one sister have diabetes mellitus. Her mother died of hypertension and a stroke. Except for easy fatigability, nocturia, and drinking three to six glasses of water daily, the rest of the history is negative. She takes no medication.

Logic So far we have an obese, somewhat hirsute

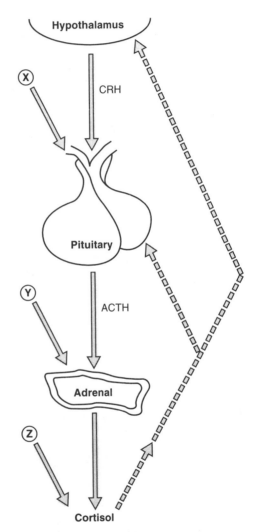

Hypothalamic Pituitary Adrenal Axis

▶ **Figure 13.4.** Hypothalamic pituitary adrenal axis. Solid arrows = stimulation; dashed arrows = inhibition; x = ectopic corticotropin releasing hormone; y = ectopic adrenocorticotropic hormone; z = exogenous steroids; CRH = corticotropin releasing hormone; ACTH = adrenocorticotropic hormone.

woman with nocturia, polydipsia, menstrual irregularities, possible infertility, and past episodes suggestive of hypoglycemia. This is a complex constellation and requires much more information for its solution. The possibilities range from trivial to serious and from rare to common.

However, on the basis of the data so far obtained, you may begin to ruminate over possibilities and likelihoods. Are we dealing with one rare disease or a combination of common ones?

Even though myxedema and Cushing's disease are associated with obesity in the minds of many, few patients with these diseases are grossly overweight. They may even be thin. In myxedema, the facial appearance, skin color, voice, and affect are critical features. In Cushing's disease, truncal obesity with thin extremities, plethora, purple striae, and other features are the crucial determinants (Table 13.2).

The patient's hirsutism is only mild, she is Mediterranean, and she does not so far appear to be virilized, so it is likely that what she considers excess hair is not pathologic but only cosmetically unacceptable to her. Her headaches, weakness, and fatigue are of little discriminatory value, but the family history of diabetes may be significant in view of her polyuria and polydipsia. The weak spells years ago could represent the hypoglycemia of early diabetes, although episodes of this type could be psychosomatic, insignificant, and nondiscriminatory; and it is important to realize that amenorrhea is sometimes seen in patients who gain or lose much weight rapidly.

Data Physical examination reveals a grossly and diffusely obese woman in no acute distress. There is no moon facies, buffalo hump, central obesity, or violaceus striae. The blood pressure is 185/100 in both arms lying and standing; the weight is 192 lb; and the height is 64 in. She has no stigmata of hypothyroidism, is not plethoric, and her facial and body hair are as described in the history. There are no signs of virilization, and the visual fields are grossly intact. A few pale pink striae measuring 0.5-cm wide are noted on the breasts and abdomen. The reflexes are brisk and have a normal rate of return. Pelvic examination reveals normal-sized ovaries and uterus. There are no other positive or pertinent negative findings.

Logic Hypertension is now added to the pattern. The striae are simple stretch marks caused by obesity. Cushing's disease is unlikely in view of the absence of other usual findings. Polycystic ovaries (Stein-Leventhal syndrome) as a cause of hirsutism, obesity, and irregular menses cannot be ruled out even in the presence of normal-sized ovaries, because the ovaries are normal in 25% of cases. Had the ovaries been enlarged, that diagnosis would have been much more likely. Hyperthecosis of the ovaries, a variant of this syndrome, is often accompanied by hypertension and diabetes, so it is still possible. A masculinizing ovarian tumor (arrhenoblastoma) is unlikely because it was not palpated, and the patient is not masculinized.

Normal visual fields and the absence of other evidence of hypopituitarism with multiglandular hypofunction weigh against a space-occupying lesion of the pituitary, third ventricle, or hypothalamus.

Adrenal virilizing tumors that combine the

TABLE 13.2. Cushing's Syndrome—Clinical Features

GENERAL FEATURES	INCIDENCE	SPECIFIC FEATURES
Truncal obesity	.90	Thin limbs, buffalo hump, supraclavicular pads
Diabetes	.88	—
Skin changes	.85	Atrophy, bruises, striae, acne, hyperpigmentation
Hirsutism	.80	—
Gonadal dysfunction	.75	Amenorrhea in females, decreased libido in males
Muscle weakness	.60	Catabolism, steroid myopathy, electrolyte disturbance
Osteoporosis	.60	Back pain, fracture
Hypertension	.50	—
Psychologic disturbances	.40	Depression, confusion, emotional changes

features of virilization and Cushing's syndrome are now most unlikely. Numerous diagnostic possibilities seem to be eliminated, but laboratory studies are needed for confirmation.

A review of the patient's photographs from recent years may help you identify cushingoid features not recognized earlier.

Data The complete blood count and electrolytes are normal. Urinalysis shows 4+ glycosuria and the fasting blood glucose is 220 mg/dL. The serum is grossly lipemic; after standing overnight in the refrigerator, the lipemia does not clear, and a creamy layer is noted on top of the serum. T_4 and TSH test results are normal. The urine vanillylmandelic acid (VMA), metanephrines, and cortisol (5μg/dL) are normal. The plasma total and free testosterone as well as the cortisol level are normal. The chest and skull radiographs are normal.

Logic The laboratory studies are conclusive. Diabetes mellitus is present. Normal cortisol levels in plasma and urine serve as excellent tests to exclude Cushing's syndrome. Effectively ruled out are adenomas in and around the pituitary gland and adenomas of the adrenal cortex and medulla. Further search for an aldosteronoma is not warranted because of the normal potassium. Ovarian diseases (thecosis, tumor, or polycystic disease) causing some or all of the cluster of clues are further ruled out by the normal testosterone level. The lipemic nature of the serum probably indicates type V hyperlipoproteinemia, a common accompaniment of uncontrolled diabetes.

Instead of having one uncommon disease that causes all her problems, this woman has a concurrence of several common diseases. She is simply an obese, slightly hirsute woman with diabetes and hypertension. Although most women with idiopathic hirsutism have slight elevation of plasma testosterone levels, remember that roughly one-fourth do not. The spells several years ago may well have been related to the hypoglycemia of early diabetes. Her failure to become pregnant needs further investigation, including a study of her mate's gonadal function. The recent severe weight gain may be related to her marital problems, and the amenorrhea is probably secondary to the rapidly acquired obesity.

Even though the patient has four cardinal features—hypertension, obesity, diabetes, hirsutism—it is not surprising that she does not have Cushing's syndrome. These clinical features are

TABLE 13.3. Incidence of Clues in a Population Subset with and without Cushing's Disease

CLUE	CUSHING'S DISEASE	NON–CUSHING'S DISEASE
Hypertension	.50	.20
Obesity	.90	.30
Diabetes	.88	.08
Hirsutism	.80	.10

common, as well as commonly seen together in the subset of 30- to 60-year-old women (Table 13.3). Bayesian calculations that consider disease prevalence, the product of probabilities, and likelihood ratios would substantiate the clinical conclusion reached in this case.

Data Problem list:

1. Exogenous obesity
2. Idiopathic hirsutism
3. Essential hypertension
4. Diabetes mellitus
5. Amenorrhea
6. Depression
7. Divorce

Appropriate treatment and superficial psychotherapy were given. The patient lost weight, diabetes was controlled, hypertension was adequately lowered, and electrodesiccation successfully removed hair from her face. The menses returned. Perhaps her husband will too.

Logic Consider the diagnostic pathway if one or more of the tests had turned out differently. If the VMA level was high, a search for pheochromocytoma would be indicated. If the serum potassium level was low, aldosteronoma would enter into consideration. But most important in this case, if the plasma and urine cortisol levels were high, there would then be need to decide whether Cushing's syndrome was caused by pituitary or adrenal disease. Treatment would hinge upon this decision.

In that event, additional studies would include:

• Dexamethasone suppression test (DST) to distinguish between a micro- or macroadenoma of the pituitary gland and an adenoma or carcinoma of the adrenal cortex

- Magnetic resonance imaging with gadolinium contrast, which is best for the detection of microadenomas of the anterior pituitary gland
- Computed tomography to detect adrenal tumor
- Inferior petrosal vein (IPV) sampling to measure ACTH concentration as compared to ACTH concentration in peripheral (P) venous blood—significant if IPV: P > 2, and especially if >3 after stimulation with CRH

These are the tests used to distinguish various members of the Cushing family. But it must be borne in mind that *nonfunctioning* adenomas of the pituitary and especially of the adrenal cortex are not uncommon. Therefore the finding of an adenoma by imaging study does not guarantee that the clinical findings are its direct consequence. And always ready to confuse the diagnostician are the facts that MRI detects only 60 to 70% of pituitary microadenomas (30 to 40% FN rate) and that there is a 1 to 8% incidence of biologically inactive adrenal cortical adenomas.

COMMENT The author started with two key clues—obesity and hirsutism—each of which had its own list of possible causes. Overlap in the two lists was immediately noted. Gradually, the two clues were built into a larger pattern that could be explained by either a rare disease or a concurrence of several common ones. The latter situation turned out to be correct in this case.

Proof was obtained mainly by exclusion of all other possibilities. Some bits of irrelevant or possibly misleading information, such as headaches, "eating nothing," weak spells, and depression, had to be suppressed in order to narrow the clues to a more wieldy cluster.

Psychosocial factors were strongly related to the clinical picture, and it was often necessary to separate the functional from the organic. These factors included obesity, eating habits, sterility, divorce, and depression. Family history and racial traits helped to decide the significance and causes of hirsutism, diabetes, and hypertension.

The crucial and decisive bits of evidence in this case were the normal values for plasma and urine cortisol. *(P.C.)*

Suggested Readings

Derkson J, Nagesser SK, Meinders AE, et al. Identification of virilizing adrenal tumors in hirsute women. New Engl J Med 1994;331(15):968–973.

Orth DN. Cushing's syndrome. New Engl J Med 1995;332(12):791–802.

Watson RE, Bouknight R, Alguire PC. Hirsutism: Evaluation and management. J Genet Intern Med 1995;10(5):283–292.

Yanovski JA, Cutler GB Jr. Glucocorticoid action and the clinical features of Cushing's syndrome. Endocrinol Metab Clin N Am 1994;23(3):487–509.

CASE 16

NERVOUSNESS AND WEIGHT LOSS

Paul Cutler

Data A 42-year-old woman visits her physician because of severe nervousness and weight loss for the past 3 months. She has always considered herself to be a nervous person, but since the death of her mother she has been more so, cries easily, is jumpy and fidgety, and her hands tremble.

Logic This combination is not specific. You consider severe anxiety, menopause, and hyperthyroidism. Furthermore, the nervousness and weight loss may not be part of the same process; in fact, she may be losing weight because she is nervous, or she may be nervous because she is losing weight. Either symptom, separately, has its own list of causes.

Data Further questioning reveals that she feels warm all the time, dresses lightly even though it is winter, and argues frequently with her husband who wants the windows shut. Her appetite has remained good; she consumes more than her usual fare, yet claims to have lost 15 lb in 3 months according to her bathroom scale. She notes frequent palpitations, and her legs and thighs fatigue easily, especially on walking up steps. Her menses had become scant and stopped completely 2 months ago.

Logic The picture is taking on a different complexion. It transcends simple nervousness and anxiety. Menopause can include almost all the symptoms, although she is quite young for that. Cessation of menses speaks for menopause, although this may stop if there are severe emotional disturbances and also if hyperthyroidism is present. Heat intolerance is a key point favoring an overactive thyroid gland. The combination of *good appetite* and *weight loss* points to the latter diagnosis too. This duet is seen mainly in three conditions: severe diabetes, hyperthyroidism, and malabsorption. On the other hand, *weight loss* and *anorexia* indicate a totally different and usually more serious spectrum of chronic infection, malignancy, or depression.

Data There is no cough, dyspnea, orthopnea, nocturia, frequent urination, or unusual thirst. She has had two to three formed bowel movements daily during the past few months, but the stools are not foul or greasy and do not float. She does not drink alcohol, consumes five cups of coffee, and smokes five to ten cigarettes each day. Her clothes have become too large, and she needs another wardrobe; this depresses her and gives her more anxiety. Although her mother died of a heart condition, she had had some kind of thyroid disease for many years.

Logic Not much is added. Malabsorption and diabetes mellitus as causes for some of her symptoms are now most unlikely. Her bowel pattern is compatible with excessive thyroid activity. Hyperthyroidism has a familial tendency and is far more common in women; these are significant facts in this case.

Data Examination discloses a lean nervous woman in no distress. Her skin is thin, velvety, warm, and moist; this is especially noticeable on handshake. A fine rapid tremor is noted on the outstretched hands. The vital signs are: temperature, 37.5°C; pulse, 120 and irregular; respirations, 20; and BP, 160/70. Her eyeballs are prominent, and sclera is noted between the upper lid and cornea (Fig. 13.5). Lid lag is present when she lowers her eyes, and she has infrequent blinking and inability to converge her eyes on a near object. Her hair is fine, silky, and scant. The thyroid gland is diffusely although only moderately enlarged, and no nodules are palpated. A systolic bruit is heard over each lower pole of the thyroid gland and a venous hum is heard in both supraclavicular areas. The heart rate is 138 and is grossly irregular, and a third heart sound is discernible at the apex. The apex beat is forceful, the left ventricular impulse is strong, and the lower portion of the neck is felt to pulsate with each heartbeat.

Logic The diagnosis is now beyond question. She has hyperthyroidism. Tremor, tachycardia, thyromegaly, and eye signs make an incontrovertible tetrad. But, in addition, there is also the characteristic nature of the hair and skin, evidence of high cardiac output, and high blood flow to and from the thyroid gland. The atrial

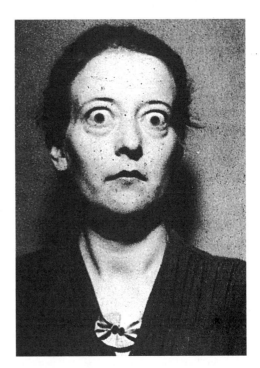

▶ **Figure 13.5.** Hyperthyroidism. Exophthalmos is obvious. Note mild diffuse thyromegaly.

fibrillation (with pulse deficit) is a common signpost. Warm sweaty hands mean hyperthyroidism, whereas cold sweaty hands mean anxiety. All the physical findings point in one direction.

Data The T_4 is 16.4 μg/dL (normal 4–12); TSH is 0.00 μU/mL: serum cholesterol is 98 mg/dL, postprandial glucose is 180 mg/dL; complete blood count, urinalysis, chest radiograph, and ECG are normal except for atrial fibrillation with a ventricular rate of 132. The 18-test chemistry profile is normal except as noted previously.

Logic Laboratory studies confirm the clinical diagnosis. The elevated glucose level may be seen in hyperthyroidism, but it should be rechecked later. The high T_4 level has suppressed TSH production.

There is a distinct family predisposition to hyperthyroidism (Graves' disease), as noted by the increased frequency of haplotypes HLA-B8, and DRw3. The cause of Graves' disease is unknown, although it is signaled by a circulatory long-acting-thyroid-stimulator (LATS) whose origin is equally enigmatic. Because the level of T_4 is elevated in this disease, the TSH level would of necessity be low, or even absent, as in this case, and need not be tested. If the level of T_4 is unexpectedly normal in a suspected case of hyperthyroidism, measure the T_3 level; occasionally it alone is elevated.

Data   The primary care physician, the surgeon, the patient, and the family discuss the alternative forms of treatment and, for a variety of debatable reasons, the following course is chosen. After an appropriate 8-week period of methimazole, propranolol, and preoperative potassium iodide, a subtotal thyroidectomy is performed. The patient did well in the immediate postoperative period, except for transient hoarseness that cleared in a few days.

Logic   Antithyroid drugs plus surgery were chosen over drugs alone or radioactive iodine even though there was some controversy. The hoarseness resulted from minor temporary damage to a recurrent laryngeal nerve.

Data   Three days postoperatively, the patient began to complain of twitching feelings in the face and tingling of the hands. A tranquilizer did not help, and on Day 6 she had generalized tonic contractions in the arms and legs, followed by convulsions. Chvostek's and Trousseau's signs were present; the ECG showed a broad ST segment and a prolonged QT interval. The serum calcium was 6.0 mg/dL, serum phosphorus was 6.0 mg/dL, and studies were otherwise normal. Intravenous calcium gluconate had already been given, and the patient was begun on vitamin D even before the test results were obtained.

Logic   Hypoparathyroidism may result from thyroidectomy because several parathyroid glands are often buried in the thyroid, and the blood supply to the others may be impaired. Usually the disorder is minimal and transient, because the remaining glands take over full function. Such a clinical picture following thyroid surgery usually has this explanation. The ECG changes are consistent with hypocalcemia.

Data   At discharge, she felt well and was clearly euthyroid by laboratory tests and becoming so by appearance. She was given a prescription for vitamin D and a calcium supplement, and told to return in 2 weeks.

She next sees her physician 3 years later, having moved to another state in the interim. She had long ago stopped taking vitamin D and the twitchy feelings never returned. Again she complains of fatigue and weakness, but this time she has not lost weight and is not nervous. In fact,

her symptoms seem diametrically opposed to the original ones. She complains of dry skin and constipation and feels cold all the time. Her husband and she still argue about the room temperature; however, now he wants the air-conditioner on when she wants it off.

Her face is puffy and pale, the skin is dry and thickened, the hair is coarse, dry, and sparse, and the reflexes demonstrate a slow return to the normal position. She is definitely anemic, she appears to have gained weight, her speech is slow, and her wit is dimmed. The vital signs are temperature, 36.6°C; pulse, 60; respirations, 12; and BP 100/70.

Logic   The clues are typical for hypothyroidism. Cold intolerance is another highly specific symptom except in the elderly; delayed relaxation of the deep tendon reflexes is a highly specific sign. After subtotal thyroidectomy, a significant number of patients will develop insufficient thyroid function and need permanent replacement therapy. It was unfortunate that this patient did not return for follow-up treatment.

Data   Laboratory tests confirm the obvious impression. The T_4 is 1.6 μg/dL, TSH level is high—125 μU/mL, and serum cholesterol is 348 mg/dL. She is started on small doses of levothyroxine, and her dose will be titrated under careful supervision until she is again euthyroid.

Logic   The measurement of the TSH has come into very popular use. TSH elevation is a *sine qua non* for the diagnosis of primary hypothyroidism; if the TSH level is normal or subnormal, suspect that the hypothyroidism is secondary to a hypothalamus–pituitary disorder. In the patient just discussed, this determination was not necessary because by history alone the hypothyroid disorder resulted from surgery, and the TSH level would have inevitably been high. But to exclude the remote possibility that pituitary gland failure is now at fault, a TSH test was ordered.

If the clinical picture was still not clear and the tests were equivocal, an injection of thyrotropin-releasing hormone (TRH) would cause a marked elevation of TSH provided the pituitary gland was intact (and the thyroid hypofunction, therefore, the result of disease, destruction, or ablation of the thyroid gland). On the other hand, if the TSH did not rise sharply, the thyroid hypofunction would be secondary to disease of the pituitary gland.

Questions

1. You see a 28-year-old woman who has numerous signs and symptoms suggesting hyperthyroidism. Her older sister takes medication for a thyroid condition. The patient is nervous, has a tremor, rapid pulse, perspires freely, and has lost weight despite a good appetite. But her thyroid gland is not palpable. The T_4 and T_3 resin uptake are twice normal, TSH level is depressed, but the radioiodine uptake is low. You consider:
   (a) another disease.
   (b) ectopic toxic thyroid tissue.
   (c) laboratory errors.
   (d) thyrotoxicosis factitia.

2. Thyrotoxicosis in the elderly is often overlooked because cardiovascular complications tend to dominate the picture. You should be alert to this possibility if the patient has:
   (a) an enlarged nodular thyroid gland.
   (b) weakness of the shoulder and hip muscles.
   (c) atrial fibrillation with a rapid ventricular rate.
   (d) nervousness, exophthalmos, heightened activity.

3. Hypoparathyroidism can result from surgery as occurs in the patient in this case. Idiopathic hypoparathyroidism is less common but does occur. It is characterized by all the following except:
   (a) episodes of tetany.
   (b) high calcium, low phosphorus levels.
   (c) calcification of basal ganglia, cataracts.
   (d) evidences of autoimmune disease.

4. Although hypothyroidism in this patient clearly resulted from surgery, there are other causes. Which of the following clinical pictures can be associated with hypothyroidism?
   (a) Thirty-eight-year-old woman who has had no menses since her last child was born 4 years ago
   (b) Sixty-four-year-old woman exposed to radioactive iodine for the treatment of a "goiter" 20 years ago
   (c) Puffy, pale, comatose elderly woman with a temperature of 33°C
   (d) Short stature, retarded bone age, and mental retardation in a 6-year-old child

Answers

1. **(d) is correct.** It is likely that the patient is taking thyroid extract or one of its analogues; the drug is available at home, and the entire clinical picture fits, although you do not yet know the psychodynamics involved. Although laboratory errors are always possible, and it is necessary to consider another disease such

as "silent" thyroiditis, self-induced hyperthyroidism is most likely. Choice (b) could be correct, because ectopic thyroid tissue in the chest or ovary could become toxic, but this is most unusual and would require scanning elsewhere for detection.

2. **(a), (b), and (c) are correct.** Such patients do have large thyroids, proximal myopathy, and atrial fibrillation with frequently uncontrolled congestive heart failure. But the features of (d) are not usually present. In fact, these patients generally are apathetic and calm; eye signs are minimal. They are often mistaken for senile patients with end-stage congestive heart failure. Recognition and proper treatment effect profound improvement.

3. **(b) is correct because it is wrong.** The basic defect, lack of parathyroid hormone, results in low serum calcium and elevated serum phosphorus levels. Tetany and calcium deposition in bone also occur. Calcification of ganglia and cataracts result too. This disease may be seen together with other allegedly autoimmune diseases, such as pernicious anemia, thyroiditis, and Addison's disease. In addition, many patients have autoantibodies to parathyroid, which lends further credence to the autoimmune etiology for the idiopathic form.

4. **All are correct.** Choice (a) Suggests a woman with Sheehan's syndrome who suffered an infarcted pituitary gland at childbirth, and then developed hypogonadism and hypothyroidism. Choice (b) The incidence of hypothyroidism after radioiodine treatment increases annually and approaches 100% with advancing age. The patient in (c) probably has myxedema coma, an advanced stage of hypothyroidism. And the child in (d) has juvenile myxedema.

COMMENT Problem solving was simple here. The diagnoses were fairly evident as the information unfolded. A sequence of hyperthyroidism, hypoparathyroidism, and hypothyroidism was unquestionable—the cause and effect relationship being so very obvious. Each diagnosis was proved by characteristic clusters of clues derived from all portions of the data base. *(P.C.)*

Suggested Readings

Finucane P, Anderson C. Thyroid disease in older patients. Diagnosis and treatment. Drugs Aging 1995; 6(4)268–277.

Singer PA, Cooper DS, Levy EG, et al. Treatment

guidelines for patients with hyperthyroidism and hypothyroidism. JAMA 1995;273(10):808–812.

Smith SA. Commonly asked questions about thyroid function. Mayo Clin Proc 1995;70(6):573–577.

POLYURIA AND POLYDIPSIA

David J. Kudzma

Data The patient is a 33-year-old professional lepidopterist whose relentless quest for the winged rare and beautiful has, during the past 3 months, been hampered by a too frequent need to urinate and drink water. This need exists throughout the waking day (every 2 hours) and awakens him three times nightly. Each time, the voided volume seems to be a "bladderful." There is no pain, burning, or difficulty with urination, but he is finding the problem wearisome. He has noted increasing thirst, and is aware that his fluid intake is generous; after most nocturnal trips to the bathroom he drinks a glass of water.

Logic The distinctive problem here is polyuria, and its possible causes are multiple. It is apparent that his urinary frequency is caused by the formation of a large volume of urine rather than by the need to void small amounts frequently. Therefore he does not have common simple frequency resulting from infection or obstruction. He is too young for prostatic hypertrophy, the most common cause of obstruction in men, nor does he have the usual symptoms that go with obstruction or infection. The nocturia of congestive heart failure can easily be eliminated, because he has daytime frequency also and because patients with congestive heart failure would have symptoms of dyspnea and fatigue rather than nocturia. Furthermore, none of these situations (obstruction, infection, congestive heart failure) causes thirst because there is no increase in total urine volume. Renal disease with waning renal function may cause a compensatory increase in urine volume, but not to this degree.

We are left with the various *polyuric-polydipsic syndromes*: (1) diabetes mellitus, (2) central diabetes insipidus (DI), (3) nephrogenic DI, (4) psychogenic polydipsia, (5) hypokalemia, (6) hypercalcemia, and (7) the use of a diuretic.

DM causes an osmotic diuresis. Central DI is caused by a lesion of the hypothalamus or posterior lobe of the pituitary gland, resulting in insufficient antidiuretic hormone. Nephrogenic DI results from renal unresponsiveness to antidiuretic hormone.

Even at this point, the surreptitious use of a diuretic is unlikely for a number of reasons: the effect of mild diuretics is limited to a number of days, and although potent diuretics are effective for longer periods, such patients would have critical volume depletion, syncope, and shock rather than polyuria alone. Low potassium and high calcium levels do not cause such severe water turnover. More historical data are needed.

Data There is no family history of DM or any other polyuric syndrome. He takes no medication, drinks ethanol infrequently, and does not smoke. There is no history of renal stones, gastrointestinal symptoms, or conjunctival irritation. His health has remained good, he feels well, has lost no strength, and his appetite and weight have remained normal. There is neither headache nor visual symptoms.

Logic The hypercalcemia of hyperparathyroidism or a non-parathyroid tumor is not suggested because there have been no stones, gastrointestinal symptoms, or symptoms of conjunctival irritation due to deposition of calcium salts. Moreover, his general health has been good. DM as a cause of polyuria and polydipsia is unlikely in the absence of weight loss, weakness, polyphagia, and family history. The absence of weakness weighs against kaliopenic nephropathy with resultant polyuria, and there is no other apparent cause for low potassium. The possibility of DI due to a pituitary of hypothalamic tumor is less likely in the absence of headache and visual disturbances. But special studies are needed to explore this diagnosis more fully. Several possibilities are already reasonably well excluded and only a few remain, idiopathic diabetes insipidus among them.

Data Physical examination discloses a healthy-looking young man. The vital signs are normal, and there are no significant orthostatic changes in pulse and blood pressure. He weighs 163 lb and is 70 in tall. With the exception of a left varicocele, everything is normal. Specifically, visual fields, tissue turgor, and mucous membranes are normal. Band keratopathy is not present.

Logic Note the absence of evidence of weight

loss, blood volume contraction, or dehydration. You would expect severe DM or potent diuretic abuse to cause them. The juxtacorneal calcium salt deposits resulting from prolonged or severe hypercalcemia are not present. Normal strength, normal deep tendon reflexes, normal blood pressure, absence of gastrointestinal symptoms, and the non-use of medications are all points that weigh against hypokalemia and some of its principal causes. The varicocele is not significant. Although laboratory tests are now needed, we have already reasonably excluded most of the causes listed for the presenting cluster.

Data Studies: urinalysis is completely normal, but specific gravity is 1.002; blood count, urine culture, ECG, and chest radiograph are normal; serum sodium, potassium, bicarbonate, chloride, glucose, creatinine, calcium, and phosphorus are all normal; serum cholesterol is 298 mg/dL.

Logic So much for DM, hypokalemia, and hypercalcemia! Also, renal disease in general is virtually eliminated. Although hypercholesterolemia may be an important problem, it is of no consequence in this diagnostic deliberation. The often ignored urine specific gravity is significantly very low, and in the context of this patient, a dilute urine directs us toward central DI, psychogenic polydipsia (PP), or nephrogenic DI. The controlled environment of a hospital is required to explore these possibilities.

Data The patient is hospitalized. A first-voided morning urine specimen has a specific gravity of 1.001. The 24-hour fluid intake is 7600 mL, and the concomitant 24-hour urine output is 6800 mL. MRI of the brain, specifically of the sella turcica and suprasellar area, is normal.

Logic Polyuria, polydipsia, and hyposthenuria are confirmed. There is no evidence of a tumor in the sellar area. Further discriminatory tests are needed.

Data Water is rigorously withheld from 10 pm to 6 am. At 10 pm, the body weight is 160 lb; at 6 am, the body weight is 156 lb. Measurements of plasma AVP (arginine vasopressin), plasma osmolality, and urine osmolality are made concurrently every 2 hours during the 8-hour period of water deprivation. By 6 am, plasma osmolality was 298 mOsm/kg, and urine osmolality was 470 mOsm/kg (up from 85 mOsm/kg at 10 pm). Plasma AVP steadily rose from 1 to 5 pg/mL from 10 pm to 6 am (see data that follow).

	10 PM	6 AM
Weight (lb)	160	156
Urine osmolality mOsm/kg	85	470
Plasma AVP pg/mL	1	5

Logic The marked rise in plasma AVP furnishes evidence that posterior pituitary function is intact. The equally marked rise in urine osmolality offers evidence that the kidneys are indeed responsive to AVP and are able to concentrate urine. Thus both central DI and nephrogenic DI are virtually ruled out.

Central DI may be partial or complete. Symptoms of AVP deficiency do not arise until 80 to 90% of the AVP-secreting cells of the posterior pituitary gland are destroyed. Partial deficiencies may occur, resulting in only mild symptoms and modest increases in 24-hour urine formation, for example, 3000 mL. Such cases may be difficult to diagnose and further tests with synthetic AVP analogues might be in order.

Although most cases of central DI are idiopathic, some result from pituitary tumors, parasellar tumors, metastatic tumors (often breast), and generalized diseases such as the histiocytoses, sarcoidosis, and other granulomatous diseases. These diseases may be located in the hypothalamus, the pituitary stalk, or in the pituitary gland itself.

None of the specific causes is evident here. The abrupt onset of symptoms and craving for ice water are characteristic of central DI; these clinical clues are not present here either.

Thus, the presenting polyuria and polydipsia are most likely explained by psychogenic factors, the reasons for which should be explored with the assistance of psychiatric consultation.

The patient is asked to restrict his fluid intake to eight glasses per day, including all types of liquids, and he will need careful watching. PP and DI are often mistaken for each other—even after studies. Should symptoms continue, more detailed investigation may be needed.

Questions

1. Which of the following diagnostic procedures would give the most valuable information in evaluating a patient with a 4-week history of polydipsia and polyuria?
   (a) Oral glucose tolerance test

(b) Urinalysis

(c) Fasting blood glucose

(d) Twenty-four-hour urine collection for volume and osmolality

2. Which of the following clues most strongly suggests DM as the cause of a 4-week history of polydipsia and polyuria?

(a) Weight loss

(b) Absence of nocturia

(c) Anorexia

(d) Bradycardia

3. Suppose the patient in Case 17 with severe polyuria and polydipsia becomes lethargic and irritable, and has neither edema nor signs of dehydration. Immediate study reveals the serum sodium to be 119 mEq/L. Otherwise, everything, including the urinalysis, is unchanged. He has a low serum sodium level that is causing mental abnormalities. The patient is critically ill because of:

(a) inappropriate antidiuretic hormone secretion.

(b) renal salt-wasting.

(c) diabetes insipidus.

(d) compulsive water drinking.

4. Assume that our patient had responded to a test dose of DDAVP (des-amino-D-arginine vasopressin [a synthetic AVP analogue in common use as antidiuretic hormone therapy]), with a rise in urine osmolality to 900 mOsm/kg and disappearance of polydipsia. Which of the following is/are correct?

(a) Plasma level of antidiuretic hormone would be high.

(b) Although the response is consistent with central DI, this diagnosis is unlikely because of his age.

(c) You would expect to find DI in other members of the family.

(d) Mild cases can exist where the urine volume is only 2000 to 3000 mL/24 h.

Answers

1. **(b) is correct.** If there is no glucose in the urine, DM can be excluded as a cause of the symptoms. The specific gravity provides useful information regarding the concentrating ability of the kidneys. Other urine abnormalities may suggest primary renal disease. The glucose tolerance test is not of much value because, even if abnormal, heavy glycosuria is required to cause the clinical picture; this is detected by the urinalysis. For the same reason, the blood glucose is of limited value. Answer **(d)** fails to consider DM, the most common cause of the presenting symptom complex.

2. **(a) is correct.** Involuntary weight loss associated with the two prominent symptoms indicates DM, unless proved otherwise by an immediate urinalysis. Because polyuric patients who have DM have nocturia and increased appetite, **(b)** and **(c)** are incorrect. The pulse rate is probably of little help, although under these circumstances it is more apt to be rapid than slow.

3. **(d) is correct.** Compulsive water drinking may sometimes result in a dilutional hypo-osmolar syndrome with low sodium, resulting mental changes, and even convulsions. Such patients who drink themselves into water intoxication are unusual. The urine findings are such as to exclude renal disease and salt-wasting. In DI, the patient drinks a lot because he or she urinates excessively, whereas the patient with PP (psychogenic polydipsia) urinates a lot because he or she drinks too much; the serum sodium level is normal or slightly high in DI. Inappropriate antidiuretic hormone secretion causes low serum sodium, but it is not associated with the polyuria and polydipsia; such patients have normal or low output.

4. **(d) is correct.** The dramatic response (exceeding the response to overnight water restriction) confirms the diagnosis of central DI. This is not an *"all or none"* disease; the deficiency of antidiuretic hormone may be mild, and symptoms may be similarly so. The plasma antidiuretic hormone level is high in nephrogenic DI, but this diagnostic possibility is disproved by the response to vasopressin. Furthermore, central DI can occur at any age, and it is not familial.

COMMENT The skilled busy physician would solve the polyuria–polydipsia cluster with alacrity. He or she knows the statistical likelihoods, the clues associated with these likelihoods, and how to reach the target quickly. The absence of urinary obstructive symptoms and the patient's age weigh against prostatic disease; further, because the total urine output does not change, thirst does not result. Good health and stable weight and appetite disqualify DM. We are now left only with the unusual.

A quick urinalysis, serum glucose, and electrolytes rule out hypercalcemia, hypokalemia, florid kidney disease, and DM. The low urine specific gravity and osmolality are helpful. You know he has dilute urine and the field is narrowed to three possibilities. The response of urine osmolality and urine output to water deprivation and a sometimes used DDAVP injection makes the distinction between nephrogenic DI, central DI, and compulsive water drinking.

All you've done is ask five or ten questions, examine the urine, get three blood chemical tests, and do two simple noninvasive procedures. *Et voilà!* You have the answer, and you haven't even touched the patient. *(P.C.)*

Suggested Readings

Blevins LS Jr, Wand GS. Diabetes insipidus. Crit Car Med 1992;20(1):69–79.

Fujiwara Tm, Morgan K, Bichet DG. Molecular biology of diabetes insipidus. Annual Rev Med 1995; 46:331–343.

Hotzman EJ, Ausiello DA. Nephrogenic diabetes insipidus: Causes revealed. Hosp Prac (Office Ed) 1995;29(3):89–93, 97–98.

Robertson GL. Diabetes insipidus. Endocrinol Metab Clin N Am 1995;24(3):549–572.

CASE 18

HYPERCALCEMIA

Paul Cutler

Data During his routine annual health examination, the 48-year-old vice-president of Strato Airways was found to have a serum calcium concentration of 11.5 mg/dL.

Logic High serum calcium values have been among the most frequent abnormalities detected on routine laboratory screening procedures. Although there is some variation in the normal ranges found in various laboratories, a serum calcium of 11.5 mg/dL in the presence of normal serum albumin undoubtedly would be classified as definite, albeit modest, hypercalcemia.

Dietary calcium is absorbed from the small intestine under the control of the vitamin D analogue—1,25-dihydroxy-vitamin D (calcitriol). To maintain calcium homeostasis in the body, the amount ingested must equal the amount excreted. Eighty percent of ingested calcium is excreted in the stool, and 20% in the urine. The level of serum calcium is kept fairly constant within narrow margins by vitamin D, which regulates the amount absorbed, and by PTH, which determines the amount resorbed from bone and excreted by the kidney.

In the blood, 55% of calcium is bound to albumin, and 45% circulates as ionized calcium—$Ca++$—the physiologically active moiety. The interpretation of what is "normal" for the blood calcium level must take into account varying levels of serum albumin. "Normal" must be adjusted by .8 mg/dL for each 1 g/dL of albumin below normal (4 g/dL). If the albumin is 2 g/dL, the normal serum calcium is 1.6 mg less than what is usually regarded as normal.

Serum calcium ($Ca++$) plays multiple roles: the secretion of many hormones; muscle contraction; blood coagulation; release of neurotransmitters; activation of enzymes; intracellular second messenger; deposition of bone; and so forth.

The more common causes of hypercalcemia in the general adult population, in approximate order of frequency, are:

1. Cancer, including multiple myeloma, lymphomas, leukemia, and various solid tumors with or without skeletal metastases
2. Primary hyperparathyroidism
3. Sarcoidosis
4. Hyperthyroidism
5. Use of thiazide diuretics
6. Milk-alkali syndrome
7. Vitamin D intoxication
8. Immobilization-induced acute bone atrophy

Ninety percent of cases of hypercalcemia are caused by items 1 and 2.

To this list of diseases must be added spurious hypercalcemia, which is relatively uncommon and easily eliminated from consideration. This is a result of:

- Blood drawn after leaving a tourniquet in place for an excessively long time. This may be avoided, even in the patient with "difficult" veins, by removing the tourniquet after venipuncture and allowing re-establishment of normal blood flow before withdrawing the sample.
- Contact of the blood or serum with cork. Cork is rarely used as a test tube closure in chemistry laboratories today and should no longer be a source of contamination.
- Laboratory error: Relatively small errors are present with most procedures for calcium measurement in common use today. Repeat

analysis should suffice to rule out this problem.

Data History taken from the patient failed to disclose any recent illnesses, obvious symptoms, or medications. He denied any unusual food habits.

Logic It is therefore reasonable to exclude milk-alkali syndrome, thiazide diuretics, and intoxication with vitamin D. Incidentally, some health food faddists may ingest excessive amounts of vitamin D (and/or A, which may also cause hypercalcemia). In addition, that fact that our patient has not been ill obviously eliminates immobilization-induced acute bone atrophy. Despite the apparent absence of symptoms, none of the other listed diseases can be ruled out.

Hypercalcemia occurs in approximately one sixth of all patients with hyperthyroidism as a direct effect of thyroid hormone's increasing bone resorption, but it is not often symptomatic or clinically troublesome. The absence of any of the usual symptoms aids in eliminating the diagnosis of hyperthyroidism, but it may be relatively asymptomatic, and appropriate laboratory tests should be performed. In most cases, a serum T_4 determination should be sufficient. (Results were normal in this patient.)

Data A more comprehensive and detailed history disclosed some pertinent information. The patient had passed three kidney stones during the past 10 years, but had hesitated to admit to his employer that he was ill for fear it might jeopardize his career. Two of the episodes were associated with pain in the left flank, and one with pain in the right. These stones had passed spontaneously and were not saved for examination, although the patient thought that they were tan or brownish in color. In addition, the patient reluctantly admitted that he regularly used an electric cart on the golf course because for the last 2 years or so he had noticed lethargy and easy fatigability. Some years earlier he had been the "boy wonder" of Strato Airways, with boundless energy and enthusiasm. Recently, however, he just did not have his old pep and had been passed over for the presidency of the company as a result of his apparent inability to make important decisions quickly.

Logic Now we are beginning to get somewhere. Although there are many causes of renal calculi, such a long history (10 years) in association with current hypercalcemia leads one to think of primary hyperparathyroidism (HPT). The passage of stones from both kidneys helps rule out a congenital or acquired ureteral lesion that might predispose to stone formation by obstructing normal urine flow.

The absence of symptoms of acute urinary tract infection, however, does not eliminate the possibility of chronic pyelonephritis as a predisposing factor, because the latter may be totally silent while destroying the kidneys. It would have been helpful to examine and analyze the stones; they are usually calcium oxalate, apatite, or brushite in primary HPT. Magnesium ammonium phosphate stones, on the other hand, would indicate infection. The tan to brownish appearance of the stones is not necessarily helpful, because this coloration might have represented small amounts of blood collected on the surface of the stones as they passed with difficulty through the ureters.

There are many causes of kidney stones, any one of which could have a chance association with any of the causes of hypercalcemia. It is worth noting, however, that renal stone has been one of the most frequent presenting features of primary HPT and may continue for many years before detection of hypercalcemia. It has been estimated that 5 to 10% of patients with urolithiasis have primary HPT. Incidentally, patients with HPT who have stones usually do not have clinically significant nephrocalcinosis.

The characteristic symptoms of mild hypercalcemia are lethargy, easy fatigability, weakness, loss of energy, and aprosexia (inability to concentrate). These symptoms are often so gradual in onset that the patient may be unaware of their presence. Furthermore, they are so nonspecific as to be of little diagnostic value. With increasing severity of hypercalcemia, symptoms may include anorexia, constipation, and drowsiness or stupor. Polyuria and nocturia may be noted because hypercalcemia antagonizes the action of antidiuretic hormone and thus leads to a loss of renal concentrating ability.

Prolonged hypercalcemia can lead to metastatic calcification in the skin, cornea, conjunctiva, and kidneys—nephrocalcinosis.

HPT, therefore, can be seen by the physician in any one or more of a variety of ways: (1) an abnormal asymptomatic laboratory result; (2) vague symptoms; (3) kidney stones; (4) back pain and crush fractures resulting from long-standing osteoporosis; and (5) hypercalcemic crisis, consisting of polyuria, dehydration, psychosis, obtundation, and coma.

The pathophysiologic sequence of events that result from the increased secretion of PTH in HPT is:

1. Excretion of excessive amounts of phosphate in the urine
2. Lowered serum phosphate as a consequence thereof
3. Elevated serum calcium level to maintain the solubility product of calcium phosphate
4. Calcium resorption from bone into blood—PTH-mediated
5. Hypercalcemia results in hypercalciuria and stones.

Data On physical examination, the patient appears to be healthy. The only abnormal physical findings were mild hypertension and some whitish granular deposits in the cornea bilaterally, just medial and lateral to the limbus. Subsequent examination by slit lamp confirmed band keratopathy.

Logic There are no physical findings characteristic or pathognomonic of primary HPT. Only rarely can even a large parathyroid adenoma be felt. The fact that the patient appeared well is compatible with that diagnosis, however, and does not support the possibility of an advanced malignancy.

The various malignant disorders previously mentioned as possible causes for hypercalcemia do so mainly by elaborating peptides that behave like but are not identical to PTH. These peptides are known as "parathyroid hormone-related protein" (PTH-rP) and can be distinguished from true PTH by radioimmunoassay techniques. But it should be noted that malignancies may also cause hypercalcemia by bone-destroying metastases.

There is no physical evidence for any of these malignant diseases such as wasting, enlarged lymph nodes, or pallor. The long history of renal calculi weighs against their being caused by the hypercalcemia of malignant disease. Hyperthyroidism is most unlikely in the absence of thyromegaly, exophthalmos, tachycardia, and tremor.

Hypertension has come to be recognized as a fairly common finding in patients with primary HPT. But because of the frequency with which it occurs in the general population, its presence is of little or no diagnostic value. Hypertension may occur in any form of hypercalcemia and has even been observed during infusion of calcium lasting only a few hours. The cause for this relationship is not known.

Detectable band keratopathy with only modest hypercalcemia suggests that hypercalcemia has been present for a long time and helps further to make the diagnosis of cancer less likely. Band keratopathy is the deposition of calcium salts in the cornea, sclera, and conjunctiva (Fig. 13.6). It is sometimes appreciated by the patient as an irritation of the eyes or conjunctivitis. More often it is asymptomatic and appears as fine white granules in the cornea and sclera just medial and lateral to the limbus and usually separated slightly from it. On casual inspection it may be mistaken for arcus senilis. Two features distinguish band keratopathy, however: granularity and the absence of deposits from the superior and inferior aspects of the eye. Band keratopathy can appear slowly in patients with long-standing but minimal to moderate elevations of serum calcium; or it can develop rapidly in patients with severe hypercalcemia.

Data Examination of other routine laboratory data disclosed the following pertinent results:

Normal: hemoglobin, hematocrit, leukocyte count, differential; erythrocyte sedimentation rate; urinalysis; serum creatinine and urea nitrogen;

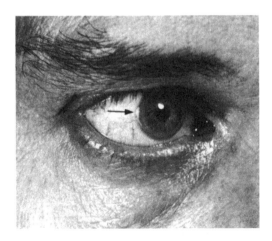

▶ **Figure 13.6.** Band keratopathy. Deposits of grayish-white calcium salts at cornea-scleral junction.

serum protein electrophoresis; serum sodium, potassium, bicarbonate; and liver function tests.

Abnormal: serum phosphorus (inorganic phosphate) 2.3 mg/dL; serum chloride 109 mEq/L; serum uric acid 9 mg/dL; serum alkaline phosphatase 100 IU/L; and urinary calcium excretion 320 mg/24 h.

Logic It is always reassuring to find normal values for hemoglobin, hematocrit, leukocyte count, sedimentation rate, urinalysis, and the serum protein electrophoresis, because they virtually rule out a host of malignant diseases: myeloma, lymphoma, leukemia, and widespread carcinomatosis. Admittedly, a relatively small and inconspicuous malignant tumor (such as a hypernephroma or bronchogenic carcinoma) could produce enough of its hypercalcemic hormone to cause hypercalcemia without otherwise appearing to affect the patient. In fact, at this time the tumor may be resectable. Therefore, some investigators suggest that hypercalcemia and other hormonal effects be used as tumor markers to identify early malignant disease.

The abnormal laboratory values shown are quite typical for primary HPT. But such values could also result from a malignant tumor that secretes parathyroid hormone or a closely related peptide. This situation is sometimes called ectopic hyperparathyroidism or pseudohyperparathyroidism for obvious reasons. Some studies have indicated that a relatively high serum chloride level (107 mEq/L) or a high ratio of chloride to phosphorus (30) strongly favors the diagnosis of primary HPT, whereas the reverse favors malignancy. The ratio in this case is 47 (109/2.3).

Hyperuricemia is a common accompaniment of primary HPT but may occur coincidentally in any hypercalcemic disorder.

Minimal elevation of the serum alkaline phosphatase is often seen in primary HPT and suggests that radiograph evidence of osteitis fibrosa may be found. It may also be increased in malignant disease due to bone involvement or hepatic metastases. Chemical distinction between alkaline phosphatases of skeletal and hepatic origin can be made in some laboratories and may be helpful.

Urinary excretion of calcium is particularly likely to aid in distinguishing primary HPT from sarcoidosis and vitamin D intoxication. In the latter diseases, secretion of parathyroid hormone is greatly decreased, so long as there is no significant impairment of renal function (or at least of the glomerular filtration rate). The hypercalcemia of vitamin D intoxication, and probably of sarcoidosis as well, is due to the effects of a high blood concentration of one or more active metabolites of vitamin D. When the serum calcium increases, secretion of parathyroid hormone is inhibited. Because parathyroid hormone is a potent factor in the renal tubular reabsorption of calcium, its relative absence would be expected to permit urinary excretion of a higher fraction of filtered calcium. Because the filtered load of calcium is the product of plasma ultrafiltrable calcium (approximately 55 to 60% of the total) and the glomerular filtration rate, urinary excretion of calcium is higher (at any given level of serum calcium) in sarcoidosis and vitamin D intoxication than in HPT, at least when renal function is normal. Urinary calcium rarely exceeds 500 mg/d in HPT; it often does so in the other two diseases.

One must be particularly wary in milk-alkali syndrome, which is usually due to excessive ingestion of milk and calcium carbonate. As originally described, this syndrome consists of hypercalcemia, normophosphatemia, azotemia, normocalciuria, and often alkalosis. The normophosphatemia and normocalciuria, however, are probably a result of renal insufficiency and therefore could occur in HPT complicated by renal insufficiency. In fact, milk-alkali syndrome may be superimposed upon HPT, as was the case in several patients of the initially reported series, presumably due to overzealous treatment of peptic ulcer (symptoms of which are common in primary HPT).

Data Radiographs of the skull, hand, clavicles, pelvis, spine, and long bones were obtained. There were no lytic lesions suggestive of metastases or myeloma. The skull was thought to show a finely stippled pattern suggestive of numerous minute areas of bone resorption. The radial aspects of several fingers showed cortical thinning, small intracortical cysts and tunneling, and subperiosteal resorption. The cortex of the distal third of each clavicle was very thin, producing an almost cystic appearance. Both bony margins of the acromioclavicular joint, but especially the clavicle, were irregular and frayed.

Logic These findings are characteristic of osteitis fibrosa, the skeletal lesion of HPT. Only rarely will a patient with ectopic HPT be found to have the characteristic radiograph features of osteitis fibrosa, presumably because the course of the disease is usually too rapid for the bone disease to become manifest. Even though our patient did not have any "brown tumors" (osteoclastomas) or cysts, enough radiograph evidence of bone disease was present to make the presumptive diagnosis of osteitis fibrosa.

At this point, therefore, the diagnosis of primary HPT seem most likely, with cancer becoming more remote. Sarcoidosis seems equally well ruled out by the normal chest radiograph, absence of lymphadenopathy, absence of characteristic cystic changes in the phalanges, normal serum protein electrophoresis, normal liver function tests, and normal renal function. High serum concentrations of 1,25-dihydroxy-vitamin D, the most potent natural metabolite of vitamin D, have been found in hypercalcemic patients with sarcoidosis or other granulomatous diseases. This suggests the possibility that the granulomas are in some way responsible for uncontrolled synthesis of this metabolite. However, measurement of this metabolite is not necessarily of diagnostic value because its levels are sometimes elevated in patients who have primary HPT. On the other hand, the combination of a high 1,25-dihydroxy-vitamin D level and a low parathyroid hormone level would be very supportive of sarcoidosis or another granulomatous disease.

Data For added assurance, it was considered advisable to obtain measurement of the serum PTH concentration. This was markedly elevated (620 pg/mL); normal (10–65), further confirming the diagnosis of primary HPT. Surgery was thought to be indicated. On careful dissection, a pea-sized adenoma of the parathyroid gland was found behind the right lobe of the thyroid and excised.

Logic Eighty to ninety percent of cases of primary HPT are caused by a single adenoma. Ten to fifteen percent of cases are related to hyperplasia of all four glands, mostly within the context of multiple endocrine neoplasia syndromes, and less than 1% are caused by parathyroid carcinomas.

Measurement of the serum concentration of PTH is not always required for diagnosis, but it is often helpful in less clear-cut situations than the present one. Some endocrinologists have found that measurement of total urinary excretion of cyclic adenosine monophosphate (cyclic AMP), or of the nephrogenous portion only, is

easier to interpret with consistency. Excretion of this substance generally parallels the serum concentration of PTH.

In this patient, the need for surgical removal of the parathyroid adenoma was clear. In addition to modest hypercalcemia, the patient had radiographic evidence of osteitis fibrosa. Some authors have suggested, however, that "chemical" HPT, that is, HPT without clinically apparent involvement of target organs such as bone and kidney, need not be treated surgically and needs only periodic confirmation that no change has occurred. This seems a rather risky position, because a hypercalcemic crisis can occur quite unexpectedly in these patients, and the development of bone disease or kidney impairment cannot be predicted. In fact, it has been reported as a result of a 10-year prospective study that it was impossible in retrospect to find any clues that would indicate which patients would subsequently require surgery. Especially with the capability of locating even rather small adenomas before surgery through the use of high-resolution ultrasonography, CT, and MRI, there seems to be little justification for withholding definitive cure (Fig. 13.7).

Quite a different case can be made for *familial hypocalciuric hypercalcemia,* a syndrome of still unknown dimension that may be confused with HPT. It has a strong familial occurrence with autosomal dominant transmission. There are few symptoms and signs, no morbidity, and no clear-cut cause. This newly described entity needs further clarification. But it must be considered when hypercalcemia is found.

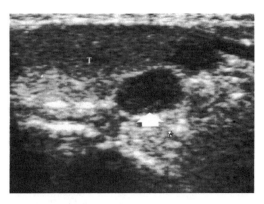

▶ **Figure 13.7.** Parathyroid adenoma detected by ultrasound—longitudinal view (magnified) T, thyroid.

COMMENT Another asymptomatic laboratory abnormality—or so it seemed at first! Vague nonspecific symptoms and a history of renal stones pointed the problem solver in the right direction. Although the major causes of hypercalcemia were quickly established and each member of the list given consideration, all were eliminated by the absence of highly sensitive clinical features, save one: parathyroid adenoma. This one was then proved by decisive data—band keratopathy and PTH elevation.

While surfing through the sea of pathophysiology incurred in the solution of this case, the author, in "think-along-with-me" style, covered calcium measurement and metabolism, the sensitivity and specificity of various clues, and multiple cause-and-effect relationships. *(P.C.)*

Suggested Readings

Bilezikian JB. Management of acute hypercalcemia. N Engl J Med 1992;326:1196.

Broadus AE, Mangin M, Insogna KL. Humoral hypercalcemia of cancer. N Engl J Med 1988;319:556–563.

Consensus Development Conference. Diagnosis and management of asymptomatic primary hyperparathyroidism. Ann Intern Med 1991;114:593.

Lafferty FW, Hubay CA. Primary hyperparathyroidism: A review. Arch Intern Med 1989;149:789–796.

 C A S E 19

COMPOUNDED CONFUSION

Barry J. Goldstein

Data You are called to the emergency department to see a 72-year-old man who was brought in by his wife because of mental confusion for several hours. He is a retired salesman who is in generally good health, except for mild hypertension that is treated with hydrochlorothiazide once daily, and glaucoma that is managed with eye drops and three acetazolamide pills daily.

He had been spending his days playing golf and tennis a few times a week until 3 weeks ago when he began to have episodes of heart *palpitations* and *sweating* associated with some *confusion*. He felt hungry and anxious during these episodes and the symptoms were relieved within a few minutes by eating some cookies or drinking fruit juice. The episodes were becoming more frequent and during the past week were occurring almost daily, especially just before his usual mealtimes.

This morning he was awakened by a similar spell at 5 am; it was not relieved by cookies or orange juice.

Logic The patient is experiencing what seems to be symptoms of adrenergic discharge. This aggregate may be seen in hypoglycemia, pheochromocytoma, and stimulant drug abuse, although similar pictures may also be caused by hyperthyroidism (which is not episodic), anxiety reaction, and panic disorders.

You are struck by the association of his symptoms with fasting or the pre-meal period, and the fact that they can be relieved by eating a snack. Whipple's triad for the diagnosis of hypoglycemia, proposed in 1938, establishes the following criteria:

1. Spontaneous blood glucose <50 mg/dL
2. Characteristic symptoms at time of hypoglycemia
3. Relief of symptoms by glucose administration

Hypoglycemia is associated with a characteristic set of signs and symptoms depending on the absolute value of the lowered blood glucose level (Table 13.4). The brain is dependent on glucose for its normal functioning. As the blood glucose is lowered, the body reacts initially by activating the adrenergic system. Later, as the glucose level falls further to a critical level, mentation is affected and with increasing severity, symptoms ranging from confusion to coma can occur. Combinations of these two sets of symptoms can be observed, but it is possible that neuroglycopenic symptoms alone may predominate, especially if the patient is taking a beta-blocker.

TABLE 13.4. Signs and Symptoms of Hypoglycemia

ADRENERGIC	NEUROGLYCOPENIC
Palpitations	Diplopia or blurred vision
Sweating	Confusion
Anxiety	Fatigue
Hunger	Amnesia
Tremor	Seizures
	Coma

Data Review of systems reveals that he has gained approximately 5 lb in the last month or so, whereas his weight (185 lb with a height of 5'11") had previously been stable for the past 10 years. He has been having occasional dull headaches on awakening, which are also unusual for him. He found that he could no longer engage in physical activities and was becoming house-bound. He has not had any generalized weakness between episodes and does not have other systemic symptoms, such as a rash, arthritis, or fevers. He drinks only a few beers on the weekends.

He had a general checkup with his primary care physician 2 months ago and was found to be in good health. A general hematology and chemistry screen was unremarkable at that time. He has never taken insulin or drugs such as sulfonylureas that can cause hypoglycemia and, other than his wife who is an insulin-taking diabetic, no one else at home or in his immediate family has diabetes or uses these types of medications. Psychologically he is very stable and according to the family there would be no apparent reason for him to be injecting himself with insulin that he does not need for medical reasons (factitious hyperinsulinemia).

Logic The mild weight gain is consistent with the increased food intake that was necessary to alleviate his symptoms, and to bring his blood glucose into a normal range. Increased physical activity will increase glucose uptake by skeletal muscles and further potentiate the lowering of his blood glucose, thus worsening the frequency or the intensity of his "spells."

The major causes of fasting hypoglycemia to be considered in this patient include increased abundance or action of circulating insulin (hyperinsulinism), drug effects, organ failure, hormonal deficiencies, and certain tumors (Table 13.5). In a pediatric population, a series of inborn errors of glucose metabolism would also need to be included. Among these possibilities, non-beta-cell tumors are unusual causes of hypoglycemia. These tumors are often large retroperitoneal masses that produce insulin-like growth factors that cause hypoglycemia by stimulating the insulin receptor and mimicking insulin action. There is nothing to suggest adrenal insufficiency or hypopituitarism—conditions that are more likely to lead to hypoglycemia only in younger patients. The possibility of major organ

TABLE 13.5. Causes of Fasting Hypoglycemia

Endogenous hyperinsulinism
Pancreatic beta-cell disorders, autoimmune hypoglycemia
Drug effects
Insulin, sulfonylureas, ethanol, and others
Organ failure
Hepatic, renal, sepsis, inanition
Hormonal deficiencies
Cortisol, growth hormone, glucagon
Non–beta-cell tumors
Inborn errors of glucose metabolism

failure or a poor nutritional state that prevents gluconeogenesis because of a poor substrate availability has been largely excluded by his recent normal medical evaluation. Autoimmune hypoglycemia is also unlikely; anti-insulin antibodies rarely occur in patients who have never received insulin, and anti-insulin receptor antibodies that mimic the action of insulin in the tissues are usually found in patients with other autoimmune diseases, such as lupus erythematosus or lymphoma.

Data On examination, the patient is a confused elderly man lying in bed and unable to tell you where he is or what year it is. His vital signs and the remainder of the physical examination were unremarkable except for the mental status changes and lethargy. The neurologic examination was otherwise non-lateralizing and within normal limits.

Initial laboratory results including complete blood count, electrolytes, and 12-channel chemistry screening panel were normal except for a plasma glucose of 23 mg/dL. The patient was immediately given 25 mL of a 50% dextrose solution intravenously, which resulted in a transient improvement in his mental state. The glucose level and his response to glucose infusion satisfied Whipple's diagnostic triad. He was then begun on an intravenous infusion of 10% dextrose at a rate sufficient to maintain his blood glucose in the 90 to 100 mg/dL range. He became more coherent and oriented to place and person and was able to eat meals. His symptoms appeared to be completely resolved by the next morning.

Logic The simple measurement of the blood glucose has confirmed your suspicions that the patient has hypoglycemia. You now need to sort out the underlying reason for his low blood glucose.

Some of the diagnostic considerations mentioned in the table have been excluded by information obtained from the history and examination. For example, he drinks very little alcohol, is well-nourished, has no overt hepatic or renal disease, and has no symptoms or physical evidence of Addison's disease (pigmentation and hypotension), pheochromocytoma (high blood pressure), arrhythmia, or hyperthyroidism (enlarged thyroid, tachycardia, tremor).

The most likely remaining possibilities are (1) neoplasm of the pancreatic beta cells (insulinoma); (2) drug effects leading to hypoglycemia; and (3) retroperitoneal tumor that produces *insulin-like* growth factors and was missed on examination (non-beta-cell tumors).

A most important diagnostic consideration at this point is whether the patient has a level of circulating insulin that is inappropriately high for the low glucose level.

In normal physiology, insulin, epinephrine, and glucagon work in concert to closely monitor the blood glucose level. Insulin lowers blood glucose by promoting its uptake and storage in the liver as glycogen, and in the peripheral tissues. Epinephrine and glucagon elevate blood glucose by promoting the breakdown of liver glycogen (glycogenolysis) and by fostering the production of glucose from substrate precursors (gluconeogenesis). Because a stable glucose level is required by brain tissue, the pancreatic beta cells are finely tuned to respond to a low blood glucose level by drastically reducing their secretion of insulin, thus allowing counter-regulatory hormones to effectively promote glucose release from the liver.

In a patient with true hypoglycemia (glucose < 50 mg/dL), a simultaneous insulin level should be ≤ 6μU/mL.

Data The insulin level drawn during the hypoglycemic episode, when the patient was first seen in the emergency department, returns at 65 μU/mL, an extraordinarily high level for a blood glucose of 23 mg/dL.

Logic *Inappropriate hyperinsulinemia* is present. The diagnostic possibilities include a pancreatic insulinoma, the surreptitious administration of insulin, or the ingestion of a sulfonylurea drug.

At this point, determination of the C-peptide level is helpful to distinguish between these possibilities. In order to produce insulin, enzymes in the pancreatic beta cells cleave the proinsulin molecule into insulin itself and the connecting or "C"-peptide, which are both present in the insulin granules and released in equimolar amounts when insulin is secreted into the bloodstream. If the insulin level in the blood is high because of a pancreatic tumor that is secreting insulin in an unregulated fashion, both the C-peptide and the insulin level will be elevated, because they are released together. Ingestion of a sulfonylurea drug potentiates the secretion of insulin by the beta cells, which also leads to increases in both the insulin and C-peptide levels. In a patient who is injecting insulin surreptitiously, the beta-cell function is normal, and the release of endogenous insulin as well as C-peptide is suppressed by the low circulating glucose level. These patients have high insulin levels due to the subcutaneously injected insulin and their C-peptide level is uncorrespondingly low. Sulfonylureas stimulate the beta cells to form and release insulin. These considerations are summarized in Table 13.6.

Data The C-peptide level, also determined from a blood sample drawn *during the episode of hypoglycemia,* was 8.0 nmol/L. C-peptide levels determined with a glucose less than 50 mg/dL should be less than 0.2 nmol/L.

TABLE 13.6. C-Peptide and Insulin Levels in Hypoglycemic Conditions with Hyperinsulinemia

LEVELS	INSULINOMA	SULFONYLUREA INGESTION	SURREPTITIOUS INSULIN INJECTION
Insulin	⇑	⇑	⇑
C-peptide	⇑	⇑	⇓

Logic The markedly elevated C-peptide value excludes the diagnostic possibility of surreptitiously injected insulin as the cause of the low blood glucose. To test for administration of sulfonylureas, a drug screen of blood and urine was performed.

Data These results revealed that the patient had ingested chlorpropamide, a potent and long-acting hypoglycemic medication. You further investigate the medications the patient has been taking. On inspection of his pill bottles brought in by his wife, you find that he renewed his prescriptions a month ago. Instead of receiving acetazolamide (Diamox), however, he was mistakenly given chlorpropamide (Diabinese), which he was faithfully taking three times daily thinking it was a generic form of acetazolamide.

Now back to the hospital . . . . After 36 hours of 10% dextrose infusion, the patient was eating his meals regularly and had no recurrence of symptoms of hypoglycemia. The infusion was tapered and stopped, and his blood glucoses were consistently greater than 80 mg/dL. He was given a new prescription for acetazolamide, and after his discharge from the hospital, he had no further hypoglycemic episodes.

Logic The scenario depicted in this case presentation is not unusual. A survey of mixed-up prescriptions performed by Huminer and his colleagues in 1989 revealed that both generic and brand names of commonly prescribed medications can be confused with sulfonylurea hypoglycemic drugs. Examples of drug substitutions that have resulted in clinical hypoglycemic episodes are indicated in Table 13.7. With its long half-life of 36 hours, inadvertent ingestion of chlorpropamide by a non-diabetic individual can cause the most serious clinical hypoglycemia, as experienced by the patient in this case.

TABLE 13.7. Examples of Erroneous Dispensing of Oral Hypoglycemic Drugs

INTENDED DRUG	SUBSTITUTED HYPOGLYCEMIC AGENT
Acetazolamide (Diamox)	Chlorpropamide (Diabinese)
Acetazolamide (Diamox)	Acetohexamide (Dymelor)
Chlorpromazine	Chlorpropamide
Tolmetin (Tolectin)	Tolazamide (Tolinase)
Aluminum hydroxide (Dialume)	Chlorpropamide (Diabinese)

COMMENT Problems of this sort seen in today's emergency departments would be quickly solved by a few questions, a focused examination, and a stat capillary blood glucose determination. If the patient is a known diabetic taking insulin or an oral agent, the problem is solved without further action. If the patient is not diabetic, blood drawn during the episodes is sent for measurement of insulin, C-peptide, cortisol, and drug analysis (especially sulfonylureas and alcohol). A separate sample is frozen for subsequent tests—proinsulin, carnitine, insulin antibodies, and lactate.

Distinction must always be made between episodes of hypoglycemia that are either *fasting* or *postprandial* in their times of occurrence. Fasting hypoglycemia occurs many hours after a meal, if a meal is missed, or during the night and early AM. Postprandial hypoglycemia always occurs in response to a meal, usually 2 to 3 hours afterward; it does not happen during the night or if a meal is missed. Each of these categories conjures up a different differential diagnosis. *(P.C.)*

Suggested Readings

Huminer D, Dux S, Rosenfeld JB, et al. Inadvertent sulfonylurea-induced hypoglycemia. A dangerous, but preventable condition. Arch Intern Med 1989; 149:1890–1892.

Hypoglycemia. Endocrinol Metab Clin N Am 1989; 18(1).

Service FJ. Hypoglycemic disorders. N Engl J Med 1995;332:1144–1152.

CASE 20

AMENORRHEA AND GALACTORRHEA

Barry J. Goldstein

Data A 26-year-old school-bus driver consults you because her menstrual periods slowed down, then stopped, and she has been having discharge from both breasts. She thought she might be pregnant.

Menses began at age 11 and appeared like clockwork at monthly intervals until approximately 8 months ago when the flow became scanty and the intervals increased; she has not had a period for 2 months.

The discharge from both nipples has been increasing during the past 2 months; its color is pale whitish-gray. She has had to put pads in her bra in order to prevent occasional seepage through her blouse. This has not happened since she had been pregnant.

Five years ago she delivered a healthy baby girl. Her menses resumed shortly after the delivery, and she was able to nurse the child without any difficulty. She is married, is sexually active, and uses a barrier method of birth control.

Logic The patient is a generally healthy young woman who has experienced a gradual cessation of menstrual periods. *Secondary* amenorrhea is the loss of menstrual periods after they had occurred at the normal time of puberty and had been regular for some time. Its most frequent cause is *pregnancy*. Although she does not have any apparent signs or symptoms of pregnancy, it is imperative that a pregnancy test be performed before further testing or drug therapy is initiated.

Other considerations for secondary amenorrhea include behavioral changes such as significant weight loss, anorexia nervosa, excessive exercise, and psychologic illness or stress. Also in the differential diagnosis are a series of endocrine disorders that include ovarian failure, ovarian tumors that produce sex steroids and suppress the gonadal axis in the pituitary, and primary pituitary or hypothalamic lesions that include tumors, trauma, or infiltrating diseases.

Data The patient has not dieted or lost significant weight during the past year and is not a marathon runner or a ballet dancer. In fact she is 20% over her ideal body weight (5'4", 152 lb) and gets little exercise. She is not under any particular psychologic stress, and her home situation is apparently comfortable. There is no history of serious medical illness and a review of all systems reveals no additional problems.

She does not take any medications except an occasional acetaminophen tablet for headaches she has been having for the past 3 or 4 months. The headaches occur every few days; they are dull and are generally relieved by the tablet, although sometimes she needs to lie down.

Logic An endocrine disorder now seems likely. The headaches make you at least consider an intracranial process as the cause of her two presenting complaints—amenorrhea and galactorrhea. It is reassuring that she does not have any visual changes but you can't help but think she may have a pituitary or hypothalamic lesion that has caused suppression of gonadotropins and excessive secretion of prolactin. A purely ovarian or uterine problem that may cause cessation of menses is less likely because the galactorrhea would remain unexplained.

Data On examination she is a well-dressed, talkative woman who is alert and oriented. The pulse is 80 and the blood pressure is 118/68. She has full ocular movements, and there are no visual field defects noted by gross confrontation. Fundoscopy shows sharp optic disk margins. The thyroid gland is palpable, not nodular, and of normal size. Except for the breast examination, the rest of the physical as well as the neurologic examination is normal. There are no breast lumps or masses but you are able to elicit easily a slightly milky fluid on mild compression of both breast areolae. Pelvic examination shows no abnormalities of the external genitalia; the uterus is palpable and normal, and the ovaries are difficult to feel.

Because there are no special positive clues in the physical examination, except for confirmation of the galactorrhea, a serum prolactin level is obtained. It reads 320 ng/mL (normal 0–20). The results of a rapid urine test for pregnancy are negative.

Logic The serum prolactin level confirms the suspicion that the patient has hyperprolactinemia. Its major causes are indicated in Table 13.8. In most physiologic or drug-induced hyperprolactinemias the serum prolactin level does not rise above 50 to 100 ng/mL. And, other than for pregnancy, postpuerperal breast-feeding, and nipple stimulation, once hypothyroidism and drugs are excluded as causes for galactorrhea, a pituitary tumor becomes a likely diagnosis. Bear in mind that one fourth of normal women who have been pregnant in the past may have some nipple secretion, and that not infrequently the cause of galactorrhea remains obscure.

Endocrine causes of hyperprolactinemia include a pituitary adenoma that secretes prolactin; this is a likely possibility in a patient with headache and a level greater than 200 ng/mL. The level often corresponds to the size of the tumor, and one would suspect that if a tumor exists it is moderately large; some prolactinomas produce levels of several thousand ng/mL.

CHAPTER 13 Endocrine Problems 207

TABLE 13.8. Causes of Hyperprolactinemia

1. Physiologic

   Stress, sleep, exercise, pregnancy, lactation, nipple stimulation

2. Pharmacologic

   Phenothiazine, haloperidol, imipramine, benzodiazepines, metoclopramide, cimetidine, methyldopa, reserpine

3. Pathologic

   Microprolactinoma (<1.0 cm), macroplactinoma (>1.0 cm), primary hypothyroidism

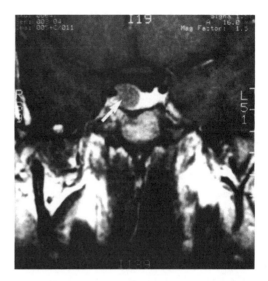

▶ **Figure 13.8.** Coronal magnetic resonance image enhanced by injection of gadolinium showing a 2.5-cm mass in the pituitary gland. The mass is causing upward doming of the diaphragma sellae toward the optic chiasm.

Amenorrhea in this case may result either from the fact that prolactin inhibits the elaboration of gonadotropic hormones and/or a prolactinoma may anatomically impinge upon and even destroy part or all of the pituitary gland and its gonadotropic hormones.

Indeed, the complex interrelationships between the hypothalamus, thyroid-releasing hormone, prolactin-releasing hormone, anterior pituitary and its gonadotropins, the thyroid, the ovary, dopamine and dopamine inhibitors—and their roles in the lactation story—have not yet been completely clarified.

The precise way in which hypothyroidism causes hyperprolactinemia and galactorrhea is equally muddy. Nevertheless one does produce the other, and it is always necessary to rule out hypothyroidism in this or in any such case.

Data Other than the acetaminophen, the patient takes no medications whatsoever—prescription, over-the-counter, or recreational. There are no symptoms of hypothyroidism such as cold intolerance, dry hair or skin, or constipation, and on examination there was no goiter or bradycardia, and the relaxation phase of the reflexes was normal. To be certain, T_4 and TSH determinations are ordered; the results are normal.

Magnetic resonance images of the pituitary gland and surrounding tissue are obtained. They show a 2.5-cm tumor that is bulging through the right upper border of the sella turcica but not yet impinging on the optic chiasm (Fig. 13.8). The patient has a macroprolactinoma. Because of the tumor, visual fields are formally tested; they are normal.

Logic A baseline delineation of visual fields will serve to help you follow the patient's future progress. One of the great advances in the treatment of endocrine tumors is the recognition that *bromocriptine* can cause a prolactinoma to stop growing and in many cases can shrink it significantly. Bromocriptine is a dopamine agonist that exerts an influence on the prolactin-secreting cells to stop not only their growth but also their secretion of prolactin itself.

It is notable that prolactinomas are by far the most common tumors in and around the pituitary gland; most are microadenomas.

Data The patient is started on a low dose of bromocriptine that is gradually increased every few days up to a dose of 7.5 mg/d. You then wait several months to recheck the prolactin level.

After 8 weeks the prolactin level is 30 ng/mL, close to the upper limit of normal range and very significantly reduced from the value first measured.

After 6 months, a repeat MRI study shows a 50% shrinkage of tumor size. The patient notes a return of menses and disappearance of both the headaches and the galactorrhea. She is delighted to avoid transphenoidal surgery.

Logic Because prolactin suppresses the secretion of pituitary gonadotropins and disrupts the normal gonadotropic-ovarian axis, the normalization of the serum prolactin level by bromocriptine restores normal dynamics, and the patient begins to ovulate and have normal menstrual periods.

She should be cautioned that her fertility has been restored and that she should be careful about becoming pregnant. Although it is safe and possible to become pregnant while the prolactin level is suppressed by bromocriptine, as soon as pregnancy is detected, the bromocriptine is usually stopped, and the patient is followed up clinically, and with visual field examination and MRI if necessary.

Questions

1. Because men do not have menstrual irregularity as an early symptom of hormonal imbalance, prolactin-secreting tumors are often discovered only after they have reached a large size. Besides evidence of local tumor invasion, which of the following is (are) the most common hormone-related endocrine symptom or symptoms of hyperprolactinemia in men?
   (a) Bradycardia, puffy face, delayed Achilles reflex
   (b) Decreased libido and testicular atrophy
   (c) Galactorrhea
   (d) Increased libido and testicular enlargement

2. A moderate-sized pituitary tumor is discovered on a head CT scan of a 46-year-old man who was in an automobile accident. The attending physician wants to know if the tumor is hyperfunctional, destructive of pituitary function, or both. A history and physical examination are performed. Which of the following tests or endocrine assays may solve the problem in each of the following derived clinical pictures?
   (a) Increased hat and shoe size, carpal tunnel syndrome
   (b) Loss of libido, testicular atrophy
   (c) Diabetes, hypertension, acne, muscle weakness
   (d) Severe thirst, frequent urination, good appetite, stable weight
   (e) Pallor, puffy face, obesity, BP 90/70, temperature 97°F
   (f) Loss of libido, diarrhea, weakness, postural dizziness
   (g) Weak, sweaty, shaky episodes, loss of libido, testicular atrophy
   (h) Negative history, normal physical examination findings

Tests and Assays

1. T$_4$	8. Cortisol
2. TSH	9. ADH
3. LH	10. GH
4. FSH	11. Serum calcium
5. ACTH	12. Blood glucose
6. Prolactin	13. Urinalysis
7. Insulin	14. Water deprivation test

Answers

1. **(b) is correct.** As in women, hypersecretion of prolactin will suppress the production of pituitary gonadotropins by its action on the hypothalamus. Thyrotropin is not affected and the absence of glandular breast tissue precludes galactorrhea. Choices (a), (c), and (d) are thus incorrect. The loss of testicular stimulation leads to a decrease in circulating testosterone, resulting in decreased libido and clinical changes compatible with a hypogonadal state. This includes diminished body hair, a decreased need for shaving, and a decrease in the size of the testes.
2. (a)-(10)—acromegaly
   (b)-(6) or (2 and 3)—prolactinoma or hypopituitarism
   (c)-(5) and (8)—Cushing's syndrome
   (d)-(9, 12, 13, 14)—diabetes insipidus or diabetes mellitus
   (e)-(1, 2)—hypothyroidism
   (f)-(5, 8)—secondary hypoadrenocorticism and hypogonadism
   (g)-(7, 11)—hypercalcemia will denote MEN type I.
   (h)—some would do nothing and repeat CT in 1 year; others would do most tests listed.

Comment In this case, where the patient had both amenorrhea and galactorrhea, each symptom by itself conjured up a separate list of diagnostic contenders. Other than in some cases of pregnancy, the single diagnosis common to both subsets is the presence of a prolactinoma.

Although not usually the cause of *both* presenting symptoms, hypothyroidism and primary ovarian failure, as well as the use of certain drugs and life styles had to be excluded.

With the current ability to assay hormones at 10^{-12} molar concentrations, and with the use of modern imaging procedures such as CT and MRI, has come the knowledge that prolactinomas are by far the most common of all pituitary tumors.

That hyperprolactinemia causes galactorrhea is clearly understood. But the precise mechanism whereby hyperprolactinemia suppresses gonadotropins—and it clearly does—remains obscure.

Less obscure are the mass effects that large prolactinomas may cause, such as headaches from expansion into the bony sella and its diaphragm, visual field defects if the tumor impinges on the optic chiasm, and hypopituitarism by direct destruction of anterior pituitary tissue. *(P.C.)*

Suggested Readings

Bevan JS, Webster J, Burke CW, et al. Dopamine agonists and pituitary tumor shrinkage. Endocrinol Rev 1992;13:220–240.

Blackwell RE. Hyperprolactinemia: Evaluation and management. Endocrinol Metab Clin N Am 1992; 21:105–124.

Cunnah D, Besser M. Management of prolactinomas. Clin Endocrinol 1991;34:231–235.

CASE 21

WEAK AND SHAKY SPELLS

Barry J. Goldstein

Data A 28-year-old graduate student is finally convinced by her family to seek your advice about her episodic "spells." She has been exercising regularly at the university gymnasium several times a week during the past year, but recently she had to stop on three occasions because of episodes lasting 15 to 20 minutes; these began with dizziness and a feeling of weakness, and were soon followed by palpitations, a throbbing headache, and a feeling of impending doom. Last week, she had an episode while walking home from class. They were not associated with fasting or meals and were not relieved by eating. She tells you she was treated at a hospital for cocaine abuse 5 years ago, and she is worried that these episodes are related to her past drug use. Since her treatment, she says she has not used any street drugs and is not taking any other medicines.

Logic This patient is experiencing classic symptoms of adrenergic hormone release that occur in discrete attacks at irregular intervals and are at times associated with exercise. Transient release of epinephrine or norepinephrine into the bloodstream can account for each of the described components of the "spells." Your task is to acquire further clinical data that will establish this possible diagnosis on biochemical grounds, and to differentiate the cause of the recurrent production of epinephrine or norepinephrine. The presentation suggests a pheochromocytoma, a tumor of the adrenal medulla that causes periodic adrenergic hormone discharge. The hormone release can be triggered by exercise, as might be happening in this case. Other possible diagnoses to consider include cocaine (or other stimulant drug) abuse, acute anxiety, panic disorder, migraine headache, hyperthyroidism, hypoglycemia, and paroxysmal atrial tachycardia, because each of these conditions may have a presentation with some similar features.

Although you have no reason to suspect that the patient is lying when she says she has not been using cocaine, she does have a history of drug abuse, and this may be a sensitive area that she does not want to discuss. Anxiety reactions or panic attacks are characterized by spells similar to those described previously; they are triggered by psychologic influences that activate the sympathetic nervous system. Migraine headaches can also be associated with systemic symptoms with features of adrenergic activation. Hyperthyroidism is also a possibility, but it would be less episodic and would manifest persistent metabolic, cardiac, and hyperadrenergic features. Hypoglycemia can cause adrenergic discharge as a counter-regulatory mechanism that serves to increase blood glucose by glycogen breakdown and glucose synthesis in the liver. The fact that this patient's symptoms do not occur with fasting (as in insulinoma) or after meals (postprandial hypoglycemia), and are not relieved by eating makes this possibility less likely. An episodic, rapid cardiac arrhythmia is possible, but it would be unlikely to be associated with headache, and other features of the hyperadrenergic state, other than through associated anxiety.

Data On your review of systems, you find out she had mild hypertension of 135/95 when she was examined for graduate school admission 18 months ago and was told to watch her salt intake and lose some weight. In fact, she notes that she has lost 15 lb during the past year, although she did not change her diet at all. She has not experienced heat intolerance, tremulousness or irritability between the episodes. There is no history of palpitations or heart murmur in the past, and there is no family history of endocrine disease or hypertension.

Logic Now you have obtained some really useful information for the differential diagnosis. In approximately two thirds of cases, a pheochromocytoma can cause persistent hypertension because the release of catecholamines into the bloodstream is increased even between episodes; the hypertension is usually exacerbated during a symptomatic paroxysm when catecholamine levels are greatly increased. The lack of heat intolerance or tremors argues against hyperthyroidism. Because you are always trying to explain a symptom complex with a single unifying diagnosis, you have gained further support for the diagnosis of pheochromocytoma, and less enthusiasm for other diagnoses under consideration.

Weight loss without a reduction of the caloric intake suggests a hypermetabolic state that can be associated with increased circulating catecholamines or thyroxine. Both of these agents will increase skeletal muscle metabolism and increase the amount of calories used in the resting state. Catecholamins in particular will promote glycogen breakdown and glucose synthesis that can lead to excessive utilization of synthetic precursors from muscle protein. This can lead to the feeling of muscle weakness. Keep in mind, however, that hyperthyroidism can also cause a myopathy with muscle aches and symptomatic weakness, especially in a proximal distribution.

Data On physical examination, you find a thin, relaxed woman who is asymptomatic at the moment. She is 5'6" and weighs 118 lb, is afebrile, and the respiratory rate is 20. Lying down, her pulse is 88 and regular and the blood pressure is 145/95. On sitting up, her pulse rises to 112, her blood pressure falls to 120/76, and she feels lightheaded for a few seconds. Her skin and hair are normal. There is no proptosis and the funduscopic examination does not show hypertensive changes. The thyroid gland is of normal size and has no nodules. There is no adenopathy and neck masses are not palpated. The axillae are moist. Heart examination shows a regular rhythm without murmurs and the lungs are clear. There are no vascular bruits. The reflexes are symmetric with a normal relaxation phase. There is no tremor of the outstretched hands. Proximal muscle strength is normal. The remainder of the examination is unremarkable.

Logic The examination corroborates the history

that she has lost weight and may have a hypermetabolic state because she is actually underweight for her height. At 5'6", you would expect her to weigh approximately (100 lb for 5') + (5 lb × 6 in over 5') = 130 lb. This finding argues against hypoglycemia due to insulinoma, because such patients typically gain weight; they overeat to offset the low blood glucose reactions that occur during periods of excessive insulin release.

You also confirm that she has moderate hypertension and note that she is volume depleted, with a significant blood pressure drop and pulse increase on assuming a sitting position. This "orthostatic change" in blood pressure is significant if the systolic pressure falls >20 mm Hg, especially when associated with an increase in the pulse rate. This characteristic finding results from a decreased plasma volume and blunted sympathetic reflexes. Of all the possible diagnoses considered thus far, this important physical finding is found only in pheochromocytoma. Hyperthyroidism is less likely in a patient with no ocular changes, no thyroid goiter, and normal stretch reflexes.

Data At this first office visit, you draw blood for a fasting glucose level and thyroid function tests (Table 13.9). The patient is also given a container to collect urine for a 24-hour period, beginning just after the occurrence of one of the attacks. If the release of catecholamines is highly episodic, some patients will have normal urine studies on days when they do not have a symptomatic episode; this can lead to a missed diagnosis in a patient who actually harbors a tumor.

Logic The elevated glucose level is surprising because the patient did not describe symptoms of polyuria and polydipsia that you would associate with diabetes mellitus. In pheochromocytoma, however, a state of glucose intolerance can exist because the excessive circulating catecholamines counterbalance the effectiveness of circulating insulin and can cause a mild form of insulin-

TABLE 13.9. Laboratory Data for Patient in Case 21

TEST	PATIENT RESULT	NORMAL VALUES
Glucose (fasting)	160 mg/dL	75–115 mg/dL
Total T$_4$	7.8 µg/dL	4.5–11.0 µg/dL
TSH	2.3 µU/mL	0.4–4.6 µU/mL

T$_4$ = thyroxine; TSH = thyroid stimulating hormone.

TABLE 13.10. Twenty-four-hour Collection Results for the Patient in Case 21

TEST (24-H URINE)	PATIENT RESULT	NORMAL VALUES
Creatinine	990 mg	1g/24 h
Drug screen for cocaine and amphetamines	Negative	Negative
Metanephrines	2560 µg	<900 µg
Catecholamines		
Epinephrine	550 µg	<100 µg
Norepinephrine	320 µg	<100 µg
VMA	14.2 mg	<7 mg

VMA = vanillylmandelic acid.

resistant diabetes. The high fasting glucose level also argues against hypoglycemia as a cause of the presenting symptoms.

Data The patient returns 2 weeks later, with her 24-hour urine collection that she began immediately after an episode of headache and palpitations that was brought on by exercise (Table 13.10).

Logic The creatinine is measured in the urine to evaluate how complete a sample was collected. Typically, approximately a gram of creatinine is expected in a 24-hour urine specimen, and the patient's value assures you that the sample is essentially complete. The negative results from the drug screen are also helpful in excluding the possibility that the episodes are related to illicit drug use.

Documentation of increased catecholamines and their metabolites in the urine fully substantiates your impression that the episodes are due to excessive catecholamine secretion, most likely from an adrenal medullary tumor. All other diagnostic possibilities have been effectively excluded.

In 90% of cases, the pheochromocytoma is found in one of the adrenal glands; 10% of the time the tumors are bilateral. Occasionally the tumor is found outside of the adrenal along the sympathetic chain, in the organ of Zuckerkandl, or in the urinary bladder.

Data An abdominal CT scan shows a 5.5-cm left adrenal tumor (Fig. 13.9). After preparing the patient with full doses of α- and β-adrenergic blocking agents, she is cured by a left adrenalectomy performed by a surgeon using a laparoscopic approach.

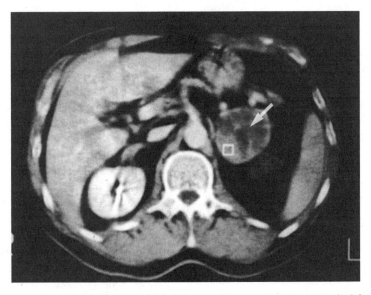

▶ **Figure 13.9.** Contrast-enhanced CT image of the abdomen, showing a 5.5-cm mass in the left adrenal gland (arrow). White box indicates the position of the cursor used to measure the radiographic density of the tumor.

Questions

1. It is potentially dangerous to initially treat a patient with pheochromocytoma with *only* β-adrenergic blocking agents because:
   (a) loss of β-adrenergic receptor stimulation alone can slow the heart and cause syncope.
   (b) loss of β-adrenergic receptor stimulation can lead to hypoglycemia.
   (c) excessive stimulation of α-adrenergic receptors in a volume-depleted patient can cause hypotension.
   (d) unopposed excessive catecholamine stimulation to the α-adrenergic receptors can lead to marked worsening of the hypertension.

2. In the course of screening for possible gallbladder disease, an ultrasound study discovers a 2.0-cm adrenal mass. The next step should be:
   (a) immediate laparoscopic excision of the tumor.
   (b) Iodine 131-metaiodobenzylguanidine (MIBG) scan to rule out pheochromocytoma.
   (c) blood pressure readings, serum potassium level determination, and 24-hour urine collection for cortisol and catecholamine measurements.
   (d) needle biopsy for cytologic analysis.

3. What additional testing should be performed in a patient with a known pheochromocytoma in order to screen for the possible occurrence of a MEN syndrome?
   (a) MRI of pituitary gland
   (b) Endoscopic ultrasound of pancreas
   (c) Serum growth hormone and prolactin levels
   (d) Serum calcium and calcitonin levels

Answers

1. **(d) is correct.** In the peripheral circulation, α-adrenergic stimulation leads to vasoconstriction, whereas β-adrenergic stimulation causes vasodilatation. If β-blocking drugs are used in a patient who has excessive circulating catecholamines of both types, the balance between α and β stimulation will be disrupted; unopposed stimulation of α-adrenergic receptors may lead to dangerous levels of hypertension.

2. **(c) is correct.** The mass is an "incidentaloma." By virtue of its size alone, it is apt to be benign. However, it is important to know if it is functioning at the biochemical level, even if it is not causing symptoms. Diagnostic possibilities include pheochromocytoma, aldosteronoma, and adrenal Cushing's syndrome. These are assessed by blood pressure measurements and catecholamine excretion in the case of pheochromocytoma,

low serum potassium in the case of an aldosteronoma, and elevated urine cortisol level in the case of Cushing's syndrome. An MIBG scan detects a functioning pheochromocytoma. Such a mass is typically followed by repeating the imaging study in 6 months to see whether it has enlarged. If so, it might prompt a biopsy or repeated biochemical evaluation.

3. **(d) is correct.** There are two main classifications of MEN syndromes. MEN type I syndrome is a disease complex consisting of a pituitary adenoma, hyperparathyroidism, and a pancreatic islet cell adenoma. MEN type II syndrome includes pheochromocytoma, medullary thyroid carcinoma (calcitonin-secreting tumor), and hyperparathyroidism. A subgroup of MEN syndrome (called IIB) also has the morphologic findings of a marfanoid habitus and mucosal neuromas.

Suggested Readings

Ross NS, Aron DC. Hormonal evaluation of the patient with an incidentally discovered adrenal mass. New Engl J Med 1990;323:1401–1405.

Shapiro B, Fig LM. Management of pheochromocytoma. Endocrinol Metab Clin North Am 1989;18:443–481.

Stein PP, Black HR. A simplified diagnostic approach to pheochromocytoma. Medicine 1991;70:46–66.

CASE 22

A FAT PROBLEM

M. James Lenhard

Data A 52-year-old professional musician is brought to the emergency department after completing a performance. For the past few months, he has had frequent urination, severe thirst, and weight loss despite a good appetite. One week ago he developed a skin rash, and for the past few hours he has had severe disabling abdominal pain.

Logic Other than for possible diabetic ketoacidosis, this constellation of symptoms does not suggest one unifying disorder. Whereas the more chronic symptoms are suggestive of new-onset severe diabetes mellitus, diabetes insipidus, or perhaps only prostatic hypertrophy, the severe abdominal pain requires consideration of an acute abdominal problem such as intestinal obstruction, perforated peptic ulcer, cholecystitis, or pancreatitis.

Data A more detailed history is difficult because he has extreme discomfort and is now vomiting. He says that the abdominal pain is sharp and stabbing, radiates straight through to the back, and is most intense in the mid-epigastric area and when he is supine. He has had no previous indigestion and his last bowel movement was only that morning.

Examination reveals an obese, somewhat dehydrated man in moderate to severe distress. The vital signs are BP,100/60; pulse, 120; respirations, 22; temperature, 38.0°C. At the time of entry he weighed 262 lb. The lungs are clear; the abdomen is distended and extremely tender and moderately rigid all over; and bowel sounds are scant.

Logic The examination suggests acute pancreatitis or perforated duodenal ulcer. Although there is no ulcer history or previous symptoms of indigestion, radiographs are needed to verify or negate the presence of free air under the diaphragm. Findings are not limited to the right upper quadrant, thus making acute cholecystitis unlikely. The absence of colicky pain weighs against obstruction, although it is still possible. Urgent laboratory tests are indicated.

Data Flat and erect radiographs of the abdomen show no evidence of free air, radiopaque calculi, or dilated loops of small intestine. The hemoglobin and hematocrit are normal; there are 15,000 WBCs per mm^3 with a normal differential; the amylase level is elevated to 712 IU/L; liver enzymes are normal; the BUN and creatinine levels are mildly elevated; and the blood glucose is 812 mg/dL. The vomitus and stool test results are negative for occult blood, and the urinalysis shows 4+ glucose and no acetone.

Logic The diagnosis of acute pancreatitis is confirmed by the markedly elevated amylase level, although its cause is not yet clear. Most cases are associated with the presence of gallstones or a history of chronic alcoholism. Normal liver enzymes suggest that biliary tract disease is unlikely but certainly not excluded. There are no historical data yet available to support other causes for acute pancreatitis such as hypertriglyceridemia, infection, or medications such as azathioprine, sulfonamides, or pentamidine.

Although stress or inflammation of the pancreas can elevate the blood glucose level to a mild degree, because of the magnitude of the glucose elevation, type II diabetes mellitus is probably also present.

Data The patient is treated with analgesics, intravenous fluids, and gastric suction, and begins to recover. Ultrasound of the gallbladder and biliary ducts fails to disclose any calculi. Further questioning reveals that although he has a predilection for hallucinogenic street drugs, he largely abstains from alcohol. There is a family history of type II diabetes and hypercholesterolemia.

Logic Based on this information, hypertriglyceridemia should be considered as a possible cause for the pancreatitis. Less than 20% of cases of acute pancreatitis are caused by elevated triglyceride levels, and many of these cases overlap with those that are alcohol-induced. Measurements of the triglycerides, total cholesterol, low-density lipoprotein (LDL), and high-density lipoprotein (HDL) are important because they will determine diagnosis, treatment, and prevention of future problems. Whereas the total cholesterol, and perhaps the HDL, are accurate in a fasting or fed state, the triglycerides and LDL must be obtained in a fasting state to ensure accuracy.

Data A fasting lipid profile is obtained. The total cholesterol is 429 mg/dL, LDL 334 mg/dL, HDL 42 mg/dL, triglycerides 4389 mg/dL. A blood alcohol level from blood obtained on admission is zero.

Logic Acute illness can cause an elevation in triglycerides but not to the levels found for this patient. Triglyceride levels greater than 1000 mg/dL will occasionally cause pancreatitis, but levels greater than 2500 or 3000 mg/dL are usually required. The mechanism whereby hypertriglyceridemia causes pancreatitis is unknown. Hypertriglyceridemia-induced cellular damage and subsequent activation of proteolytic enzymes has been proposed.

Data Further examination reveals the presence of lipemia retinalis. Arcus corneae is present, and xanthelasmas are noted around the eyes (Fig. 13.10).A skin examination reveals the presence of red morbilliform lesions over the elbows, knees, and buttocks (Fig. 13.11).Tendinous and tuberous xanthomas are not present.

Logic These findings are a part of the physical examination of a patient with hyperlipidemia.

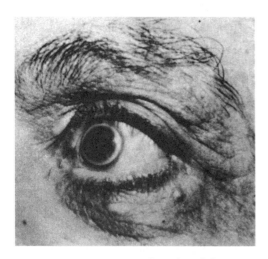

▶ **Figure 13.10.** Arcus senilis and xanthelasma. Note grayish-white band surrounding the iris and off-white fatty deposits in the inner canthus.

Generally, patients with hypertriglyceridemia may have lipemia retinalis and eruptive skin xanthomas. Periodic abdominal pain and pancreatitis are common, and hepatomegaly and hypersplenism, from accumulation of fat-laden cells, may occur. The finding of tendinous or tuberous xanthomas is almost pathognomonic for familial hypercholesterolemia, with xanthomas found most frequently on the extensor surface of the hands and on the Achilles and patellar tendons. Arcus corneae is commonly seen with hypercholesterolemia, whereas xanthelasma around the eyes is a nonspecific finding that is very often associated with it. The laboratory values and the physical examination support the presence of elevated levels of both triglycerides and cholesterol.

Data The patient's pancreatitis resolves. He is seen in follow-up after his discharge. Laboratory tests are repeated. Total cholesterol is now 440 mg/dL, the LDL is 342 mg/dL, the HDL is 44 mg/dL and the triglycerides are 1986 mg/dL. A fasting blood glucose is 202 mg/dL. He is not taking any medications.

Logic The evaluation of a patient with a lipid disorder may be broken down and thought of in an orderly fashion. Two questions should be investigated each time. First, which lipid is present in abnormal quantities? There are generally only three choices: LDL, very-low-density lipoprotein (VLDL), or both. The primary abnormality

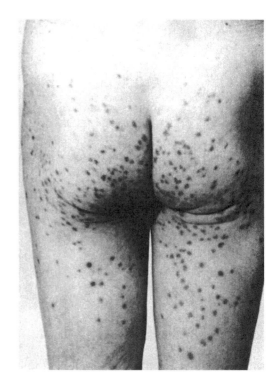

▶ **Figure 13.11.** Eruptive xanthomas over the buttocks are characteristic of hyperlipoproteinemia (seen with diabetes mellitus).

in hypercholesterolemia is an elevation of LDL. Elevated levels of triglycerides imply that VLDL is elevated, although VLDL is very rarely measured directly. An elevation of both LDL and VLDL can be present at once.

The second question to be addressed concerns the cause of the elevation. Again, there are three choices: the elevation can be *primary* (inherited, diet influenced), *secondary* to some underlying disorder such as diabetes, or *both*. The method of treatment will depend on the answers to these questions. In this patient, it appears that levels of both LDL (total cholesterol) and VLDL (triglycerides) are elevated. If levels of both lipids are elevated, which lipid abnormality of the two is the most urgent? Acute pancreatitis secondary to hypertriglyceridemia can be recurrent, and is the most important and threatening abnormality for this patient at this time.

Data His father and paternal uncle both died of myocardial infarctions in their 50s. Both were being treated for elevations in cholesterol, but the patient does not know of any problems with elevated levels of triglycerides. His mother and brother have type II diabetes.

Logic The family history is important because many lipid abnormalities are familial. This patient's history suggests that he may have an element of familial hypercholesterolemia. He clearly has hypertriglyceridemia, so his diagnosis would be mixed hyperlipidemia. A search for secondary causes should be undertaken.

Data The patient denies any history of hepatic or renal disease, known hypothyroidism, and again denies alcohol ingestion. He smokes two packs of cigarettes per day.

Logic Diabetes in poor control is a known secondary cause of hypertriglyceridemia, as are alcohol ingestion, uremia, estrogens, and nephrosis. Common secondary causes of hypercholesterolemia include hypothyroidism, cholestasis, nephrosis, and anorexia nervosa.

Data Laboratory tests are run, including liver function, BUN, and TSH. They are all normal. The patient's glycosylated hemoglobin (hemoglobin A$_{1C}$) is 12.9% (normal range 4.3 to 6.1), which is consistent with poorly controlled diabetes.

Logic He appears to have mixed hyperlipidemia, with both primary and secondary causes. The common forms of *primary* dyslipidemias are listed in Table 13.11(this does not include secondary causes, as cited in the text). Therapy should be started to prevent recurrent pancreatitis and to prevent coronary artery disease.

Data He is started on a sulfonylurea for his diabetes. Self-monitoring of his blood glucose is encouraged, but he is resistant because he believes it would interfere with his guitar playing. Weight loss and better meal planning are encouraged, and he is referred to a registered dietitian for assistance. The dietitian advises him to follow an American Heart Association Step One diet, as well as caloric restriction for his diabetes.

Logic A Step One diet comprises less than 300 mg cholesterol per day. Appropriate therapy of hyperlipidemia is very difficult without curtailing the dietary intake of fats. Except in cases of extreme hyperlipidemia, where acute injury is possible, the first step should always be dietary fat restriction. After 6 months of meal planning, pharmacologic therapy can be added. The Step Two diet is similar to the Step One diet, except the daily total of cholesterol is limited to 200 mg/d.

Data After 6 months, the patient returns. His weight is down to 220 lb. A fasting lipid profile reveals a total cholesterol of 296 mg/dL, an LDL of 228 mg/dL, an HDL of 36 mg/dL, and triglycerides of 218 mg/dL. The glycosylated hemoglobin (hemoglobin A$_{1C}$) is down to 7.1%

Logic Through management of the secondary cause of his hypertriglyceridemia, and through reduction of fat intake, the patient was able to control his hypertriglyceridemia. The lipid profile now reveals a significantly elevated LDL level. This seems to be due to primary hypercho-

TABLE 13.11. Common Primary Forms of Dyslipidemias

OFFICIAL NOMENCLATURE	WHAT IT REALLY MEANS	CLINICAL FINDINGS*
Familial hypertriglyceridemia	Triglycerides are elevated	Lipemia retinalis, eruptive cutaneous xanthomas, pancreatitis; some patients have associated hyperglycemia, hypertension, insulin resistance, and obesity.
Familial combined hyperlipidemia	Triglycerides and LDL are both elevated	Same as for familial hypertriglyceridemia; xanthelasma may also be present.
Familial hypercholesterolemia	LDL is elevated	Tendinous xanthomas, premature death from coronary artery disease, xanthelasmas; LDL is often above 350 mg/dL.
Polygenic hypercholesterolemia	LDL is elevated	Absence of tendinous xanthoma; LDL is usually lower than 350 mg/dL; the disorder is polygenic, and quite variable.
Familial hypoalphalipoproteinemia	HDL is decreased	Premature death occurs from coronary artery disease.

LDL = low-density lipoprotein cholesterol; HDL = high-density lipoprotein cholesterol.
*Clinical variation exists; all of the clinical findings may not be present.

lesterolemia, and is associated with an increased risk of myocardial infarction. Further treatment is dependent on his risk factors for an MI.

The National Cholesterol Education Program (NCEP) has recommended the following as risk factors: diabetes, cigarettes, hypertension, peripheral vascular disease, age (men > 45 years, women > 55 years), HDL cholesterol < 35 mg/dL, and a positive family history of heart disease (MI in a male first-degree relative < age 55 or a female first-degree relative < 65). A beneficial factor (subtract one risk from analysis) is an HDL cholesterol level greater than 60 mg/dL. Obesity is no longer considered a risk factor, but commonly occurs with those listed.

Data Perhaps because he is a traveling musician, he has made little progress in quitting cigarettes. His blood pressure has been repeatedly normal.

Logic Recommendations for therapy in hypercholesterolemic adults are based on LDL levels and the number of risk factors for coronary heart disease. This patient has a very high LDL level and four risk factors—diabetes, cigarette smoking, age, and family history. Accordingly, a treatment regimen is indicated.

There are five classes of lipid-lowering medications currently available: HMG CoA reductase inhibitors, fibric acid derivatives, bile acid sequestrants, niacin, and probucol. In addition, estrogen replacement therapy in postmenopausal women should be considered if the LDL level is elevated, and the levels of triglycerides are not. Patient compliance, side effects, cost, and comorbid medical conditions need to be weighed carefully when choosing a lipid-lowering drug.

Data After consultation with his physician, the patient had an HMG CoA reductase inhibitor added to his meal plan. He reported no obvious side effects and was able to take his medicine regularly except on days that he gave concerts. Three months later, a fasting lipid profile reveals a total cholesterol of 202 mg/dL, an LDL of 136 mg/dL, and triglycerides of 209 mg/dL.

Logic He has had an excellent response to lipid-lowering therapy. The values are not completely within the NCEP guidelines, but they are close. Further reinforcement of meal planning and weight loss will be needed.

Data Several months later, the patient calls from the Mars Hotel in San Francisco, where he is playing a concert. His weight is increasing despite dietary compliance, and he has had problems with constipation, fatigue, leg cramps, and muscle weakness.

Logic The symptoms described could be a side effect from his medication, but they also sound like symptoms of thyroid disease. In addition to looking for possible side effects of the medication, thyroid function tests are needed. An evaluation by the band's traveling physician is recommended. The physician orders blood tests including thyroid function tests.

Data Electrolytes are normal, as are liver enzymes and muscle enzymes. The TSH level is elevated to 77 mIU/L, the T_4 is 3.9 μg/dL, and the T_3U is 20%. The total cholesterol has increased to 246 mg/dL, whereas the triglycerides have not changed. This confirms the diagnosis of hypothyroidism, and thyroid hormone replacement is prescribed. After several weeks of therapy with thyroid replacement hormone, the patient's symptoms disappeared.

Logic In this case, a new secondary cause was likely responsible for the increase in the cholesterol level. Hypothyroidism occurs more frequently in persons who have diabetes, and diabetic patients with an elevated level of LDL cholesterol should be tested for it. Laboratory testing for secondary causes should be performed every 1 to 2 years in patients with known severe hyperlipidemia.

Questions

1. All of the following are often found in association with hypertriglyceridemia except:
   (a) Hypothyroidism
   (b) Type II diabetes mellitus
   (c) Hypertension
   (d) Obesity
   (e) Atherosclerotic coronary artery disease

2. Which of the following statements regarding the effects of medications on lipid levels is false?
   (a) Estrogens may cause a decrease in triglyceride levels.
   (b) Ethanol may cause an increase in HDL cholesterol levels.
   (c) Insulin may cause a decrease in triglyceride levels.
   (d) Estrogen may cause a decrease in LDL cholesterol levels.
   (e) Testosterone may cause a decrease in HDL cholesterol levels.

3. A 63-year-old woman is seen by her physician for a long overdue checkup. She is concerned about her risk of a myocardial infarction, because her 52-year-old diabetic brother had just died from this. She has no previous history of any health problems. A physical examination reveals an upright blood pressure of 168/94, and her weight is 80 kg. An absence of sensation to soft touch is noted in both feet. Which of the following is incorrect?

(a) She has a high likelihood of having diabetes.

(b) Without any further information, the lipid value that is statistically most likely to be abnormal is an elevation in triglycerides.

(c) She has at least three risk factors for heart disease.

(d) Her obesity may be related to hypercholesterolemia.

(e) A screening test for hypothyroidism should be considered.

4. A 53-year-old man is seen by his physician for evaluation of hypercholesterolemia. A physical examination reveals carotid bruits, tendinous xanthomas in the Achilles and patellar tendons, and arcus corneae. His total cholesterol level is 394 mg/dL, and his triglyceride level is normal. Which of the following is incorrect?

(a) The patient should have a measurement of his HDL cholesterol.

(b) He may have asymptomatic atherosclerotic vascular disease at the present time.

(c) This is a rare disease; the odds of his children having a similar dyslipidemia are very low.

(d) He probably has heterozygous familial hypercholesterolemia.

(e) Normalization of cholesterol levels can be achieved in most compliant patients.

Answers

1. **(a) is correct.** The remainder of the choices listed are commonly found together in the same patient. This constellation of findings has been attributed to insulin resistance, which has been found in association with choices (b) through (e). Hypothyroidism may rarely cause an increase in triglycerides, but it is classically associated with an increase in LDL cholesterol.

2. **(a) is correct because it is false.** Estrogen may cause an increase in triglyceride levels, and a decrease in LDL cholesterol levels. Ethanol may lead to a modest increase in HDL cholesterol levels. Insulin activates lipoprotein lipase, thereby promoting triglyceride clearance and lowering blood levels. Androgens such as testosterone may lead to a decrease in HDL cholesterol levels.

3. **(d) is correct because it is false.** The presence of symmetric neuropathy suggests a systemic disease such as diabetes or hypothyroidism, both of which can develop gradually. Hypertriglyceridemia is probably the most prevalent lipid abnormality, and triglyceride levels are more closely correlated with body fat than are LDL cholesterol levels. Although obesity is commonly found in association with other risk factors for heart disease, cholesterol itself is not known to be associated with obesity. Her risk factors include age > 55, hypertension, and a positive family history. Diabetes, if present, would be another risk factor.

4. **(c) is correct because it is incorrect.** A serum cholesterol in excess of 350 mg/dL in the presence of tendinous xanthomas is very suggestive of heterozygous familial hypercholesterolemia. Patients with the homozygous form tend to succumb to atherosclerosis at a young age. Eighty-five percent of men with heterozygous familial hypercholesterolemia will have a myocardial infarction before age 60. The cholesterol levels can often be normalized with diet and medication. One half of all first-degree relatives are affected, and a careful family history as well as laboratory analysis of relatives is recommended.

COMMENT This patient developed a chain of events in which there were implied or clear-cut pathophysiologic relationships. First came severe diabetes mellitus, then acute pancreatitis, hypertriglyceridemia, and last hypothyroidism.

During the development of the case logic, it was necessary to discuss the simultaneous presence of two diseases at the outset, then arrive at a cause for the acute abdomen, later pinpoint the reason for the pancreatitis.

Subsequent clinical reasoning revolved about the various causes for lipid disorders, their distinguishing physical signs, and their management.

It is notable that biochemical responses to treatment were good until an additional unrelated disease entered the picture—hypothyroidism.

More and more over the past few decades, both the medical profession and the public have become increasingly aware of the existence of various disorders of lipid metabolism. Yet a precise and durable classification has not been established. Yesterday's nosology has been replaced with today's, and even now a new classification is in preparation. *(P.C.)*

Suggested Readings

American College of Physicians. Guidelines for using serum cholesterol, high-density lipoprotein cholesterol, and triglyceride levels as screening tests for preventing coronary heart disease in adults. Ann Intern Med 1996;124:515.

Brown BG, et al. Lipid lowering and plaque regression: New insights into prevention of plaque disruption and clinical events in coronary disease. Circulation 1993;87:1781.

Expert Panel on Detection, Evaluation, and Treatment of High Blood Cholesterol in Adults. Summary of the second report on the National Cholesterol Education Program (NCEP) Expert Panel on Detection, Evaluation and Treatment of High Blood Cholesterol in Adults (Adult Treatment Panel II). JAMA 1993;269:3015–3023.

Rosenson RS. Beyond low-density lipoprotein cholesterol. Arch Intern Med 1996;156:1278.

CHAPTER 14

Cardiovascular Problems

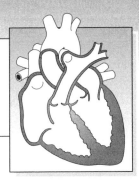

Heart diseases number in the hundreds, and it takes a 2000-page textbook to describe them all. Yet the ways in which patients who have cardiac diseases are first seen by the physician comprise a short list:

- Incidental findings
- Early chamber failure
- Florid congestive heart failure
- Embolus
- Arrhythmia
- Chest pain
- Syncope
- Infection
- Combinations of the aforementioned

In recent years, more and more patients without cardiac symptoms are coming to the doctor because of abnormalities detected elsewhere on routine examination or in the course of other illnesses. These abnormal findings include murmurs, cardiac enlargement or contour abnormality seen on the chest radiograph, or any of dozens of electrocardiogram (ECG) abnormalities. Many of these findings may never cause symptoms.

Beginning chamber decompensation or early congestive heart failure (CHF) brings many patients to the physician. Often the patient never knows he or she has a cardiac problem until the left ventricle or right ventricle begins to fail and causes symptoms. Sometimes the patient knows of hypertension or a heart murmur that has existed for years. Although the causes of congestive heart failure are many, the symptoms are generally the same. The history, physical examination, and studies will differ somewhat depending on the underlying cause for the failure and on the chamber that fails. Left ventricular failure (LVF) is by far most common, and it results in dyspnea and fatigue on exertion, orthopnea, and night cough. Mitral stenosis results in "left atrial failure," which has the same presentation of symptoms as LVF, although palpitations may be more prominent because of atrial irritability. Right ventricular failure (RVF) causes distended neck veins, right upper quadrant discomfort, indigestion, and swollen legs.

Florid CHF with all the signs and symptoms of bilateral chamber failure is seen in the unusual patient who does not heed the earlier warnings, in the patient who is inadequately treated, or in the patient at the end of his or her illness. LVF usually precedes and is the most common cause of RVF. However, florid textbook CHF is not so common as in the past, because patients are treated better, and the full picture is often suppressed until death occurs from a complication. But, on the other hand, as arrhythmia therapy improves, we are beginning to encounter more patients who survive despite the presence of severe myocardial dysfunction. So if the patient lives long enough, and avoids thromboemboli, pneumonia, arrhythmias, and infarctions, severe CHF is the common end point of most forms of heart disease.

An embolus may be the first indication that a cardiac problem exists. The sudden onset of a stroke, or flank pain and hematuria, or a cold, painful, pulseless limb may on further study reveal mitral stenosis, atrial fibrillation, infective endocarditis, or recent unnoticed myocardial infarction (MI)—all sources of arterial emboli.

Any sort of arrhythmia may augur heart disease. The patient may come to the physician complaining of palpitations, skipped beats, or fluttering in the chest. These may be momentary, continuous, or repetitive. Correct identification can be achieved by an ECG, superimposed exercise, or even long-term monitoring.

But further examination of the heart may disclose the cause (early CHF, mitral stenosis, Wolff-Parkinson-White [WPW] syndrome, Barlow's syndrome, coronary artery disease, hyperthyroidism) or may reveal no heart disease at all.

A common presentation is chest pain caused by angina pectoris or myocardial infarction. Bear in mind that subclinical coronary disease may often become symptomatic because of anything that might suddenly or subtly further worsen anoxia to an area of already ischemic heart muscle. This includes a paroxysm of tachycardia, gastrointestinal hemorrhage, gradually developing severe anemia for any reason, worsening of chronic obstructive lung disease, or pneumonia. The same holds true for patients with heart disease who are bordering on CHF. They can suddenly go into congestive heart failure with the advent of a paroxysmal tachycardia, a small myocardial infarct, a gastrointestinal hemorrhage, pneumonia, rapid transfusions or saline infusions, or sudden severe physical or emotional strain.

One or more syncopal attacks may unveil the presence of paroxysmal tachyarrhythmia, paroxysmal bradyarrhythmia, complete heart block, sinus node disease, aortic stenosis (AS), coronary disease, or even an atrial thrombus or myxoma.

Infection as a presenting problem refers principally to infective endocarditis, viral myocarditis, or pericarditis. Here the clinical picture varies. In endocarditis, the patient may seek help because of fever, lassitude, and embolic manifestations. Viral myocarditis usually results in arrhythmias and heart failure with dyspnea, orthopnea, and edema. Pericarditis, with or without effusion, usually has a presentation of chest pain, at times dyspnea, and fever, depending on the underlying cause.

Combinations of any of the common presentations may occur at the same time. A patient can be seen with chest pain, LVF, and arrhythmia simultaneously. In instances of this sort, you always have to determine which came first, because any one condition could precipitate the other two. If severe aortic stenosis is present, syncope, LVF, and angina can and often do coexist.

Remember that many healthy patients are seen because they only think they have heart disease. A vague chest pain, a "skipped heartbeat," a sighing deep breath, or the sudden death of a friend or relative may prompt a visit to the doctor's office.

As in other areas of medical diagnosis, most patients with symptoms referable to the cardiovascular system can be managed with the time-honored modalities of a good history and a well-done physical examination—perhaps too with the addition of a chest radiograph and an electrocardiogram.

However, for more complex cases, recent advances in imaging technology—that invoke the more intelligent use of roentgen waves, sound waves, computers, catheters, magnets, linear accelerators, radioisotopes, and contrast agents—have given the clinician a broad armamentarium of procedures that may offer virtual diagnostic certainty when simpler clinical means fail to do so.

Especially today, when almost 100% certainty is required before performing coronary artery bypass grafts, intracoronary thrombolysis, percutaneous angioplasty, stents, laser ablation, valve replacement, atherectomies, and subendocardial resections, the newer array of procedures must be thoroughly accurate and dependable. No longer can we tolerate false-negative and false-positive results.

The high-technology tests of today include the use of ultrasound with Doppler color flow, radionuclide imaging, superfast computed tomographic (CT) scans, cine-magnetic resonance imaging (MRI) scans, and positron emission tomography (PET) scans. Despite cardiac motion, some of these procedures can deliver serial slices that depict anatomic and functional detail in a way not dreamed of 10 to 20 years ago. Thrombi, aneurysms, dissections, valve defects, ischemic areas, wall thickness, motility, and viability are all clearly demonstrable.

Various diagnostic strategies are currently in transition, especially because even newer imaging methods are now on the research table. The aim is to eventually replace invasive procedures with noninvasive ones.

For the moment, however, for the precise definition of coronary artery anatomy and pathology—perhaps the most common of all cardiac diagnostic problems to be solved—transfemoral cardiac catheterization and coronary arteriography is still the gold standard test. *(P.C.)*

ABNORMAL ECG

Paul Cutler

Data After a routine insurance examination, a 56-year-old man was told that because there was something wrong with his ECG, he should consult his private physician. A repeat ECG shows a left ventricular hypertrophy (LVH) pattern. Thereupon you proceed to ask questions and examine simultaneously.

Logic To solve this problem, you could easily depart from the trunk of the diagnostic tree, fol-low a branching pattern, and quickly arrive at a cause for the ECG abnormality. First, note the wisdom of repeating the ECG to make sure the abnormality and the patient match. True, there are negative T waves in leads I, aVL, and V_4 to V_6, high voltage, and left axis deviation; a left atrial abnormality is also noted. You can deduce that the left ventricle is strained and hypertrophied and that the left atrium is secondarily so (Fig. 14.1).

As you study the ECG, you think of the common disorders that can strain the left ventricle, especially in a man this age: hypertension, coronary heart disease, aortic stenosis, aortic regurgitation (AR), mitral regurgitation (MR), and car-

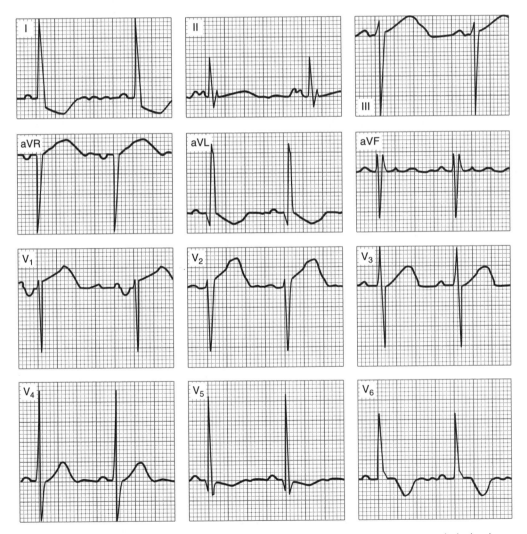

▶ **Figure 14.1.** Left ventricular and left atrial hypertrophy. Left axis deviation; QRS = .10 seconds; high voltage; negative T waves in leads I, aVL, V_5, V_6; diphasic P waves with prominent negative component in lead V_1.

diomyopathy. These should be easily discernible by history and examination.

If hypertension is the cause, there may be a history of this condition, and it will be apparent in the fundi and blood pressure (BP) measurement. Although essential hypertension (EH) is the usual variety, secondary causes of hypertension, like chronic bilateral renal disease, unilateral renal ischemia, primary aldosteronism, and pheochromocytoma, must also be considered if the blood pressure is found to be high. Remember that it takes moderate to severe sustained and prolonged hypertension to strain the heart. Also bear in mind that hypertension is so common that it may exist, yet not be the only cause of the patient's LVH; further examination is needed even if the BP is high.

Data The BP is 136/58 in the right arm and 132/60 in the left arm. Ophthalmoscopy shows no evidence of present or past hypertension. Furthermore, the patient tells you that he has never had high BP on previous examinations, and nobody in his family has ever had it.

Logic So much for that! Wisely, the BP was checked in both arms because atherosclerotic occlusion or musculoskeletal deformity can make it falsely low in one arm. Next you consider another common cause for LVH: coronary heart disease. For this to be considered as the cause, there must be a history of having had a coronary occlusion or ECG evidence thereof, or angina pectoris. Diffuse ischemic cardiomyopathy may exist without any of these three being present, but it is rare.

Data The patient has never had any chest pains, never had a heart attack that he knows of, does not have diabetes, and his ECG shows no evidence of infarction.

Logic The two most common causes of LVH have been eliminated. You are about to go to the next diagnostic decision point, when you realize you have not determined whether his heart is enlarged (in keeping with his ECG), nor have you decided if he is compensated or in beginning congestive heart failure.

Data The apex beat is diffusely felt between the left midclavicular line and the anterior axillary line in the fifth and sixth intercostal spaces. A slight left ventricular heave is also noted. But there are no basal rales, neck veins are not distended at 45 degrees, and the patient has no dysp-

nea on exertion, sleeps flat, and has no night cough. A quick examination of the heart reveals no murmurs, gallops, thrills, or abnormalities of S_1 and S_2.

Logic The heart is indeed enlarged, but there is no evidence of even beginning congestive heart failure, because P_2 is not loud, and there are no gallops, pulmonary congestion, or symptoms. You are becoming a bit concerned because the absence of murmurs weighs against rheumatic heart disease, which is another common cause of LVH. The cause of the LVH pattern is not readily apparent.

Knowing that some rheumatic valvular murmurs are often overlooked, you decide to reexamine the heart more carefully. However, you have a bad cold, your nose is clogged, and you are not hearing too well that day. So first you think awhile; more examinations and questions will come later.

Aortic stenosis can be congenital or rheumatic in origin and supravalvular, valvular, or infravalvular in location. If significant stenosis is present, there is usually at least a grade 3/6 systolic ejection murmur heard at the base of the heart radiating into the carotid arteries, an S_4, a palpable thrill, and a slow carotid upstroke. Often, S_2 is paradoxically split and an ejection sound is heard.

Aortic regurgitation (AR) is caused chiefly by rheumatic heart disease, but infective endocarditis, syphilis, chest trauma, rheumatoid arthritis and its variants, and aortic dissection can cause it too. Uncommon hereditary diseases (Marfan, Ehlers-Danlos, and Hurler's syndromes) would be seen in a much younger age group but could also be associated with AR. Signs of regurgitation include a wide pulse pressure and a high-pitched diastolic decrescendo murmur starting with S_2 and radiating from the aortic valve auscultatory area down to Erb's point and along the left sternal border. Confirmatory signs—such as water-hammer pulse, a Quincke's pulse, and Duroziez's sign—may be present.

Mitral regurgitation results from rheumatic heart disease, old myocardial infarction with papillary muscle dysfunction, and the rare hereditary diseases that also cause AR. Its hallmark is a high-pitched pansystolic murmur at the apex radiating to the left axilla or base of the heart. An S_3 or short mid-diastolic flow murmur is often present, and S_2 may be widely split because aortic closure is early.

Data You reexamine the heart and again hear no murmurs, gallops, or abnormal splits. There is no history of alcoholism, and the patient does not know how long his heart has been enlarged. The tongue is not enlarged, lymph nodes are nowhere palpable, and the liver and spleen are not enlarged.

Logic The last common consideration—cardiomyopathy—seems unlikely. Even though this large group of diverse diseases can be caused by hereditary obstructive and restrictive muscle hypertrophy, alcohol, systemic disorders, such as sarcoidosis, amyloidosis, vasculitis, and viral infections, so far there is no evidence for any of these. Because it is often difficult to identify and verify a specific cause precisely, and because you realize cardiomyopathy is a catchall diagnosis, you may have to accept this etiology and observe the patient.

On a final review of the data, you again note that the pulse pressure is slightly widened. So you instill nose drops in your nose, blow it, and inflate your middle ear with a Valsalva's maneuver. Then you change stethoscopes, because you note a crack in the diaphragm you have been using. Now you can hear better.

Data On applying the diaphragm of the new stethoscope firmly to the chest in the area of Erb's point—with the patient sitting up, leaning forward, and at the end of expiration—you hear a grade 2/4 soft, high-pitched, diastolic decrescendo murmur starting with S_2. On rechecking the BP, you find it to be 130/30 in both arms. Earlier, when your hearing was not so good, you entered the fifth Korotkoff phase too soon (Fig. 14.2).

Logic Aortic regurgitation is clearly present. Do not berate yourself, because this murmur is easily missed if not carefully auscultated. What is the cause of the AR?

Data There is no history of acute rheumatic fever or symptoms thereof (prolonged fever, chorea, joint pains, nosebleeds, lengthy bed rest as a child). The Venereal Disease Research Laboratory test results are negative, and the patient was never treated for syphilis. Hereditary defects are manifested at an early age. A chest radiograph merely shows moderate cardiac enlargement (cardiothoracic ratio = 18:30) but no

pulmonary congestion or widening of the ascending aorta.

Logic No cause was found for the valvular lesion. Because rheumatic heart disease is the most common cause, and because many patients who have chronic rheumatic valvular disease report no history of a previous acute episode, this remains the presumptive diagnosis. No urgent treatment is indicated at the moment, although you might consider Doppler ultrasound studies to quantitate the regurgitation in anticipation of valve replacement (Fig. 14.3).

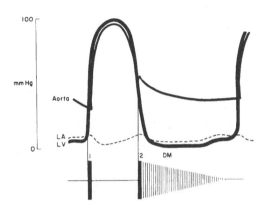

▶ **Figure 14.2.** The murmur of aortic regurgitation is high-pitched, decrescendo in shape, and begins with S_2.

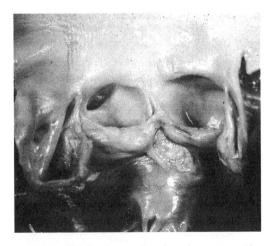

▶ **Figure 14.3.** Aortic valve of another patient with aortic regurgitation. Cusps are stiff, thickened, and commissures are widened, which results in valvular incompetence.

Questions

1. Assume that the same patient has a grade 3/6 mitral regurgitant murmur, a grade 3/6 systolic ejection murmur and thrill over the aortic valve, a slow carotid upstroke, and a BP of 160/100 in both arms. The fundi are normal. His electrocardiographic LVH pattern is most likely caused by:
   (a) essential hypertension.
   (b) aortic stenosis.
   (c) mitral regurgitation.
   (d) two of the aforementioned.

2. If the ECG abnormality had been right ventricular hypertrophy (RVH), each of the following would be possible except which one?
   (a) Mitral stenosis
   (b) Tricuspid stenosis
   (c) Pulmonic stenosis
   (d) Multiple pulmonary emboli

3. Change the patient's data a bit. The fundi show exudates, hemorrhages, and arteriovenous nicking, and the BP is 220/110 in both arms. Leg pulses are strong. Two distinct murmurs are heard: a grade 2/6 systolic ejection murmur in the right second intercostal space next to the sternum, and a grade 2/6 pansystolic high-pitched murmur at the apex radiating to the left axilla. A distinct S_4 is present, and the apex beat is strong, diffuse, and displaced to the left. The cause of the patient's LVH pattern is probably:
   (a) essential hypertension.
   (b) coarctation of the aorta.
   (c) aortic stenosis.
   (d) mitral regurgitation.

Answers

1. **(d) is correct,** although the answer could be "all of the aforementioned." The hypertension is mild, probably not of long duration, and at most is contributing little to the LVH. The patient clearly has aortic stenosis as indicated by the findings. Mitral regurgitation may be present as a separate valvular lesion, but it could also result from functional insufficiency secondary to altered left ventricle geometry. Aortic stenosis would tend to make the mitral regurgitation worse. Each of the conditions in (a), (b), or (c) could cause LVH. It is probable that at least two of the lesions are operative here.

2. **(b) is correct** because it is the only lesion not associated with RVH. The obstruction is proximal to the right ventricle, and only the right atrium hypertrophies. Mi-

tral stenosis causes RVH after many years of left atrial hypertrophy; eventually pulmonary congestion and pulmonary hypertension affect the right ventricle. Choices (c) and (d) are obvious causes of RVH. Note that mitral stenosis does not cause LVH for the same reason that tricuspid stenosis does not cause RVH.

3. **(a) is correct.** Severe long-standing hypertension is present. Secondary forms of hypertension are statistically unlikely. Coarctation is ruled out by strong leg pulses. The aortic murmur is more characteristic of hypertension than aortic stenosis. The mitral murmur is mild and probably results from inability of the valve leaflets to coapt properly. Hypertrophied enlarged hearts often have mild mitral regurgitant murmurs regardless of the cause of the hypertrophy. S_4 is heard in any condition where the left ventricle is stiff, thick, and noncompliant.

COMMENT A large number of problem-solving techniques were used in this case. First, a list of common possibilities was established. Positive and pertinent negative clues gave continued guidance as diagnostic contenders were eliminated one by one. As each bit of information was acquired, the line of inquiry could have veered in one of two directions—the correct diagnosis or further information. The possible presence of rheumatic valvular disease in the absence of acute rheumatic fever invoked a negative syllogism. One clue—the slightly wide pulse pressure—led the author to zero in on the correct diagnosis in Holmesian fashion.

The flowchart of data acquisition required to solve this case was as follows: repeat the ECG, corroborate LVH by physical examination and radiograph, rule out congestive heart failure, take the BP, listen for murmurs, and rule out angina and infarct; consider cardiomyopathy if all other test results are negative. If any step is positive (severe hypertension, characteristic murmur, and so forth), the search may end. In fact, proper auscultation of the heart could have solved the problem in one step. *(P.C.)*

PROBLEM-BASED LEARNING The simple problem just discussed requires that you master a wealth of material that will subsequently be of great value in solving many cardiac problems. For example, to get the most from this case study, you should know about:

- Electrocardiographic criteria for LVH (while learning this, also learn the P, Q, R, S, and T's for *right* ventricular hypertrophy)
- Pathophysiologic causes of LVH
- Hypertension, its criteria and physical signs, the primary and secondary causes thereof, and the symptoms, signs, and other confirmatory evidence for each possible cause
- Aortic stenosis, its various anatomic types and causes, the symptoms, signs of each cause, and how to prove each type conclusively
- Mitral regurgitation, its causes, physical signs, means of confirmation, and consequences
- Aortic regurgitation, its various causes and associated diseases, their physical signs, and their confirmation
- Coronary heart disease as it may relate to LVH
- Cardiomyopathy, its classification and causes, and how it may selectively affect the left ventricle
- Heart murmurs, gallops, and thrills, and their understanding based on mastery of the Wiggers diagram and the complete cardiac cycle
- Relationship of congenital and acquired defects to: the causation of valve dysfunction, restrictive and obstructive cardiomyopathies, and their resultant LVH
- The vanishing but still present specter of syphilis in causing aortic regurgitation
- Chest radiographic evidence of LVH and the measurement of the cardiothoracic ratio

Learn all of this, and cardiology becomes much simpler.

Suggested Readings

Barletta GD Donato M, Baroni M, et al. Left ventricular remodeling in chronic aortic regurgitation. Int J Cardiol Imag 1993;9(3):185–193.

Carabello BA. The relationship of left ventricular geometry and hypertrophy to left ventricular function in valvular heart disease. J Heart Valve Dis 1995;4(suppl)2:132–138.

Tornos MP, Olona M, Permanyer-Miralda G, et al. Clinical outcome of severe asymptomatic chronic aortic regurgitation: A long-term prospective follow-up study. Am Heart J 1995;130(2):333–339.

CASE 24

SEVERE SUBSTERNAL TIGHTNESS

Michael H. Crawford

Data After 1 hour of continuous tight substernal pain, a 53-year-old accountant is brought to the emergency department. He had been treated for hypertension for 10 years but did not adhere to his regimen nor did he see his physician regularly. Three years ago he was found to have adult-onset diabetes mellitus. He was treated with some success by diet alone but had difficulty losing weight. For the past year he has had recurrent episodes of tight substernal discomfort occurring two or three times per week. These were provoked by emotional stress or severe exertion and relieved in approximately 1 to 2 minutes by a sublingual nitroglycerine tablet or by rest. He limited his activities to avoid these episodes.

This pattern remained stable until a month ago when he observed his chest pain becoming more severe, more prolonged, and more easily provoked. He needed two or three nitroglycerin tablets for relief. One week before admission he was experiencing chest pain four to five times daily. The pain during the present attack was worse than usual, radiated to the neck and down the left arm, and was unrelieved by three nitroglycerin tablets. He felt ill and was nauseated and in a cold sweat, so he came to the hospital.

Logic Chest pain may originate from any one of various structures in the chest. However, the information gotten about the nature of the pain, and what causes and relieves it, points directly to coronary artery disease. He has a new pattern of crescendo angina pectoris that seems to have resulted in a myocardial infarction (MI). There are two well-established risk factors here for this disease: hypertension and diabetes. Other important risk factors yet to be determined in this patient are tobacco abuse, hereditary background, and serum cholesterol. There is also evidence that sedentary occupation, obesity, dietary fat intake, and personality type may be risk factors.

Angina pectoris results from an imbalance between myocardial oxygen supply and demand. When severe coronary artery disease is present, the supply of oxygenated blood to the heart muscle is limited. During exercise or emotional tension, demand increases, but supply cannot match it. This imbalance results in myocardial ischemia and chest pain.

Worsening angina may be caused by increasing demand: more emotional stress, more physical exertion, or rising blood pressure. It may also worsen if oxygen availability is decreased either by the progression of coronary artery lesions, coronary artery spasm, decreased oxygen supply (chronic lung disease), or decreased oxygen-carrying capacity of the blood (anemia).

Data Further questions reveal that the patient had decreased his activity and exposure to emotional tension during the past month. He has never smoked and has no other significant symptoms. The family history, however, is notable for a high frequency of coronary disease, hypertension, and diabetes.

The physical examination was completely normal except for the vital signs and heart: BP, 160/95; pulse, 85 beats per minute, with frequent premature beats; temperature 37.1°C; respirations, 18 per minute. The lungs, jugular venous pressure, and carotid pulses were normal. The apical impulse was in the fourth and fifth left intercostal spaces just lateral to the midclavicular line and was approximately 5 cm in diameter. A prominent presystolic wave and a sustained outward systolic thrust were palpated. On auscultation, S_1 was soft, S_2 was normal, and there was a soft S_3 and a loud S_4. No murmurs were heard.

Logic The family history adds another potent risk factor. The lateral displacement and enlargement of the apical impulse may be due to left ventricular hypertrophy from long-standing hypertension or systolic expansion of a noncontractile segment resulting from the new MI. The presystolic pulsation and loud S_4 are common in both these conditions and are synchronous with the atrial infusion of blood into a noncompliant ventricle. The soft S_1 and the S_3 signify early myocardial decompensation.

Data The ECG showed marked ST-segment elevation in leads V_1 to V_4, ST depression in leads III and aVF, and frequent premature ventricular beats (VPBs) (Fig. 14.4). Blood was drawn for cardiac enzymes, complete blood count, routine chemistries, and partial thromboplastin time (PTT). Further history was negative for recent bleeding, surgery, or central nervous system symptoms. Thus, intravenous tissue plasminogen activator (tPA) and 325 mg aspirin were given. He was admitted to the coronary care unit.

Logic It is now certain that the patient has an acute MI and that his worsening angina was probably related to plaque rupture and impending coronary thrombosis. In addition, he has the most common

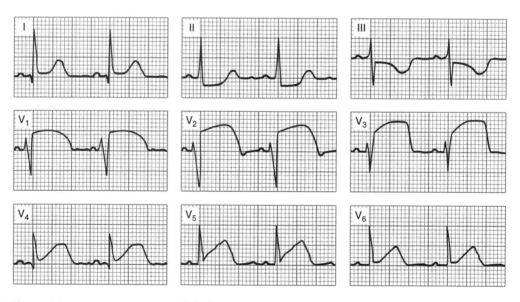

▶ **Figure 14.4.** Acute anterior myocardial infarction. ST segments markedly elevated in leads I and V_1 to V_5; ST segment depressed in leads II and III. Premature ventricular beats not noted in this tracing.

complication of MI—an arrhythmia. The multiple VPBs result from abnormal electrical currents in the ischemic tissue. However, other causes for VPBs that may be operant are hypoxia, electrolyte imbalance, anxiety, acidosis, alkalosis, and certain drugs (e.g., "diet pills").

Acute MI with ST elevation on the ECG is almost always due to thrombosis in a coronary artery. Thus, if there are no serious risks of bleeding (e.g., recent stroke or active gastrointestinal bleeding), thrombolytic therapy is indicated within the first 6 to 12 hours. Recent trials have shown that tPA is somewhat more effective than streptokinase in terms of short-term arterial patency and mortality. However, tPA more frequently causes hemorrhagic stroke, and its cost is 10 times that of streptokinase. Also, because of rebound thrombotic effects, tPA should be used with heparin, whereas heparin is less important when streptokinase is used. In this young individual with a large anteroseptal MI (probably due to left anterior descending coronary artery occlusion) and who has signs of LV dysfunction (S_3), tPA is believed to have the lowest risk-benefit ratio. Immediate angioplasty is also a consideration for rapidly opening the coronary artery, but it is effective only if it can be done without significant delay.

Data Pain subsided rapidly, and the patient appeared much improved. The temperature rose to 37.7° C, the pulse stayed at 90 beats per minute, and the S_4 persisted. Results of serum electrolytes, blood gases, blood pH, complete blood count, urinalysis, and other blood chemistries were all normal, except for the blood glucose, which was 160 mg/dL, and a serum magnesium of 1.5 mg/dL (below normal). The patient was taking no drugs. The VPBs increased in frequency, and there were salvos of 2 to 4 VPBs. Intravenous magnesium was begun and the VPBs disappeared. After the tPA was given and the PTT had fallen to ≤ 100 seconds, intravenous heparin was begun. Repeat ECG showed decreased ST elevation. Blood pressure remained elevated, so he was given 5 mg metoprolol 3x. Serum creatine kinase (CK) at 12 hours rose to 1096 mIU/1 (normal is 25 to 120), 16% of which was the MB isomer (specific for myocardium).

Logic The subsidence of chest pain, decrease in ST-segment elevation, early CK peak, and decrease in arrhythmias suggest that recanalization and reperfusion were accomplished. It is difficult to interpret the disappearance of chest pain because he was receiving intravenous nitroglycerin. The decrease of arrhythmias is an unreliable marker of reperfusion; this patient did have a low magnesium level and was given magnesium sulfate. However, the early peak CK is highly suggestive of rapid wash-out in an open arterial system and the decrease in ST elevation is an excellent sign of reperfusion.

Data The patient remained pain-free for 48 hours. Because arrhythmias were absent, the magnesium infusion was stopped at 24 hours. VPBs did not recur. At 48 hours the heparin was stopped and the nitroglycerin drip was tapered off over 3 hours. Metoprolol 50 mg bid and 325 mg aspirin daily were continued. An ECG showed distal apical-septal akinesis, but overall left ventricular function was normal (ejection fraction 55%). The blood pressure was initially controlled on intravenous nitroglycerin and metoprolol but increased to 165/100 after the nitroglycerin was stopped. Thus, an angiotensin-converting enzyme inhibitor (ACEI) was started.

Logic Nitroglycerin therapy is largely for pain control, but it can supplement blood pressure and heart failure treatment. Thus, once pain and blood pressure were controlled for 48 hours, it was stopped. The duration of heparin post-thrombolytic therapy is not clearly defined, but 48 to 72 hours is typical, with aspirin continued indefinitely. Beta-blockers (metoprolol) have been shown to reduce mortality in acute MI patients and are excellent antihypertensive agents. This therapy was used for both reasons in this case. The mortality benefit of β-blockers wanes after 2 years. ACEIs have been shown to reduce mortality and improve left ventricular function in post-MI patients, especially those with low ejection fractions (< 40%). Consequently, it is a good choice for controlling his blood pressure.

Data Despite control of his blood pressure, the patient had recurrent chest pain during ambulation on day four. Coronary angiography was done and showed a 50% stenosis of the left anterior descending coronary artery. It was elected to treat him with antianginal medications, institute risk factor control, and recommend rehabilitation. The patient did well and chest pain did not recur.

Logic Recurrent myocardial ischemia, reduced LV function, and previous MI are clear indications for coronary angiography. Other reasons are more controversial. Many studies have shown that a noninvasive evaluation with stress tests results in the same patient outcomes as does a policy of coronary angiography in all MI survivors. Coronary angiography is reserved for persons with markedly positive results from their stress tests. This patient had single vessel disease with a non-critical lesion ($\leq$ 50% diameter narrowing); the MI was probably due to rupture of this plaque and subsequent thrombus formation. Thus, this patient's eventual regimen consisted of medical therapy, risk factor reduction, and a rehabilitation program.

It is important to note that he was first seen with a typical MI from the standpoint of both history and physical findings. Many infarctions are atypical. They can have a presentation of syncope, weakness, acute pulmonary edema, or an arrhythmia. Often there are no symptoms whatsoever and the infarct is discovered later on a routine ECG. The physical examination may vary from no abnormal physical findings to pulmonary edema and shock, depending on the size of the infarct.

COMMENT Here the diagnosis is easily recognized by a pattern of worsening angina in a patient with diabetes and hypertension, culminating in an acute MI. With the given risk factors, coronary disease and MI are to be expected. The sequence of events is unmistakable. The ECG is specific, although it may not be highly sensitive until hours have elapsed. Elevation of the creatine kinase and its MB isomer is both very specific and very sensitive. The principles of cause and effect are thoroughly used in determining the causes for VPBs and worsening angina.

Not usually done in this book, treatment is discussed in detail, mainly because it brings into focus the interplay of various pathophysiologic events—enzyme release, arrhythmia, ST-segment elevation, the role of magnesium, blood pressure elevation, washout principle, reperfusion, and left ventricular function. *(P.C.)*

Suggested Readings

Califf RM, Ohman EM. The diagnosis of acute myocardial infarction. Chest 1992;101 (4 [suppl]):106–115.

Murata GH. Evaluating chest pain in the emergency department. West J Med 1993;159(1):61–68.

Murray C, Alpert JS. Diagnosis of acute myocardial infarction. Curr Opin Cardiol 1994;9(4):465–470.

Rozenman Y, Gotsman MS. The earliest diagnosis of acute myocardial infarction. Annu Rev Med 1994; 45:31–44.

CASE 25

SYSTOLIC MURMUR

Paul Cutler

Data During an examination for a life insurance policy, a healthy 28-year-old man was found to have a heart murmur. He consulted his private physician who confirmed the presence of a grade 2/6 midsystolic ejection murmur in the aortic and pulmonic areas but noted no other abnormalities. Symptoms of cardiac disease had not been present. Chest radiograph and ECG results were normal.

Logic When a murmur is unexpectedly found in presumably healthy person, you must decide whether it is functional and without significance, or a manifestation of subtle underlying cardiac disease that can cause trouble in the future.

It is important to know how long the murmur has been present. If heard at or shortly after birth, congenital lesions are suspected. But if first heard at age 28, as in this patient, it may be an acquired lesion—unless the patient had never been carefully examined in the past.

Care should be taken to establish the presence or absence of cardiac symptoms, such as chest pain, syncope, dyspnea, orthopnea, paroxysmal nocturnal dyspnea, edema, or palpitations. A history of rheumatic fever must be sought by name or by its common manifestations. Inquiries should also be made about any family history of cardiac disease.

The physical examination is of paramount importance. If a murmur is functional, the vital signs, jugular venous pulse, arterial pulse, and apical impulse should be normal, and the lungs should be clear. Abnormal precordial lifts, cyanosis, edema, and clubbing should be absent. Chest deformities must be noted; either pectus excavatum or straight back syndrome can cause murmurs because of narrowing of the anteroposterior diameter of the chest. A third heart sound is normal only if the patient is under 20 years of age. A fourth heart sound often reflects decreased ventricular compliance, but it can be normal in those past age 55 or those who exercise vigorously. S_2 should be physiologically split and the pulmonic component audible only in the pulmonic area.

Data In this case the history was entirely negative, the murmur was the only physical finding of note, and because the chest radiograph and ECG were normal, no further tests were deemed necessary. Based on these data, the physician informed the patient that the murmur appeared to be functional but recommended a yearly examination to see if any new findings might appear.

Logic In reference to murmurs it should be noted that diastolic murmurs are almost always pathologic. Only systolic murmurs may be innocent or functional. If the murmur is holosystolic, high-pitched, and plateau-shaped, it is more apt to be organic, and mitral regurgitation, tricuspid regurgitation, or ventricular septal defect should be considered (Fig. 14.5). These conditions are unlikely in this patient because the murmur was of the ejection type and was heard at the base.

Ejection murmurs are shorter, usually diamond-shaped, and of medium pitch. They can be functional or organic. Basal ejection murmurs may be associated with many disease states, such as aortic or pulmonic stenosis, systemic or pulmonary hypertension, high flow through the pulmonary artery as in atrial septal defect, and high flow through both sides of the heart (high output states) as in chronic anemia, beriberi, hy-

perthyroidism, and Paget's disease. The systolic murmur of the click-murmur syndrome is best heard at the apex in late systole and is preceded by a click.

Each of these disease states has its accompanying characteristic physical findings. Because none were present here, the murmur was considered to be innocent or functional. But the physician wisely recognized that evidence of disease might appear later and recommended rechecks.

Data The patient elected not to return, and he continued to be asymptomatic until 20 years later. At age 48, while chasing an intruder on his property, he suddenly passed out for approximately 1 minute. He ignored this incident, but on two subsequent occasions during the next year and a half, he had similar episodes of syncope during strenuous exertion.

He began to deliberately avoid vigorous activity, but during the next 6 months he experienced numerous episodes of substernal pressure lasting 1 to 3 minutes. These came on with mild exertion, especially after meals. For the past few days he has had difficulty in getting a deep breath when sitting and watching television. Disturbed by these symptoms, he consulted a physician.

On examination he was found to have a blood pressure of 105/90, with a resting pulse rate of 90 beats per minute. The carotid and brachial artery pulses were noted to have a prolonged upstroke. The apical impulse was normally positioned but was diffuse and had a powerful, prolonged, heaving quality. A thrill was palpable in the aortic area. The first sound was normal, the second was paradoxically split, and a prominent fourth sound was present. A harsh grade 3/6 systolic ejection murmur was heard; it was loudest in the aortic area and radiated to both carotid arteries (Fig. 14.6). There were no rales. On the chest radiographs, a dense calcification was noted in the vicinity of the aortic valve, the lungs were clear, the aorta was prominent, and the left ventricle appeared to be either normal or slightly enlarged. The ECG showed left ventricular hypertrophy and "strain." An echocardiogram demonstrated thickening and diminished movement of the aortic valve leaflets.

Logic The findings are classic for aortic stenosis (AS). Reduced pulse pressure, prolonged or slow ejection noted at the apex and carotid artery, a heaving left ventricle, the murmur, thrill, and

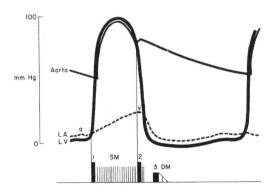

▶ **Figure 14.5.** Murmur of mitral regurgitation. The murmur is plateau-shaped, begins when the mitral valve is supposed to close, and ends after the second heart sound when the mitral valve opens.

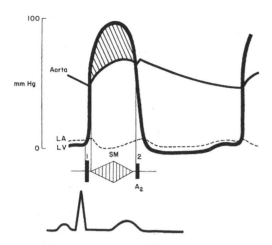

▶ **Figure 14.6.** Murmur of aortic stenosis. The murmur begins when the aortic valve opens and ends when it closes. Its diamond shape corresponds to the aortic-ventricular gradient.

fourth heart sound are all the result of a hypertrophied left ventricle laboring to eject blood through a stenotic valve orifice.

Syncope, angina, and left ventricular failure, either singly or in combination, are the usual presenting symptoms in AS. Only the first two are present here. Commonly, dyspnea and fatigue on exertion appear first. This patient's "dyspnea" makes you wonder. It sounds more like hyperventilation than organic dyspnea because it occurs at rest, is characterized by deep single breaths, and there are no signs of failure. He is probably anxious about his newly acquired symptoms.

In general, the cluster of a typical murmur and thrill is enough to diagnose AS. But thrills are not so common as once thought, because the disease is now discovered earlier, and there may be concomitant chronic obstructive lung disease obscuring the abnormal vibrations. Furthermore, the murmur may sometimes be best heard at the apex, and both thrill and murmur may be difficult to detect if severe congestive heart failure supervenes. Perhaps a more reliable cluster would be a typical murmur plus a slow carotid upstroke.

Abnormality of S_2 is almost always present in advanced AS. Paradoxical splitting occurs because of a prolonged left ventricular ejection time, so that aortic closure is delayed beyond pulmonic closure; with inspiration, P_2 catches up with A_2. Sometimes A_2 is inaudible because the valve is calcific and immobile. The S_4 results

from decreased ventricular compliance due to the left ventricular hypertrophy. An ejection sound may precede the murmur.

Calcification in the aortic valve is common. Left ventricular hypertrophy is almost always present in the ECG. The causes of AS are congenital (bicuspid valve commonly) and rheumatic. Calcific AS in the elderly is in most cases probably the end result of a congenital bicuspid valve. Bicuspid valves usually develop stenosis, regurgitation, or both, although some never do. Concomitant coronary disease may also be present. However, angina often occurs in aortic stenosis with normal coronary arteries because a Venturi effect just beyond the narrowed valve tends to reduce coronary flow, and ventricular hypertrophy increases the amount of oxygen needed by the myocardium.

The genesis of symptoms is easy to understand. They occur on exertion because the heart is unable to increase its stroke volume when called upon to do so.

You begin to wonder about the cause of AS in this patient. As far ar you can determine by history, no murmur was noted before age 28. This does not mean it was not present, because he rarely saw a physician, and it may have been missed when he did. Even if no murmur had been present in childhood, stenosis of a bicuspid valve may take years to develop. The absence of a history of rheumatic fever does not in the least exclude it as a diagnostic possibility. If the mitral valve were also diseased, you would lean toward rheumatic infection, but this is not the case here.

Data The physician recognized that aortic stenosis was present. He advised cardiac catheterization and explained that if, as he suspected, very advanced AS were present, surgical replacement of the aortic valve with a prosthesis would be recommended. The patient refused all procedures.

He had no difficulties except occasional angina-like pain until 1 year later, when he began to notice that he would awaken from his sleep sweating profusely. He had chilly sensations or feelings of warmth during the day and had a general feeling of malaise. After 4 weeks with these symptoms, he awoke one evening with severe shortness of breath and was taken to a hospital.

At the hospital, the pulse was 120 beats per minute; respirations, 40 per minute; BP, 100/40; and temperature, 38.8°C. Rales were diffusely present in both lung fields. The neck veins were markedly distended. The carotid and brachial pulses were full and bounding with a rapid upstroke. The apical impulse was diffuse and located in the sixth intercostal space 10 cm from the midsternal line. S_1 was barely audible, S_2 was narrowly split, an S_3 was heard at the apex, and S_4 was not audible. The systolic murmur was present as before. A grade 3/4 high-pitched, blowing, diastolic murmur was present in early and mid-diastole along the left sternal border. A grade 2/4 short, low-pitched, mid-diastolic rumble was noted at the apex. Blood cultures drawn soon after admission grew *Streptococcus viridans* 2 days later.

Logic The picture was drastically changed. He had developed classic findings of aortic regurgitation in addition to the AS. This was shown by the wide pulse pressure, water-hammer pulses, and new murmurs. A high-pitched, decrescendo, early diastolic murmur along the left sternal border in association with a wide pulse pressure is virtually diagnostic of aortic regurgitation.

Pulmonary regurgitation would have no effect on the peripheral pulse and blood pressure. The mid-diastolic murmur at the apex (Austin Flint murmur) is caused by the regurgitant stream striking the mitral valve leaflet, resulting in relative mitral stenosis. The S_3 indicates either failure or rapid early diastolic filling.

However, the heart has now enlarged and both left and beginning right ventricular failure are present. In view of the sudden onset of aortic regurgitation, left and beginning right ventricular failure, fever, sweats, and malaise, you must think first in terms of cusp erosion 2nd valve destruction by bacterial endocarditis (BE) (Fig. 14.7). This was confirmed by blood culture, and appropriate treatment against *S. viridans* was begun. A cardiovascular surgeon was consulted.

You have no idea what caused the endocarditis, because there was no history of dental procedures of oral surgery—the usual causes when a mouth organism is involved. Perhaps vigorous toothbrushing can be implicated.

He had none of the other common findings of infective endocarditis, such as embolic phenomena, petechiae, enlarged spleen, and clubbing. These are often absent although they should be sought.

If the clinical picture had been obscure, Doppler ultrasound could have helped to clarify it.

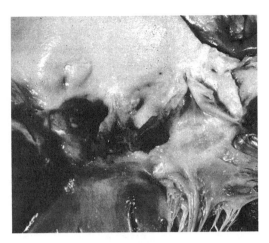

▶ **Figure 14.7.** Bacterial endocarditis superimposed on stenotic aortic valve. Ulcerated valve permits regurgitation (different patient).

Questions

1. You find a grade 2/6 systolic murmur in the aortic area of a 42-year-old asymptomatic man. The murmur is audible in the neck. No lifts or thrills are present. The carotid pulses and the first and second heart sounds are normal. There is no third or fourth heart sound. You suspect AS. Which of the following is correct?
   (a) A functional murmur is likely.
   (b) AS or pulmonic stenosis is present.
   (c) Rheumatic heart disease is probably present.
   (d) If no murmur was present in childhood, a bicuspid aortic valve could not be present.

2. Assume that a 16-year-old asymptomatic high school student is sent to you because his school physician has noted a murmur. You suspect an atrial septal defect (ASD) because he has a grade 2/6 ejection murmur at the base, a wide fixed split S_2, and a right ventricular lift. If your suspicion is correct, which of the following is least likely to be present?
   (a) A soft diastolic murmur at the left lower sternal border
   (b) A normal chest radiograph
   (c) Anomalous pulmonary veins
   (d) rSr' in V_1 of the ECG

3. An asymptomatic 33-year-old man is found to have a grade 4/6 blowing murmur, loudest at the apex and well heard in the left axilla. The murmur begins immediately with S_1 and continues through A_2 without varying in pitch or amplitude (plateau type). It does not

vary with respiration. Jugular venous and carotid pulses are normal. Aside from a 3-month illness at age 9, during which he was kept out of school because of pain and discomfort in his upper and lower extremities, he has been well. The most likely diagnosis is:

(a) idiopathic hypertrophic subaortic stenosis.
(b) functional murmur.
(c) aortic stenosis.
(d) mitral regurgitation (Table 14.1).

4. The patient described in this logic session had aortic stenosis, aortic regurgitation, left ventricular failure, and bacterial endocarditis. These conditions occurred in which of the following pathophysiologic time sequences?

(a) AS-AR-LVF-BE
(b) AS-BE-LVF-AR
(c) AS-BE-AR-LVF
(d) AS-LVF-BE-AR

Answers

1. **(a) is correct.** The absence of a slow upstroke in the carotid pulse and the absence of abnormalities of S_2 rule out significant AS. Pulmonic stenosis is unlikely in view of the location and radiation of the murmur and the lack of a wide splitting of S_2. There is no history of rheumatic fever or evidence of mitral involvement to support a diagnosis of rheumatic disease. A congenital bicuspid valve can result in AS or aortic regurgitation, and if these lesions develop, the murmur may first appear during adult life. However, because all of the findings noted can be normal, a functional murmur is the most likely diagnosis. But, as in the case discussed in the protocol, what is thought to be functional today may prove to be organic years later.

2. **(b) is correct.** The chest radiograph in ASD has prominent hilar shadows and prominent distal vasculature in most cases because of the high pulmonary blood flow. The systolic murmur is caused by high flow across the pulmonic valve, and not by blood traversing the septal defect. The diastolic murmur is due to high flow across the tricuspid valve and occurs when the shunt is large. Anomalous pulmonary veins are present in approximately 25% of patients with secundum type ASD. In most centers, more than 90% of postpuberty patients with ASD have the secundum type lesion, in which an incomplete right bundle branch block is common.

3. **(d) is correct.** The murmur is holosystolic and is heard best at the apex; it radiates to the axilla and does not vary with respiration. This is the usual finding in mitral regurgitation. The childhood illness was most likely rheumatic fever, which is the most common cause of severe mitral valve disease. Holosystolic murmurs are not functional. The clinical features of aortic valve stenosis were discussed in the case study. Idiopathic hypertrophic subaortic stenosis is a disease that involves a functional obstruction of the aortic outflow tract below the aortic valve due to muscular hypertrophy and a supernormal contraction of the ventricular muscle. Its murmur is crescendo or crescendo-decrescendo in type, tends to be long although not holosystolic, and is often heard best at the apex; radiation to the axilla is uncommon. The carotid upstroke is often rapid, and the carotid pulse is bifid; S_2 is paradoxically split, although A_2 remains well heard. The echocardiogram is distinctive; it shows a markedly hypertrophied interventricular septum and an abnormal movement of the mitral valve during systole.

4. **(c) is correct.** The sequence was clearly AS, eventually BE, which in turn caused destruction of a valve leaflet and acute AR; the regurgitation brought on the LVF. Not uncommonly, LVF will be the first manifestation of AS—but not so in this case.

TABLE 14.1. Causes of Major Systolic Murmurs

	AORTIC STENOSIS	MITRAL REGURGITATION
Timing	Ejection	Pansystolic
Shape	Diamond	Plateau
Pitch	Medium	High
Location	Base	Apex
Radiation	Neck	Axilla
Other	S_4	S_3

COMMENT The patient was seen with an asymptomatic finding that was detected on routine examination. A heart murmur became the key clue. The various causes of plateau and ejection murmurs were listed, and each was eliminated by the absence of associated findings. But after a number of years, a reliable cluster formed to make the diagnosis of AS. This cluster included symptoms and physical signs, each of which exhibited varying specificity and sensitivity; but when grouped together, the weight of evidence made the diagnosis unmistakable. The thrill is specific but not sensitive; the slow carotid upstroke is both specific and sensitive; the S_4 and paradoxically split S_2 are sensitive but not specific.

Considerable overlap of three clinical presentations (LVF, angina, syncope) can occur with AS. A patient can be seen with one, two, or three of these manifestations. This patient had only two. The third, LVF, was not present; dyspnea was caused by hyperventilation and could have been misleading.

Bacterial endocarditis then developed, and it was diagnosed in the absence of many signs that are often present. Sequence of events and a series of causes and effects portrayed the pathophysiologic development of AS-BE-AR-LVF. Note too how the clinical picture changed when a new disease was superimposed (BE upon AS) and that BE and AS combined to cause one effect, which in turn caused another. *(P.C.)*

Suggested Readings

Constant J. How to differentiate ejection murmurs from systolic regurgitant murmurs. Keio J Med 1995;44(3):85–87.

Grayburn PA. Hemodynamic assessment of aortic stenosis. Am J Med Sci 1992;303(5):345–354.

Harvey WP. Cardiac pearls. Dis Mon 1994;40(2):41–113.

CASE 26

HIGH BLOOD PRESSURE

Timothy N. Caris

Data A 43-year-old essentially asymptomatic black man comes to you for care. He is a self-employed gardener, and several weeks ago he had his blood pressure checked by a screening group in a shopping center. He was told it was 210/122. Subsequent daily recordings at a neighborhood clinic were 180/110, 192/108, 200/114, and 182/106.

Logic At the onset, you recall that the prevalence of hypertension in this country approaches 20% of the adult population. High blood pressure is a major risk factor for stroke, congestive heart failure, renal failure, and coronary heart disease. You recall also that the ravages of hypertension are more likely to occur in blacks than in whites, and in men than in women. Your patient, then, is in a high-jeopardy category.

Eighty-nine percent of patients with high blood pressure suffer essential or primary hypertension (EH), 6% have secondary causes for the elevation such as chronic renal parenchymal disease, and a final 5% have potentially surgically correctable secondary causes such as renal ischemic disease, coarctation of the aorta, pheochromocytoma, Cushing's syndrome, or primary aldosteronism.

You therefore proceed with the remainder of your evaluation keeping appropriate categorization in mind.

Data The patient has been in excellent health and, as a consequence, has not undergone medical examination in years. When he was discharged from the army at age 20, he was asked to lie down for 3 hours, and his blood pressure was checked every 30 minutes. He was told the pressure was high initially but returned to normal with rest. The patient was raised by a nonrelative, so family history is not obtainable. He has occasional occipital headaches late in the day that get worse as evening approaches; they usually respond to aspirin. He has not had exertional dyspnea, orthopnea, paroxysmal nocturnal dyspnea, palpitations, easy fatigability, chest discomfort, or chest pain. There have been no episodes of unsteady gait, memory defects, muscle weakness, sensory loss, difficulty in coordination, or visual disturbances. The remainder of the past history and history by systems was not contributory.

Logic The natural development of essential hypertension includes lability of blood pressure during the second and third decades. Fixed hypertension usually appears in the 30s. Your patient fits this facet of the clinical picture. EH tends to occur in families, but this fact is of no help in this situation.

EH is an insidious, painless disorder for many years—until target organs (heart, brain, kidneys) are significantly involved. Symptoms such as headaches, tinnitus, dizziness, fainting, and epistaxis that commonly have been ascribed to high blood pressure are nonspecific, and their incidence is found to be the same in normotensives as in hypertensives. Also, headaches occurring in the hypertensive patient are not temporally related to the height of the blood pressure. A pounding occipital headache that is present in the morning and wears off as the day progresses does occur in some persons with hypertension. This patient is describing a "tension" headache that may occur in anyone.

By history, he has no suggestion of left ventricular decompensation, myocardial ischemia, or cerebral ischemia. Pheochromocytoma is not likely because there is no history of paroxysmal headaches, sweating, racing of the heart, palpitations, tremulous sensation, or lightheadedness after arising abruptly from a seated or lying position.

Data The physical examination reveals a well-developed, moderately obese black man (72 in tall, 224 lb). The pulse rate is 76 beats per minute and regular, there are no bruits in the neck, and all the peripheral pulses are present, equal, and strong bilaterally. The remainder of the physical and neurologic examinations is completely normal, except for the fundi, which show narrowing of the arterioles and arteriovenous crossing defects as well as hemorrhages and exudates. Blood pressure is 204/116 in the right arm and 200/114 in the left with the patient lying down. Blood pressure in the left arm is 200/116 when the patient is sitting and 194/118 when standing. Auscultation reveals a fourth heart sound at the apex and no bruits over the abdomen.

Logic The ophthalmoscopic changes indicate long-standing hypertensive vascular disease. Patients with pheochromocytoma are likely to be hypermetabolic with tremor, tachycardia, and lean habitus; the lack of orthostatic drop in blood pressure also helps exclude this possibility. The absence of bruits in the neck is a point against significant carotid or vertebral atherosclerosis. Less than 20 mm Hg disparity between the blood pressures in the arms excludes the complications of aortic arch disorders such as occlusive atherosclerosis, dissecting aneurysm, or atypical coarctation. The diagnosis of ordinary coarctation of the aorta depends in part on diminished femoral pulses compared with the carotids. You can dismiss this possibility in your patient. The fourth heart sound indicates that concentric hypertrophy of the left ventricle has already begun—target organ involvement.

The absence of an abdominal bruit is important. In individuals less than 50 years old, a bruit is the most discriminatory clinical finding for renovascular ischemic disease causing secondary hypertension. Although abdominal bruits may be heard in up to 5% of patients with EH they are present in 50 to 60% of patients with renovascular hypertension in this age group.

To distinguish the bruit of renovascular stenosis from the innocent bruits commonly heard over the aorta, the nature of the bruit, its location, and the technique of auscultation are important. Aortic bruits in older persons and in those with EH are soft, low-pitched, purely systolic, and heard in the epigastrium. The bruit caused by renal artery stenosis is high-pitched, continuous or systolic and diastolic, and is best heard in the subcostal margin and laterally into the flank; moderate pressure must be applied to the diaphragm of the stethoscope.

The characteristic central fat distribution of Cushing's disease or syndrome is not present in this patient. If you further consider the absence of ecchymoses, plethora, purple abdominal striae, and muscle weakness, this endocrine disease can be excluded.

Data Selected laboratory data needed to solve this problem are: urinalysis, normal; hematocrit, 44%; serum creatinine, 0.8 mg/dL; serum potassium, 4.2 mEq/L; fasting blood glucose, 80 mg/dL; normal chest radiograph; and ECG showing early left ventricular hypertrophy.

Logic Normal results from urinalysis help exclude renal parenchymal disease as a source of secondary hypertension, whereas a normal serum creatinine level speaks for good renal function. Primary aldosteronism is unlikely in the presence of a normal serum potassium. Neither history nor physical examination leads to the suspicion that coarctation of the aorta, pheochromocytoma, or Cushing's syndrome is the cause of the blood pressure elevation in this man. The normal blood glucose is another point against the last two.

Renal artery disease producing renal ischemia is the most common correctable cause for secondary hypertension. In this event, the elevated blood pressure tends to occur earlier in life and is of greater severity, and the course is more rapidly progressive than in the patient under discussion. But renal ischemic disease may closely mimic EH.

The absence of abdominal bruits is helpful but does not absolutely exclude renal artery disease. Some feel that despite the lack of clinical clues of renal artery stenosis, all patients should undergo a rapid infusion, rapid sequence intravenous pyelogram. Unequal size of kidneys, delay in visualization, or hyperconcentration of the contrast material on one side is considered indicative of renal vascular disease. Although still controversial, the present consensus is not to include intravenous pyelography in the initial evaluation of a hypertensive patient.

On the other hand, one must always consider and exclude renal artery disease if the patient has sustained hypertension and is less than 30 years old, if the patient is elderly and has severe elevation of blood pressure (i.e., sustained diastolic pressures of 130 mm Hg or greater), or if the patient has the documented sudden onset of fixed hypertension, rapidly worsening hypertension, or hypertension with an abdominal bruit.

There is no assurance that all patients with secondary hypertension will be identified; a very small number will slip through. If patients fail to respond to appropriate treatment for EH, these few should be reassessed. A more exhaustive diagnostic approach including a renal arteriogram, magnetic resonance angiography, renal vein renin measurements, urinary metanephrines and vanillylmandelic acid (VMA), plasma aldosterone and plasma renin activity determinations, angiotensin blocking agents, and the dexamethasone suppression test might be undertaken at this point despite lack of clinical clues.

Recall that when first facing a patient with hypertension your main task is to decide whether this is garden variety EH or hypertension resulting from an endocrine disorder, renovascular disease, or renal disease. Doing so is most important because treatment is based primarily on this differentiation. EH is controllable, but not curable, and requires treatment for life. The hypertension caused by renal disease is only partially controllable and needs treatment during a curtailed life. But hypertension resulting from endocrine disorders and renovascular ischemia offers a good chance for cure.

Also, note that in deciding on the type of hypertension your patient may have, you are using both a multivariate analysis and an algorithmic technique that include critical factors such as age, gender, race, family history, rapidity of onset and severity of hypertension, and response to drug treatment.

The 90% with EH usually have a positive family history; their hypertension begins in the 30s and 40s and becomes progressively worse.

However, this type usually responds to diligent resourceful treatment.

Endocrine diseases associated with hypertension can be excluded by the clinical picture and a few well-selected tests.

Renovascular ischemic hypertension results mainly from either an atherosclerotic plaque causing 50% or more obstruction of a renal artery or fibromuscular dysplasia of one or both renal arteries. The former occurs mostly in men older than 50, and the latter occurs in women younger than 35 years old. The common denominator is a marked decrease in perfusion pressure in the afferent arteriole of the glomerulus; this causes a release of renin, which in turn invokes the renin-angiotensin-aldosterone mechanism. Hypertension results from the pressor action of angiotensin II abetted by the volume expansion caused by aldosterone. Somewhere between 1 and 5% of hypertensives have renovascular ischemic disease. Therefore, the following diagnostic pursuit applies only to a small minority of all hypertensive patients.

Once you suspect the presence of this problem, it must be proved—for surgery may be the treatment of choice. There are many diagnostic procedures, but each has its limitations.

Inevitably you must come to the rapid sequence intravenous pyelogram. The criteria for test positivity result in 75% sensitivity and 89% specificity (11% false positives). Although this is a fairly good distinguishing test because it is performed on a patient who is already highly suspect of having renovascular hypertension—$P(D) = .50$ or more—it is not reliable enough to hang your surgical gloves on.

If your suspicion is still high, two additional procedures must be done. First comes renal arteriography, which is invasive although productive in the detection of a stenotic lesion. But stenosis may exist yet not be the cause of the hypertension. Therefore, the definitive test is done by sampling the blood in both renal veins via a catheter introduced into the femoral vein. Plasma renin activity (PRA) is measured in both renal veins. The PRA in the vein coming from the ischemic kidney should be much higher than the PRA coming from the nonischemic kidney. This difference is accentuated by the fact that the excessive secretion from the affected kidney suppresses the secretion from the normal one.

The presence of bilateral renal ischemia complicates the situation, although one side is usually more ischemic than the other. In effect, the arteriogram decides if stenosis exists, and venous sampling decides if the stenosis is the cause of the hypertension. These two studies will identify the 90% of those whose hypertension will be cured by surgery.

Recently, many techniques of renal artery imaging for the evaluation of possible renovascular disease have been developed and show promise of clinical usefulness in the future. These include captopril-enhanced radionuclide renography, digital subtraction angiography, magnetic resonance angiography, and duplex ultrasound scanning of renal arteries. These procedures do present various degrees of technical difficulty, are expensive, and will require more experience to become validated.

There was no evidence nor clues to suggest secondary forms of hypertension in this patient, and no additional studies were done beyond the initial ones.

Data During the ensuing 8 years, the patient was treated medically for EH. Because he felt well, he failed to take his medication regularly and visited his physician only rarely for acute minor problems. The blood pressure remained high, his heart got larger, albumin appeared in his urine, and more hemorrhages were noted in his fundi.

At age 51, he suddenly developed severe chest, back, and abdominal pain requiring hospitalization. The ECG and enzymes remained normal, but he continued to be critically ill. Both legs became cold and pulseless, urine formation ceased, and he developed an aortic diastolic murmur and abruptly died.

Logic Poor patient compliance is common. Target organ involvement was becoming more noticeable (heart, kidneys, fundi). His terminal event was a dissecting aortic aneurysm, not uncommon in hypertensives or patients with disorders like Marfan syndrome and cystic medial necrosis. The dissection was extensive, involved and occluded the circulation to the legs and kidneys, then dissected retrograde to include the aortic valve and cause regurgitation. Probably dissection into the pericardial sac with tamponade caused sudden death (Fig. 14.8).

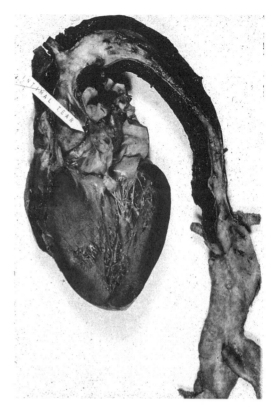

▶ **Figure 14.8.** Dissecting aneurysm. Arrow indicates point of rupture into pericardial sac.

Questions

1. Your patient is an asymptomatic 26-year-old woman whom you are examining for the first time. You note arteriovenous nicking on ophthalmoscopic examination, and the BP is 220/132. She is hospitalized for an in-depth evaluation, which includes renal arteriography, because you also find:
   (a) family history of hypertension.
   (b) four to five white blood cells per high-powered field on urinalysis.
   (c) she is not using any oral contraceptives.
   (d) a faint bruit in the left subcostal area that has short systolic and diastolic components.

2. The urinalysis from the patient in Question 1 shows 4+ glucosuria, and a subsequent fasting blood glucose is 200 mg/dL. Which of the following is not causally related to hyperglycemia in a hypertensive patient?

(a) Diabetes mellitus
(b) Fibromuscular dysplasia of the renal artery
(c) Pheochromocytoma
(d) Cushing's syndrome

3. A patient with fixed hypertension has a serum potassium level of 2.8 mEq/L. Which one of the following would have no bearing on this electrolyte disorder?
(a) Patient is a chronic daily user of laxatives.
(b) Patient is taking hydrochlorothiazide daily.
(c) Patient may have primary aldosteronism.
(d) Patient jogs 3 miles daily.

4. An 80-year-old asymptomatic man is referred to you because repeated blood pressure determinations in a neighborhood screening clinic have ranged from 180 to 200/70 to 80. Except for this finding, your physical examination reveals no abnormalities. The most likely explanation is:
(a) beginning essential hypertension
(b) aortic insufficiency
(c) renal artery occlusive disease
(d) atherosclerosis of the aorta

Answers

1. **(d) is correct.** A young woman with severe hypertension and an epigastric bruit must be regarded as having hypertension secondary to renovascular ischemic disease until proved otherwise. Positive family history of hypertension does not relate to renal artery occlusive disease. Pyuria may suggest infection, but not renal artery disease. Choice (c) merely excludes estrogen-containing pills as the cause of her hypertension.

2. **(b) is correct.** There is no relationship between hyperglycemia and fibromuscular dysplasia of the renal artery. The latter notably occurs in young women and may cause unilateral renal ischemia. Diabetes mellitus is a strong consideration, and its incidence is higher in hypertensives than in normotensives. Increased catecholamine levels result in transformation of glycogen stores in the liver to circulating blood glucose, and pheochromocytoma can be excluded if the catecholamine, metanephrine, and VMA levels in a 24-hour urine specimen are normal. Cushing's syndrome is related to adrenal hypercorticism, and hyperglycemia is a common manifestation of such a state because of excessive gluconeogenesis.

3. **(d) is correct.** There is no relationship between increased musculoskeletal activity and hypokalemia. Patients who are chronic daily laxative users deplete body potassium stores via the gastrointestinal tract. A 24-

hour urine potassium determination would probably show less than 30 mEq, which indicates that the body is truly attempting to conserve potassium. Thiazides cause excess potassium excretion as well, particularly in the presence of the high-salt diet that is common in Americans. This drug should be discontinued for 4 weeks, and the serum potassium levels should then be re-evaluated. The patient may well have primary aldosteronism. If so, the 24-hour urine potassium level will be greater than 30 mEq despite hypokalemia, plasma renin activity will be low, and the aldosterone level will be high.

4. **(d) is correct.** The atherosclerotic aorta has lost its compliance. Absence of aortic distention with systolic expulsion of blood leads to high systolic pressure. The diastolic pressure remains normal. EH includes elevation of both systolic and diastolic pressures. There is no murmur to suggest aortic insufficiency. Renal ischemic disease that leads to hypertension includes diastolic pressure elevation as well.

COMMENT The high incidence of hypertension, the especially high incidence of the disease and its ravages in black men, and the fact that only 5% of hypertensives have possibly surgically correctable lesions influence your thoughts and management. The reliability of an abdominal bruit as a decision point is outlined.

An orderly stepwise approach in this case would be: (1) obtain family history for hypertension; (2) check BP in arms and legs; (3) seek evidence of target organ involvement; (4) study the urine, creatinine, potassium, VMA, ECG, and chest radiograph; (5) look for clues for renovascular hypertension; and (6) treat medically if none are present; do further studies if renal ischemia is suspected. The latter may include an intravenous pyelogram, arteriogram, other new imaging procedures, and PRA measurements from both renal veins. Each procedure has fairly well-established sensitivity and specificity, and the $P(D)$ is altered by the results obtained by each one. If all procedure results are positive, you approach the 100% certainty that is desirable before surgery is performed. You have pinpointed the cause, evaluated the damage, and decided on treatment in six steps.

A decision tree, algorithm, or flowchart is ideally adaptable to the diagnostic process in this instance. *(P.C.)*

Suggested Readings

Emovon OE, Klotman PE, Dunnick NR, et al. Renovascular hypertension in blacks. Am J Hyperten 1996;9:18–23.

Hillman BJ. Imaging advances in the diagnosis of renovascular hypertension. AJR 1989;153:5–14.

Joint National Committee on Detection, Evaluation, and Treatment of High Blood Pressure. The fifth report. Ann Intern Med 1993;153:154–184. [Here is the consensus of national authorities on the diagnostic and therapeutic approaches to patients with hypertension.]

Olin JW, Piedmonte MA, Young JR, et al. The utility of duplex ultrasound scanning of the renal arteries for diagnosing significant renal artery stenosis. Ann Intern Med 1995;122:833–838.

Turnbull J. Is listening for abdominal bruits useful in the evaluation of hypertension? JAMA 1995;274:1299–1301.

CASE 27

DYSPNEA ON EXERTION

Paul Cutler

Data   A 58-year-old overweight married homemaker was rushed to the emergency department at 2 AM because of the sudden onset of severe shortness of breath. She was markedly dyspneic, orthopneic, and cyanotic, so immediate treatment with oxygen and morphine sulfate was given before further history could be obtained.

While waiting for her to improve, a quick examination revealed BP, 240/120; respirations, 26/min; pulse, 120 beats per minute; temperature, 37°C; cyanosis; neck vein distention 5 cm vertically above the sternal angle; fine and coarse inspiratory rales at the lung bases; loud inspiratory and expiratory wheezes; and a large heart with a diffuse forceful apex beat. No further heart detail was obtainable because of noisy breathing.

Logic   Sudden dyspnea in the presence of severe pulmonary congestion, hypertension, and a large heart suggests a cardiac emergency such as acute left ventricular failure with pulmonary edema, or a myocardial infarction. Were it not for the quickly obtained physical findings, sudden dyspnea might also have made you think of bronchial asthma, pneumothorax, pulmonary embolus, pleural effusion, atelectasis, or acute hyperventilation.

Data   The patient felt better in 10 minutes. Additional history revealed dyspnea and fatigue on exertion for several months. However, for the past few weeks she found it necessary to go to sleep on several pillows in order to breathe more easily, and on several occasions she awoke breathless and coughing and had to sit on the side of the bed or go to the window for relief. On the night of admission to the hospital, the dyspnea did not subside rapidly as usual but got steadily worse.

She attributes her recent difficulties to cigarette smoking as she gives a 45 pack-year history. In fact, for years she has had a morning cough productive of small amounts of grayish-white sputum. Hypertension had been present for more than 10 years, during which time she received intermittent treatment. She had difficulty adhering to a careful therapeutic regimen and, in addition, was unable to lose weight.

Both her mother and sister were hypertensive, and her mother died of a stroke. There is no history of acute rheumatic fever, joint pains, or murmur; no contact with tuberculosis or history of hemoptysis; no childhood asthma or other allergies; no chest pain or palpitations; no episodes of severe pounding headache and tremulousness; and no deep sighing breaths associated with numb sensations and lightheadedness. She takes no medication and is on no particular diet.

Logic   It now appears that the patient has a chronic problem that seems to have culminated in an acute episode. Although hypertension and left ventricular failure (LVF) seem to be responsible for the picture, other concomitant or alternate possibilities must still be considered.

As for the heart, hypertension may not be the only problem; she might easily have coronary disease, valvular disease, or cardiomyopathy in addition. Her clinical course is typical of gradually worsening LVF. But the history can also be explained by a chronic progressive lung disease with a superimposed acute complication, such as pleural effusion, pneumothorax, or atelectasis. Although severe anemia can cause dyspnea on exertion, it cannot account for orthopnea and the sudden acute episode.

You are left mainly with the possibilities of LVF or chronic lung disease with an acute complication. The presence of a large heart favors a cardiac etiology. But it is possible that both diseases coexist, and you must decide which is contributing principally or totally to the picture. Although severe hyperventilation based on anxiety can have a presentation of what seems to be acute dyspnea, its recognition is simple, and there would not ordinarily be any evidence of heart or lung disease. The absence of certain symptoms in the system review weighs against tuberculosis, asthma, coronary disease, pheochromocytoma, and hyperventilation—in that order.

Data Physical examination done after marked improvement showed obesity and normal vital signs, except for a BP that was 210/110 in both arms with no orthostatic changes. Cyanosis was no longer present, and her color was good. The fundi showed arteriolar tortuosity, arteriovenous nicking, a few exudates, and a rare round hemorrhage. Neck veins were no longer distended at 45 degrees. Faint bilateral expiratory wheezes and a few fine basilar rales were still present, but there was no dullness or flatness, the trachea was in the midline, and fremitus was normal. The diaphragm moved 2 to 3 cm on deep inspiration. The apex beat was forceful and diffuse in the fifth and sixth intercostal spaces at the left anterior axillary line. There was a left ventricular heave, a grade 2/6 systolic ejection murmur at the base, and a barely audible S_3. Two components of S_2 were clearly discernible, and the first component (aortic closure) was loud. The rest of the examination was normal.

Chest radiographs (posteroanterior and lateral views) showed normal lungs except for mild basilar congestion; the left ventricle was markedly enlarged. The abdominal radiograph revealed normal-sized kidney shadows. The ECG demonstrated left ventricular hypertrophy and "strain" plus a left atrial abnormality. Complete blood count, urinalysis, and 18-test blood chemistry profile were normal. Serum creatine kinase (MB isomer) was normal.

Logic The patient clearly has LVF, as evidenced by the radiograph, rales, enlarged heart, and S_3. The failure is caused by prolonged severe hypertension. There are no valve defects; the systolic murmur is mild and probably relates to hypertension, not to aortic stenosis, as there is no ejection click and the aortic component of S_2 is well preserved. There is no evidence by history, ECG, or enzyme changes for acute coronary disease. Cardiomyopathy could exist in addition to

hypertension, but there are no clinical features of the hypertrophic, restrictive, or congestive forms of this entity, nor are there any etiologic factors evident.

The positive family history of hypertension, normal leg pulses, normal renal size, normal urinalysis, and normal serum potassium, and the absence of symptoms to suggest pheochromocytoma, are all indications of essential hypertension rather than hypertension secondary to another disorder.

No doubt the patient also has mild-to-moderate chronic obstructive pulmonary disease as denoted by the history of cough and expectoration, excessive smoking, faint expiratory wheezes, and insufficient diaphragmatic motion. The loud wheezes on admission may have been due to interstitial fluid compressing the bronchioles; the faint ones heard later may have resulted from her chronic obstructive pulmonary disease. At any rate, lung disease is probably contributing little, if at all, to her present acute problem. Pulmonary function tests will be done later.

Data Cardiac enzyme levels and ECG did not change during the next 2 days. In the meantime, the patient was treated with digitalis, diuretics, antihypertensive medication, and a salt-restricted diet; improvement was marked and rapid. At discharge, the seriousness of her situation was carefully explained, and she was impressed with the need to give up smoking and adhere strictly to a drug and diet regimen.

She visited her physician at regular intervals and seemed to be doing quite well. After having missed two scheduled visits, she returned feeling weak and anorexic. Further, she complained of fainting spells, leg cramps, and not feeling "clear" in her mind at times, although she insisted that she was religiously observing her prescribed treatment plan. Her examination was the same as on previous visits, except that the 150/90 BP dropped to 80/60 when she stood up.

Immediate studies showed: blood urea nitrogen, 42 mg/dL; serum sodium, 118 mEq/L; and serum potassium, 2.6 mEq/L. The ECG was the same, except for widening of the QT interval, prominent U waves, and multiple ventricular premature depolarizations (Fig. 14.9).

Logic Indeed the patient had adhered quite well to her physician's treatment plan—even too well! Salt had been completely eliminated from her

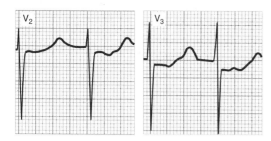

▶ **Figure 14.9.** Hypokalemia as revealed by electrocardiogram. Wide QT interval and prominent U wave.

diet, and she was taking a potent diuretic (furosemide). As a result, she had become volume, sodium, and potassium depleted. Volume depletion caused the hypotension and prerenal azotemia; sodium and potassium depletion caused the cramps, mental changes, weakness, and ECG changes. Premature beats resulted because hypokalemia made the heart more susceptible to the toxic effects of digitalis.

Data She was given a milder diuretic, supplemental potassium salts, and a diet less restricted in sodium; she returned in several days feeling much better. This was documented by improved blood chemistry determinations, loss of symptoms, and absence of orthostatic BP changes. Pulmonary function tests at that time showed evidence of mild-to-moderate obstructive disease.

Two years later, the patient returned with severe dyspnea and peripheral edema. She was being treated by her husband's physician. He was not so "strict" with treatment, and her family had convinced her to change physicians. At this time she was in severe biventricular failure, was dyspneic, orthopneic, and had generalized anasarca. The BP was 220/120 and, in addition to the signs of LVF that she originally had, she also exhibited neck veins distended 8 cm vertically above the sternal angle when sitting, a large tender liver, and 4+ edema up to the midabdomen.

Logic When severe persistent LVF occurs, secondary aldosteronism resulting from decreased renal blood flow causes sodium and water retention, but peripheral edema does not ordinarily occur until right ventricular failure eventually supervenes. Then the increased capillovenous pressure works in tandem with sodium and water retention to cause edema. This patient is now

in florid congestive heart failure (CHF) because of inadequate treatment, the natural course of her disease, or complicating factors such as anemia, pulmonary emboli, and so forth.

Data The ECG was unchanged from the original one; chest radiograph disclosed marked cardiomegaly, severe pulmonary congestion, and bilateral pleural effusions (right greater than left) (Fig. 14.10). Chemical studies showed blood urea nitrogen 45 mg/dL, sodium 122 mEq/L, potassium 3.5 mEq/L, chloride 84 mEq/L, and bicarbonate 30 mEq/L.

Logic Hyponatremia is again present, but this time for another reason. With severe edema and advanced CHF, the low sodium represents dilutional hyponatremia and not depletion of body sodium. Although the total body sodium is excessive, disproportionately more water is present, because the kidneys somehow lose their ability to excrete water; so the sodium concentration is far below normal. This, too, needs treatment.

Data She is placed at rest, severe fluid restriction is imposed, and the other components of therapy remain unchanged. Marked generalized improvement occurs as diuresis ensues, edema diminishes, and the weight comes down by 2 lb daily. After 2 weeks the patient is much better according to both symptoms and signs.

Suddenly she becomes dyspneic and cyanotic. Her legs are still slightly swollen although not tender. Chest radiograph shows cardiomegaly,

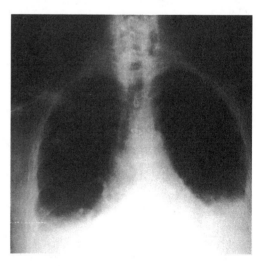

▶ **Figure 14.10.** Congestive heart failure. Enlarged heart and bilateral pleural effusions.

absence of the previously noted effusions, and no infiltrates. A pulmonary ventilation–perfusion scan discloses a large area with absent perfusion and normal ventilation in each lung. Intravenous heparin is begun, but the patient suddenly dies the next day.

Logic Even though her CHF was improving, she developed clinical findings compatible with multiple pulmonary emboli and no doubt died from the last one. Emboli notoriously occur in patients who are incapacitated with severe CHF. The clinical picture and ventilation–perfusion scan are incontestable.

Questions

1. As mentioned in the case study, there are many reasons why patients with CHF get worse. Which of the following are possible causes?
   (a) Excessive physical or emotional strain
   (b) Superimposition of another disease causing anoxemia
   (c) Excessive sodium in the diet
   (d) Inappropriate medication
2. The diagnosis of pulmonary emboli was not difficult to make in this case discussion. But it is often overlooked because its manifestations may be different. All of the following statements regarding pulmonary emboli are true except which one?
   (a) Pleuritic pain, cough, and hemoptysis may be the presenting symptoms.
   (b) Think of emboli in a bedridden patient who has unexplained low-grade fever and tachycardia.
   (c) Consider emboli if the patient is persistently dyspneic, yet is otherwise improved from his/her CHF.
   (d) A perfusion lung scan is highly specific for emboli.
3. You suspect a pulmonary embolus, but you are not sure. The perfusion lung scan is suggestive. You are considering the use of anticoagulants because the patient is seriously ill and might not tolerate a second embolus. But the patient also has a relative contraindication to the use of heparin. In order to make sure of the diagnosis, your most specific and sensitive test would be:
   (a) Ventilation-perfusion scan
   (b) Serial enzyme studies (lactate dehydrogenase, serum glutamic-oxaloacetic transaminase)
   (c) Pulmonary arteriography
   (d) Physical examination

4. A 64-year-old man who has both severe chronic obstructive lung disease and severe biventricular failure is initially seen with a wide array of symptoms and signs. Which of the following clues is/are specific for one condition or the other?
   (a) Markedly distended cervical veins
   (b) Orthopnea and paroxysmal nocturnal dyspnea
   (c) Leg edema and liver 5 cm below the costal margin
   (d) S_3 at the apex and pulsus alternans

Answers

1. **All are correct.** In choice (a), the heart is forced to work harder. The patient who develops worsening obstructive lung disease or anemia for any reason (ulcer, cancer) will decrease the heart's work-capacity by virtue of progressive anoxemia. Excessive sodium intake may occur if the patient does not care or does not understand. He or she may not know which foods and household remedies contain large quantities of sodium (bacon, canned soups, baking soda, and so forth). As for medication, errors abound regarding too much or too little digitalis, diuretics, and potassium supplementation. Other causes for apparent worsening include unidentified multiple pulmonary emboli, masked hyperthyroidism, unnoticed myocardial infarction, and an arrhythmia.
2. **(d) is untrue.** A perfusion scan is not specific because pneumonia, infiltrates, or effusions may also show decreased perfusion; it is, however, sensitive because emboli with infarcts usually show perfusion defects. In doubtful cases, a ventilation-perfusion scan will differentiate between infarct and other causes for infiltrates where both perfusion and ventilation may be impaired. Choices (a), (b), and (c) are all different presentations for pulmonary emboli. This many-faced disease can also have a presentation as pulmonary hypertension with right ventricular failure, sudden severe coronary-like chest pain, or pleural effusion. The source of the emboli (the leg veins) may become apparent before, during, or after the embolus—but more frequently never at all.
3. **(c) is correct.** The delineation of an arterial obstruction is both highly specific and sensitive, although invasive. In this case, it may well be the procedure of choice. Choice (a) is much more informative than a simple perfusion scan although probably not so informative as arteriography. Admittedly, some clinicians might prefer choice (a) in this situation. Enzyme studies are not specific and take several days. Examination is not apt to be of much definitive help even should a friction rub develop.

4. **(d) is correct.** A third heart sound and pulsus alternans are specific for CHF. They result from a high left ventricular end-diastolic pressure, decreased ventricular compliance, and alternating end-diastolic fiber length. On the other hand, choices (a), (b), and (c) can be seen in either condition. The patient with severe chronic obstructive pulmonary disease must often sit up to move his chest more easily, or secretions may clog his airways at night, causing him to get up. His liver is pushed down by a low diaphragm, and his legs are often swollen because his dyspnea makes him sit most of the time.

COMMENT The presence of heart disease and lung disease in the same patient needed careful sorting in order to decide which disease was causing the acute problem and which clues belonged to each of the two diseases. Considerable overlap existed because the symptoms and signs for both are similar. With the sudden onset of dyspnea as the key clue, the author rapidly built an unmistakable pattern for hypertensive cardiovascular disease with LVF. Note that urgent treatment was given even before a diagnosis was made.

"Cause and effect" was extensively utilized as the two causes for hyponatremia were encountered and as the causes for worsening CHF were detailed. Also, the reader had the opportunity to follow a patient with CHF from its inception to its termination, observing the cause-and-effect relationships through a series of intermediate complications.

In detailing the many presentations of pulmonary embolism, the author had to consider the specificity and sensitivity of various diagnostic clues. *(P.C.)*

Suggested Readings

Leier CV, Dei Cas L, Metra M. Clinical relevance and management of the major electrolyte abnormalities in congestive heart failure: Hyponatremia, hypokalemia, and hypomagnesemia. Am Heart J 1994;128(3): 564–574.

Levy D, Larson MG, Vasan RS, et al. The progression from hypertension to congestive heart failure. JAMA 1996;275(20):1557–1562.

Seamens CM, Wrenn K. Breathlessness. Strategies aimed at identifying and treating the cause of dyspnea. Postgrad Med 1995;98(4):215–216, 219–222, 225–227.

CASE 28

COMA AND T-WAVE INVERSION

Chul Joon Choi and Hiroshi Yamasaki

Data After a neighbor found her poorly responsive and on the floor, this 73-year-old woman was brought to the emergency department. No further history was obtainable at the time.

Logic Such presentations are frequently seen. Causes are varied and range from drug reactions to attempted suicide, alcohol, heart attacks, strokes, infections, renal failure, metastatic malignancies, and others. The field of diagnostic possibilities is wide open. Much initial reliance must be placed on the physical examination because little history is available.

Data The patient was confused, restless, and semi-stuporous. Blood pressure was 180/110, pulse 66 and regular, temperature 36.8°C, and respirations 20/min. Pupils were of moderate size and with prompt light reflexes. Fundi showed grade 2 hypertensive retinopathy without hemorrhages or papilledema.

The jugular venous pressure, carotid pulses, and lungs were normal. There were no bruits in the neck. The apex beat was forceful and was felt in the sixth intercostal space between the midclavicular and anterior axillary lines. Other than a grade 2 systolic ejection murmur at the base of the heart, there were no murmurs, thrills, or gallops, S_1 was normal and the first component of S_2 was loud. Abdominal examination was normal, there was no edema of the lower extremities, and distal pulses were full and symmetric.

Neurologic examination could not be accurately assessed because of the patient's condition, but as far as could be determined, cranial nerves were normal, all four limbs had normal tone and were mobile, and deep tendon reflexes were normal and equal. There was some equivocal stiffness of the neck, but she did not wince; the test for Babinski's sign elicited downward flexion of the toes on the left foot, but the big toe did not move upward. Muscle strength could not be assessed.

Logic As evidenced by the blood pressure, fundi, enlarged heart, and murmur, hypertensive cardiovascular disease was present. The neurologic examination was difficult to interpret with certainty. The paucity of background clinical information made this case challenging to the treating physician. On such occasions, proper interpretation of the initial ECG often plays a crucial role in subsequent decision making.

Data The ECG (Fig. 14.11) showed normal sinus rhythm with diffuse T-wave changes and prolongation of the QT interval.

Logic The differential diagnosis of T-wave inversion on an ECG is broad. It normally occurs in leads aVR and V_1, occasionally in lead aVL (when the heart is positioned vertically), and in leads III and aVF (especially with a horizontal orientation). *Normal* T-wave variants may be seen as a persistent juvenile pattern, in response to anxiety or fear, or with hyperventilation.

Additionally, numerous physiologic and pathologic conditions have been associated with T-wave inversions on the ECG.

Coronary artery disease (CAD) causing ischemia or infarction is a common cause of T-wave inversion. Any alteration in the coronary supply/demand relationship, however, as seen with coronary artery spasm, tachycardia, shock, exercise, hyperthyroidism, aortic valve disease, anemia, or with hypertension may also produce inverted T waves in the absence of significant CAD. Myocardial ischemia and infarction generally affect localized areas of the heart; therefore, the resulting T-wave changes are usually seen in *well-defined areas* on the ECG.

When the extent of ischemia is wide and/or multiple vessels are involved, however, *diffuse* T-wave changes may result. This is also the rule with myocarditis, pericarditis, and systemic and/or extracardiac conditions. Pulmonary embolism can cause localized T-wave inversion especially in leads II, III, aVF, and V_1 to V_3. Finally, "secondary" T-wave changes (non-ischemic) occur with left ventricular hypertrophy in leads I, aVL, and V_4 to V_6, but they are typically asymmetric.

It appears that more information is needed in order to narrow the field of diagnostic contenders and establish a reasonable differential diagnosis. A knowledge of the previous medical history and current medications often yields helpful clues.

Signs and symptoms of myocardial ischemia or infarction in the elderly are often atypical, and CAD should still be high on the list, especially in view of the enlarged heart and the blood pressure

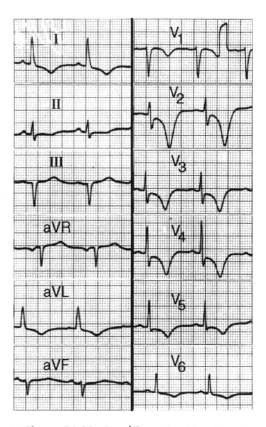

▶ **Figure 14.11.** Broad T-wave inversions in most leads.

elevation. The possible neck stiffness and equivocal Babinski offer added concerns.

Data A daughter living nearby was contacted, and it was found that the patient had a history of hypertension, arthritis, and non–insulin-dependent diabetes. There was no history of previous myocardial infarction (MI), angina, syncope, or neurologic disorders. Current medications included verapamil, a diuretic, and glyburide.

Blood pressure was controlled with intravenous nitroglycerine and a repeat ECG showed no significant changes. Chest radiograph, arterial blood gases, toxicology screening test, complete blood count, platelet count and prothrombin time, electrolytes, cholesterol and triglycerides, renal and liver function tests, and the first CK were normal.

Transthoracic echocardiogram revealed mild left ventricular hypertrophy (LVH) without wall motion or valvular abnormalities, intracardiac or pericardial masses, shunts, or pericardial effusions.

Logic Normal ventricular wall motion during persistent ECG abnormalities suggests that ongoing myocardial ischemia or infarction is unlikely. The essentially normal echocardiogram also excludes other potential diagnoses such as structural abnormalities of the heart. No evidence of electrolyte, acid-base disorders, or other systemic disease was found and there were no medications that would cause T-wave inversion.

The LVH noted on echocardiography is probably secondary to long-standing hypertension and is unlikely to cause diffuse, symmetrical T-wave inversions. For these reasons, a central nervous system (CNS) disorder should be strongly considered as possibly causing this clinical picture.

Intracranial disease may cause significant ECG changes of the T wave, U wave, ST segment, and QT interval. Its common presentation is that of inverted T waves associated with marked T-wave widening, minor degrees of ST-segment depression, and prolongation of the QT interval. These changes often closely resemble those seen with myocardial ischemia. Familiarity with this clinical picture is therefore valuable in managing patients with combined CAD and central nervous system disorders.

Data CT scan of the head showed a moderate-sized subarachnoid hemorrhage (Fig. 14.12). An ECG obtained days later showed normalized T-wave morphology. The MB fraction of the CK enzymes remained within normal limits. Later, a previous ECG was obtained from her primary care physician's office that showed no diffuse T-wave inversions as seen at initial presentation.

Logic T-wave changes are a common post-stroke ECG finding and appear most often in the setting of intracranial hemorrhage and hypertension. It has been shown that in 100 patients with subarachnoid hemorrhage, 80% had abnormal ECGs, in whom T-wave inversion (34%), bradycardia (32%), abnormal U waves (28%), and prolonged QT interval (21%) were seen with decreasing frequency.

Large, inverted, or upright peaked T waves usually appear immediately after a stroke, although they may be delayed for up to a week. Sometimes, within hours after admission, the T-wave changes disappear or shift from an inverted to an upright morphology or vice versa. Although they may persist for months, the T-waves usually tend to return to normal rather

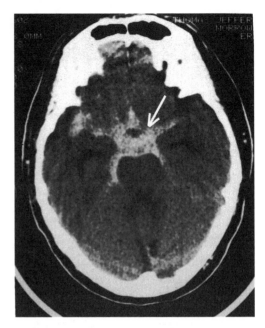

▶ **Figure 14.12.** Computed tomographic scan shows blood filling the basal cistern and extending into both sylvian fissures.

quickly as the condition of the patient improves. There is an interesting debate over whether these ECG abnormalities represent true myocardial damage or if they are merely a reflection of the CNS disturbance. The general consensus, however, is that they are caused by altered autonomic tone and are not due to ischemia.

It is important to note that stroke and other CNS disorders cause various changes on the electrocardiogram that closely mimic patterns observed with myocardial ischemia. This can lead to serious errors of over- and under-diagnosis of underlying heart disease in a stroke patient. Erroneously interpreting the ECG as showing an acute coronary event often leads to anticoagulation and/or thrombolytic therapy that may worsen the patient's stroke syndrome.

Data The patient's usual medications were continued, and she was given only supportive treatment for the vascular accident. She recovered rapidly, and her sensorium cleared by the 4th day. Neck stiffness disappeared, and Babinski's sign never materialized. She required ibuprofen for mild headaches and told of the "the worst headache of my life" suddenly striking her as she became ill and lost consciousness.

Logic Twenty percent of all strokes are hemorrhages, of which one half are subarachnoid and one half are intracerebral. Of those that are subarachnoid, the large majority result from a ruptured berry aneurysm in an artery at the base of the brain. Others are caused by arteriovenous malformations that are usually over the hemispheres, and some are the result of a vasculopathy or a coagulopathy.

Loss of consciousness occurs in more than 50% of patients when the intracranial pressure approaches perfusion pressure and cerebral blood flow diminishes. The headache described by the patient is characteristic. Photophobia and vomiting are common but did not occur in this case. Usually there are no focal neurologic changes, unless subsequent vasospasm occurs.

Non–contrast CT is the diagnostic modality of choice. It detects blood within the basal cisterns, in the sylvian fissure, or over the hemisphere in almost all cases. After several days have passed, it is not so reliable because blood breakdown products become isodense. MRI has a lower index of accuracy.

If the results of CT are negative, yet the clinical picture suggests subarachnoid hemorrhage, lumbar puncture must be done. It will show blood in the spinal fluid in all cases.

If the results of CT are positive for hemorrhage, the same study will often locate the offending aneurysm, and at this stage consideration for surgical clipping is indicated. Ten percent of patients with ruptured aneurysms die with the first event; another 25% will rerupture within 3 months, of whom more than half will die. This is a serious disease.

Before surgery, four-vessel angiography must be done. This study will delineate the precise anatomy and will pinpoint the bleeding source 80 to 90% of the time, as well as identify the 30% of patients who have more than one aneurysm.

Data The pros and cons of surgical treatment were discussed with the daughter and subsequently with the patient. Included in the decision tree were the statistics and likelihoods of recurrence, of death from disease, of surgical failure, of death from surgery, and the generally impaired health of the patient.

All opted to control the diabetes and hypertension by medical means, to deny surgery, and to hope for the best.

Questions

1. Which of the following clinical situations might result in a subarachnoid hemorrhage with diffusely inverted T waves?
   (a) Sixty-five-year-old man taking warfarin sodium for atrial fibrillation
   (b) Forty-two-year-old woman with recent onset of double vision and headaches
   (c) Thirty-eight-year-old woman with anemia, heart murmurs, and petechiae
   (d) Twenty-two-year-old man, unconscious as a result of an automobile accident
   (e) Forty-seven-year-old woman with purpuric eruption and nosebleeds
2. Inverted T waves can be found in each of the following clinical situations except which one?
   (a) Healthy obese patient with horizontal heart
   (b) Patient with swollen leg and chest pain
   (c) Diabetic patient with severe chest pain
   (d) Patient in diabetic coma who receives intravenous potassium
   (e) Patient with congestive heart failure receiving a potent diuretic

Answers

1. **All choices are correct.** They represent (a) overtreatment with warfarin sodium; (b) aneurysm at base of brain impinging on either cranial nerve III or VI at its exit from the brain; (c) infective endocarditis with a mycotic aneurysm; (d) traumatic hemorrhage; and (e) thrombocytopenic purpura.
2. **(d) is correct.** It represents hyperkalemia, a dangerous situation; the T waves are tall and peaked. The patients in choices (a), (b), (c), and (e) may all have negative T waves due to altered axis of repolarization, pulmonary embolus, myocardial infarction, and hypokalemia, respectively.

COMMENT The distinction between a heart attack and a stroke should be easy and simple based on history alone. Not so in this case. History was initially not available and physical examination was inconclusive. The key clue was the ECG showing inverted broad T waves in all leads. Such diffuse abnormalities in the presence of normal myocardial motility suggested a search for a cause outside the myocardium and perhaps inside the cranium. Even without this line of reasoning, a CT scan would have been the decisive clue for it is almost invariably performed in today's emergency departments when an old, disoriented, and semi-stuporous patient arrives. *(P.C.)*

Suggested Readings

Broderick JP. Heart disease and stroke. Heart Dis Stroke 1993;2(4):355–359.

Lidgren A, Wohlfart B, Pahlm O, et al. Electrocardiographic changes in stroke patients without primary heart disease. Clin Physiol 1994;14(2):223–231.

Oppenheimer SM, Hachinski VC. The cardiac consequences of stroke. Neurol Clin 1992;10(1):167–176.

CASE 29

SHARP CHEST PAINS

Paul Cutler

Data After successfully concluding a malpractice suit, a 39-year-old attorney had an episode of sharp stabbing left chest pain lasting several minutes. He sat down on the steps of the courthouse until it subsided and then directly visited his physician. Within the past month he had noted six similar although milder episodes, each lasting 30 to 40 seconds. Several episodes occurred while he was sitting at his desk, and some while walking home from work.

Logic A problem of recurrent left-sided chest pain is always a challenge. The principal task is to separate coronary heart disease from a multitude of benign conditions. Careful inquiry must be made into all the characteristics of the pain: when it comes, what it feels like, where it is, where it radiates, what causes it, and what relieves it. Today, when so many individuals are heart conscious, they usually come to the physician with sundry types of chest pains; the majority do not have serious organic disease.

Chest pain can consist of one severe episode or multiple smaller ones. In the former instance, you think of myocardial infarction, pulmonary embolus, dissecting aneurysm, ruptured esophagus, acute pericarditis, acute pleuritis, pneumothorax, and even subdiaphragmatic events like acute pancreatitis, perforated ulcer, and acute cholecystitis. By the nature of the history so far, none of these is likely because each tends to be a single event. Pericarditis and pleuritis can last for

a while, but the pain is usually worse on breathing, coughing, or positioning, and the underlying cause and associated clues are evident.

Causes for recurrent chest pains include angina, musculoskeletal disturbances, intercostal neuralgia, postherpetic neuralgia, bone involvement by hematologic and other malignancies, hiatal hernia, peptic esophagitis, psychosomatic disorders, and breast conditions.

Musculoskeletal pain is probably the largest group and includes cervical discs, cervical and thoracic osteoarthritis, exercise of untrained muscles, fibromyositis, inflammation of the costochondral or chondrosternal articulations (Tietze's syndrome), cervical ribs, and thoracic deformities.

Remember the very important relationships of musculoskeletal pain to motion, esophageal pain to swallowing, pleuritic pain to breathing, and coronary pain to exertion.

Data Further history reveals that the episodes of pain are sharp, involve the left upper and lower parts of the chest, do not radiate, and are not related to strenuous physical activity, swallowing, eating, mealtimes, breathing, or changes in position. He continues to play two sets of singles tennis a few times weekly and gets no pain at those times. The pain is not accompanied by dyspnea, palpitations, or a cold sweat. He has no chronic indigestion, heartburn, or any other symptoms.

Logic Much has been learned. Coronary pain unrelated to exertion is unlikely, unless the disease is so bad that the patient gets it even at rest; but then he would get it on exertion too, and certainly could not play tennis. Lack of relationship to the other activities mentioned weighs against the variety of conditions that were just set forth.

It is incorrect to assume that only coronary pain radiates to the left arm. Although coronary disease is the most common cause, this type of radiation occurs occasionally with esophageal, pleuropericardial, diaphragmatic, and musculoskeletal diseases. The complexities of nerve supply and neurotomes determine the site of pain. Another important point to remember is that both coronary disease and musculoskeletal disease are very common and frequently coexist in the same individual. On careful questioning it may become apparent that the patient has two types of pain. And next, don't necessarily associate chest pain with an incidental hiatal hernia, a nonspecific

ECG abnormality, or some spurs seen on the cervical or thoracic spine radiograph.

Data The patient has never had previous chest pain and has had a yearly physical examination and ECG that were normal. He is the youngest of three brothers and there is no heart disease in his siblings or his parents, who are still living. Neither is there a family history of hypertension, diabetes mellitus, strokes, or blood lipid abnormalities. The patient is generally under tension and smokes one to two packs of cigarettes per day, but he stays lean and does not have a high intake of dairy products or meat.

Recently, he has been working under great stress on an important case. This has involved long hours of work, irregular meals, and a reduced amount of sleep. A reason for his immediate concern is that a senior law partner died of a heart attack not long ago after suffering from angina for several years.

Logic There are no risk factors for coronary disease except for the cigarette smoking. The negative family history is significant too. His high degree of tension influences you. Although some believe that environmental or emotional stress increases the risk of coronary disease, it is more likely that unusual stresses may cause a morbid preoccupation with mild discomforts that would otherwise be ignored. And the nature, location, and timing of his pain make it unlikely that he has coronary disease. But what does he have?

Data Complete physical examination is normal. The blood pressure is 120/80, the fundi are normal, the thyroid is not enlarged, the lungs are clear, and the heart is not enlarged and has no murmurs, ectopic lifts, S_3, or S_4. Movements of the neck and shoulders do not elicit pain. There are no areas of tenderness anywhere in the chest, including the rib cartilages and their articulations. The abdomen and the rest of the examination are normal.

Logic The normal blood pressure rules out an additional coronary risk factor; the absence of murmurs weighs against valvular stenoses, which can cause angina-like pain; and the absence of an S_4 weighs somewhat against coronary disease. Tietze's syndrome is unlikely because there is no chondral tenderness; although the pain of this disease is often misleading in that it can be sharp and darting or a dull precordial ache, the affected areas should be tender. Failure of neck motions to cause pain weighs against cervical radiculitis or disk.

Data Chest radiograph is normal; a cervical rib is not present. Radiographs of the cervical and thoracic spine are normal. The resting ECG is normal and unchanged from previous tracings. Blood count, urinalysis, erythrocyte sedimentation rate, and blood chemistries are all normal.

Logic Normal complete blood count and erythrocyte sedimentation rate are reassuring when a patient has undiagnosed pain and you are considering a possible malignancy. Radiographs rule out spondylogenic causes, and the normal ECG is comforting too. The normal serum glucose, cholesterol, and triglycerides eliminate other coronary risk factors.

Although you are reasonably assured that the patient has no serious disease, you still cannot explain the pain. However, it seems safe to conclude that the pains are related to his state of tension, to an undiagnosed but nonserious musculoskeletal condition, or to "gas under the diaphragm" associated with a splenic flexure syndrome or spastic colon.

Data You inform the patient of the findings and your conclusions, reassure him that he has no serious problem, and advise him to reduce his working hours, slow his pace of living, reduce or preferably discontinue cigarette smoking, and return in 6 weeks.

Logic In view of the almost complete absence of risk factors, the unimpressive nature of the pain, the negative family history, and the normal examination, you are comfortable in reaching this conclusion. Further tests are not indicated.

Data The patient unexpectedly returns 2 weeks later. He has followed your advice but has had three more episodes of pain. They are similar to but not exactly the same as the other attacks. One episode came during an argument, and the other occurred while he was walking up steps; each lasted approximately 30 seconds.

Examination remains the same. A graded exercise treadmill test is done and a thallium scan is performed at the conclusion of exercise and several hours later. (Present evidence indicates that more than 90% of patients with serious coronary atherosclerosis have this condition detected by thallium exercise tests.) All results are normal, and there is no evidence of coronary disease or myocardial ischemia. You reassure the patient again and reschedule his visit.

He does not return at the scheduled time, and you therefore assume he is well. Two months later you read his obituary notice in the newspaper, and learn that he suddenly dropped dead in court during a heated argument.

Logic This is a shocking bit of news. On reviewing his records, you feel completely justified in your conclusions. Was there a relationship between the chest pains and his demise? There was not a single bit of evidence for coronary disease. All test results were negative, yet false negatives do occur. Should another patient with the same picture come to see you, you would do the same thing. Here is a situation where all the evidence pointed in one direction—yet the opposite turned out to be the case.

Questions

1. Had there been indication of the existence of coronary disease in this patient and had it been urgent to establish the diagnosis, the specific thing to do would have been:
   (a) trial of nitroglycerine for pain.
   (b) long-acting nitrate for prevention of pain.
   (c) coronary arteriography.
   (d) echocardiography.

2. A 49-year-old man complains of chest pains that frequently waken him from his sleep and occasionally occur during the day. It is a deep, burning type of pain and is relieved by antacids. At times, swallowed food seems to get stuck in his lower chest, and he has considerable heartburn. To prove what you suspect, do:
   (a) upper gastrointestinal radiograph.
   (b) Bernstein test.
   (c) esophagoscopy.
   (d) gastric analysis.

3. As for the various types and causes of chest pain, which one of the following statements is incorrect?
   (a) Pericardial pain is usually caused by inflammation of surrounding structures. The pain of pericarditis may be worse with breathing, motion, cough, or swallowing; it may be crushing in type, or synchronous with each heartbeat; or combinations of these types may exist.
   (b) Chest pains related to emotional disorders can occur anywhere, can last any length of time, are associated with fatigue, and bear no relationship to activity or exercise.
   (c) Persistent although intermittent long-standing pain girdling the left chest can be the result of a previous known or unnoticed herpes zoster infection.
   (d) The chest pain of pulmonary embolus is of two types. Immediately there may be severe substernal coronary-like pain. Twelve to twenty-four hours later, as an infarct forms, pleuritic pain on breathing may occur.
   (e) Chest pain following a severe emotional disturbance is psychosomatic in origin.

Answers

1. **(c) is correct.** Nothing is more specific than the invasive procedure of coronary arteriography. Nitroglycerine relieves many things, and prophylactic nitrates are either not helpful or inconclusive. An echocardiogram might show a poorly contractile area, so choice (d) might be done, too, but the positive yield for choice (c) should be greater.

2. **(a), (b), and (c) are correct.** The Bernstein test is specific for what you expect to be present: peptic esophagitis. Acid reflux is common in the reclining position. A drip of dilute hydrochloric acid into the lower esophagus will reproduce the pain. Radiographs may be helpful in delineating a stricture or an often accompanying hiatal hernia. A fiberoptic look may also be of help to rule out another obstructing lesion. The gastric analysis will add nothing of great value.

3. **(e) is correct.** It is the only wrong statement. Chest pain following an emotional disturbance may very well be coronary in origin, because the release of catecholamines may elevate the blood pressure and also make the heart work harder. Thus, the myocardial need for oxygen rises, and if sclerosis exists, the oxygen supply may not be increasable. The other statements are all correct and serve to characterize a variety of chest pains.

COMMENT Solving the problem of chest pain can be very simple for typical pictures but difficult for atypical ones. Generally the clinician can establish a reasonably precise disease probability—$P(D)$—on the basis of the history. The presence or absence of risk factors helps. The ECG is only approximately 50% sensitive.

Patient or doctor anxiety, or the need for

more precision, may warrant additional studies, such as a treadmill test, thallium scan, and, in some cases, coronary arteriography. Digital subtraction and magnetic resonance offer promise of lending greater assistance at less risk in the near future.

But always remember that all test results may be negative, yet the patient may have a variant or atypical form of angina—Prinzmetal's angina. In that case, coronary artery *spasm* occurs either at the site of a fixed atherosclerotic lesion or in a normal coronary artery. The cause for spasm remains obscure, and the angina usually occurs at rest. But the results of spasm—angina, infarction, or death—are well known. Such may have been the case in the patient just discussed. *(P.C.)*

Suggested Readings

Richter JE. Overview of diagnostic testing for chest pain of unknown origin. Am J Med 1992;92(5A): 418–458.

Shima MA. Evaluation of chest pain. Back to the basics of history taking and physical examination. Postgrad Med 1992;91(8):155–158.

Vantrappen G. Critique of the session on diagnostic testing. Am J Med 1992;92(5A):818–835.

 CASE 30

SWOLLEN LEGS

Michael H. Crawford

Data A 47-year-old Mexican woman was brought to the hospital by her family because of progressive weakness and swollen legs. The patient was visiting from Mexico, and the family knew very little about her medical history. Not realizing the further need for an interpreter, the family left. Therefore, the physical examination was done first because there were no bilingual persons immediately available.

The vital signs were: pulse 90 and regular, blood pressure 107/65, respirations 26 and labored, and temperature 37.1°C. Severe pitting edema was present up to the midabdomen. The jugular veins were distended to the angle of the jaw at 45 degrees, and there was a prominent "a" wave. Carotid pulses were weak. Chest expansion was decreased, and there was poor diaphragmatic movement. Diffuse rales and wheezes were

auscultated over the lung fields. There was a sustained lower left sternal border systolic impulse and a systolic pulsation in the second left intercostal space. The left ventricular apex could not be felt. The first heart sound was easily heard and the second component of the second heart sound was loud. Further clarification of the cardiac examination was impossible due to the excessive pulmonary noises.

Examination of the abdomen was difficult because of pitting edema of the lower abdominal wall; but liver dullness extended 15 cm from top to bottom in the right midclavicular line, and the right upper quadrant was tender. There was anterior abdominal and flank distention, but no definite fluid wave or shifting dullness was noted. Peripheral pulses were weak but equal. Otherwise, the physical examination was normal.

Logic Two pathophysiologic events are immediately apparent: severe pulmonary hypertension (sustained right ventricular lift, palpable pulmonary artery pulsation, and loud pulmonary component of S_2) and right ventricular failure (neck vein distention, hepatic engorgement, edema, and probable ascites).

Hypertension in any vascular bed is due to an imbalance between flow and resistance. Excessive blood flow through a normal-caliber vascular channel can cause a mild increase in pressure, but more marked hypertension can be caused only by an increase in resistance to flow. Therefore, this patient must have increased resistance to blood flow somewhere downstream from the main pulmonary artery.

Some of the possibilities, in anatomic order, include: (1) pulmonary artery branch stenosis; (2) pulmonary arterial constriction (e.g., hypoxia from any cause); (3) pulmonary arterial obstruction (e.g., multiple pulmonary emboli); (4) chronic pulmonary diseases that obstruct or destroy the arteriolar-capillary bed (e.g., chronic obstructive pulmonary disease or pulmonary fibrosis); (5) mitral valve stenosis; and (6) left ventricular failure from any cause. The last item is the most common cause of pulmonary hypertension and right ventricular failure in the adult.

Pulmonic valve stenosis is not a viable consideration because of the patient's age and the presence of physical evidence of pulmonary artery hypertension. Pulmonary artery branch stenosis is not likely, because no systolic murmur was heard, and it is rare. The low blood pressure, weak pulses, and tachycardia suggest that the patient may have low cardiac output. In such a situation the murmur of mitral stenosis may be markedly diminished to the point where excessive respiratory noises might obscure it. However, the lung findings suggest that the pulmonary hypertension may be due to primary pulmonary disease.

Data To further clarify the patient's problem, an ECG and chest radiograph were done. The ECG exhibited normal sinus rhythm with right ventricular hypertrophy and left atrial abnormality (Fig. 14.13). The chest radiograph was of poor quality due to an inadequate inspiration but showed generally hazy lung fields. Cardiac size or specific chamber enlargement could not be reliably evaluated.

Logic This information is very important in narrowing the possibilities. Absence of both hyperaeration and a flat diaphragm weighs against the presence of chronic obstructive lung disease, a common cause of pulmonary hypertension in adults. The presence of left atrial abnormality and the absence of left ventricular hypertrophy or myocardial infarction on the ECG places the obstruction at the mitral valve and not downstream from the left ventricle. Therefore, mitral valve stenosis is the most likely diagnosis.

Data After treatment with oxygen and diuretics, the patient's respiratory rate decreased, and pulmonary wheezes and rales were no longer audible. Cardiac auscultation at this time revealed a normal first heart sound and a physiologically split second heart sound with a loud pulmonary component (P_2). No opening snap was audible, but at the apex there was a grade 2/4 rumbling decrescendo diastolic murmur that started just after P_2 and was loud enough to be heard at the apex. This murmur was best heard in the left lateral decubitus position with the bell of the stethoscope.

At the base of the heart there was a high-pitched decrescendo diastolic murmur that started with the second heart sound and was audible only during the first one-third of diastole. This murmur was best heard along the left sternal border but could also be faintly heard at the right second interspace (aortic area).

After the congestion cleared, a repeat chest radiograph showed no evidence of chronic pul-

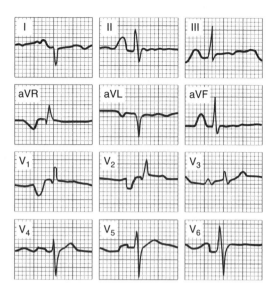

▶ **Figure 14.13.** Electrocardiogram demonstrates advanced mitral stenosis: left atrial hypertrophy (prominent negative P wave in leads V_1 and V_2); right ventricular hypertrophy (right axis deviation, prominent R wave in leads V_1 and V_2, deep S wave in leads V_5, V_6); right atrial hypertrophy (tall P waves in leads II, III, and aVF).

monary disease; the heart appeared to be moderately enlarged, and straightening of the left cardiac border and prominence of the pulmonary vasculature were noted (Fig. 14.14).

More history was obtained through an interpreter. The patient denied any knowledge of acute rheumatic fever or previous heart disease. She had two children in her early 20s without complications. She has not seen a doctor since then and felt well until the last year, when she began noting progressive fatigue, dyspnea on exertion, and, more recently, swelling of her lower extremities and abdomen.

Logic The low-pitched diastolic murmur at the apex is characteristic of mitral valve obstruction and confirms the suspected diagnosis. However, the clinical evaluation does not clarify the etiology of this obstruction. Only 50% of patients with rheumatic heart disease give a history of a prior illness compatible with acute rheumatic fever. Although the murmur of mitral regurgitation may appear during the acute attack, mitral stenosis does not develop until many years later. Ordinarily there is a latent period of approximately 10 years before the auscultatory findings

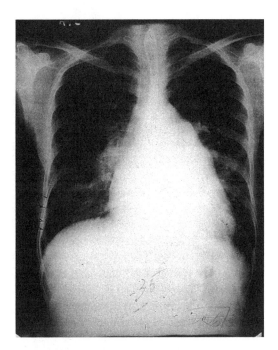

▶ **Figure 14.14.** Severe mitral stenosis. Note convexity of left cardiac border resulting from prominent pulmonary vasculature and an enlarged left atrium. Cardiac enlargement results from right ventricular hypertrophy.

of mitral stenosis can be appreciated. At this time the patient is usually asymptomatic but may become symptomatic during periods of cardiovascular stress, such as pregnancy. The asymptomatic period lasts another 10 years, and then the symptoms begin in the third decade of the disease. Symptoms progress until death ensues during the fourth decade as a result of pulmonary congestion and low cardiac output.

The patient does not fit this classic description of rheumatic mitral stenosis. There is no history of prior acute rheumatic fever, and her symptoms are only recent. Also, the lack of an opening snap on physical examination raises the possibility that she has some other form of mitral valve obstruction. Another cause of such obstruction is left atrial myxoma. This pedunculated tumor attaches to the interatrial septum and obstructs the mitral valve during diastole and then moves back into the left atrium during systole. Approximately 25% of patients with left atrial myxoma suffer from a systemic illness with fever and arthralgias. The short duration of our

patient's symptoms and the severity of the pulmonary hypertension would favor this diagnosis.

The high-pitched basal diastolic murmur is characteristic of regurgitation through a semilunar valve. In this particular case, the murmur could represent Graham Steell's murmur of pulmonary regurgitation associated with pulmonary hypertension; this murmur is commonly heard in severe mitral stenosis. However, Graham Steell's murmur is usually confined to the left sternal border and is rarely heard in the aortic area. Our patient's murmur was heard in the aortic area, which suggests that it is of aortic valvular origin. Rheumatic valvular disease often strikes more than one valve, the mitral and aortic valves being the most common. Thus, the presence of an aortic diastolic murmur would favor a rheumatic etiology for the mitral valve disease.

Data The patient responded well to therapy in the hospital and excreted 1 kg overnight. However, the next morning she complained of numbness of the left leg. It was cold and blue from the midthigh to the toes. The left femoral pulse was no longer palpable, and the patient's pulse was irregularly irregular at a rate of 130. Atrial fibrillation without other changes was documented by ECG.

Logic An embolic occlusion of the femoral artery has occurred. The most likely source for this embolic material would be the heart, presumably the left atrium, because the occlusion was accompanied or preceded by the development of atrial fibrillation. It is common for patients who have mitral stenosis, especially those in atrial fibrillation, to develop thrombi in the left atrium or its appendage; these thrombi can dislodge as emboli into the peripheral circulation. Such emboli are usually small and resolve without any difficulties, but occasionally they occlude large vessels and cause severe organ damage.

The diagnosis of rheumatic mitral stenosis has yet to be firmly established. Large vessel peripheral emboli are frequent in left atrial myxoma too. Emboli often occur from the valvular vegetations of bacterial endocarditis, and, finally, acute myocardial infarction can lead to mural thrombi that may also cause embolization. There is no clinical evidence to support the latter two possibilities in our patient and the choice remains between rheumatic heart disease and left atrial myxoma.

Data Femoral embolectomy was rapidly performed under local anesthesia. Pathologic examination of the removed specimen was consistent with thrombic material without evidence of myxomatous tissue. An echocardiogram showed a thickened, poorly mobile mitral valve and an enlarged left atrium that supported the diagnosis of rheumatic mitral stenosis; there was no evidence for a myxoma. There also was mild thickening of the aortic leaflets without stenosis.

The right heart chambers were mildly enlarged and the estimated right atrial pressure based upon the size and lack of expansion of the inferior vena cava was 15 mm Hg. Doppler evaluation estimated the mitral valve area at 0.6 cm². The presence of silent moderate tricuspid regurgitation allowed the estimation of a pulmonary artery systolic pressure of 70 mm Hg. Mild aortic regurgitation was also present.

Cardiac catheterization revealed: pulmonary artery pressure 70/26 mm Hg, mean pulmonary capillary wedge pressure 35 mm Hg, and left ventricular end-diastolic pressure 10 mm Hg. The mean diastolic mitral valve gradient was 21 mm Hg and cardiac output was 2.0 L/min, resulting in a calculated mitral valve orifice of 0.5 cm². At surgery the mitral valve was found to be thickened, calcified, and immobile; this probably explains the lack of an opening snap and the lack of a loud first heart sound (Fig. 14.15). The coronary arteries were normal. Mitral valve replacement was accomplished without difficulty, and the patient has done well since then.

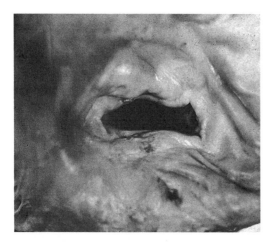

▶ **Figure 14.15.** Stenotic mitral valve viewed from the left atrium. Note marked narrowing and distortion of orifice and fibrosis as well as calcification of the leaflets.

Questions

1. A 26-year-old woman complains of fatigue. Physical signs of pulmonary hypertension and right ventricular hypertrophy are present. Chest radiograph exhibits enlargement of the right atrium, right ventricle, and central pulmonary arteries. Systemic arterial blood gas levels are normal. At right heart catheterization, the following pressures are found: mean right atrium, 12; right ventricle, 80/15; pulmonary artery, 80/30; and mean pulmonary capillary wedge, 7 mm Hg. Which of the following diagnoses is/are most likely?
   (a) Multiple pulmonary emboli
   (b) Primary pulmonary hypertension
   (c) Restrictive pulmonary parenchymal disease
   (d) "Silent" mitral stenosis

2. In the natural course of mitral stenosis, a variety of situations can occur. Which one of the following is least likely?
   (a) Dysphagia and hoarseness
   (b) Sudden episodes of collapse
   (c) Sustained left ventricular lift at the anterior axillary line
   (d) Acute pulmonary edema

3. Which of the following clinical situations can be associated with right ventricular hypertrophy and failure (RVF), with resultant leg edema?
   (a) A 350-lb man who has a normal chest radiograph
   (b) A 26-year-old woman who has a systolic basal murmur since birth, wide fixed splitting of S_2, and marked prominence of the pulmonary arteries as revealed by radiograph
   (c) A 48-year-old beauty parlor operator with 6 months of progressively more severe dyspnea on exertion and diffuse reticular markings of the lungs as revealed by chest radiograph
   (d) A 60-year-old heavy smoker with chronic cough, expectoration, and worsening dyspnea

Answers

1. **(b) is correct.** Multiple small pulmonary emboli and primary pulmonary hypertension are very difficult to separate clinically, but multiple emboli usually cause a decreased PO_2. Both conditions occur more frequently in young women; birth control pills increase the incidence of emboli. Both exhibit enlarged central pulmonary arteries with smaller peripheral vessel "cut-offs" seen on chest radiograph or pulmonary angiography. Most restrictive lung diseases result in pul-

monary fibrosis, which is detectable on chest radiograph and impairs oxygen transport, leading to decreased arterial oxygen saturation. The normal pulmonary capillary wedge pressure excludes mitral valve obstruction.

2. **(c) is correct and least likely to occur.** The obstruction at the mitral valve limits left ventricular filling, and thus this chamber is usually smaller than normal. Dysphagia and hoarseness can occur because of esophageal and recurrent laryngeal nerve compression by an enlarged left atrium. A large left atrial thrombus may act as a ball valve and intermittently obstruct the stenotic mitral valve, which leads to sudden cessation of cardiac output and collapse. The change in body position moves the clot away from the orifice, and circulation resumes. Excessive pulmonary venous pressure may cause fluid transudation into the pulmonary alveoli. This often occurs during pregnancy in otherwise asymptomatic women with mitral stenosis because of an obligate increase in vascular volume during this condition. It also occurs when left atrial pressure rises rapidly, as in tachycardias with decreased diastolic ventricular filling time.

3. **(a), (b), (c), and (d) are all correct.** Tremendous obesity can cause hypoxia and hypercarbia because of mechanical difficulty with breathing (pickwickian syndrome). Chronic hypoxia results in pulmonary hypertension and RVF. Choice (b) describes a patient with atrial septal defect whose right ventricle is under chronic strain from circulatory overload. The beauty parlor operator probably has pulmonary fibrosis (hair spray- related?), which causes obstruction of pulmonary capillaries and pulmonary hypertension. Choice (d) is the classic presentation of a patient with chronic obstructive pulmonary disease. Numerous other clinical situations can cause RVF too.

COMMENT The traditional order of data gathering was necessarily reversed and the physical examination was done first. RVF was evident and all the causes for RVF were listed. Almost all were eliminated by an absence of confirmatory clues. Only mitral stenosis and atrial myxoma remained. There are considerable overlap of signs, although some of the features (absence of opening snap, short duration of illness, severe pulmonary hypertension) favored the much less common disease—atrial myxoma. But two highly specific

and highly sensitive clues (the absence of myxomatous tissue in the embolus and the echocardiogram) proved the far more common diagnosis (mitral stenosis) to be the correct one.

Not having a history, the diagnostician was at a disadvantage. Ordinarily, this case would be solved simultaneously with treatment in 24 to 48 hours. Pulmonary hypertension and right ventricular failure in the absence of previous pulmonary symptoms quickly narrow the choices. At this point, an ECG, chest radiograph, and ultrasound study would deliver the diagnosis with the same speed as rapid diuresis and the detection of typical murmurs—perhaps sooner. A more aggressive problem solver might request immediate pulmonary arteriography, Swan-Ganz catheter placement with pressure studies, and a ventilation-perfusion isotope scan. But most physicians would consider the latter studies unnecessary, wasteful, or ill-timed. *(P.C.)*

Suggested Readings

Abbo KM, Carroll JD. Hemodynamics of mitral stenosis: A review. Cath Cardiovasc Diagn 1994;2(suppl): 15–25.

Feldman T. Rheumatic mitral stenosis. On the rise again. Postgrad Med 1993;93(6):93–94, 99–104.

MacNee W. Pathophysiology of cor pulmonale in chronic obstructive pulmonary disease. Part One. Am J Respir Crit Care Med 1994;150(3):833–852.

MacNee W. Pathophysiology of cor pulmonale in chronic obstructive pulmonary disease. Part Two. Am J Respir Crit Care Med 1994;150(4):1158–1168.

Rigolin VH, Robiolio PA, Wilson JS, et al. The forgotten chamber: The importance of the right ventricle. Cath Cardiovasc Diagn 1995;35(1):18–28.

CASE 31

PALPITATIONS

Paul Cutler

Data A 38-year-old obese salesman consults his physician because he has had recurrent brief episodes of "fluttering of the heart." These have been present for several years, used to occur infrequently, but more recently have been coming almost weekly and last from 1 to 10 minutes. You, the doctor, elicit more information.

Doctor: Tell me more about these episodes.

Patient: They seem to come for no particular reason and at no special time. My heart starts to pound, I get a sinking feeling in my chest and feel a little lightheaded, but I never faint. Nothing I do seems to help. Whether I walk, sit, lie down, drink something, or eat—they just go away when they want to.

Doctor: Do the attacks seem to start and stop suddenly? (You are thinking of paroxysmal atrial tachycardia, which begins and ends with a sudden "click.")

Patient: I'm not sure. I suddenly become aware of them, and when they stop I feel better, but my pulse stays fast for a while.

Doctor: If you feel your chest or take your pulse, can you tell whether the pounding is regular like a clock or irregular in timing? (The doctor taps first regularly and then irregularly on his desk.) And how fast are they?

Patient: I've never noticed the timing, and I couldn't count them.

Doctor: Do you get short of breath or do you have chest pain with these attacks?

Patient: No! It's as I told you—I get lightheaded and a little anxious, but I don't even faint. Once they're over, I feel just fine.

Doctor: Tell me about some of your habits. Do you drink Cokes and coffee? Are you taking any medications? And how are your nerves?

Patient: Well, I guess I'm an easy-going guy. Nothing seems to really bother me, and I don't have any financial or family troubles. I don't take any medication at all now. Once a doctor gave me something to lose weight but it didn't help, so I quit. By the way, you didn't ask, but I never drink any alcohol, and I haven't smoked in years. Only one cup of coffee a day and no Cokes!

Doctor: What about your general health? Do you or any members of your immediate family have any illnesses?

Patient: Aside from being a little fat (chuckle), I guess I'm in pretty good shape. A few years ago I had some indigestion and a doctor told me he thought I had a hiatal hernia, but I doubt it. It doesn't ever bother me, anyway. Maybe I've got gallstones like my mother. Dad has diabetes, but nobody else in the family does. Both my parents are still doing well, though, and they're pushing 80.

Doctor: Have you seen a doctor for this rhythm problem before?

Patient: Yes, I did, about a year ago. He told me I was OK as far as he could tell. He took an electrocardiogram and said it was probably my nerves. But I didn't really believe him. I've got nerves like steel.

Logic This 3-minute exchange has elicited much useful information. The physician knows he is dealing with a paroxysmal arrhythmia. It is not simple sporadic ventricular or atrial premature beats because it lasts too long. In order of commonness, the patient is most apt to have (1) paroxysmal atrial tachycardia (PAT), (2) paroxysmal atrial fibrillation (PAF), (3) paroxysmal ventricular tachycardia (PVT), or (4) paroxysmal atrial flutter (PAFl). Sinus tachycardia cannot be ruled out.

PAT is the most common; PAF is a close second; PVT is a distant third; and PAFl is only one tenth as frequent as PAF. If the patient is truly healthy you are most likely dealing with PAT, and if he has heart disease, you could be dealing with any. But even in heart disease, PAT and PAF are most common.

You know that he does not have heart disease serious enough to give him coronary insufficiency or left ventricular failure when the rapid rate comes on. The lightheadedness could result from mild cerebral ischemia due to decreased cardiac output. Furthermore, there are no precipitating events like fright, excitement, or trauma, and he takes no possibly causative agents like excessive caffeine, nicotine, alcohol, amphetamine, or digitalis. There is no evidence for anxiety factors, either. The likelihood of sinus tachycardia is diminished.

Because PAT often starts and stops with the suddenness of a click, this negative information was of no help. Moreover, the patient was unable to tell you whether the heart is regular, slightly irregular, or very irregular. Some patients can do so, and it helps distinguish PAT, PVT, and PAF.

Data Complete physical examination is essentially normal except for moderate obesity (height 68 in, weight 184 lb). In particular, the vital signs are normal; there are no heart murmurs, clicks, snaps, or gallops (except for a possible grade 1/6 short midsystolic ejection murmur over the pulmonic valve). The heart rhythm is normal and the rate is 80/min. There is no abdominal tenderness.

While performing the physical examination, the physician fills in the rest of the history as he examines each system. No additional positive or helpful information is obtained.

A blood-count, urinalysis, 6-test chemistry profile, chest radiograph, gallbladder ultrasound, upper gastrointestinal series, and ECG are obtained. They are all normal; in particular, the PR interval is not short, and the QRS complex is not prolonged.

Logic On the basis of all the evidence, the patient can be reassured with reasonable certainly that he has no heart disease. The very faint murmur appears to be benign, especially because there are no concomitant findings of heart disease. There is no evidence of mitral stenosis, hyperthyroidism, or click-murmur syndrome, each of which is notorious for causing paroxysmal arrhythmias.

Although the ECG is normal and gives no positive clues, at least it rules out the Wolff-Parkinson-White and Lown-Ganong-Levine syndromes. These two disorders of anomalous conduction are most often associated with PAT. Both are characterized by a short PR interval, and there is a wide QRS complex in the first and a normal QRS in the second.

The gastrointestinal and gallbladder radiographs were obtained to verify whether or not an ulcer or gallstones were present, although this might be considered unnecessary by some. But there are those who think diseases in these two systems may be reflexly associated with arrhythmias.

Data Your patient is informed that there is no evidence for any significant heart disease and that his arrhythmias are almost certainly benign paroxysms of atrial tachycardia. He is further told that it would be helpful to have documentation of this fact by an ECG recording taken during an attack, before proper therapy can begin. The matter of hospitalization is raised. You both decide it would be poor hospital utilization because his attacks come only once a week, and even if he were monitored for 24 hours by Holter monitor, or for 3 days in an intensive care unit, the chance of obtaining the needed information is not great. Furthermore, it is understood that hospitalization for such a purpose would not be authorized. He is therefore advised to lose weight and come to see you or visit the nearest emergency department at the next attack.

Logic After he leaves, you reexamine the possibilities. PAT comes and goes abruptly, is usually benign, has a ventricular rate of 150 to 250/min, and is often stopped by carotid sinus pressure or induced vomiting.

PAF has an irregularly irregular ventricular rate ranging from 90 to 150, is usually associated with heart disease, and is only uncommonly benign. Carotid sinus pressure may slow the ventricular rate somewhat but doesn't change the rhythm.

PVT and PAFl may be slightly irregular and are almost always associated with heart disease. Carotid sinus pressure and other vagal stimulants such as holding one's breath or the Valsalva maneuver don't stop PVT, may briefly stop ventricular contractions in PAFl, and may even cause PAT to revert to a normal rhythm.

You are anxious to know exactly what is going on, and you consider the use of a trans-tele-phonic cardiac events recorder. With this portable device the patient can obtain electrogram recordings while symptoms occur—a more agreeable and more cost-effective mechanism than the Holter monitor. You plan to obtain the equipment, but it will take 1 to 2 weeks to reach you.

Data Four days later, the patient returns. He has had two attacks during this time, but each one stopped before he could get to you or to a hospital. Although he thinks the heart rhythm was regular and the rate approximately 180/min, he is not sure. In the meantime, he has heard of a person with similar symptoms who "dropped dead," and he is now much more concerned about heart disease.

Logic Because you have not completely ruled out coronary heart disease with PVTs, and because the patient is now becoming very worried, you decide to do noninvasive procedures that should further strengthen your opinion—an exercise tolerance test to evaluate him for possible coronary disease and an echocardiogram to detect mitral valve prolapse (Barlow's syndrome). Both are associated with paroxysmal arrhythmias.

Data After 15 minutes of increasing exercise, the pulse rate having reached maximal levels for some time, the test is discontinued. There were no symptoms except for mild shortness of breath, no arrhythmias, and no ECG abnormalities to suggest coronary disease. An echocardiogram done with adjunctive amyl nitrite fails to detect evidence of mitral valve prolapse.

The significance of both tests and the small incidence of false negatives is explained to the patient. He feels reassured. So do you.

Three days later, you receive a telephone call from the emergency department of a hospital on the other side of town. (Your own pulse quickens.) The intern tells you, "Doctor, your patient is having an ECG-documented attack of paroxysmal atrial tachycardia. What would you like me to do?"

After a sigh of relief, you say—"Don't do anything. It will go away in a few minutes. If it doesn't, call me back. If it does, have him see me in the morning with a copy of his ECG. I'll put him on prophylactic medication. Thank you very much!" (Fig. 14.16)

Logic If the initial ECG taken on this patient had shown evidence of the Wolff-Parkinson-White syndrome, no further problem-solving would have been required. A short PR interval (<.12 sec), a prolonged QRS complex (> .12 sec), and the presence of a delta wave (slurred upstroke) in the initial portion of the QRS indicate the presence of an accessory conduction pathway between the right atrium and the ventricle, bypassing the AV node (Fig. 14.17). In this setting, an appropriately timed premature contraction can initiate a circus-like conduction of the electrical impulse down one pathway and up the other, thus creating a paroxysm of rapid arrhythmia. Atrial tachycardias are most common, although ventricular tachycardia and atrial fibrillation are also seen. Conduction through the normal pathway or through the accessory bundle can usually be either anterograde or retrograde.

PAT can arise by a similar mechanism in which two separate conduction pathways exist within the AV node, one conducting the impulse in a different direction from the other. The interval ECG is normal. This is probably the mechanism invoked in the case discussed here.

The prolonged QT syndrome is characterized by a prolonged QT interval, usually in excess of .5 sec, that results from delayed repolarization (see Fig. 14.17). This genetic defect would be detected on an initial ECG and expresses itself with congenital deafness, episodes of ventricular tachycardia, and sudden death.

COMMENT Several things are worth noting in the solving of this problem. The interview started with open-ended questions that got more closed as the

Normal

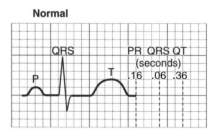

Wolff-Parkinson-White Syndrome

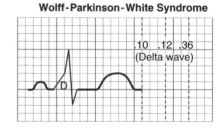

Prolonged QT Syndrome

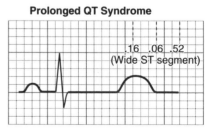

1 space = .04 seconds

▶ **Figure 14.17.** Electrocardiogram abnormalities associated with major arrhythmias. Normally, PR = 0.12 to 0.20 seconds, QRS = .06 to .08 seconds, and QT = up to 0.36 seconds. In Wolff-Parkinson-White syndrome, pre-excitation of the ventricle shortens the PR interval and lengthens the QRS complex. The ST segment is prolonged in the wide QT syndrome, which is also a cause of arrhythmias.

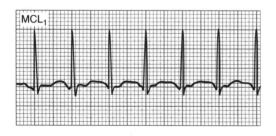

▶ **Figure 14.16.** Paroxysmal atrial tachycardia, 150 beats per minute.

dialogue proceeded. Furthermore, the history pursued only one subset; the rest of the history was obtained while doing the physical examination. The remainder of the data base was obtained in a somewhat branched manner, too, because pursuit of the arrhythmia was the principal issue.

Note that the physician first listed each possibility, then searched for clues of each. The weight of evidence grew for the presence of PAT and the absence of organic heart disease. Nonpertinent information, such as possible gallbladder disease, possible hiatal hernia, and slight heart murmur, had to be suppressed.

And last, Bayesian probabilities were considered. PAT is the most frequent tachyarrhythmia, and it is percentage-wise even more common in the set of persons who do not have demonstrable heart disease. So for the most part it is a benign arrhythmia. In this case, the decisive clue was the ECG taken during an attack. *(P.C.)*

Suggested Readings

Clair WK, Wilkinson WE, McCarthy EA, et al. Spontaneous occurrence of symptomatic paroxysmal atrial fibrillation and paroxysmal supraventricular tachycardia in untreated patients. Circulation 1993;87(4):1114–1122.

Haines DE, DiMarco JP. Current therapy for supraventricular tachycardia. Curr Probl Cardiol 1992;17(7): 411–477.

Kinlay S, et al. Cardiac event recorders; a controlled clinical trial. Ann Intern Med 1996;24:1, 16–20.

Manz M, Luderitz B. Supraventricular tachycardia and pre-excitation syndromes: Pharmacological therapy. Eur Heart J 1993;14(suppl)E:91–98.

SOMNOLENCE AND SWOLLEN LEGS

Richard P. Borge, Jr, and Edward K. Chung

Data A 55-year-old obese man complains that he can't sleep at night and that he is sleepy all day long. For the past few months his legs have been quite swollen.

Logic Three symptoms automatically register in the doctor's mind: insomnia, hypersomnolence, and swollen legs. Are they separate, unrelated conditions? Is there a common denominator? Is he sleepy all day because he doesn't get a good night's rest? Or does he have insomnia because he naps during the day? Why is his circadian rhythm seemingly reversed?

Data The patient goes on to describe lower extremity edema that has progressed over several years and has gotten gradually worse. He has had mild dyspnea on exertion, although there has been no chest pain, cough, paroxysmal nocturnal dyspnea, or orthopnea.

His most troublesome problem, however, is that he has slept poorly through the years, wakes up frequently, and doesn't seem to get enough rest. He wakes up with a morning headache, and then is sleepy, drowsy, and irritable the rest of the day.

The patient smokes a pack of cigarettes daily, drinks several mixed drinks during the day and one at bedtime, has no coffee or caffeinated beverages, and other than lorazepam at bedtime to help him sleep, takes no medications or over-the-counter drugs.

Logic *Insomnia* is said to exist when one has difficulty in falling asleep; or wakes early and can't return to sleep; or wakes frequently. Sometimes a patient wakes because he has to urinate; in other instances, he urinates because he happens to awaken. Causes for insomnia include worry, depression, or anxiety, sometimes brought on by situational stress, but in other cases by a true psychiatric disorder. Persistent insomnia is harmful in that it can impair daytime function, cause daytime sleepiness, result in mood disturbances, and increase the risk of auto accidents. Caffeine, alcohol, and nicotine may be contributory factors.

Narcolepsy is a severe form of daytime sleepiness associated with involuntary episodes of sleep and sudden episodes of weakness and loss of muscle tone (cataplexy). Although an identifiable stress may precede the onset of symptoms, this disorder may have a genetic basis, for all true narcoleptics have a positive test result for human lymphocyte antigen DR2. It does not appear that this patient has true narcolepsy as the cause of his daytime somnolence.

Swollen legs have a clearly definable pathophysiology that invokes an understanding of plasma oncotic and hydrostatic pressures within the capillary bed. These interactions, commonly referred to as Starling forces, facilitate the movement of large amounts of fluid while maintaining volume neutrality. When these forces are unbal-

TABLE 14.2. Causes of Edema

1. Decreased colloid osmotic pressure (low serum albumin)
   (a) cirrhosis of liver
   (b) nephrotic syndrome
   (c) malnutrition
2. Increased hydrostatic pressure (venous flow impeded or obstructed)
   (a) right ventricular failure
      1. left ventricular failure
      2. chronic obstructive pulmonary disease
      3. multiple pulmonary emboli
      4. primary pulmonary hypertension
      5. obstructive sleep apnea
   (b) venous occlusion—thrombophlebitis
3. Miscellaneous
   (a) hypothyroidism
   (b) pregnancy
   (c) certain drugs

Hydrodynamics of Edema Formation

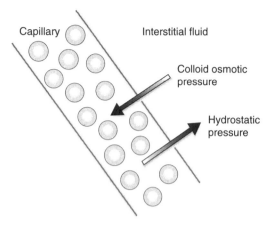

▶ **Figure 14.18.** Hydrodynamics of edema formation.

anced, volume remains in the interstitial space and edema results.

Edema can be caused by a wide range of conditions, each with different clinical implications (Table 14.2). Right ventricular failure with subsequent increase in venous pressure is the most common cause. It often results as a consequence of left ventricular failure, but may occur independently as a result of chronic obstructive pulmonary disease, multiple pulmonary emboli, primary pulmonary hypertension, obstructive sleep apnea, and other less common abnormalities of the cardiovascular system, all of which are associated with pulmonary arterial hypertension and right ventricular strain.

Diseases associated with a marked decrease in plasma proteins, such as cirrhosis of the liver, nephrotic syndrome, and severe malnutrition result in edema because the plasma oncotic pressure is lowered (Fig. 14.18).

In all of these situations, fluid accumulates in a general distribution but more so in dependent parts and where the interstitial fluid pressure is lower. On the other hand, thrombophlebitis and lymphatic obstruction cause localized edema due to decreased venous and lymphatic drainage from the affected area.

Miscellaneous causes of edema include hypothyroidism, pregnancy, and certain drugs (e.g., calcium channel blockers).

Data His wife tells you he snores loudly and excessively, that at times she must wake him and have him turn to another position in order to stop or decrease the snoring. Sometimes she goes to bed in the guest-room so she herself can get some sleep. She has noticed recent personality changes in him—irritability, forgetfulness, and not being quite "with it."

At times she watches him sleep and notes that he seems to stop breathing for periods of time, sometimes for up to ten seconds, awakens suddenly with deep, heavy breathing, and then falls asleep and begins to snore again.

Logic A good history, whether from patient and/or family members, often narrows the differential diagnosis and permits the physician to list the diagnostic contenders in order of likelihood.

Snoring is produced by vibrations of the soft tissue of the nasopharynx that result from turbulent air flow through a narrowed airway. During sleep, the soft palate and pharyngeal muscles relax, especially if the person lies supine, and the upper airway narrows. Thirty to fifty percent of those older than 50 snore, and snoring has become the theatrical symbol for sleep, the signature for some television commercials, the subject of social comment by humorists, and a cause of domestic unrest.

This man's symptoms are suggestive of obstructive sleep apnea (OSA), which can produce pulmonary hypertension, right ventricular failure, and peripheral edema. But because he has some risk factors for coronary artery disease and ischemic or alcoholic cardiomyopathy, as well as hepatic cirrhosis, other diseases must still be excluded. Finally, hypothyroidism bears consideration, as it can cause obesity, edema, and personality changes.

Data The patient is an obese, lethargic man in no distress. Blood pressure is 185/105 in both arms, pulse is 100 and regular, respirations 18 and normal in character. He weighs 190 lb and is 68 in tall. His neck is burly with full neck veins. The lungs are clear despite distant breath sounds.

The cardiovascular examination revealed a right ventricular lift at the lower left sternal border, a grade 2/6 holosystolic murmur at the lower right sternal border that increased with inspiration, and a loud pulmonic second sound. Although there was some tenderness in the right upper quadrant, the lower edge could not be clearly felt, and there were no signs of hepatic failure such as spider angiomata, palmar erythema, jaundice, or splenomegaly. Two-to-three-plus bilateral lower extremity pitting edema was present up to the level of the knees. Deep tendon reflexes were normal.

Logic Critical items in the examination were obesity, systemic hypertension, and evidences of pulmonary artery hypertension, right ventricular hypertrophy, tricuspid regurgitation, and right ventricular failure. Liver disease as a cause of edema is excluded. Normal reflexes make hypothyroidism less likely.

Data Laboratory tests were: hemoglobin 18 g/dL (elevated); serum albumin and electrolytes, renal and thyroid function tests normal; alkaline phosphatase and transaminases 20% above normal. Arterial blood gases on room air were: pH, 7.37; $PCO_2 = 51$; $PO_2 = 61$; $HCO_3 = 28$; O_2 saturation = 88%. Chest radiograph revealed clear lungs and an enlarged cardiac silhouette.

Logic The patient's laboratory values are notable for mild hypercapnia, hypoxia, and polycythemia. Liver function tests are consistent with hepatic congestion. At this point, pulmonary hypertension with subsequent right ventricular failure (cor pulmonale) secondary to OSA seems the most likely diagnosis. A chest radiograph showing clear lungs and an enlarged heart adds further evidence

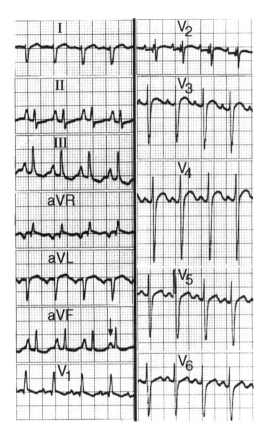

▶ **Figure 14.19.** Electrocardiogram showing right atrial and right ventricular strain. Arrow in lead aVF denotes atrial premature contraction.

to this diagnosis. Because other forms of heart disease are still possible, although unlikely, a 12-lead ECG is done to narrow the field (Fig.14.19).

Data The ECG reveals: (1) sinus tachycardia at 120 beats per minute; (2) atrial premature contractions (APC); (3) right atrial enlargement (P pulmonale—tall peaked P waves in leads II, III, and aVF); (4) right ventricular hypertrophy (RVH), as manifested by right axis deviation, tall R waves in lead V_1, and deep S waves in leads I, V_5, and V_6.

Logic The ECG evidence of RVH and right atrial enlargement adds credibility to the clinical impression of pulmonary hypertension and right ventricular failure.

Data A transthoracic echocardiogram is notable for moderate tricuspid regurgitation and pulmonary hypertension (70 mm Hg estimated). A formal sleep study (polysomnography) demonstrated 30 to 40 apneic episodes per hour, associated with arterial oxygen desaturation despite continued respiratory effort.

Logic   The pieces of the puzzle fit neatly together. *Obstructive sleep apnea* is defined as the intermittent cessation or marked decrease of airflow at the level of the nose and mouth during sleep due to oropharyngeal collapse. It occurs most commonly in overweight, middle-aged men who snore heavily. Systemic hypertension is often present.

The basic pathophysiologic defect consists of long-standing, inadequate pulmonary ventilation, resulting in hypoxia and hypercarbia. Frequent and repeated episodes of hypoxia cause pulmonary arteriolar vasoconstriction, pulmonary hypertension, and eventual right ventricular failure, as well as compensatory polycythemia. Morning headaches and personality changes result mainly from hypercarbia.

An appropriate diagnosis of OSA may be made if five or more episodes of apnea occur per hour of sleep, if the episodes last for ten seconds or more, and if oxygen saturation decreases by 4% or more during the apnea. These events arouse the patient, who breathes heavily for a few seconds, then falls back to sleep.

Narrowing or closure may take place at many sites in the upper airway, but especially during REM sleep when the muscles and tissues around the pharynx and palate are particularly relaxed. Craniofacial abnormalities and soft-tissue anomalies may play a role.

Questions

1. Match the ECG hypertrophy patterns to the diseases:
   (a) Mitral stenosis   (1) LA + LV
   (b) Mitral regurgitation   (2) RA + RV
   (c) Pulmonary hypertension   (3) LA + RV
   (d) Systemic hypertension   (4) RA
   (e) Tricuspid regurgitation   (5) RA + LA
   (f) Tricuspid stenosis   (6) RA + LV
2. Arrange the following events in pathophysiologic sequence.
   (a) Edema of legs
   (b) Increased right ventricular end-diastolic pressure
   (c) Systolic liver pulsation
   (d) Increased pulmonary artery pressure
   (e) Decreased PO_2
   (f) Tricuspid regurgitation

(g) Snoring, apneic episodes, daytime hypersomnolence
(h) Increased right atrial systolic pressure
3. Which of the following produce(s) localized (non-generalized) edema?
   (a) Hepatic cirrhosis
   (b) Superior vena cava obstruction
   (c) Femoral artery thrombosis
   (d) Nephrotic syndrome
   (e) Femoral vein occlusion

Answers

1. (a)-(3), (b)-(1), (c)-(2), (d)-(1), (e)-(2), (f)-(4)
2. (g), (e), (d), (b), (f), (h), (c), (a)
3. **(b) and (e) are correct.** The former causes edema of the head and both arms; the latter causes swelling of the affected limb. Cirrhosis and nephrosis cause generalized edema because of low serum albumin levels in each instance. Arterial occlusion does not cause edema.

COMMENT   Snoring, somnolence, and swollen legs were woven together into a classic case of obstructive sleep apnea (OSA)—not a rare disease, although often unrecognized. Each symptom was carefully explored for its possible causes and a common denominator was sought and found. The diagnosis of OSA was clearly established by linking a series of related pathophysiologic events. Alternative diagnoses were eliminated by pertinently negative clues on a one-by-one basis.

In the absence of left ventricular disease and chronic pulmonary disease, think of OSA as one of the causes of right ventricular failure and edema.

And in the case of the fat man who snores and has daytime somnolence, a detailed overnight study that analyzes the respiratory rate, heart rate, oxygen saturation, and sleep cycles remains the gold standard diagnostic test. *(P.C.)*

Suggested Readings

Bonsignore MR, Marrone O, Insalaco G, et al. The cardiovascular effects of obstructive sleep apneas: Analysis of pathogenic mechanisms. Eur Respir J 1994;7:786–805.

Colt HG, Haas H, Rich GB. Hypoxemia vs. sleep fragmentation as a cause of excessive daytime sleepiness in obstructive sleep apnea. Chest 1991;100: 1542–1548.

Rosen RC, Rosekind M, Rosevear C, et al. Physician education in sleep and sleep disorders: A national survey of U.S. medical schools. Sleep 1993;16:249–254.

Stroll PJ Jr, Rogers RM. Obstructive sleep apnea; pathophysiology, diagnosis and treatment. N Engl J Med 1996;334(2):99.

CHAPTER 15

Pulmonary Problems

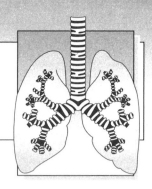

The symptoms of lung diseases are few: cough, expectoration, hemoptysis, wheeze, dyspnea, pleurisy, and fever. Scores of pulmonary diseases share one or more of these symptoms, so that overlap and nonspecificity exist. A patient with cough and expectoration may have any of many diseases.

Dyspnea on exertion (one symptom) can result from the decreased partial pressure of oxygen in inspired air, decreased oxygen-carrying capacity of the blood, or disease and malfunction of any intervening structure. This includes obstruction anywhere from the nasopharynx to the bronchioles; loss of functioning alveoli due to edema, disease, or destruction; diffusion defects between the alveoli and capillaries because of infiltrative diseases; and perfusion defects resulting from disease in the pulmonary arterial-capillary system. Therefore, high altitudes, obstruction, destruction, ventilation-diffusion-perfusion defects and mismatches, and severe anemias can all cause the same symptom. The disease processes that can create these conditions are myriad.

Physical findings are equally nonspecific. Rales, wheezes, consolidation, atelectasis, and effusion give you some conception of the underlying anatomic-physiologic derangement. But many diseases can share a single physical finding. A portion of solid lung can be caused by pneumonia, fibrosis, collapse, cancer, or tuberculosis. Pulmonary function tests tell only the physiologic derangement, not the cause of the disease. Blood gas measurements survey alveolar ventilation, and radionuclide scans assess ventilation and perfusion, but these studies offer no specific diagnoses either. An exception is the almost certain diagnosis of pulmonary embolus if a well-ventilated area is poorly perfused.

Diagnosis must often be made by more specific indicators, such as chest radiograph, special radiographic techniques, comparison with former radiographs, pulmonary function tests, computed tomographic scan, magnetic resonance imaging, fiberoptic bronchoscopy, cell or bacterial identification, and biopsy.

Although symptoms and physical signs may not offer many specific clues, the family history, occupational history, geographic history, and exposure history are often of great help. A diagnosis may hinge on a very small bit of evidence hidden in the patient profile.

A family history of asthma may suggest that the patient's chronic cough is the beginning of asthma. Tuberculosis in another member of the immediate family is always worrisome. A history of lung disease during childhood in other family members leads you to consider Kartagener's syndrome, congenital bronchiectasis, mucoviscidosis, or agammaglobulinemia.

The occupational history is extremely important because so many lung diseases are caused by the inhalation of microparticulate irritating substances. Such job hazards include exposure to silica, asbestos, beryllium, sugar cane, nitrogen dioxide, and numerous other chemicals and molds. It is not enough to inquire about the patient's occupation. You must know the patient's entire job history: how long he or she has worked at each job, exactly what he or she did, and whether the ventilation was adequate. The occupation this year may be harmless, but for the previous 10 years the patient's inhalation hazard may have been appreciable. The job may seem hazardous yet not be, and vice versa. Heavy exposure for a short time is as bad as moderate exposure for a long time.

Talc, hair spray, polluted air, and, above all, cigarette smoke are dangerous inhalants. The latter noxious agent is the worst offender insofar as lung disease is concerned. An exact smoking history must be obtained—not just what the patient is or is not smoking this month since the cough developed. Remember the hazard of inhaling somebody else's smoke.

The geographic history is important if you suspect a fungal disease. Coccidioidomycosis is endemic in central California and the Southwest; histoplasmosis is seen in the Ohio and Mississippi basins and the middle Atlantic states; and blastomycosis has considerable overlap with the latter. Histoplasmosis may be caused by exposure to the excreta of birds, bats, turkeys, and chickens—on roofs, in caves, and on poultry farms. Newly acquired domestic or tropical psittacine birds can cause a bacterial pneumonia; the villain may be spotted in a cage in the living room.

The great majority of patients who have lung disease come to the physician for one of the following reasons: (1) abnormal chest radiograph, (2) sudden dyspnea, (3) gradually worsening dyspnea, (4) pleuritic chest pain, (5) chronic cough and expectoration, (6) hemoptysis, (7) cough and fever, (8) wheeze and dyspnea, (9) cough, expectoration, and dyspnea, (10) weakness, weight loss, and anorexia, or (11) combinations of the foregoing.

Although large numbers of lung diseases are described in the textbooks, for practical purposes, when confronted with a patient, only common ones need be considered first. These include chronic bronchitis, acute respiratory tract infections (tracheobronchitis and pneumonia), asthma, chronic obstructive pulmonary disease, tuberculosis, and cancer.

Remember, too, that certain diseases like tuberculosis, cancer of the lung, and sarcoidosis may have a broad spectrum of presentations and can affect organs all over the body as well as manifest themselves differently in the lung. Hemiplegia may be the first omen of lung cancer. *Pneumocystis carinii* pneumonia may be the first clinical manifestation of the acquired immunodeficiency syndrome (AIDS). Pulmonary tuberculosis can be asymptomatic or overwhelming; it may cause partial bronchial obstruction, atelectasis, fibrosis, bronchiectasis, abscess or cavity, pneumonia, effusion, pneumothorax, or an infiltrate with low-grade fever and anorexia—each with a different clinical picture, different physical findings, or different radiographic finding. *(P.C.)*

CASE 33

RADIOGRAPHIC ABNORMALITY

Paul Cutler

Data   During a routine employment examination, a 52-year-old male roofer was found to have an abnormal chest radiograph, and he comes to you for advice. He had always been in good health, had the "usual childhood diseases," pneumonia at 24, and an appendectomy at 44.

You decide to solve this problem quickly by a decision path or dendrogram approach with a series of stepwise questions.

Data   What is the abnormality? The chest radiographs (posteroanterior [PA] and lateral views) are repeated, and you see a single round 2-cm nodule in the right upper lobe. It seems partially hidden behind the second rib, has smooth borders, and is surrounded by normal parenchyma. No calcium or cavitation can be seen within it. You are sure it is in the lung because it is there in both views and because you cannot feel any soft-tissue lumps on the chest wall that might mislead you (Fig. 15.1).

Logic   The description is that of a solitary pul-

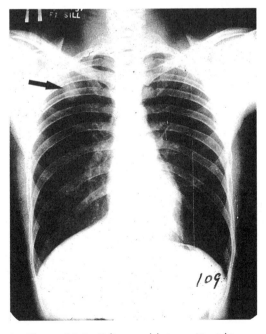

▶ **Figure 15.1.** Solitary nodule (arrow) in right upper lobe.

monary nodule (formerly called a "coin lesion"). These are most commonly caused by cancer (one third), granulomas (one third), and congenital hamartomas (less than one third); miscellaneous causes such as an arteriovenous fistula and bronchogenic cysts make up the rest. The respective incidences of these categories vary with the population subset under consideration. Sixty-year-old male smokers skew the percentages toward cancer; 30-year-old male nonsmokers with nodules have a very low incidence of cancer. Granulomas include mainly tuberculosis, histoplasmosis, coccidioidomycosis, and nocardiosis.

Careful inspection of the simple chest radiograph may solve the riddle. If the nodule is round, smooth, sharp, and has calcification patterns well known to the radiologist, it is a hamartoma or granuloma. But if the nodule is irregular and fuzzy-edged, has small irregular radiating projections, and has no calcification, it is likely to be malignant. The nodule size is a variable to be considered. The larger the lesion the more likely is cancer, but smallness does not justify complacency.

Further decision nodes and branching will establish which disease exists in this patient. However, your principal concern is not to establish a precise diagnosis, but to decide if this is cancer, and if it is resectable. Little else matters.

Data 2 Has a previous chest radiograph been taken, and what did it show? The patient says that the results of a radiograph taken 2 years ago were negative. He cannot recall the doctor's name, so the radiograph is unobtainable for personal review and comparison.

Logic This is important although insufficient information. It would be better to have an official report rather than hearsay evidence—better yet to have the radiograph itself, because you could compare sizes and spot small lesions that are easily overlooked.

When comparing two such radiographs, any one of four situations can exist: (1) the nodule was not present before, (2) the nodule is now smaller, (3) the nodule is the same size, or (4) the nodule is larger. If the nodule is now smaller or the same size, concern for malignancy is minimal. But if the nodule was not present before, concern is high. Difficulty arises when the lesion has enlarged and you must now concern yourself with *doubling time.* Cancers of the lung double their *volume* in 1 to 15 months (mean, 4 months);

such comparative measurements are made by cubing the diameters. Thus, a nodule that increases its width from 1.0 to 1.3 cm has more than doubled it volume. The assumption is made that growth is equal in all three dimensions.

If it is determined that the doubling time is less than 1 month (very rapid growth), the lesion is apt to be inflammatory. But if it takes more than 15 months to double its size (very slow growth), the lesion is likely to be a granuloma or hamartoma. On the other hand, if the doubling time is 4 to 6 months, cancer is likely. Rare exceptions occur, especially with some metastatic tumors.

Data 3 Are there any symptoms of cancer or tuberculosis? This includes questions about weakness, weight loss, anorexia, cough, expectoration, hemoptysis, night sweats, and fever. But tuberculomas, histoplasmomas, and hamartomas rarely become large enough to cause symptoms. Because cancer can be metastatic, a review of other systems (genitourinary, gastrointestinal, and so forth) for evidence of a primary lesion is in order too. All the answers are negative.

Logic Absence of symptoms rules out nothing. Any of the aforementioned diseases can and does exist without symptoms in the early stages. Primary cancer elsewhere might be asymptomatic too.

Data 4 How many cigarettes does the patient smoke? The answer is two packs a day for the past 30 years.

Logic This constitutes a heavy smoking history (60 pack-years) and weights our judgment toward cancer. It is unusual to see carcinoma of the lung in nonsmokers, and a high percentage of patients with lung cancer have a strongly positive smoking history. Obviously, not everyone who smokes heavily gets lung cancer.

Data 5 Where does the patient live, where has he lived, and where has he visited? The patient lives in South Dakota and has never been in any other part of the country, except when he once visited Des Moines.

Logic We are interested in establishing contact with *Histoplasma capsulatum* or *Coccidioides immitis,* which are endemic in the Ohio-Mississippi basin and the Southwest, respectively. Both can cause granulomas. Although he has never been in these two geographic belts, strict geographic boundaries are not completely applicable and spillovers occur.

Data 6 Are the patient's occupation and habits such that he might have contracted one of the two aforementioned fungus diseases? He is a roofer and works where bird droppings are abundant.

Logic Bird and bat droppings contain the spores of these fungi. So being a roofer, pet store owner, or spelunker might be helpful clues. But the patient does not inhabit an area where these diseases prevail, so these possibilities become less likely. Were he in South Texas where both of these disease belts cross, the question would be more relevant. But remember that bird migrations do not respect geographic boundaries.

Occupation is also important in that some occupational contacts increase the incidence of lung cancer—asbestos, uranium, chromium, cobalt, nickel, arsenic, and any type of radioactivity.

Data 7 Has the patient had prolonged contact with family members, acquaintances, or co-workers who cough a lot or who are known to have or have had tuberculosis? The answer is no.

Logic This is only somewhat dependable. Had the answer been "yes," your concern for tuberculosis would heighten. Hospital personnel are subject to contact of this sort without being aware of it. Many persons have annual purified protein derivative (PPD) skin tests done, and it would be helpful to know when and if conversion had already taken place.

Data 8 Are there physical signs of any of the suspected diseases? A lesion as small as the one under discussion would not be likely to give physical signs of itself. However, you would look for evidence of metastasis (large liver, hard supraclavicular lymph node), and signs and symptoms of a primary lesion elsewhere (breast, thyroid, lymph nodes, testicles, prostate, abdominal mass). Fever might indicate an active tuberculous process. Clubbing and distal periostitis might suggest cancer of the lung. *The complete physical examination is normal.*

Logic You now have a 52-year-old man who smokes heavily; he has an asymptomatic nodule in his lung that he says was not present 2 years ago. The probability is that he has cancer and will need surgery. However, further studies must first be done.

Data (1) Intermediate strength PPD skin test result is 15-mm wide; (2) coccidioidin skin test result is negative; (3) complete blood count (CBC), urinalysis, and sedimentation rate are normal; (4)

computed tomography (CT) with thin sections through the nodular lesion shows no calcification and no cavitation; (5) there is no sputum, but morning gastric washings do not show any acid-fast bacilli; and (6) fiberoptic bronchoscopy is performed. No abnormalities are noted. Washings in the suspected area are sent to the laboratory for tumor cell, tubercle bacilli, and fungus studies. All study results are negative; you must wait 6 weeks for the results of the tuberculosis cultures.

Logic The value of computed tomography lies in its ability to define better the density and configuration of tissue within the nodule, to detect satellite lesions, to note special patterns of calcification within the lesion, and to observe mediastinal lymphadenopathy.

The positive PPD result is not helpful because it is common in the absence of a tuberculoma. A negative test result would have more meaning in this patient. Fungal skin tests are basically not helpful. Histoplasmin skin tests are contraindicated because they increase blood antibody titers and invalidate subsequent serologic tests for this disease; this skin test is useful only in epidemiologic studies. Coccidioidin skin test results are positive in exposed persons but may become negative with active dissemination, so they are of limited help. Positive blood titers (complement fixation) indicate either past or active infection and, unless very high, do not assist in determining the nature of a lesion. When negative, these results are of diagnostic acid.

The study of gastric washings in patients without sputum is probably not reliable. Many saprophytic mycobacteria are present. It would have been better to try to induce sputum formation with ultrasonic saline nebulization. But even when sputum is present, the true positive yield is low.

The normal sedimentation rate merely tells us there is no active inflammation in process. Had CT shown calcification or cavitation, you would have leaned toward a granuloma, but these findings can occur in cancer also, although rarely. So this too is nonspecific. Bronchoscopy was not helpful. Surgery seems imminent.

Data Results of liver, brain, and adrenal gland computed tomographic scans are normal. Isotopic skeletal survey reveals no metastases. Liver function test results are normal. Blood count is normal, and stools tests negative for occult blood. The results of the electrocardiogram (ECG) are normal.

Logic Several data sets were just explored. The results of either set may stay the surgeon's hand, and they concern themselves with:

- If the lung lesion is cancer, are there metastases present?
- Is the lung lesion metastatic from another source?
- Is the patient operable?

First, there is no evidence for metastases to liver, bone, adrenal gland, or brain—common sites for spread from lung cancer. Second, there is no evidence for a primary carcinoma elsewhere resulting in a solitary lung metastasis. This was reasonably well proved by the previous normal physical examination and the absence of blood in the urine and stools. Third, the normal ECG, negative history, and normal physical examination establish that the patient is a good risk for surgical intervention.

Many do not consider such extensive preoperative screening necessary and would do only liver function tests. Bone, brain, and liver scans are done only if there are bone pains and tenderness, neurologic symptoms or signs, and an elevated alkaline phosphatase and/or an enlarged liver.

The various studies provided little help with the crucial question: Cancer? Yes or no? In certain instances, when you wish to be *more certain before proceeding with surgery,* you aim for histologic identification first. Oat cell carcinoma accounts for the 3 to 5% of solitary malignant nodules; if biopsy can establish the presence of this cell type, surgery should not be performed because this disease is invariably generalized. Then too, if the patient has other diseases that substantially *increase his surgical mortality risk* to 5 to 10%, greater diagnostic certainty is desirable before thoracot-omy is done.

Under these circumstances, choose between *flexible fiberoptic transbronchial biopsy* and *percutaneous transthoracic thin-needle biopsy.* The former method is most effective for central larger lesions. The latter is preferable when the lesion is peripheral, but it has a higher complication rate. Neither method is highly sensitive, false negatives are common if the lesion is missed, specific diagnoses are not made with great regularity, and frequent reports of "chronic inflammation" do not instill confidence.

Because negative biopsy results are not dependable, when surgery seems likely, the physician often goes directly to thoracotomy, open biopsy, frozen section, and excision. This approach is as close to 100% specific and 100% sensitive as is possible—a gold standard test.

On occasion, mediastinoscopy is performed first when enlarged hilar nodes are suspected by previous radiographic procedures. Its risk is low, metastases may be confirmed, and a high-risk patient may be spared an operation whose mortality is much higher than the possible harm of this diagnostic procedure. Affected nodes are unlikely, however, if the lesion is small and peripheral, and mediastinoscopy is not indicated if tomography shows no enlarged mediastinal nodes.

Data On the basis of the entire clinical picture, surgery is deemed advisable. The nodule and a segment of adjacent lung are removed. The pathologic diagnosis is tuberculoma. No evidence of tuberculous activity is noted, although a Ziehl-Neelsen stain shows some tubercle bacilli at the center of the nodule.

Logic The decision for surgery was wise, even though cancer was not found. Evidence for malignancy was strong—age, heavy smoking, an allegedly normal radiograph 2 years before, plus no indication that the lesion might be infectious. You do not know if the nodule is recent or was simply obscured on the previous radiograph. The latter situation is more likely.

Test Your Judgment

Devise a clinical strategy for each of the following patients described in a brief case presentation. A set of options is provided; the strategy should consider and include one or more of the stated options in proper sequence. The author's choices and explanations follow. Do not be disturbed if you disagree. Oncologists sometimes do, too. And strategies may be revised in the future as more data are obtained about various diagnostic procedures.
1. **Do nothing**
2. **Recheck in 1 to 2 months**
3. **Do a CT scan**
4. **Do transbronchial biopsy**
5. **Do percutaneous biopsy**
6. **Do mediastinoscopy**
7. **Do metastatic screen**

8. Do open biopsy
9. Do lobectomy if option 8 yields positive results for cancer

Patient 1. A 26-year-old man is seen for a 2-cm nodule in the right upper lung field. He has lived in Sacramento, California, all his life and smokes one pack of cigarettes daily. The lesion has a ring of calcium. There are no symptoms or signs, and the results of routine tests, smears, and cultures are normal or negative. All skin test results are positive. No previous radiographs are available.

Patient 2. Consider the same patient. The lesion is in the right midlung field near the hilum and it is not calcified. A radiograph taken 2 years ago shows the same lesion, but its diameter was 1.5 cm. All else is the same.

Patient 3. This is a 56-year-old man who smokes two packs daily. He has a 2-cm nodule in the right midlung field. It shows no calcification by conventional radiography. However, the right upper hilar nodes are questionably enlarged. No previous radiographs are available. PPD skin tests shows 15-mm erythema after 48 hours, and he lives in New Mexico. Results of bronchoscopic examination, brush cytology, and stains for acid-fast bacilli and fungal spores are all negative. He is otherwise quite well.

Patient 4. A 75-year-old man with moderately severe coronary artery disease and mild congestive heart failure has a 2-cm nodule in the right midlung field equidistant between the hilum and the pleura. Previous radiographs are unavailable. He has never smoked. CT shows no calcification and no enlarged hilar nodes. Skin test results are negative except for mumps and *Candida* antigens.

Answers to Test Your Judgment

1. Do nothing. This is an obvious granuloma, probably a histoplasmoma.
2. This case is more difficult. The lesion has grown but probably too slowly to be considered malignant; its doubling time is slightly less than 2 years. Yet it is not calcified. It may be asking too much to expect a 28-year-old to live with even a 3% specter of cancer. As always, the patient must enter the decision-making process. I would do a CT scan hoping to find calcification. If not found, and no mediastinal nodes were noted, I would bypass options 4, 5, and 6, do a minimal 7 (alkaline phosphatase), and go directly to 8—open biopsy. Others may disagree. What would you do?
3. The patient's age, smoking, and noncalcified nodule far outweigh the distractions of his habitat and positive PPD skin test. In addition, hilar adenopathy is worrisome but does not necessarily preclude surgical cure. Do 6, 7, 8,

and 9, each step depending on the results of the previous one. If the results of mediastinoscopy and node biopsy are negative for cancer, do a metastatic screen; if the screen shows no metastases, proceed with open biopsy and surgery if biopsy results are positive. There is no unanimity of opinion if mediastinal biopsy results are positive. Most would stop at this point and begin radiotherapy and/or chemotherapy. A few would not consider hilar node involvement a contraindication to extensive surgery and would continue with steps 7, 8, and 9.

4. This patient has a high risk for complications from thoracotomy (approximately 10%). Therefore, be sure he has cancer without metastases before performing surgery. Options 4 or 5 or both are in order. Although these procedures have risk, the risk is small compared with option 8. A tissue diagnosis assumes first priority. If 4 or 5 is positive for cancer, proceed with 7, 8, and 9 unless metastases are found. Lung cancers are seen in nonsmokers too. But if 4 and 5 are fruitless, consider 2 or 8. When all studies are equivocal in a high-risk patient and some clinical features suggest this may not be cancer (e.g., no smoking, positive PPD skin test, splelunking history, and so forth), you may justifiably wait and recheck the patient in 2 months. Even if it were cancer, considering the doubling time, the disease has already existed for a few years and a short wait would have no great impact on the outcome. Others would disagree and see nothing to gain by waiting. Most would proceed with steps 7, 8, and 9 as indicated. Decision analysis and the construction of a decision tree using the patient's values and your researched data might be helpful here. Doubt may be preferable to surgery.

The last word! Individual cases with variant clinical pictures may not be so neatly categorized as the four prototype patients just described. There are many instances where management decisions are closer calls—sometimes even tossups.

Question

1. A 2-cm diameter pulmonary nodule is noted in retrospect to have had a 1-cm diameter 1 year ago. What is its doubling time? Is it probably malignant?

COMMENT Despite newer technologies, the diagnostic approach to the sort of problem seen in the patient in Case 33 is much the same in the 90s as in the 60s. Better out than doubt!

The road we have just traversed is simply an academic exercise, because we want to know mainly if this is a primary cancer, and if it is operable. For, given a lung nodule in an otherwise healthy man, unless *obviously* long present or *clearly* caused by a granulomatous disease, intermediate procedures may be omitted, and open biopsy with possible additional surgery *must be done*. It's fast, it's relatively safe, it often cures, and it eliminates doubt and observation.

For the problem solver who seeks the middle road between avoiding surgery and missing a curable lesion, the approach to each case must be individualized and tailored at least in part to the informed patient's values.

It should not be necessary to remove 20 benign lesions to find one that is malignant. But in *this* case, a benign lesion was justifiably removed. Solving the problem here lent itself handily to using many techniques. First, bits of information were gathered via a decision path invading only the pulmonary subset of the data base. This patient had an asymptomatic presentation for which such a technique can be readily used. Clues of all types were present—negatives (absence of certain expected features) and false positives (heavy cigarette smoking, yet no cancer). Some clues were misleading (occupation and "negative radiograph" 2 years ago). Geography, occupation, and contact history were considered but were of limited help. Tuberculosis was present despite no history of contact, no symptoms, and no specific radiographic evidence.

The specificity and sensitivity of clues were an integral part of logic as we considered various points in the history and modes of testing. According to probability theory, this patient was likely to have cancer. But probabilities did not provide a correct solution in this case. Boolean logic and Venn's set theories were frequently invoked when considering the overlap of smokers, nonsmokers, and cancer; the reliability of fungal tests; the significance of positive and negative PPD test results with tuberculosis; the existence of diseases with and without symptoms or signs; and the presence of nodules with or without calcification.

The operating characteristics of various procedures and the concept of imperfect information were explored as each diagnostic modality was considered and its value placed into proper perspective. And in this era of cost containment, the rationale of using so many procedures was bared for debate.

Hanging like an invisible shroud over the entire diagnostic process in this case were the Bayesian theorems of probability and probability revision plus newer notions of medical decision making. *(P.C.)*

PROBLEM-BASED LEARNING To learn all about this patient and his type of presentation, the student should read texts referable to the following subjects:

- How to interpret a chest radiograph
- Other chest radiographic abnormalities that may be asymptomatic
- Causes and prevalence of each cause of pulmonary nodules and their associated clinical manifestations, including a large array of uncommon disease (e.g., Osler-Weber-Rendu's disease with a pulmonary arteriovenous fistula), in addition to the common ones described in the text
- Lung cancer, its cell types, relationship to cigarettes, and the broad spectrum of its clinical presentations
- Very special paraneoplastic syndromes associated with specific types of lung cancer
- Pulmonary tuberculosis, its clinical manifestations, PPD skin test interpretation, and its varied modes of presentation
- Pulmonary mycoses: their clinical features and laboratory diagnosis
- Hamartomas
- Simple tests such as sputum smears, cultures, and cytology
- Indications for and limitations of bronchoscopy (rigid and flexible); bronchography;

mediastinoscopy; transbronchial, percutaneous, and open biopsy; and computed tomographic scan

- When, if, and how to confirm extrapulmonary metastases

All this information will add another 5% to your rapidly expanding knowledge base.

Suggested Readings

Lillington GA, Caskey CI. Evaluation of management of solitary and multiple pulmonary nodules. Clin Chest Med 1993;14:111.

Midthun DE, Swenson SJ, Jett JR. Approach to the solitary pulmonary nodule. Mayo Clin Proc 1993; 68:378.

Webb WR. Radiologic evaluation of the solitary pulmonary nodule. AJR 1990;154:701.

WHEEZE AND DYSPNEA

Juan A. Albino and W. G. Johanson, Jr

Data A 28-year-old man became acutely dyspneic while vacationing in the mountains with his family. The dyspnea was associated with cough and wheezing and a local physician was consulted.

Logic Wheezing indicates airway obstruction. It is important that the physician identify the site of obstruction and the nature of the obstructing process. The location of the obstruction may be in the *upper, central,* or *peripheral airway.*

Upper airway obstruction in the region of the epiglottis and larynx may produce wheezing. Such lesions mainly cause inspiratory obstruction and result in stridor, a crowing noise during inspiration, but may result in expiratory obstruction as well. Stridor is typically caused by inflammatory processes in infants and by trauma, allergy, infection, or carcinoma in adults.

Central obstruction involving the trachea or major bronchi may be due to foreign bodies, tumors (benign or malignant), infiltrative diseases (sarcoid), trauma, and cicatricial stenosis (after endotracheal intubation and/or tracheostomy). Foreign body aspiration in adults is usually associated with a known or suspected episode of aspiration; such episodes are frequently less obvi-

ous in children or in obtunded alcoholics. Central airway obstruction due to a foreign body or tumor may mimic the physical findings of peripheral airway disease and must be carefully considered in all patients with the new onset of wheezing. The obstruction is usually relentless, leading to persistent symptoms unless relieved by therapy.

Obstruction of peripheral airways is by far the most common cause of dyspnea with wheezing and is usually due to asthma, chronic obstructive pulmonary disease (COPD), or left ventricular failure. Rarely, the acute onset of dyspnea with wheezing is caused by viral bronchiolitis (children, atopic adults), toxic fume exposure, or pulmonary embolism (predisposed adults). Bronchoconstriction with asthma occurs in the peripheral airways at the level of the bronchioles (airways < 1 mm with no cartilage) where smooth muscle spasm can act as a sphincter and where the narrowing effects of inflammation (edema, cellular infiltrate, and excess mucus) can have their most prominent effects (Fig. 15.2).

Data The patient worked as a book editor, had never smoked, and had previously enjoyed excellent health. None of his family members had experienced fever or other symptoms of respiratory tract infections. He did recall nasal congestion and sneezing since arriving in the mountains. He had asthma each autumn as a child while living in the Midwest but the episodes had ceased after age 12 when he and his family moved to the Southwest.

On physical examination the patient was in

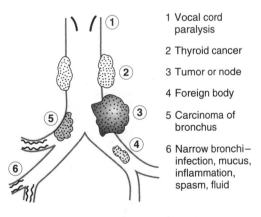

▶ **Figure 15.2.** Sites of airway obstruction.

moderate respiratory distress, but had normal vital signs. The nasal mucosa was boggy and bluish in hue, and a thin watery discharge was present. Examination of the chest revealed bilateral expiratory wheezes. The cardiac examination, including auscultation in the left lateral decubitus position, was entirely normal. A chest radiograph and electrocardiogram were also within normal limits. A smear of the nasal mucosa showed numerous eosinophils. The peripheral blood leukocyte count was 7500/mm^3 with 12% eosinophils.

Logic The absence of smoking, chronic cough, and impaired exercise capacity is strong evidence against chronic obstructive pulmonary disease (COPD). The normal blood pressure, cardiac examination, chest radiograph, and ECG rule out the presence of any cardiac disease that might present with pulmonary congestion. Mitral stenosis may be difficult to detect by auscultation alone, but the absence of a history of rheumatic fever and the normal chest radiograph and ECG do not support this diagnosis. Rather, the patient demonstrates typical findings of acute bronchial asthma.

Bronchial asthma is a condition of widespread airway narrowing that changes rapidly in severity either spontaneously or as the result of treatment. Reversibility of obstruction is the key diagnostic feature of asthma, and airway inflammation is the pathologic hallmark (eosinophilic bronchitis). Patients with asthma have *hyperactive airways* that serve to separate them from normal individuals and, to a large extent, from patients with COPD.

Immediate hypersensitivity, mediated by immunoglobulin E (IgE) and the release of mediators from mast cells, is the common mechanism triggering asthma attacks.

However, besides the early acute phase of airway obstruction, there is a late phase occurring 6 to 8 hours later, which is characterized by an influx of inflammatory cells. A genetic predisposition to atopic disorders, manifested by rhinitis, asthma, or eczema, is usually present in other family members. Episodes of asthma occur predictably upon exposure of a patient to the agent or agents to which he is sensitive, that is, to which he has formed specific IgE antibody. Such episodes may be explosive in nature, as with anaphylaxis, or more gradual in onset, as was the case in this patient.

Data The physician prescribed inhaled bronchodilators (β-agonists), and the patient improved. The next day he and his family left the mountains and returned home where he consulted his own physician. Physical examination at that time revealed a few scattered expiratory wheezes, although the patient felt he had returned to normal. Spirometry results were obtained (Table 15.1).

Logic These results were interpreted as showing moderately severe airway obstruction, with significant ($>$ 12%) improvement in forced vital capacity (FVC) and/or forced expiratory volume in 1 second (FEV$_1$) following bronchodilator administration. Objective measurement of airway obstruction with spirometry or peak expiratory flowmeter is very useful in the diagnosis and management of asthma. Airway obstruction in asthma is multifactorial and caused by: (1) bronchospasm from contraction of bronchial smooth muscle, (2) edema and inflammation of airway walls that encroach on the bronchial lumen, and (3) retention of tenacious secretions within the airways.

Our patient had been on no prior therapy and improved quickly just with β-agonist inhalers, although he continued to have obstruction. Because the β-agonists mainly relieve the bronchoconstric-

TABLE 15.1. Spirometry Results: Before and After Bronchodilator Therapy

MEASUREMENT	PREDICTED NORMAL VALUE	BEFORE BD	AFTER BD
FVC	5.72 L	4.50 L (79%)	5.50 L (96%)
FEV$_1$	4.47 L	2.50 L (56%)	4.20 L (94%)
FEV$_1$/FVC	0.78	0.56	0.76

BD = bronchodilators; FVC = forced vital capacity; FEV$_1$ = forced expiratory volume in one second.

tion due to smooth muscle contraction, additional therapy aimed at airway inflammation is indicated. Corticosteroids are the first line agents for this purpose. The patient's subsequent therapy will also depend on the physician's assessment of the cause of his asthma attack.

Based on the presence of previous allergic disorders, the absence of infection, and the lack of exposure to known nonspecific irritants (cold air, fumes, air pollution, cigarette smoke, strong odors), it was reasonably presumed that the attack was due to exposure to an allergen to which the patient was sensitive, and he was referred to an allergist for further evaluation.

Data Skin testing was performed with a number of likely antigens, and flare and wheal reactions occurred to many. A brisk reaction developed to an extract of mountain cedar pollen that had been in season at the time the patient had visited the area. In light of the prompt response of the patient to avoidance of this antigen and to symptomatic therapy, it was decided not to undertake hyposensitization injections.

Logic Avoidance of the offending antigens is without doubt the ideal management of allergic disorders. When the patient's symptoms are due to well-defined agents, such avoidance may be readily accomplished. Unfortunately, in many patients, symptoms are produced by a number of antigens, exposure to which can be reduced but frequently not altogether eliminated. Immunotherapy, or "allergy shots," is of proven benefit for some patients with allergic rhinitis, although its benefit is less well documented in most patients who have asthma.

Data Maintenance therapy with regularly scheduled inhaled corticosteroids and β-agonists on an "as-needed" basis was continued for several weeks, and the patient remained asymptomatic. Spirometry performed 1 month after the attack showed entirely normal findings, which confirmed the diagnosis of asthma and ruled out COPD. It was concluded that the patient's asthma was due to hypersensitivity to mountain cedar. With continued avoidance of this antigen, he remained well, and therapy on a regular basis ceased.

Two years later the patient became ill with an upper respiratory tract infection accompanied by cough, dyspnea, and wheezing. During an episode of coughing he experienced a sudden increase in dyspnea associated with sharp pain in the right chest. Alarmed by his extreme air hunger, his wife called an ambulance that arrived quickly and transported the patient to a nearby hospital.

Logic The sudden onset of dyspnea is an uncommon symptom that indicates a catastrophic derangement in cardiopulmonary function. It may occur in asthmatic patients as a result of widespread bronchospasm triggered by exogenous agents. In any patient with excessive airway secretions, acute worsening may be a manifestation of plugs of material moving centrally from the periphery of the lung, thus obstructing a greater fraction of the total airway. Such movement of secretions occurs commonly during recumbency in patients with COPD, resulting in episodes of nocturnal dyspnea that simulate episodes of left ventricular failure. Cardiovascular events, including myocardial infarction or pulmonary embolism, may produce sudden severe dyspnea. Last, a pneumothorax may cause symptoms that vary from only mild chest discomfort to severe dyspnea and death. The occurrence of chest pain suggests that diagnosis but does not rule out other possibilities.

Data On arrival to the hospital, the patient's vital signs were: pulse, 140/min; BP, 60/40; and respirations 40. He was cyanotic and in obvious severe respiratory distress. A rapid examination revealed distended neck veins, tracheal shift to the left, tympany, absent breath sounds, and absent respiratory movements of the right hemithorax. Heart sounds were inaudible due to wheezing and rhonchi over the left lung. A clinical diagnosis of tension pneumothorax on the right was made, and a 15-gauge needle was inserted through an intercostal space. Gas under pressure quickly escaped, and the patient's blood pressure improved. A portable radiograph was obtained, and a chest tube was inserted with prompt improvement in the patient's dyspnea, cyanosis, and heart rate. The radiograph showed approximately 90% collapse of the right lung at the time of chest tube insertion, with a shift of the mediastinum to the left (Fig. 15.3).

Logic Spontaneous (nontraumatic) pneumothorax results when the visceral pleura ruptures, exposing the pleural space to air within the lung. Spontaneous pneumothoraces occur most commonly in healthy young men with tall asthenic physiques or in patients who have emphysema. In the former case, pneumothorax is usually due

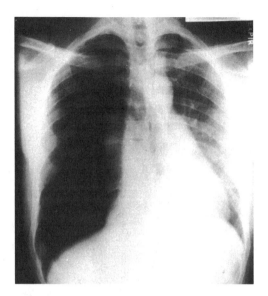

▶ **Figure 15.3.** Pneumothorax. Ninety percent collapse in right lung. Shift of mediastinum to left.

to rupture of a thin-walled bleb at the lung apex. In emphysema, pneumothorax is due to the rupture of bullae formed as part of the disease process. Pneumonias due to necrotizing organisms, such as *Staphylococcus aureus,* can form pneumatoceles that can rupture and lead to a pneumothorax. In asthma, a valve type obstruction of a small bronchiole may lead to progressive hyperinflation of a region of lung and ultimate rupture. Spontaneous pneumothorax most commonly occurs in association with exercise or cough but may occur at rest or even during sleep.

A special category of pneumothorax is that associated with a rise in pleural pressure above atmospheric pressure: a tension pneumothorax. The positive pleural pressure impairs venous return, leading to circulatory collapse as well as collapse of the lung. A tension pneumothorax develops when the communication between the intrapulmonary air spaces and the pleura contains a valve-like mechanism preventing reentry of air from the pleural space into the lung but allowing further accumulation in the pleural space during inspiration.

Data Examination of the patient's sputum revealed numerous neutrophils, a few eosinophils, and small pleomorphic gram-negative organisms. *Haemophilus influenzae* was isolated in the sputum culture. Treatment with β-agonists via

nebulizer, intravenous corticosteroids, and cefuroxime was initiated and the asthma rapidly improved. The medications were then changed to β-agonists and steroids via metered dose inhalers (MDI) and oral cefuroxime. Intravenous steroids were replaced by tapering doses of oral prednisone; inhaled steroids were started again when the daily dose of prednisone was decreased to 20 mg/d.

Logic Whereas the previous attack had been precipitated by a specific allergen, this attack followed a respiratory tract infection. Differentiation of attacks due to infections from those due to allergens or other irritant exposures may be difficult but can usually be made on the basis of the history and examination of the patient's sputum.

Data Following an uneventful course in the hospital the patient was discharged, the chest tube having been removed on the third hospital day. Prednisone was tapered over the ensuing 2 weeks, and he was maintained on inhaled steroids with β-agonists to be used as needed pending his next visit to his physician.

Questions

(More than one answer may be correct.)

1. Shortness of breath, wheezing, and production of purulent sputum in a 14-year-old female with asthma:
   (a) usually indicates acute bronchitis due to a viral infection.
   (b) occurs episodically and will disappear without treatment.
   (c) requires a chest radiograph for proper evaluation.
   (d) may be due to either allergy or infection.

2. A 50-year-old businessman has noted persistent cough and wheezing since he choked on a mouthful of popcorn at a ball game 1 week ago. His symptoms can be attributed to bronchial irritation alone when:
   (a) his chest radiograph is shown to be free of infiltrates.
   (b) physical examination is found to reveal diffuse and nonlocalized wheezing.
   (c) his chest examination results are found to be normal.
   (d) bronchoscopy fails to reveal a foreign body, and the chest radiographic findings are normal.

3. Arterial blood gases during asthmatic attacks:
   (a) usually show mild hypoxemia and hypocarbia during mild-to-moderate attacks.
   (b) show hypercarbia early in the attack.

(c) may show decreases in PaO$_2$ following bronchodilator therapy.

(d) show hypoxemia refractory to oxygen therapy.

Answers

1. **(d) is correct.** It is important to know that increases in the number of either eosinophils or neutrophils in sputum will cause purulence due to the enzymes contained in these cells. Thus, either infection (neutrophils) or allergy (eosinophils) could be responsible for the patient's symptoms. A smear of the sputum will be more informative than the chest radiograph, especially in the absence of fever. Although fever and sputum examination will probably identify a pyogenic lower respiratory tract infection, and the physical examination will help to localize it, a chest radiograph will reliably confirm the presence of pneumonia (infiltrate) and distinguish it from bronchitis, particularly if a subtle atypical pneumonia is present, or physical signs are not clear.

2. **(d) is correct.** Foreign bodies may not be radiopaque and may not completely obstruct bronchi. Their presence may be heralded by only cough, occasionally by wheezing. With the history provided, it would be mandatory to examine the patient's tracheobronchial tree endoscopically to be certain that a foreign body is not present.

3. **(a) and (c) are correct.** Blood gases in asthma display rather characteristic changes—alveolar hyperventilation (low PaCO$_2$) and mild hypoxemia early on, with CO$_2$ retention and severe hypoxemia occurring only when airway obstruction is extremely severe. In a significant percentage of patients, bronchodilator therapy causes worsening hypoxemia, apparently due to the release of the pulmonary arterial vasoconstriction caused by regional hypoxia, thus worsening the ventilation-perfusion (V/Q) mismatch. Hypoxemia in asthma is usually due to V/Q mismatching and responds readily to oxygen therapy.

COMMENT Although a wheeze may result from situations as diverse as the aspiration of a peanut, the inhalation of a noxious dust, emboli from leg veins, lung cancer, or pulmonary vein congestion—by far the most common causes are bronchial asthma and chronic obstructive pulmonary disease.

The common denominator for all wheezes is obstruction somewhere in the airways, and other than for readily apparent local causes such as cancer and foreign body, the bronchial lumina may be diffusely narrowed by spasm, edema, inflammation, and infection of their walls. Because the resistance to flow through a narrow tube is inversely proportional to the fourth power of the radius (Poiseuille), narrowed airways result not only in wheezes but in the increased work of breathing and consequent dyspnea.

Key decision points for the solution of the patient who wheezes include: (1) age; (2) associated symptoms (cough, dyspnea, orthopnea, expectoration, chest pain, hoarseness); (3) the mode of onset and course of the clinical picture; (4) the role of specific allergens and respiratory tract infections; and (5) the elimination of congestive heart failure. Patients with asthma demonstrate complete remissions; they have no symptoms and their pulmonary function tests are normal between attacks. On the other hand, patients with COPD are chronically and progressively ill; they always have symptoms and altered function tests.

Bronchial asthma is a common, recurrent, lifelong disease, treatment is only partially successful, and emergency departments usually harbor one or more asthmatic patients at any single time. Either the patient gets well in a few hours, spends the night in a holding area—or is admitted to the hospital if treatment doesn't help, if the PCO$_2$ rises, or if he or she becomes exhausted. For the most part, asthmatic patients can be successfully managed on an ambulatory basis. *(P.C.)*

Suggested Readings

Creticos PS, Reed CE, Norman PS, et al. Ragweed immunotherapy in adult asthma. N Engl J Med 1996;333:501–506.

Emerman CL, Cydulka RK. Effect of pulmonary function testing on the management of acute asthma. Arch Intern Med 1995;155:2225–2228.

McFadden ER, Jr, Elsanadi N, Dixon L, et al. Protocol therapy for acute asthma: Therapeutic benefits and cost savings. Am J Med 1995;99:651–661.

 CASE 35

COUGHING OF BLOOD

Paul Cutler

Data After coughing up a cupful of bright red blood, a 48-year-old female office worker is brought to the emergency department. For the previous 3 months she has had a chronic cough productive of whitish-gray mucoid sputum that had become slightly blood streaked for the past few weeks. She also noticed increasing fatigability, dyspnea on exertion, and difficulty in sleeping for a few months.

Logic Hemoptysis is usually a serious presenting symptom and invariably brings the patient to the physician. You wonder why this patient did not come in sooner, considering the variety of symptoms. Initially you think of the common causes of hemoptysis:

1. Carcinoma
2. Tuberculosis
3. Bronchiectasis
4. Bronchitis
5. Heart failure
6. Pulmonary infarct
7. Mitral stenosis

Less common causes include pneumonia, abscess, parasites, fungi, anticoagulant drugs, Goodpasture's syndrome, Wegener's granulomatosis, and periarteritis nodosa. We are no doubt dealing with hemoptysis rather than hematemesis or nasopharyngeal bleeding because of the associated pulmonary symptoms.

The distinction between hemoptysis and hematemesis is sometimes not simple. If the amount of blood is large, the patient may not know if it was coughed or vomited. In hemoptysis the blood is frothy, red, and alkaline. Vomited blood is usually darker red, acid, and may contain food particles. If in doubt, gastric intubation helps you decide.

In view of the chronic cough and expectoration, diagnoses 1, 2, 3, and 4 are all serious considerations. Congestive heart failure is also suggested by the additional symptoms of fatigue, dyspnea on exertion, and difficulty in sleeping. Cancer or tuberculosis could cause these symptoms too if there were destruction of much tissue or an associated pleural effusion. At this point it is not known if the sleeping problem is from orthopnea, severe cough, or ordinary insomnia.

Data The patient has smoked two packs of cigarettes daily for the past 30 years and drinks 8 to 10 cups of coffee a day, but she had no known medical illnesses. She had a hysterectomy for fi-

broids, cholecystectomy for stones, and a subsequent laparotomy for adhesions. The last operation was 5 years ago. Her appetite has been excessive. She gained 60 lb in the past 5 years and now weighs 230 lb. She attributed her many symptoms to obesity and smoking and did not seek medical care until she coughed a large quantity of blood. There have been no chest pain, night sweats, or fever.

Logic Such a cigarette history always raises the specter of cancer. The coffee intake is not significant here. No relationship can be established between the three surgical procedures and the patient's present problems. Too much time has elapsed for the existence of emboli, and there has been no pleuritic pain. Weight gain plus hearty appetite tend to negate cancer and tuberculosis. Heavy smoking might relate to chronic bronchitis or chronic obstructive lung disease. This, plus the additional burden of severe obesity and its resulting alveolar hypoventilation, might explain the fatigue and dyspnea. Do not infer that all obese patients have alveolar hypoventilation. Occasionally, in extreme obesity, massive accumulations of fat prevent adequate mechanical ventilation, and hypoxemia and hypercarbia may result.

Data Further history reveals that her father died of tuberculosis at 56 when she was 20, and that one of her close co-workers developed a "chest condition" 6 months ago for which she was hospitalized and is still under treatment. (Pulmonary tuberculosis is still a common cause of hemoptysis and must always be seriously considered, especially in those living in inner cities and in recent immigrants from Haiti and southeast Asia.) There has been no history of leg injury or a recent long automobile trip, and she takes no birth control pills.

Logic You now know that she has had close contact with tubercle bacilli and that there is no obvious reason why she should have leg vein thrombosis with emboli. But remember that visceral carcinoma can increase the propensity toward venous thromboemboli. So can wheelchair or bed confinement, congestive heart failure, postsurgical status, leg trauma, and a history of thrombophlebitis—none of which is present in this patient.

Data A review of systems reveals nervousness, headaches, insomnia, occasional ringing in the ears, rare double vision, bad taste and dryness in the mouth, nocturia 3×, occasional burning on urination, painful menses, slight vaginal discharge, constipation, worsening of her cough at night, and the need to sleep on three pillows for comfort. Her mother died in an automobile accident many years ago; she has no siblings, and she has three well children, ages 25, 21, and 18.

Logic The multiplicity of symptoms needs weeding out. She gives many positives, most of which are unrelated to her main problem. In fact, some are clearly psychosomatic and others are what anybody might have from time to time. They should, however, be closely checked, because additional problems may exist. The dyspnea and orthopnea do seem genuine and suggest left ventricular failure.

Data Physical examination discloses a markedly obese woman in no acute distress, although appearing quite apprehensive. The vital signs are temperature, 37°C; pulse, 106 with slight irregularity; respirations, 18; and BP, 106/80. General inspection shows no remarkable abnormalities. In particular, there is no malar flush, no clubbing, and no hypertrophic pulmonary osteoarthropathy.

Logic A rich amount of material may often be harvested from the physical examination in patients with hemoptysis. Considering the common possibilities, you may find rales at the apex, rales at the bases, metastatic nodes, Horner's syndrome, pleural friction rub, tracheal deviation, pleural effusion, enlarged nodular liver, tender calf, or positive Homans' sign. Basal rales or rhonchi may represent aspirated blood and not pinpoint the bleeding site. The significance of each of these findings should be apparent. In this patient the apprehension and rapid pulse are understandable, although the irregularities in the pulse need clarification. A malar flush might suggest rheumatic mitral valve disease. Absence of clubbing and hypertrophic pulmonary osteoarthropathy weigh against lung cancer and bronchiectasis, although certainly do not rule them out, because only a minority of patients with these diseases exhibit such features. Absence of fever weighs against pneumonia or abscess, as is the long history of symptoms.

Data Further examination shows no lung abnormalities except for a few coarse wet rales at both bases; there are no friction rubs or wheezes.

An occasional premature beat without a compensatory pause is noted. The second heart sound is loud; its second component (P_2) is not only heard all over the precordium but it is felt over the pulmonic valve area. At the apex of the heart, an opening snap (OS) is heard shortly after S_2 (S_2-OS time = 0.05 second). This is followed by a low-pitched, rumbling, decrescendo-crescendo murmur terminating in a loud S_1. The apex beat is normally situated, and no thrill is felt. The remainder of the examination is normal. In particular, there is no neck vein distention, hepatomegaly, or leg edema. The calves are not tender and Homans' sign is negative.

Logic Mitral stenosis is well established. Premature atrial contractions denote atrial irritability, a loud P_2 suggests pulmonary hypertension, and tight severe mitral stenosis is indicated by the short S_2-OS interval, opening snap, typical murmur, and loud S_1. Obesity obscures the thrill and a malar flush is not always present. The murmur was probably present at the times of surgery, although one can only guess why it was not noted. There is as yet no evidence for right ventricular strain or failure.

The basal rales represent either pulmonary congestion from the mitral stenotic valve, blood still present in the lower airways, or concomitant lower airway bronchial disease. Bronchiectasis, chronic bronchitis, or chronic obstructive lung disease could be present too and may warrant investigation later. The absence of general or local wheezes lessens the likelihood of chronic obstructive lung disease and partial airway obstruction from a neoplasm. For the moment, one diagnosis can easily explain the entire picture.

Data The 18-test chemistry profile, blood count, and urinalysis are normal. Intermediate strength purified protein derivative skin test is negative. The sputum tests negative for acid-fast bacilli and tumor cells on three occasions. Platelet count, prothrombin time, and partial thromboplastin time are done to rule out a bleeding diathesis; they are normal. The ECG shows evidence of left atrial abnormality and occasional premature atrial contractions but is otherwise normal (Fig. 15.4). Chest radiograph demonstrates no pulmonary parenchymal lesions, a normal-sized heart, straightening of the left cardiac border with a prominent convexity at its midportion, mild pul-

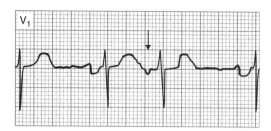

▶ **Figure 15.4.** Electrocardiogram of mitral stenosis. Diphasic P waves with prominent negative component in V_1 suggests left atrial hypertrophy. Arrow notes premature atrial contraction.

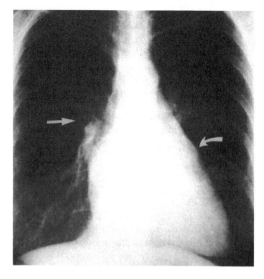

▶ **Figure 15.5.** Mitral stenosis. Straightening and convexity of left cardiac border resulting from enlarged left atrium (curved arrow). Prominent upper lobe pulmonary veins denote cephalization of blood flow (straight arrow).

monary edema, and distended upper lobe veins (Fig. 15.5).

Logic   The normal levels of serum calcium, alkaline phosphatase, and transaminases weigh against lung cancer, especially with liver metastases. The diagnosis is now certain. The radiographic and ECG findings are characteristic; negative test results help rule out other possibilities. Without doubt, the mitral orifice is small, the valve gradient is high, left atrial and pulmonary capillovenous pressure is high, pulmonary congestion exists, and a pulmonary varix has ruptured.

Before valve replacement, the patient will be encouraged to lose weight, stop smoking, and restrict activity. Cardiac catheterization and an echocardiogram will be performed to round out the picture. Fiberoptic bronchoscopy might be considered only if the patient were still bleeding and there were a need to locate the bleeding site should massive hemoptysis occur before valve surgery.

In fact, flexible fiberoptic bronchoscopy may be extremely useful in cases of this type. With it one may discover a small intrabronchial adenoma or carcinoma still too small to be visible by chest radiograph, and bronchial washings for smear, culture, and cytologic study often solve the problem when the diagnosis is not otherwise apparent. In this case it was not reasonable to search further.

With the advent of fiberoptics, bronchograms are becoming of less value but are still useful in localizing bronchiectasis amenable to resection. If repeated emboli were under consideration a ventilation-perfusion scan and pulmonary arteriography might be performed.

Questions

1. Consider the same patient with the following variations: she has signs and radiographic evidence of a large right pleural effusion. The chest radiographic findings are otherwise normal, and there is no evidence of mitral stenosis. The ECG is normal. Furthermore, she has lost weight and has anorexia. Your diagnostic spectrum shifts considerably. You should:
   (a) remove 10 mL of fluid for study.
   (b) remove all fluid and perform a bronchogram.
   (c) study sputum for tumor cells and tubercle bacilli.
   (d) remove all fluid and repeat the chest radiograph.

2. As a matter of Bayesian statistical likelihood, a 48-year-old woman who smokes heavily and has hemoptysis most commonly has:
   (a) no disease.
   (b) carcinoma of the lung.
   (c) chronic bronchitis.
   (d) tuberculosis.

3. If the data in case 35 were rearranged so that you suspected multiple pulmonary emboli, which procedure might give you the highest yield at the lowest risk?
   (a) Venogram of lower extremities
   (b) Ventilation-perfusion lung scan
   (c) Pulmonary arteriogram
   (d) Blood gases

4. Assume that your 48-year-old patient was initially seen with chronic cough and expectoration, hemoptysis, weakness, weight loss, and anorexia. She is a heavy smoker and has had exposure to tuberculosis. Chest radiograph showed an infiltrate in the right upper lobe, although the physical examination results were negative. The diagnosis would be most reliably established by:
   (a) purified protein derivative skin test.
   (b) bronchogram.
   (c) fiberoptic bronchoscopy.
   (d) isotope lung scan.

Answers

1. **(c) and (d) are correct.** The likelihood rests between cancer and tuberculosis. The long history, weight loss, and anorexia point away from repeated pulmonary emboli, although this is still a consideration. Heart failure is ruled out by the normal heart examination. Bronchitis and bronchiectasis do not give pleural effusions. Both (c) and (d) should be done. A simple sputum examination might provide the answer. But the fluid would have to be removed for therapeutic purposes as well as to study it and radiograph the underlying lung. To remove only 10 mL might give the answer, but it is almost as easy to remove it all and then do another radiograph. Bronchogram would probably be worthless, because bronchiectasis is unlikely in view of the effusion.

2. **(c) is correct,** because it is by far the most common cause of hemoptysis. Choice (a) is most unlikely in view of the clinical picture. Choices (b) and (d) are possibly correct, although less common.

3. **(b) is correct.** The positive yield is high and risk is almost nil. Venograms are formidable, time consuming, and may show nothing because the clots may be coming from sites other than the legs. Blood gases would show anoxemia, which is nonspecific. An arteriogram is invasive and not without risk, although the yield of positive information would be high. It might be done if the scan were inconclusive or if the insertion of a vena cava filter is being considered.

4. **(c) is correct.** The most likely diagnoses in these circumstances are carcinoma of the lung and tuberculosis. With fiberoptic bronchoscopy, biopsy of a visible lesion or bronchial washings for tumor cell study and acid-fast bacilli could both be obtained. Simple sputum examination might be most helpful, but it was not mentioned in the list of possibilities. A positive purified protein derivative skin test result would be of no value, although a negative result would be helpful. A bronchogram, no longer commonly done, would be of value if bronchiectasis were suspected; this is not the case here because an apical lesion was noted. A lung scan would help diagnose pulmonary embolus, not suggested by the clinical picture.

COMMENT First, we invoked the law of probabilities in dealing mainly with common diseases. Second, a large amount of information was gathered in the history, much of which was irrelevant. Then extraneous material was filtered out by suppression of information in a patient who seemed prone to answer yes to most inquiries. Pertinent negative clues were an important part of the data base—for example, absence of weight loss, night sweats, and fever; lack of clubbing; lack of pulmonary infiltrate; and negative sputum examination results. The absence of a rheumatic fever history represented a false-negative clue. False-positive clues like the contact with tuberculosis had to be dealt with. Venn diagrams and Set Theory were subconsciously employed in considering the overlap of pulmonary findings, cardiac findings, and hemoptysis.

Bayes' theorems were an integral part of the reasoning. In considering the causes of hemoptysis, we began by considering the incidence of diseases in the general population. The seven diseases first listed have a relatively high incidence in this country. However, in certain areas of the Orient, paragonimiasis would have been the prime consideration. In addition, we weighed the likelihood of hemoptysis given a certain disease and the likelihood of a disease given the symptom of hemoptysis.

This problem could probably have been very quickly solved by an experienced clinician. Presented with a patient who coughed blood, he or she would have ordered a stat chest radiograph, asked 5 or 10 pertinent questions while examining the heart and lungs, and out would have come the diagnosis of mitral stenosis. The physician would then have completed the data base at leisure, ruling out the other already unlikely possibilities, establishing concomitant diseases, and confirming the first impression. *(P.C.)*

Suggested Readings

Bakarti JB, Tashkin DP, Small GW. Factitious hemoptysis. Adding to the differential diagnosis. Chest 1994;105(3):943–945.

Cahill BC, Ingbar DH. Massive hemoptysis. Assessment and management. Clin Chest Med 1994;15(1):147–167.

DiLeo MD, Gianoli GJ. Diagnosis and management of hemoptysis. J La State Med Soc 1994;146(4):155–158.

CASE 36

COUGH, FEVER, AND CHILLS

Lisa L. Dever and W. G. Johanson, Jr

Data A 32-year-old architect comes to the physician's office complaining of awakening with fever, pain in the left chest aggravated by deep breathing, and cough productive of sputum. While eating breakfast he had a single shaking chill that lasted for 5 minutes. He had felt reasonably well up until 2 days ago, when he experienced headache, nasal congestion, and a mild cough, symptoms he attributed to a cold. The patient smokes two packs of cigarettes daily. He is single and lives with a roommate who has not been ill.

Logic This is a characteristic history for bacterial pneumonia. Many patients with bacterial pneumonia have antecedent upper respiratory symptoms for 24 to 72 hours before the development of symptoms of lower respiratory tract disease. The association of influenza with bacterial pneumonia is well documented. However, other viral infections may also be associated with bacterial pneumonia.

Data Physical examination reveals an acutely ill patient with flushed face, slight cyanosis of the nail beds and lips, and frequent episodes of cough that elicit severe left chest pains. Vital signs are: temperature, 39.4° C; pulse, 110/min; BP, 120/82; and respirations, 24/min.

The left hemithorax shows diminished expansion with dullness and increased tactile fremitus posteriorly. Breath sounds in this area are increased in intensity and distinctly bronchial in quality; whispered pectoriloquy is present. Numerous fine inspiratory crackles are heard over the lower third of the left chest posteriorly. No pleural friction rub is heard. The rest of the physical examination results are normal.

Logic The chest radiographic findings are those of consolidation with a patent bronchus. Diminished expansion is due to the combined effects of consolidation plus severe pleural pain with splinting, although physical signs of pleuritis are not present. Obstruction of a lobar bronchus with distal atelectasis leads to dullness and *absent* breath sounds, findings that mimic pleural effusion. Pneumonia is the most probable diagnosis. Examination failed to reveal signs of infection at other sites that might have been the source of the pneumonia or have resulted from it. Now the physician's problem is to determine the etiology of this pneumonia so that appropriate therapy can be given.

Data Chest radiographs including posteroanterior (Fig. 15.6), lateral, and left lateral decubitus views disclose extensive consolidation of the left lower lobe but no pleural effusion. The right lung and left upper lobe are normal. The leukocyte count is 23,500/mm^3 with 90% polymorphonuclear leukocytes (PMNs). Arterial blood gases while breathing room air reveal: pH, 7.46; PCO$_2$, 30 mm Hg; PO$_2$, 52 mm Hg; and 84% saturation. A Gram's stain of expectorated sputum shows PMNs and numerous gram-positive, lancet-shaped diplococci (Fig. 15.7). A sputum culture and two sets of blood cultures are obtained.

Logic The markedly elevated leukocyte count strongly supports bacterial infection because nor-

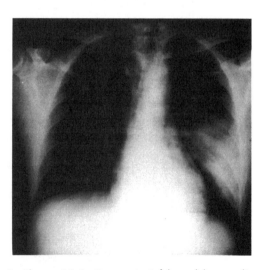

▶ **Figure 15.6.** Pneumonia. Left lower lobe consolidation.

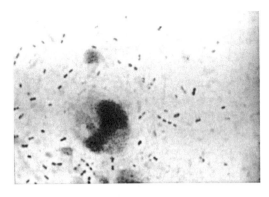

▶ **Figure 15.7.** Sputum smear. Gram-positive lancet-shaped diplococci (pneumococcus).

mal or low values are usually found in patients with viral or other nonbacterial pneumonias. Alveolar hyperventilation is present, as indicated by the low PCO_2. Hypoxemia in pneumonia is due to ventilation-perfusion mismatching and to the development of shunts in regions of alveolar consolidation that maintain some perfusion without ventilation.

A presumptive diagnosis of pneumococcal pneumonia has been made. A predisposing factor such as viral infection or underlying chronic disease is present in at least 70% of persons with community-acquired bacterial pneumonia. Although patients with HIV infection are well known to be at high risk for lung infections caused by opportunistic pathogens such as *P. carinii* and mycobacteria, they are also at increased risk for bacterial pneumonia as well. The usual organisms associated with bacterial pneumonia are *Streptococcus pneumoniae* (pneumococcus) and *H. influenzae*. Less common agents are *Moraxella (Branhamella) catarrhalis, S. aureus, S. pyogenes* (group A streptococcus), various gram-negative bacilli, particularly *Klebsiella pneumoniae,* and on occasion anaerobic bacteria. *Legionella, Mycoplasma,* and *Chlamydia* species, causative agents of so-called atypical pneumonia, must also be considered.

Influenza markedly increases the likelihood of staphylococcal pneumonia, and this agent must therefore be sought with great care in patients suspected of having an antecedent viral illness consistent with influenza. Staphylococcal pneumonia typically involves multiple lung segments, is usually bilateral, and is associated with early lung necrosis, abscess formation, and empyema. The absence of cavitation and pleural effusion, the localized nature of the process, the apparent absence of the organism in sputum, and the absence of a preceding illness consistent with influenza, argue against a staphylococcal etiology.

Pneumonia due to group A streptococcus occurs principally in young persons and typically produces an early exuberant empyema. Community-acquired pneumonias due to *H. influenzae, N. catarrhalis* or enteric bacilli such as *K. pneumoniae* are uncommon in previously healthy adults, occurring principally in individuals with chronic obstructive lung disease, alcoholism, and perhaps diabetes. Pneumonia caused by *S. pneumoniae* and *H. influenzae* are common in patients with HIV infection, even before the clinical development of AIDS. Patients should be questioned about possible risk factors for HIV infection, and the physician should be alert for findings on physical examination or laboratory evaluation, such as oral thrush or hairy leukoplakia, lymphadenopathy, or lymphopenia, that may be suggestive of HIV infection. In some patients, testing for HIV antibody may be warranted.

Data The patient is admitted to the hospital and given ceftriaxone 1 g every 12 hours, oxygen at 4 L/min, and codeine for pleuritic pain.

Logic Many patients with community-acquired pneumonia can be successfully treated with oral antibiotics as outpatients. Patients who are severely ill or have multiple risk factors for increased morbidity and mortality should be hospitalized. Among these risk factors are age greater than 65 years, chronic underlying illnesses, hypotension, hypoxemia, leukopenia or leukocytosis, and unfavorable chest radiograph findings (multiple lobe involvement, presence of a cavity or pleural effusion).

It would be comforting for physicians if the bacterial etiology of pneumonia could be determined quickly and safely. Blood cultures are positive in up to one third of patients and, if positive, provide by far the best means of establishing the bacterial agent responsible for pneumonia. Pleural fluid is the second best source, and a sample should be obtained if fluid is present. This was the reason for the lateral decubitus radiograph taken of this patient. Sputum cultures are more problematic because the rates of both false positivity and false negativity may be 25% or higher. Contamination of expectorated specimens by secretions from the oropharynx is a major cause of this problem. Transtracheal aspiration avoids the resident flora of the upper respiratory tract and typically yields fewer species of potentially pathogenic bacteria than expectorated sputum. This procedure is used to establish the causative role of anaerobic bacteria in certain infections of the lower respiratory tract, such as lung abscess. It is rarely indicated in the evaluation of patients with pneumonia as it has largely been supplanted by safer fiberoptic bronchoscopic techniques. Such techniques allow sampling of lower airways in the area of pneumonia with a protected sterile brush while avoiding contamination by organisms present in the upper airways. Transthoracic lung aspiration may also be used to obtain material directly from the lung parenchyma for stain and culture; the rate of complications with this procedure is too high to permit its use in the routine evaluation of pneumonia, at least in adults.

Pneumonia due to respiratory viruses, mycoplasma, or *Legionella* may have a similar presentation to that of this patient. However, such pneumonias are generally more diffuse, lack shaking rigors, and are not associated with numerous PMNs and bacteria in respiratory secretions. Even though pneumococcal pneumonia is suspected clinically in this patient, sputum culture was obtained to attempt to confirm the diagnosis and to detect the presence of penicillin-resistant pneumococci.

Data The patient partially improved with treatment. However, on the fourth day he still had an oral temperature of 38.3°C and complained of persistent discomfort in the left chest. Physical examination revealed flatness to percussion, absent tactile and vocal fremitus, and markedly diminished breath sounds over the left lower lobe. Radiographs confirmed the presence of a moderately large pleural effusion. Thoracentesis was performed with the removal of 1000 mL of slightly cloudy fluid containing 6000 leukocytes per mm^3, 85% of which were PMNs. Gram's stains of the fluid did not reveal organisms and both anaerobic and aerobic cultures were subsequently negative. Following aspiration of the pleural fluid, the patient's recovery was uneventful.

Logic This effusion represents a parapneumonic effusion. These are common with pneumococcal pneumonia, although, as with this patient, they usually develop after several days of treatment and are sterile. It is important to note that other bacterial agents may have been present from the onset or may have been acquired during antibiotic therapy. Empyema is particularly common with pneumonia due to staphylococci, gram-negative bacilli, or anaerobic bacteria. The patient's original sputum culture yielded only pneumococci that were fully susceptible to penicillin, and therefore also ceftriaxone; his blood cultures were sterile. Empyema due to inadequately treated lung infection produces grossly cloudy pleural fluid with leukocyte counts exceeding 25,000/mm^3; organisms are usually evident by stain and culture. Pleural fluid pH is helpful in deciding which exudative effusions will require drainage. If the pH of a parapneumonic effusion is less than 7.2, a tube thoracostomy will be necessary.

Continuing fever after 3 to 4 days of antibiotic treatment in a patient with pneumonia requires investigation. Most commonly, an incorrect choice of antibiotics is responsible, such as penicillin treatment of mycoplasma pneumonia or erythromycin for treatment of gram-negative bacillary pneumonia. A recent concern is the appearance of strains of pneumococci that are resistant to penicillin as well as other drugs commonly used to treat pneumonia. In some areas, 25% or more of pneumococcal isolates may be resistant to penicillin. This has led some experts to recommend the use of broader spectrum cephalosporins, such as cefuroxime or ceftriaxone, in the initial treatment regimen for patients with severe community-acquired pneumonia; they are active against pneumococci, including most penicillin-resistant strains, as well as *H. influenzae*. When culture results and susceptibilities are known, therapy can be adjusted accordingly. For example, this patient with a fully susceptible pneumococcus could be continued on ceftriaxone or changed to penicillin. Other causes for continued fever must also be considered and ruled out by physical examination or special procedures. These include lung abscess, pericarditis, meningitis, or other remote foci of infection. Last, "drug fever" may be responsible, although this diagnosis should not be entertained until other causes of fever have been eliminated.

Questions

1. Microorganisms that commonly cause early pleural effusions in pneumonia include:
   (a) *S. aureus.*
   (b) anaerobic streptococci.
   (c) *K. pneumoniae.*
   (d) *Mycoplasma pneumoniae.*
2. Isolation of *S. pneumoniae* from which of the following specimens would prove the etiology of a pneumonia beyond any reasonable doubt?
   (a) Expectorated sputum
   (b) Pleural fluid
   (c) Transtracheal aspirate
   (d) Blood
3. Causes of continued fever after 4 days of treatment of *H. influenzae* pneumonia with ceftriaxone include:
   (a) presence of pericarditis.
   (b) inappropriate initial selection of antibiotic.
   (c) presence of pleural effusion.
   (d) development of resistance of *H. influenzae* isolate to ceftriaxone during therapy.
4. Which of the following patients are predisposed to bacterial pneumonia caused by *S. pneumoniae?*
   (a) A 75-year-old smoker with chronic obstructive pulmonary disease
   (b) A bone marrow transplantation patient
   (c) A 40-year-old HIV-infected patient
   (d) A 19-year-old army recruit in basic training

Answers

1. **(a), (b), and (c) are correct.** Pleural effusions may occur in the course of pneumococcal pneumonia; most occur after several days of illness and are not present on admission to the hospital. However, the presence of an early pleural effusion should alert the physician to the likelihood of another etiologic agent, because such effusions are commonly found with pneumonia due to *S. aureus*, anaerobic organisms, gram-negative bacilli, and group A streptococci. Mycoplasma pneumonia may produce effusions in up to 20% of patients, but these are almost always small and usually undetected.
2. **(b) and (d) are correct.** The finding of pneumococci in sputum is difficult to interpret because the rate of false positives is approximately 25%. In a similar percentage of patients with pneumococcal pneumonia, the organism cannot be recovered in sputum cultures (false negatives); in such patients a Gram's stain of sputum may be more rewarding than the culture. Transtracheal aspiration improves the yield somewhat, but there remain yet a significant number of both false-negative and false-positive specimens. However, isolation of *S. pneumoniae* from either pleural fluid or blood is incontrovertible evidence of infection due to the organism. Pleural fluid should always be examined and blood cultures should be drawn in patients requiring hospitalization before initiating therapy.

3. **(a) and (c) are correct.** Ceftriaxone is appropriate therapy for *H. influenzae* and resistance does not develop during treatment. Continued fever after 4 days of appropriate antibiotic therapy would suggest a complicated pneumonia. The presence of a parapneumonic effusion or empyema or pericarditis could result in continued fever.

4. **(a) and (c) are correct.** Patients with underlying diseases such as chronic obstructive pulmonary disease and HIV infection are particularly susceptible to pneumonias with community-acquired bacterial pathogens. As an aside, such patients should receive pneumococcal vaccine in an effort to prevent pneumococcal infection. Hospital-acquired pneumonias are usually due to gram-negative bacilli, and patients who are seriously ill or immunosuppressed are particularly susceptible. Infection with opportunistic pathogens including fungi, mycobacteria, viruses, and *P. carinii* can also occur in severely neutropenic and immunosuppressed patients, particularly those receiving bone marrow or organ transplantations. Pneumonias among military recruits, or among other groups of healthy young persons, are generally viral, mycoplasmal, or chlamydial in etiology.

COMMENT Problem solving was simple for this patient for whom the symptoms, physical signs, and chest radiographic findings were typical for lobar pneumonia; the sputum examination clearly identified the causative organism as the pneumococcus (*S. pneumoniae*). The presenting pictures for all types of pneumonia are not so characteristic. This is especially true for viral pneumonias, legionnaires' disease, psittacosis, mycoplasmal pneumonia, and those due to more virulent bacterial organisms.

It is important to identify pneumonia quickly when it exists and to try to determine its microbiologic cause, because treatment may differ.

Distinctions are made by the clinical picture, the nature of the radiologic changes, and special laboratory procedures. Some features suggest one organism rather than another. If herpes labialis is present, suspect the pneumococcus. If bullous myringitis is present, suspect *Mycoplasma*. In an outbreak among middle-aged male smokers who attended a convention 1 month ago, suspect *Legionella pneumophila*. Think of Q fever (*Coxiella burnetii*) if there was recent contact with infected livestock. And consider aspiration pneumonia (mouth organisms) if there was a preceding episode of altered consciousness caused by alcohol, epilepsy, stroke, or drug overdose.

Cough and *fever* are generally present in all pneumonias. Other than direct identification by smear and culture (tests that have varied sensitivity and specificity depending on the source of tested material), rising titers of cold agglutinins (IgM antibodies) in mycoplasma infection and the detection of direct fluorescent antibody in *Legionella* infection may help make the diagnosis.

Always to be considered is pneumonia in the *immune-compromised host*. If the patient is a promiscuous male homosexual, has hemophilia, takes steroids for any disease, has undergone a renal transplantation with suppressed immunity, or has leukemia or lymphoma, he or she is highly eligible for developing infection. This often takes the form of pneumonia and may be caused by ordinary bacteria; but notable in these patients is the development of infection with gram-negative bacilli, *Candida, Aspergillus fumigatus,* cytomegalovirus, mycobacteria, and *P. carinii.*

Because so many antibiotics are available for treating pneumonias, you should choose the antibiotic on the basis of a clinical assumption, or better yet on the basis of direct or indirect organism identification. *(P.C.)*

Suggested Readings

Bartlett JG, Mundy LM. Community-acquired pneumonia. N Engl J Med 1995;333:1618–1623.

Fang GD, Fine M, Orloff J, et al. New and emerging etiologies for community-acquired pneumonia with implications for therapy: A prospective multicenter study of 359 cases. Medicine 1990;69:307–316.

Marrie TJ. Community-acquired pneumonia. Clin Infect Dis 1994;18:501–513.

SUDDEN SHORTNESS OF BREATH

W. G. Johanson, Jr, and Juan A. Albino

Data A 48-year-old woman noticed shortness of breath one morning while climbing a flight of stairs to her office. She had been aware of discomfort in her right chest for several days but related this symptom to chronic cigarette smoking. On further questioning the patient reported that she had enjoyed excellent health except for a fracture of the left femur sustained in an automobile accident 3 years earlier. Since that time she had experienced recurrent swelling and mild pain in the left lower extremity, aggravated by prolonged standing or walking, and relieved by rest and elevation of the leg.

Logic Dyspnea of sudden onset is usually due to a major cardiac or pulmonary event. Acute myocardial infarction with pulmonary congestion is one of the most common causes, although the patient's age, sex, and lack of angina-type pain make the diagnosis unlikely in this case. Acute left ventricular failure can occur from other causes, but is usually preceded by a long history of heart disease. Tachyarrhythmias may produce dyspnea and are usually abrupt in onset; many are accompanied by "palpitations," a sensation not experienced by our patient.

Pulmonary embolism is frequently followed by dyspnea and chest pain. Most patients with pulmonary embolism have risk factors such as cancer, surgery, congestive heart failure, prolonged immobility, abnormalities of the leg veins, leg trauma, or prior history of thrombosis. The history of unilateral orthostatic edema is suggestive of chronic venous disease and must raise the physician's index of suspicion, because the femoral fracture may have led to deep vein thrombosis and consequent venous insufficiency.

Pneumonia may certainly have the sudden onset of dyspnea, although associated symptoms of fever, cough, and sputum production usually dominate the clinical picture. Spontaneous pneumothorax may produce symptoms that vary from mild to severe depending on the extent of lung collapse, the pressure within the pleural space, and the presence or absence of underlying lung disease.

The symptoms of pleural effusion may be acute or chronic and vary widely depending on the cause of the effusion, the rapidity of its development, and the presence of underlying cardiopulmonary disease.

Data The patient's vital signs were normal except for a respiratory rate of 24 breaths per minute. Examination of the head and neck was unremarkable; the neck veins were flat with the patient elevated to 45 degrees, and the trachea was not deviated. The heart was normal in size, and auscultation was entirely normal. Examination of the chest revealed diminished expansion of the right hemithorax, diminished fremitus, and dullness to percussion to the level of the right midscapula posteriorly, and markedly diminished breath sounds over the right lower chest. There was a firm, nontender, 2-cm nodule in the upper outer quadrant of the right breast; several enlarged axillary lymph nodes were also palpable. The left lower extremity was mildly edematous and the left calf circumference was 3 cm greater than the right. Neither lower extremity was tender to palpation, venous cords were not found, and Homans' sign was absent.

Logic The physical findings indicate the presence of a large right pleural effusion that is the probable cause of the patient's symptoms. The physician must now determine the cause of the effusion in order to plan effective therapy. The most common causes of pleural effusion are shown in Table 15.2.

On the basis of history and physical examination, you can rule out all but the last four. Connective tissue disease would be unlikely in the absence of other symptoms. The physical findings provide clues that may support malignancy or pulmonary embolus. At this point, radi-

ographic studies and analysis of the pleural fluid are indispensable.

Data Radiographs of the chest were taken in posteroanterior, lateral, right lateral decubitus, and left lateral decubitus positions. The posteroanterior radiograph showed a large right pleural effusion; the cardiac and mediastinal structures appeared normal. With decubitus positions, the fluid layered out along the chest wall, which indicated that the fluid was not loculated; and the height of the fluid was 5 cm, which indicated that it was safe (>1 cm) to tap it (Fig. 15.8). The left lateral decubitus radiograph was taken to better evaluate the right lower lobe of the lung. No lesions were identified in the right lung. Thus, the patient has a pleural effusion without underlying lung infiltration. An intermediate purified protein derivative (PPD) skin test was applied.

Thoracentesis was performed in the ninth intercostal space in the posterior axillary line. Several hundred milliliters of serous fluid were easily obtained. Multiple pleural biopsies were performed in the same needle tract with an Abrams needle. These specimens were submitted for the following tests: total protein, lactate dehydrogenase (LDH), glucose, white blood cell count and differential, specific gravity, Gram's stain, fluorochrome stain, and cultures for aerobic and anaerobic bacteria, mycobacteria, and fungi. Cytologic preparations were made from the unspun

TABLE 15.2. Common Causes of Pleural Effusion

TRANSUDATIVE	EXUDATIVE
Congestive heart failure	Pneumonia
Cirrhosis of the liver	Pulmonary embolism
Nephrotic syndrome	Tuberculosis
	Cancer
	Connective tissue diseases

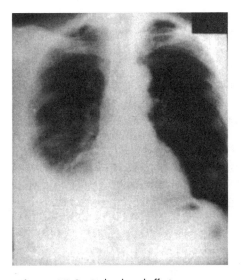

▶ **Figure 15.8.** Right pleural effusion.

fluid and a cell block was prepared from the sediment following centrifugation.

One piece of pleural tissue was homogenized and cultured for mycobacteria; the other pieces were fixed in formalin. A simultaneous blood specimen was submitted for measurement of total protein, LDH, and glucose. The resultant pleural fluid data are shown in Table 15.3.

Logic Transudates usually have low white blood cell counts and a specific gravity less than 1.015. Exudates and transudates can be distinguished more reliably on the basis of the ratio of pleural fluid to serum protein and LDH concentrations, and the absolute pleural fluid LDH concentration. A pleural exudate is defined by fluid that meets at least one of the following criteria: the pleural fluid:serum ratio exceeds 0.5 for protein or 0.6 for LDH, or the pleural fluid LDH exceeds 2/3 of the serum LDH. If none of these criteria are met, the fluid is a transudate. Total blood cell and differential counts show large variations and are of less help, except when great numbers of polymorphonuclear leukocytes are present, which indicates pyogenic infection.

Except for cases of obvious congestive heart failure, thoracentesis is almost always necessary for a diagnosis. The appearance of the fluid alone may guide you. A milky fluid (chylothorax) usually suggests lymphoma or cancer obstructing the thoracic duct. However, turbidity may be caused by lipid or leukocytes. Blood-tinged (serosanguinous) fluid results from 10^3 to 10^4 red blood cells per mm^3 and may be seen with a variety of causes. Grossly bloody fluid (hemothorax) indicates the presence of 10^5 or more red blood cells per mm^3 (or pleural fluid hematocrit > .5 blood hematocrit) and is seen in patients with cancer, trauma, and dissecting aneurysm.

The distinction between transudate and exudate is most important. Transudates occur in congestive heart failure, hepatic cirrhosis, the nephrotic syndrome, and protein malnutrition. Pleural effusions associated with malignancy, tuberculosis (TB), connective tissue diseases, pneumonia, or pulmonary infarction are generally exudative. The predominance of either neutrophils or lymphocytes has diagnostic utility, with lymphocytosis, as in this case, pointing to cancer or tuberculosis.

Data The intermediate PPD (tuberculin) skin test result was negative, resulting in only 3-mm induration after 48 hours. Gram's and fluorochrome (acid-fast) stains of the pleural fluid did not reveal organisms.

Logic The negative PPD skin test is helpful because at least 70% of immunocompetent patients who have tuberculous effusions have positive (> 10 mm) skin tests. However, many adults may have positive tests anyway, and this finding would not have proved the etiology of the patient's effusion. The pleural biopsy will reveal granulomas in approximately 40% of patients with tuberculous effusions, and another 30% of patients will have positive TB cultures from either pleural fluid or pleural tissue. Thus, a definite diagnosis of tuberculosis can be made in approximately 70% of patients; repeat pleural biopsies from other sites increases the yield even further. Similarly, malignant cells will be recovered from either pleural fluid, the sediment sectioned as a cell block, or the pleural biopsy specimen in approximately 75% of patients who have malignant effusions. In both circumstances, the pleural biopsy significantly increases the diagnostic yield from thoracentesis.

While awaiting the results of these studies, the physician still faces the possibility that a pulmonary embolism is the cause of the patient's symptoms and pleural effusion. The chemical findings in the pleural fluid would be compatible with that diagnosis, although blood-tinged fluid is more typical. Arterial blood gases usually reveal an increased alveolar-arterial oxygen gradient following pulmonary embolism. However, this finding is

TABLE 15.3. Pleural Fluid Findings*

TESTS	PLEURAL FLUID	SERUM
Total protein	4.5 g/dL	7.0 g/dL
LDH	240 IU/L	80 IU/L
WBC	800/mm³	—
	(84% lymphocytes)	—
Glucose	88 mg/dL	100 mg/dL
Specific gravity	1.021	—

*Patient's data. The pleural fluid is an exudate as noted in the text by the pleural fluid:serum ratios of protein and LDH.
LDH = lactate dehydrogenase; WBC = white blood cell count.

nonspecific and a large pleural effusion would be expected to produce hypoxemia, regardless of its etiology, due to impaired ventilation of the underlying lung.

Ventilation and perfusion lung scans can be performed rapidly with no hazard to the patient. It must be kept in mind that the effusion alone will cause diminished perfusion and ventilation to the right lower lobe. Thus, a perfusion defect in this region will not be interpretable; pulmonary emboli can be diagnosed in this situation only when multiple perfusion defects are found in areas of lung that appear normal on the chest radiographs, and especially on the ventilation scan (unmatched defects).

Data After removal of all possible fluid by thoracentesis, a perfusion lung scan showed only nonsegmental decreased perfusion in the right lower lobe, and a ventilation scan also showed diminished uptake in the same area (matched defect). Thus, anticoagulants were not begun. Doppler studies of the legs were negative for deep vein thrombosis. Mammography revealed a stellate lesion with punctate calcifications in the right breast suggestive of a malignancy. The pleural biopsy showed nests of malignant cells compatible with metastatic carcinoma of the breast. Biopsy of the right breast mass revealed a tumor with similar histology. All cultures were subsequently negative for mycobacteria. The diagnosis is now certain: carcinoma of the breast with pleural metastases.

Logic In this instance the diagnosis is clearly evident. But if the ventilation/perfusion scans were indeterminate (i.e., neither normal nor high probability), and had the pleural and breast biopsies been negative for cancer, further studies to exclude a pulmonary embolus might have been indicated, such as pulmonary arteriography. However, one could first perform Doppler studies of the legs, because if they are positive for deep vein thrombosis, anticoagulation therapy is mandatory; and angiography becomes a moot point. Should emboli recur despite adequate anticoagulation, a filter can be placed in the inferior vena cava below the renal veins. In this patient, had pulmonary emboli been found, the source was already apparent in her swollen left leg, probably resulting from chronic venous insufficiency.

Questions

(More than one answer may be correct.)
1. The mediastinum may shift:
   (a) toward the side of a large pleural effusion.
   (b) toward the side of a pneumothorax.
   (c) toward the side of pneumonia.
   (d) toward the side of atelectasis.
2. A region of decreased perfusion visualized on a perfusion lung scan:
   (a) indicates decreased capillary blood flow in that region relative to other regions of the lungs.
   (b) indicates pulmonary vascular obstruction, usually due to emboli.
   (c) suggests embolism only if no corresponding infiltrate or ventilation defect is present.
   (d) is helpful in diagnosing pulmonary embolism in the presence of emphysema.
3. In evaluating patients with pleural effusions:
   (a) therapy for the suspected disorder should be instituted promptly, and thoracentesis should be reserved for those patients who do not respond promptly.
   (b) pleural biopsy adds significantly to the diagnostic accuracy of thoracentesis.
   (c) it is advisable to obtain only small amounts of fluid initially because more can be readily obtained later if needed.
   (d) serum should always be obtained simultaneously for comparison of certain values between pleural fluid and serum.

Answers

1. **(d) is correct.** Shift of the mediastinum is an important sign that indicates either loss of volume of one lung or an increase in the volume of the other. It is detected by tracheal deviation, asymmetric chest expansion, and displacement of the apex beat. Because both a pleural effusion and a pneumothorax increase the volume of the involved hemithorax by the addition of either air or fluid, mediastinal shift, if present, should be away from the side of involvement. Such shift may be an important clue to the presence of tension pneumothorax. Despite the large effusion, the mediastinum did not shift in the patient just discussed. It may have been fixed by tumor. Shift of the mediastinum toward the involved lung indicates atelectasis of the underlying lung.
2. **(a) and (c) are correct.** Regionally depressed activity on a perfusion lung scan indicates decreased capil-

lary blood flow but does not clarify the reason for such a decrease. A decreased capillary bed (as in emphysema) or regional alveolar hypoxia with vasoconstriction (as in airway disease, pneumonia, or atelectasis) can decrease capillary blood flow and mimic the vascular obstruction seen with pulmonary embolism. Such regions will usually display impaired ventilation as well. Thus, combined ventilation and perfusion scans provide the most definitive information in suspected cases of pulmonary embolism. Multiple segmental perfusion defects with normal ventilation (unmatched large defects) are highly suggestive of pulmonary emboli.

3. **(b) and (d) are correct.** Failure to obtain pleural fluid before initiating therapy may delay making the proper diagnosis and complicate interpretation of the results. Pleural fluid should always be obtained if the diagnosis is in doubt. In inflammatory conditions, pleural fluid may loculate rapidly and render subsequent attempts at thoracentesis unsuccessful. Therefore, aspiration of all obtainable fluid is advised. In the hands of experienced physicians, pleural biopsy adds only a small additional risk to the possible complications of thoracentesis itself (pneumothorax, hemorrhage, infection) and the diagnostic yield far exceeds the added risk. The comparison of pleural fluid: serum levels of protein, LDH, and glucose may provide more valuable data than the pleural fluid levels alone, because serum levels may vary widely among individuals; thus, simultaneous serum tests should always be obtained. The presence of an obvious pneumonia with an ipsilateral effusion (parapneumonic effusion) also mandates early thoracentesis to ascertain whether chest tube drainage is indicated (empyema, most complicated parapneumonic effusions) or not required (uncomplicated parapneumonic effusion).

COMMENT The principal problem-solving technique here was the use of the key clue. First it was acute dyspnea; next it was a pleural effusion. Each was pursued by considering the major causes, eliminating most by the absence of concomitant features, and proving the presence of only one. Emboli from thrombophlebitis and metastatic cancer from a palpable breast lesion became the dominant Bayesian likelihoods as the author pondered the specificity-sensitivity of the PPD skin test, the isotope lung scan, and the studies of pleural fluid and pleura. The finding of

metastatic cancer cells was the clue with the greatest three-dimensional magnitude. The presence of old thrombophlebitis and cigarette smoking were misleading positive clues. A direct approach using a chest radiograph, thoracentesis, scan, and study of the pleura and its fluid would have solved the problem quickly—no questions asked or examination done until later. *(P.C.)*

Suggested Readings

Manning HL, Schwartzstein RM. Pathophysiology of dyspnea. N Engl J Med 1995;333:1547–1553.

Sahn SA. Management of complicated parapneumonic effusions. Am Rev Respir Dis 1993;148:813–817.

Sahn SA. State of the art: The pleura. Am Rev Respir Dis 1988;138:184–234.

CHEST PAIN AND SHORTNESS OF BREATH

Paul Cutler

Data Your 65-year-old patient of long standing calls you from his home because of the sudden onset of sharp left chest pains and shortness of breath. He tells you he just returned from a 1-month business trip to the Orient and that he wasn't too well there, either. You tell him to meet you in the hospital's emergency department, because you suspect something serious.

Logic This combination of symptoms frequently augurs a major cardiopulmonary event, and with his known background, on the way to the hospital you mull over the possibilities of acute myocardial infarction, dissecting aneurysm, and pulmonary embolus. At the same time, you consider less threatening situations such as a musculoskeletal injury, spontaneous pneumothorax, and a pleuritic reaction resulting from pulmonary infection.

Data Having reviewed his records before departing, you first recall that the patient had a myocardial infarction 10 years ago from which he made a satisfactory recovery. Yet for the past few years he has had chest discomfort on walking fast or against a wind on the average of twice a month. This is promptly relieved by a nitroglycerine tablet under his tongue.

Second, you note that he has had mild-to-moderate hypertension for many years, and that despite various antihypertensive medications, his blood pressure usually hovers around 160/96 on visits to the office. And third, you see a consultation report from the patient's urologist reminding you that the patient had a prostatectomy 2 years ago for carcinoma, and that he takes diethylstilbestrol daily.

Logic The patient has coronary artery disease, an old myocardial infarction, and stable angina pectoris. This episode may well represent another infarction. It is important to know what type of pain he is having.

Long-standing hypertension can result in aortic dissection. The presence of cancer, the taking of estrogens, and the recent prolonged plane trip are all predisposing factors toward the development of pulmonary embolism.

Data Upon arriving at the emergency department, you immediately note that he is very uncomfortable, takes shallow frequent breaths, and seems to be splinting his left side. The pain is sharp, like a knife, and occurs whenever he inspires. He had several similar episodes of chest pain while in the Orient, once on the left side and twice on the right. He saw a physician who told him he had pleurisy and prescribed some antibiotics. Each time he recovered rapidly.

On his return trip, the airplane encountered turbulence while he was on the way to the restroom, and he was thrown against the side of a seat, striking the right side of his chest. It hurt for a few minutes, and there were no bruises.

Logic The pain is clearly pleuritic in nature. The dyspnea seems to be caused by the pain and is related to the fact that his breaths must be rapid and shallow to minimize the pain. Coronary chest pain is heavy, continuous, and central. The pain of dissecting aneurysm is much the same. Most pulmonary emboli do not cause pain. However, large ones that result in a high degree of obstruction may initially cause pain that resembles that of myocardial infarction because of associated generalized vasospasm and acute pulmonary hypertension. The characteristic chest pain resulting from pulmonary emboli is pleuritic in nature and comes on several hours to days after the embolic event has occurred; it results from pulmonary infarction and its associated pleuritis.

Although the patient injured himself in the airplane, this does not explain pain on the other side and the episodes that had previously occurred. Pain resulting from a musculoskeletal injury would be worse on certain body movements. And even though pneumonia may be associated with pleuritic pain and dyspnea, the presenting clinical features generally highlight cough and fever.

Data He has had no pain, swelling, or discomfort in the legs, has not been coughing, and has not felt feverish nor had chills. Other than the symptoms already described, he has felt well and has a good appetite and strength.

Logic Infectious pleuritis may be eliminated. The absence of symptoms in the legs does not exclude deep thrombophlebitis because these symptoms do not have high sensitivity. Their presence would not be highly specific, only suggestive.

Data Physical examination: temperature, 98°F; pulse, 116 and slightly irregular; respirations, 28; and BP, 180/100 in both arms. Pulses are normal everywhere and equal on both sides. The patient is in distress. Morphine sulfate is given to relieve pain. Neck veins are distended to the angles of the jaw with the patient lying at 45 degrees; there are prominent "a" waves. Premature contractions without compensatory pause are noted.

The apex beat is not felt, but there is a prominent right ventricular lift at the lower left sternal border. The second pulmonic sound is loud and is also felt in the left second intercostal space. There is an S_4 heard in the area of the ventricular lift.

Logic These findings are very helpful. The equality of pulses weighs against aortic dissection. Pulmonary hypertension with right ventricular strain and beginning failure are evidenced by the nature of the P_2, the lift, the right ventricular S_4, the prominent "a" waves, the premature contractions that are probably atrial, and the high jugular venous pressure.

The cardiac findings plus the history of repeated episodes of pleuritis point in the direction of multiple pulmonary emboli. Let's do the examination of the lungs and legs.

Data There is dullness, absent fremitus, and decreased breath sounds at both bases, especially on the left. No friction rubs or rales were heard. The calves were not tender to deep palpation and Homans' sign was negative. There is no cyanosis, clubbing, or edema.

Logic Examination of the chest suggests the presence of bilateral medium-sized pleural effusions, more on the left, although it is difficult to be sure because of splinted breathing. If a spontaneous pneumothorax had occurred, there would be tympany on the left side.

Data An immediate radiograph of the chest shows small bilateral pleural effusions and a normal cardiovascular silhouette. The ECG reveals sinus tachycardia, multiple atrial premature contractions, and an $S_1 Q_3 T_3$ pattern that may be found in the presence of acute pulmonary embolus (Fig. 15.9). CBC is normal. Arterial blood gases on room air reveal a pH of 7.50, a PCO_2 of 32 mm Hg, a PO_2 of 62 mm Hg, and an alveolar-arterial oxygen gradient of 42.

Logic A dissecting aneurysm is virtually excluded by the type of pain, the equality of pulses, the normal cardiovascular contour, and the physical findings that point elsewhere. The low PO_2 is understandable in the presence of what probably represents at least a 50% decrease in the pulmonary vascular bed. The low PCO_2 and moderate alkalosis result from hyperventilation, and the widened gradient is characteristic.

The ECG pattern in pulmonary embolus is variable. Most commonly there are no changes. Abnormalities are not specific and they may range from sinus tachycardia to atrial irritability to right axis deviation, and to the pattern observed in this patient—a picture that may be confused with an inferior wall myocardial infarction. There was no evidence of the old infarct.

Data The patient was hospitalized and immediately placed on intravenous heparin with continuous ECG monitoring. A ventilation-perfusion (V-Q) scan performed the next day showed multiple areas of mismatch, not only at the lung bases where you might expect it from the effusions alone, but also in the left and right midlung fields. Several ventilated areas were not perfused (Fig. 15.10).

The pain rapidly subsided and breathing became normal. Evidence for right ventricular strain gradually lessened. In view of the subsiding clinical picture and the initiation of highly-indicated anticoagulation, thoracentesis was deemed unnecessary and inadvisable. The blood count, blood chemistries, and cardiac enzymes were normal.

Logic The V-Q scan exhibited "high probability" and under these circumstances, heparin was imperative; high probability scans are truly positive in 97% of patients, whereas normal scans are truly negative in 96% of patients. Indeterminate or low-probability scans need additional studies if clinical suspicion is high. These may include pulmonary arteriography, which is a gold-standard test, or venous imaging of the lower extremities by Doppler ultrasound or phlebography.

Data On the fourth day of treatment, the patient

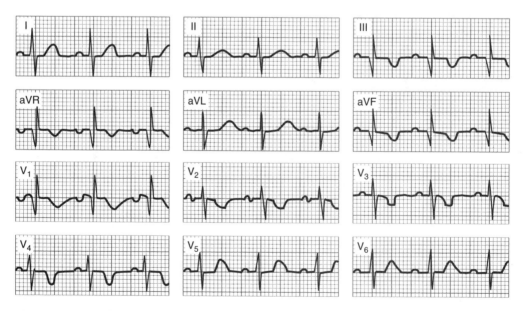

▶ **Figure 15.9.** Cardiac tracing for a pulmonary embolus. Note tachycardia, $S_1 Q_3 T_3$ pattern. Atrial premature contractions not noted in this tracing.

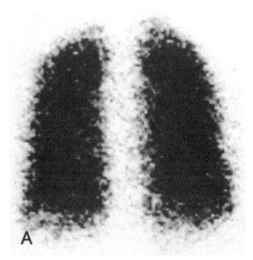

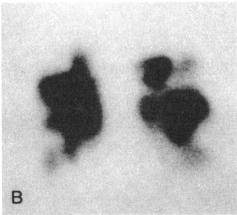

▶ **Figure 15.10. A.** Normal xenon ventilation study. **B.** Multiple large wedge-shaped pleural-based perfusion defects that are mismatched to the ventilation (defects white, perfused areas black).

suddenly and quite rapidly developed severe dyspnea. The neck veins became markedly distended; arterial pressure dropped to 70/50; there were fine rales at the bases; and heart sounds could not be heard.

Logic The acute event of the fourth day represents a hemopericardium with cardiac tamponade resulting from anticoagulant therapy—a dramatic emergency.

Data An emergency chest radiograph showed marked and diffuse widening of the cardiac silhouette. Needle aspiration of 350 mL of frank blood from the pericardial sac via an infrasternal approach resulted in rapid improvement. Heparin was stopped and consideration was given to

the placement of a vena caval filter. Imaging studies for the presence of deep iliofemoral vein thrombosis was deferred.

Logic This unfortunate complication created an ideal climate for the construction of a decision tree that compares the risks and benefits of treating this way or that, a matter that is presently not germane to this case study. However, a classification of factors that predispose to thrombus formation and increase the coagulability of blood is germane.

The risk factors for venous thrombosis include:

- *Stasis,* resulting from prolonged immobility in a bed, chair, or airplane seat; and congestive heart failure
- *Endothelial injury* resulting from pelvic or leg surgery, or leg trauma
- *Hypercoagulability* resulting from malignancies, use of oral contraceptives, and genetic deficiencies of natural coagulation inhibitors (antithrombin III, protein C, protein S)

At least three risk factors were present in this patient—stasis, estrogens, and cancer.

Questions

1. To prove the presence of thrombosis in the deep veins of the lower extremities, which is the most reliable test?
   (a) Physical examination
   (b) Impedance plethysmography
   (c) Radiolabeled fibrinogen
   (d) Doppler ultrasound (duplex)
   (e) Ascending contrast venography
2. Pulmonary emboli may arise from each of the following situations except which one?
   (a) Acute anteroseptal myocardial infarction
   (b) Post hysterectomy
   (c) Mitral stenosis
   (d) Atrial fibrillation
   (e) Post hip replacement
3. Of the pathophysiologic events that are consequent to a pulmonary embolus, which statement is incorrect?
   (a) A "dead space" occurs.
   (b) A decrease in pulmonary surfactant results in alveolar collapse in the affected area.
   (c) Pulmonary infarction is a common consequence.
   (d) Fibrinolysis begins to take place.

Answers

1. **(e) is correct.** Although discomforting and often impractical, this test is most reliable and has the highest sensitivity and specificity. It is the gold-standard test. The physical examination detects abnormalities (tenderness, cords, swelling, redness, positive Homans' sign) in less than half the patients. Impedance studies detect venous outflow obstruction and are best for thrombi in the thighs, but not in the calves. Radiolabeled fibrinogen is no longer available, but radiolabeled platelets are under investigation; these products tend to concentrate in the area of clots. Ultrasound studies are valuable, but their results are operator-dependent and their operating characteristics are not well-defined.

2. **(c) is correct.** Mitral stenosis causes clots to form in an overstretched left atrium, but these embolize to the peripheral circulation. The anteroseptal infarct may result in mural thrombi in either the left or right ventricle. Thrombi from the right ventricle, uterine veins, fibrillating right atrium (plus left), and iliofemoral veins, if dislodged, will embolize to the lung.

3. **(c) is correct.** Infarction occurs in at most 10% of patients. Lung tissue is also supplied by the bronchial circulation, and infarction with hemoptysis and bloody effusions occurs mainly in persons whose cardiorespiratory status is already impaired. The dead space occurs because ventilated tissue is not being perfused. A decrease of surfactant in the affected area results in alveolar shrinkage and decreased ventilation—perhaps a physiologic attempt to offset the dead space. The large majority of emboli will be dissolved by fibrinolysis that begins almost immediately.

COMMENT Critical to the solution of this problem was the nature of the pain and the physical findings. The presence of three risk factors for thromboembolus weighed heavily in the formulation of contending hypotheses. The "high probability" V-Q scan clinched the diagnosis. In this case, one must postulate the presence of clots in the proximal deep veins of a leg. This will have to be proved before a vena cava filter receives serious consideration. *(P.C.)*

Suggested Readings

Hull RD, Feldstein W, Stein PD et al. Cost-effectiveness of pulmonary embolism diagnosis. Arch Intern Med 1996;156:68–72.

Kelley MA, Carson JL, Palevsky H, et al. Diagnosing pulmonary embolism: New facts and strategies. Ann Intern Med 1991;114:300–306.

Moser KM. Venous thromboembolism. Am Rev Respir Dis 1990;141:235–249.

CASE 39

CHRONIC COUGH AND EXPECTORATION

W.G. Johanson, Jr, and Juan A. Albino

Data A 64-year-old unemployed alcoholic man comes to the emergency department because of a change in his chronic cough. He has had a chronic cough productive of scant mucoid sputum for more than 10 years. At least once each year he experiences episodes of acute bronchitis, characterized by increased amounts of sputum that is yellow or slightly green in color. Antibiotic therapy resulted in gradual improvement. Approximately 3 weeks ago he noted slightly increasing amounts of purulent sputum in the early morning. On two occasions, including the morning of admission, he saw streaks of blood after episodes of vigorous coughing.

Logic The patient has chronic bronchitis, which is defined as the presence of a productive cough on most days for at least 3 months during the past 2 years. Chronic bronchitis is a common disease, and as part of the more general disease entity of chronic obstructive pulmonary disease (COPD), it affects as many as 15% of adult men in some surveys. However, it should be recognized for what it is: a chronic inflammatory disease of the airways accompanied by mucous hypersecretion, and not dismissed as "smoker's cough." In terms of etiology, COPD can be viewed as one of the major complications of nicotine addiction, with lung cancer and coronary artery disease the other main complications.

Although smoking cigarettes is the most common cause of chronic bronchitis, a variety of other conditions may give rise to similar symptoms. Persistent or repeated episodes of cough may be the only symptoms of mild asthma. Chronic inflammation of the airways may result from recurrent inhalation of dust or fumes during occupational or other exposures. Hair spray may be one such offender. A frequently overlooked cause of chronic bronchitis is gastroesophageal reflux with nocturnal aspiration. Specific pulmonary diseases such as bronchiectasis, tuberculosis, or lung cancer may be manifested only by chronic cough, and these must be excluded before a diagnosis of chronic bronchitis due to smoking is made. In most patients with chronic cough and sputum production, the history, physical examination, and chest radiograph will provide an adequate evaluation.

Hemoptysis is a serious symptom that requires investigation. Although no cause other than chronic bronchitis can be identified in some patients, hemoptysis commonly heralds the presence of lung cancer, tuberculosis, lung abscess, or bronchiectasis. It is important to note that the patient's usual pattern of chronic bronchitis with acute flare-ups has changed. The current episode differs from previous episodes in that the onset was gradual, sputum purulence was not prominent, and blood streaking of sputum had occurred. These symptoms suggest the presence of a new problem complicating his chronic bronchitis.

Data The patient lives in a shelter for homeless men and was born and raised in New Jersey traveling only to New York. He has smoked two packs of cigarettes daily for nearly 50 years and drinks two quarts of wine every day. He denies homosexuality or injection drug use and has not had relations with commercial sex workers. His last chest radiograph was taken 6 months ago and was normal as far as he knew. He has lost weight during the past few months but could not estimate an amount. He has not had fever, chills, or night sweats. He admits to there being many men with the human immunodeficiency virus infection at the shelter but denies being exposed to anyone with tuberculosis. He does recall two men who had productive coughs for several months, one of whom died.

Physical examination revealed a thin, elderly appearing man in no acute distress. Vital signs were normal. Conjunctivae were not icteric. There was no thrush on the oral mucosa and no cervical or supraclavicular adenopathy. Examination of the chest disclosed an area of bronchial breath sounds and whispered pectoriloquy anteriorly beneath the right clavicle and in the right supraclavicular fossa. The trachea was shifted to the right. Scattered coarse rhonchi were heard

throughout the remainder of both lung fields and expiration was prolonged. The liver was enlarged with a vertical span of 15 cm. The spleen was not palpable. Definite clubbing of the fingers was present, and pressure over the distal radii and tibiae elicited pain. Numerous spider angiomata were seen over the upper thorax, shoulders, neck, and face. Palmar erythema was noted, but no asterixis was present. He was alert and oriented to person, time, and place but had problems recalling three objects. Except for some mild cerebellar past-pointing, he had no other focal neurologic deficits.

Logic The physical findings in the chest indicate volume loss and consolidation of the right upper lobe. The presence of pectoriloquy in this region must be interpreted with caution; although its presence usually indicates a patent bronchus, tracheal deviation may be sufficient to permit tracheal sounds to be transmitted to a segment that is totally obstructed and atelectatic. He has signs of cirrhosis of the liver as noted in the physical examination and chronic obstructive pulmonary disease, as suggested by the history.

Data Posteroanterior and lateral chest radiographs revealed a density in the right upper lobe consistent with partial atelectasis of the lobe (Fig. 15.11). The right diaphragm was elevated. Air bronchograms were not visible in the right up-

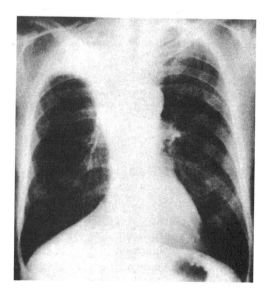

▶ **Figure 15.11.** Atelectasis right upper lobe; elevated right hemidiaphragm.

per lobe. Radiographs of the distal tibiae and fibulae revealed periosteal elevation and new bone formation. Attempts to locate the patient's previous radiographs were unsuccessful.

Computed tomographic (CT) scanning of the chest with contrast media showed mediastinal nodes in the right paratracheal and subcarinal groups whose diameters were more than 2 cm—suggestive of tumor—whereas a left periaortic node was borderline at 1.3 cm. In addition, the right upper lobe bronchus could not be traced from its take off from the right main bronchus suggesting an obstructive lesion. There was volume loss in the right upper lobe that confirmed atelectasis, but an inflammatory process could not be excluded. No lesions were seen in the rest of the lung and views of the adrenals and liver failed to show any metastatic nodules.

Logic The chest radiograph reveals focal disease in the right upper lobe (such as tumor, atelectasis, and bacterial, tuberculous, or fungal infection), and does not show more diffuse disease such as sarcoid, other interstitial diseases, or even diffuse infections, for example, infections with *P. carinii*. The absence of air bronchograms in the area of density suggests proximal obstruction such as from a tumor or a mucous plug. This chest radiograph is not helpful in distinguishing volume loss of the right upper lobe due to bronchial obstruction from that due to a chronic inflammatory process.

Tuberculosis, fungal infection, or bacterial pneumonia could have this type of presentation, although the absence of specific acute symptoms makes the latter unlikely, and the lack of travel to the Southwest and Mississippi River valley makes infection with coccidioidomycosis and histoplasmosis, respectively, unlikely. Given the possibility of tuberculosis, the patient is placed in isolation pending further evaluation. However, bronchial obstruction, most commonly due to carcinoma, remains the main possibility, especially in view of the findings on CT scan. Also, nodes greater than 1 cm are compatible with malignant spread but require confirmation via mediastinoscopy. Tuberculous nodes often demonstrate an interesting characteristic: central necrosis seen on CT as an area of lower attenuation.

Digital clubbing may be found not only in a wide variety of thoracic diseases but also in chronic liver disease, bacterial endocarditis, congenital heart disease, and inflammatory bowel disease. Occasionally, clubbing is congenital and not

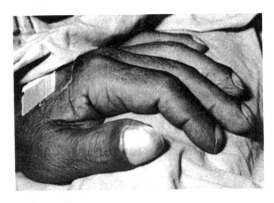

▶ **Figure 15.12.** Clubbed fingers.

associated with disease. Among the chest diseases, carcinoma of the lung and pulmonary fibrosis are common causes. Chronic obstructive pulmonary disease alone rarely causes clubbing (Fig. 15.12).

The presence of long bone tenderness, usually best demonstrated in the forearm or above the ankle, suggests periostitis due to hypertrophic pulmonary osteoarthropathy (HPO). The radiographs of the leg confirm this diagnosis. Patients with this disorder usually, but not necessarily, have clubbing as well. Chronic suppurative diseases of the lung including tuberculosis and bronchiectasis formerly were common causes of HPO; currently, the great majority of cases are due to lung cancer. It is important to recognize that extrathoracic causes of clubbing are rarely, if ever, associated with HPO. Thus, although this patient has definite signs of chronic liver disease and chronic airway obstruction, his clubbing and HPO are most likely due to the process in the right upper lobe (Fig. 15.13).

Data Skin tests were applied with intermediate strength purified protein derivative (PPD), mumps, and *Candida* antigens. Three early morning sputa were examined by Ziehl-Neelsen and fluorochrome stains and were negative for acid-fast bacilli (AFB). Three expectorated sputa were negative for malignant cells.

Logic A positive PPD skin test will not distinguish between past infection with *Mycobacterium tuberculosis* and present active disease. In fact, a negative tuberculin skin test does not exclude active tuberculosis. *Candida* and mumps antigens were used as controls to determine whether this debilitated patient's delayed hypersensitivity mechanisms were intact. Because the skin test data will be nondiagnostic, and sputum cultures for mycobacteria

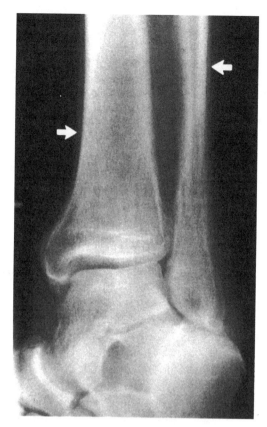

▶ **Figure 15.13.** Hypertrophic pulmonary osteoarthropathy. Periostitis can be seen along shafts of distal tibia and fibula (arrows).

will not be available for several weeks, further work-up should proceed without delay in situations in which such infections are not highly probable. Results of smears are valuable because they both allow the presumption of infectious disease (pending cultures or response to treatment) and are good indicators of the infectiousness of the patients. All three skin tests had positive results. Had the PPD skin test been negative and others positive, tuberculosis would have been unlikely, especially with negative sputum smears. However, given the negative AFB smears the patient can be taken out of isolation.

Data Fiberoptic bronchoscopy was performed with topical anesthesia. The orifice of the right upper lobe bronchus was completely occluded by a friable endobronchial mass. Biopsies of this lesion revealed squamous cell carcinoma and were devoid of granulomas. Smears were also negative for AFB and fungi.

Logic At this point, the diagnosis is established. The presence of extrathoracic manifestations of lung cancer (clubbing and HPO) does not eliminate the consideration of resection, because these represent paraneoplastic syndromes and not the metastatic spread of tumor. Other paraneoplastic phenomena include hypercalcemia with squamous cell tumors and various endocrine abnormalities associated with small or oat cell tumors such as the syndrome of inappropriate antidiuretic hormone (SIADH), and ectopic adrenocorticotropic hormone production (ACTH). All paraneoplastic manifestations of lung cancer tend to regress with effective treatment of the primary lung tumor.

In our patient, the following two issues must be addressed before his treatment plan can be finalized:

1. Is the lesion resectable? Contraindications to resection are, in general, evidence of extrathoracic metastases, contralateral mediastinal lymph node involvement, phrenic or recurrent laryngeal nerve involvement, or malignant pleural effusion. Answering this question will require sampling of the large mediastinal nodes and ultimately staging of his disease by the TNM system (size and local spread of tumor, node involvement, and metastatic spread).

2. Is the patient operable? Can he tolerate a lobectomy or pneumonectomy? From the data accumulated so far, we know that he has COPD and liver disease, and given his age and life-style, the presence of heart disease is likely. The key issue is the patient's pulmonary function, because one of our objectives is to successfully wean him off mechanical ventilation after surgery and not leave him a "respiratory cripple." Answering this question will require tests of total lung function and an assessment of regional lung contributions to overall function by isotope scanning techniques. The patient's cirrhosis alone puts him at high risk for surgery, whereas his cardiac status requires at least an ECG for evaluation.

Data ECG only showed nonspecific changes, but pulmonary function studies revealed severe airway obstruction with an FEV_1 (forced expiratory volume in 1 second) of only 0.7 L despite bronchodilator therapy. Using quantitative lung scanning, it was estimated that the right lung contributed 40% of his overall lung function. From this calculation it was deduced that a right pneumonectomy would leave the patient with an FEV_1 of less than 0.5 L, such that he would be seriously impaired postoperatively, and probably not come off mechanical ventilation. Given the patient's other medical problems, exercise testing, which would give the most reliable estimate of the patient's overall fitness, was not undertaken. It was concluded that the patient was not a candidate for resectional surgery because of underlying lung and liver disease, and further staging procedures, that is, mediastinoscopy and node biopsy, were not performed. The right upper lobe lesion and large nodes were treated with irradiation.

The final problem list is as follows:

1. Squamous cell carcinoma of the lung, probable Stage IIIb
2. COPD, severe
3. Cirrhosis of the liver
4. Alcoholism
5. Nicotine addiction (cigarette abuse)

The patient's two addictions, alcohol and nicotine, are at the root of his main problems.

Logic Because lung cancer may have as short a doubling time as 1 month, diagnostic delays must be avoided. The physician must rapidly make the diagnosis, determine the cell type, and decide on operability. The success of surgery depends on the absence of metastases and contralateral nodal spread, absence of serious visceral disease that might preclude a surgical procedure, and the patient's willingness to undergo surgery. In the great majority of patients found to have lung cancer, the disease is inoperable because of already existing metastases and/or abnormal pulmonary function tests resulting from concomitant lung disease.

It is interesting to note the varied presentations of lung cancer. Occasionally, asymptomatic patients have lung cancer detected by routine chest radiographs. Most often the initial presentation is with pulmonary symptoms of cough, expectoration, hemoptysis, and/or chest pain combined with constitutional symptoms such as weight loss. Depending on the cancer's location and extent in the lung, the symptoms and signs may vary greatly: bronchial obstruction, atelectasis, a hilar mass, rib erosion, superior vena cava obstruction, hoarseness, Horner's syndrome, brachial plexus involvement, and hemidiaphragm paralysis. Not infrequently it is a metastasis that brings the patient to the doctor: neurologic manifesta-

tions, severe backache, jaundice, and so forth. Finally, patients occasionally are seen with symptoms caused by a paraneoplastic syndrome: hypercalcemia, myopathy, neuropathy, cerebellar degeneration, periostitis, and so forth.

Autopsies on patients who die of lung cancer show metastases to lymph nodes in 70% and to brain, liver, and bone in 30 to 40%. Therefore, the search for metastases may begin with the biopsy of a palpable scalene node, mediastinoscopy if large nodes are suspected by radiographic studies or CT scans, and thoracentesis and pleural biopsy if pleural fluid is present. In evaluating the patient with symptoms, the physical examination and laboratory tests should guide the physician in investigating for metastases, particularly of the brain, bones, and other visceral organs, bearing in mind that false positives and false negatives do occur.

Assessment of pulmonary function is important. An FEV_1 that is less than 2 L or a maximal breathing capacity that is less than 50% of the predicted value are bad omens, given that the patient's obstructive disease has been maximally treated. The presence of hypercapnia ($PCO_2 > 45$ mm Hg) and a poor functional history greatly increase surgical risk. Quantitative perfusion scanning can be helpful when spirometry results are abnormal to determine what lung function will remain if resectional surgery is performed; exercise testing can be helpful in the evaluation of individuals with both cardiac and pulmonary disease.

Data The patient died several months later. The major autopsy finding is noted in Figure 15.14.

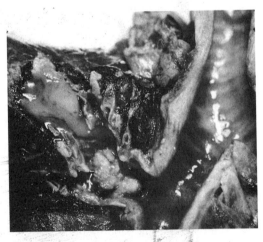

▶ **Figure 15.14.** Carcinoma of right upper lobe bronchus.

Questions

(There may be one or more than one answer.)

1. The development of digital clubbing in a 55-year-old heavy cigarette smoker:
   (a) is usually due to chronic bronchitis and/or emphysema.
   (b) if associated with lung cancer, will regress with treatment of the tumor.
   (c) is so common that extensive investigation is not indicated.
   (d) is usually not associated with pulmonary osteoarthropathy.

2. Hemoptysis occurring for the first time in a 60-year-old smoker with normal chest radiographic findings:
   (a) can be safely dismissed as being due to chronic bronchitis.
   (b) should be evaluated with repeated chest radiographs at monthly intervals.
   (c) should be evaluated with multiple examinations of sputum for mycobacteria.
   (d) should be evaluated by sputum examinations for malignant cells and fiberoptic bronchoscopy.

3. Bronchiectasis should be considered in the presence of:
   (a) recurring bacterial pneumonias.
   (b) persistent coarse basilar rales.
   (c) persistent purulent sputum.
   (d) hemoptysis.

Answers

1. **(b) and (d) are correct.** Clubbing of the digits occurs commonly in association with bronchiectasis, pulmonary fibrosis, and cancer of the lung. The development of this finding in a cigarette smoker should not be attributed to chronic obstructive pulmonary disease until other causes have been ruled out. Effective treatment of the primary lung tumor is usually followed by regression of clubbing. HPO is much less common than clubbing.

2. **(d) is correct.** Chronic bronchitis is one of the most common causes of hemoptysis, but the initial occurrence of this symptom should prompt a thorough evaluation of the patient. Carcinoma of the bronchus may not be visible on radiographs of the chest until the tumor has been present for 3 to 4 years. Because such tumors begin in the bronchial mucosa, hemoptysis may occur before any abnormality can be detected by radiography. Awaiting sufficient growth of the tumor to permit detection by radiograph makes little sense. Sputum cytology may indicate the presence of a tumor, and may in fact be positive even when the tumor cannot be visualized endobronchially. Such tumors represent in situ malignancies and, if localized by bronchial brushing or biopsy, have a high cure rate following resection. Choice (c) is reasonable, too, but (d) is obligatory.

3. **All are correct.** Compared to those patients who have bronchitis alone, most patients with bronchiectasis differ in that they expectorate persistently purulent sputum, have coarse basilar rales, and experience recurrent episodes of pneumonia. Persistent infection leads to episodes of hemoptysis.

COMMENT Hemoptysis superimposed on chronic cough and expectoration indicated a change in the nature of a chronic cluster and warranted an investigation. The most likely and most common possibilities were considered. Solving the problem was complicated by the fact that the patient did indeed have two coexistent lung diseases—cancer and chronic obstructive pulmonary disease—wherein there was a broad overlap of clues. But HPO and clubbing lay outside the zone of overlap. Probability theory (Bayes) was used to evaluate this 64-year-old heavy smoker with a cluster of symptoms and signs that statistically could mean only cancer. The decisive clues were delivered by radiograph, bronchoscopy, and biopsy—in order of their specificity. (P.C.)

Suggested Readings

O'Neil KM, Lazarus AA. Hemoptysis: Indications for bronchoscopy. Arch Intern Med 1991;151:171–174.

Pratter MR, Bartter T, Akers S, et al. An algorithmic approach to chronic cough. Ann Intern Med 1993; 119:977–983.

McCloud TC, Bourgouin PM, Greenberg RW, et al. Bronchogenic carcinoma: Analysis of staging in the mediastinum with CT by correlative lymph node mapping and sampling. Radiology 1992;182:319–323.

CASE 40

WORSENING SHORTNESS OF BREATH

Gary D. Harris and Waldemar G. Johanson

Data This 46-year-old female nurse consults her physician because of shortness of breath and cough that have been slowly progressive for approximately 6 months. Dyspnea has increased in severity to the point that she had to modify her usual daily activities, avoiding climbing stairs or carrying groceries, for example. The cough is nonproductive, but several colleagues have commented on it.

Logic This constellation of symptoms is a common mode of presentation of a variety of disease processes. The patient relates that specific activities have become increasingly difficult for her to perform, establishing the progressive nature of the process. Almost certainly this represents either chronic pulmonary or cardiac disease. One could now approach this problem in one of several ways: pursue a detailed history; go directly to a physical examination to separate the possibilities; or obtain screening tests to facilitate and guide the evaluation. Let us begin with a limited examination in this patient.

Data The vital signs are: pulse, 88 and regular; BP, 110/70; respirations, 20; and temperature, 37°C. Jugular venous pressure is normal and the heart is normal in size. Neither right nor left ventricular hypertrophy is apparent by palpation. S_2 splits normally with inspiration, but the pulmonic component is accentuated. No murmurs or abnormal sounds are present. The chest is normal by inspection and expansion is equal bilaterally. There is no dullness to percussion. Coarse mid-inspiratory crackles are present at both lung bases. Expiration is not prolonged, wheezes or rhonchi are not present, and the patient can exhale her vital capacity in less than three seconds. The rest of the physical examination results are normal.

Logic Several findings of significance are present. The increased P_2 suggests an increase in pulmonary artery pressure, although the absence of a parasternal lift indicates that this increase is not so severe as to have produced clinically detectable right ventricular hypertrophy. Pulmonary hypertension may result from left ventricular failure. However, in the absence of cardiomegaly, displacement of the apex beat, an S_3, or any cause for left ventricular hypertrophy, such failure is unlikely. Pulmonary hypertension may be caused by an increase in left atrial pressure due to mitral valve stenosis. The absence of a diastolic murmur, opening snap, and no increase in intensity of S_1 make this unlikely. Thus, cardiac disease does not appear to account for either our findings or the patient's symptoms.

Pulmonary hypertension can result from narrowing of the pulmonary arteries due to intimal and/or muscular hyperplasia. In the absence of chronic lung disease, pulmonary thromboembolism, conditions causing alveolar hypoxia, or cardiac disease, this process is called "primary pulmonary hypertension." This unusual disorder typically affects younger women, producing progressive limitation of exercise capacity and cor pulmonale. Our patient's history and physical findings are compatible with that diagnosis with two exceptions: this diagnosis would not account for the patient's crackles, and it would be unusual for primary pulmonary hypertension to produce such severe symptoms without more impressive signs of right ventricular hypertrophy on physical examination. The category of disease that fits her symptoms and findings best is interstitial lung disease; this would explain all the features of her illness—progressive dyspnea, crackles, and loud P_2. Having suspected this diagnosis, the physician will obtain chest radiographs and pulmonary function studies.

Data The radiographs reveal a diffuse process throughout both lungs, but most marked at the lung bases, characterized by accentuated linear interstitial markings and irregular small opacities (Fig. 15.15). There is no lymphadenopathy. Pulmonary function study results are shown in Table 15.4. Arterial blood gases while breathing room air

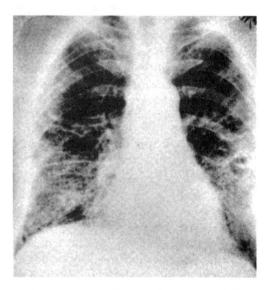

▶ **Figure 15.15.** Pulmonary fibrosis. Diffuse bilateral interstitial infiltrates.

TABLE 15.4. Pulmonary Function Study Results

MEASUREMENT	UNITS	PREDICTED NORMAL VALUE	OBSERVED
TLC	L	5.00	2.50 (50%)
FVC	L	4.01	1.52 (48%)
FEV_1	L	3.12	1.65 (53%)
FEV_1/FVC		0.78	0.86
FEF_{25-75}	L/sec	3.43	2.06 (60%)
DL_{COSB}	mL/min/mm Hg	22.10	7.70 (35%)

TLC = total lung capacity; FVC = forced vital capacity; FEV_1 = forced expiratory volume in 1 second; FEF_{25-75} = forced midexpiratory flow; DL_{COSB} = diffusing capacity, single breath, carbon monoxide.

show pH, 7.44; PCO_2, 30 mm Hg; PO_2, 76 mm Hg; and 93% saturation. During moderate exercise the PO_2 decreases to 60 mm Hg, and the saturation decreases to 88%.

Logic These studies show the following:

- Proportionate reductions in TLC, FVC, and FEV_1 indicate that the patient's lungs are abnormally small.
- Ratio of FEV_1:FVC is normal, and expiratory flow rates are reduced only in proportion to loss of lung volume, which indicate that airway obstruction is not present.
- Oxygen transport is markedly abnormal, as is shown by the decreased diffusing capacity and desaturation of arterial blood with exercise.

These findings are characteristic of diffuse interstitial disease. The reduction of lung volumes may be due to abnormal stiffness of the lung (decreased lung compliance) or to the loss of lung units due to inflammatory or fibrotic processes. The reduced diffusing capacity may result from several factors including loss of lung units, thickening of the alveolocapillary membrane, and mismatching of ventilation and perfusion.

Diffuse lung disease may be caused by a wide variety of agents. Infectious etiologies would be unlikely in this case given the absence of fever and the long duration of symptoms. However, tuberculosis must be considered in a health care worker with lingering respiratory symptoms. The major possibilities in this patient would be:

- Pulmonary fibrosis associated with a systemic disease, especially those associated

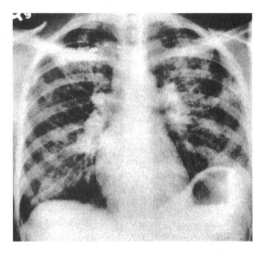

▶ **Figure 15.16.** Sarcoidosis. Interstitial infiltrates are present here, too, but note marked hilar adenopathy.

with altered immunity (such as connective tissue diseases, thyroiditis, or chronic active hepatitis)
- Hypersensitivity pneumonitis, an immunologically-mediated response to inhaled organic antigens
- Idiopathic pulmonary fibrosis (IPF)
- Sarcoidosis (Fig. 15.16)

Less common causes of this presentation would include chronic drug reactions (busulfan, methysergide, nitrofurantoin); fungal infections (either histoplasmosis or coccidioidomycosis); or lymphangitic spread of malignancy in the lungs.

Data The patient is a surgical nurse in a busy community hospital. She had not had contact with known cases of tuberculosis, either at work or elsewhere. Her tuberculin skin reaction results have been consistently negative at work, and she was last tested approximately 12 months ago. She takes no medication regularly and has not traveled to areas in which histoplasmosis or coccidioidomycosis is endemic. She is an avid gardener, maintaining a greenhouse with a wide assortment of plants, but is unable to associate her symptoms temporally with exposure to her working materials. A review of other systems reveals intolerance of fatty foods and occasional dysmenorrhea. There is no history suggestive of connective tissue disease, thyroid conditions, or liver disease in the patient or her close relatives. Her mother has non-insulin-dependent diabetes mellitus.

Logic The physician now faces a diagnostic and therapeutic dilemma. On the basis of the accumulated evidence, he is certain that the patient has a diffuse pulmonary disease and that this process is the cause of her symptoms. No other disease is apparent from the history or physical examination. Sometimes interstitial lung disease precedes the clinical appearance of an associated disease such as rheumatoid arthritis, although usually the associated condition has been present for some time.

Patients with hypersensitivity pneumonitis usually have clearly identified environmental exposures such as farmers exposed to moldy hay or persons who raise pigeons or other birds. Only approximately one half of individuals with lung disease resulting from such exposures have acute symptoms; in the rest, lung impairment develops insidiously. Hypersensitivity pneumonitis has been associated with fungal contamination of air-conditioning systems in large buildings, so this diagnosis must be considered in anyone having, as our patient did, diffuse lung disease, even in the absence of unusual exposures. Clues to the diagnosis of sarcoidosis are often found outside the lungs—in the eyes, liver, spleen, or skin. These were of no help in diagnosing this patient.

As is often the case, the history, physical, and initial laboratory findings have shed no light on the etiology of the diffuse lung disease. Now the clinician must consider how far to go in making a specific diagnosis. Selection of one procedure or another may be facilitated by high-resolution CT (HRCT) scanning of the chest. This procedure provides an excellent view of the lobular

anatomy of the lung, and it is now known that certain diseases produce characteristic patterns.

Data The HRCT scan reveals a hazy ground-glass pattern of opacity in the periphery of the lung bases; there is no fibrosis or bronchiectasis. These findings are typical of IPF. A battery of serologic tests including antibody titers against common fungal agents, *Aspergillus,* and thermophilic actinomycetes are negative. The results of an 18-test blood chemistry profile are normal except for a fasting glucose level of 140 mg/dL. Skin tests with purified protein derivative, *Candida,* and mumps antigens are applied; all test results are negative at 48 hours.

Logic The HRCT findings strongly suggest IPF. Additionally, the ground-glass appearance has been associated with cellular inflammation, not end-stage fibrosis. This finding, along with the patient's history, physical findings, and pulmonary function test results provide strong support for the diagnosis. The remaining question is whether a lung biopsy should be performed before treatment is begun. Because the initial therapy will be corticosteroids, one school of thought would argue for an empiric trial. Another school would argue that histologic confirmation is necessary in this relatively young person with a disease that is more likely than not to fail to respond well to treatment; this group believes that all uncertainty should be removed before committing the patient to a therapy with frequent and severe side effects. In no small part, the patient's wishes should play a deciding role in this decision making, after a thorough discussion of the pros and cons.

Most clinicians would recommend a lung biopsy if it were easily obtained with little or no morbidity. Bronchoalveolar lavage (BAL) is a relatively noninvasive method of obtaining cellular material from the lungs. However, BAL findings are nonspecific and unreliable indicators of the patient's future course. Transbronchial biopsy (TBB) performed via fiberoptic bronchoscopy yields small fragments of lung tissue that are adequate for the diagnosis of several diffuse diseases, including sarcoidosis and lymphangitic spread of cancer, conditions characterized by relatively uniform and widespread changes. In contrast, TBB specimens may be misleading in the diagnosis of IPF in which the pattern of lung involvement is much less uniform. Open lung biopsy, which requires a thoracotomy and the attendant hospitalization and other morbidity, has been the diagnostic procedure of choice, a fact that has deterred many physicians. However, recent experience with thoracoscopic lung biopsy has shown that adequate lung specimens can be obtained with little morbidity without a formal thoracotomy. Unfortunately, the pathology of IPF is nonspecific and not helpful in determining an etiology. However, the stage of IPF, whether cellular and inflammatory or only scarred and fibrotic, is useful for predicting the patient's response to treatment.

Data The patient was concerned that corticosteroid therapy might precipitate diabetes in her and decided that she would rather know for certain whether or not it was likely to be helpful. A thoracoscopic lung biopsy was performed without complication. Alveolar spaces were filled with mononuclear cells and alveolar septa were moderately thickened. Granulomata were not found. The serologic tests were negative and all cultures, including cultures of lung tissue, were negative for fungi and mycobacteria.

Logic Thus, we have established that the patient's problems are due to a diffuse pulmonary process, and that histologically the process is compatible with IPF. The patient was relieved to know the exact diagnosis even though no etiology could be established.

Data She was treated with long-term corticosteroid therapy and improved physiologically, radiographically, and symptomatically. Glucose intolerance did develop but was managed with an oral hypoglycemic agent.

Logic The pathogenesis of IPF is poorly understood, although it is clear that many immunologic processes may contribute. BAL has been used to document increases in acute-phase cytokines such as interleukin-1-α (IL-1-α), tumor necrosis factor-α, IL-8, and macrophage inflammatory proteins (MIP-1-α and MIP-β and MIP-2), members of the superfamily of cytokines called chemokines. Fibrogenic cytokines such as PDGF and TGF-β have also been demonstrated by BAL. Collagen synthesis by fibroblasts is stimulated by several factors found in BAL, reflecting activity in the alveolar milieu. Although the precise inciting agents are unclear, it seems certain that IPF is the result of lung defense mechanisms gone awry.

COMMENT One wonders why a patient with worsening dyspnea waits 6 months before consulting a physician. Perhaps it represents denial, reluctance, procrastination, or misinterpretation. At any rate, the chief complaint—dyspnea on exertion—is the *key clue*. A variety of alternate pathways for gathering data appeared. The physician chose to do the physical examination first, and by finding evidence of diffuse lung disease, pulmonary hypertension, and a normal heart, he pinpointed the diseased organ. A chest radiograph and pulmonary function tests narrowed the diagnostic list to *diffuse fibrosis*.

Not uncommonly, patients of this sort are given a diagnosis of "pulmonary fibrosis." But lifting the lid of the pulmonary fibrosis box releases a swarm of exotic diseases. You must now consider collagen disorders (rheumatoid arthritis, systemic lupus erythematosus, and scleroderma); drugs as previously listed; radiation exposure; hemosiderosis; histiocytosis X; alveolar proteinosis; lymphangitic carcinomatosis; idiopathic pulmonary fibrosis; Hamman-Rich syndrome; sarcoidosis; and so forth. Closely competing pictures are presented by environmental lung diseases such as those caused by asbestos, silica, beryllium, and other inhaled nuisance organic dusts.

In this situation, other aspects of the history and physical examination may offer help. For example, the presence of lymphadenopathy, polycythemia, arthritis, or clubbing may guide you. And, as always, one simple question regarding the patient's occupation may furnish the answer. You must be aware of the special roles of age, gender, race, occupation, and inhalation hazards that may serve as clues in the various diseases included under pulmonary fibrosis.

Had a chest radiograph been done first, the diagnostic possibilities would have diminished rapidly, and a specific line of data gathering could have branched from that point. Studies might have been differently sequenced, and the physician might have opted for a lung biopsy before all else.

Had the initial probe been into the history, the problem solver would have found a dearth of cardiac clues—no history of rheumatic fever, heart disease, murmur, orthopnea, or palpitations. This would have led him or her back to the lung as the disease site. As is frequently the case, the distinction between heart and lung disease as the cause of symptoms had to be made. Here it was simple. When both organs exhibit disease, it may be difficult to decide which one, or perhaps both, contributes to the chief complaint of dyspnea. *(P.C.)*

Suggested Readings

Blackmon GM, Raghu G. Pulmonary sarcoidosis: A mimic of respiratory infection. Semin Respir Infect 1995;10:176–186.

Driscoll KE. Macrophage inflammatory proteins: Biology and role in pulmonary inflammation. Exp Lung Res 1994;l20:473–490.

Lynch DA. Imaging of small airways diseases. Clin Chest Med 1993;14:623–634.

Marciniuk DD, Gallagher CG. Clinical exercise testing in interstitial lung disease. Clin Chest Med 1994;15:287–303.

Mornex JF, Leroux C, Greenland T, et al. From granuloma to fibrosis in interstitial lung diseases: Molecular and cellular interactions. Eur Respir J 1994;7: 779–785.

CASE 41

WHEEZE, COUGH, FEVER, DYSPNEA

Paul Cutler

Data While working in an ambulatory emergency department that services Medicaid patients for the Super Care HMO, the intern sees a 50-year-old man who arrives by ambulance. He is dyspneic, cyanotic, wheezes, is semi-stuporous, and feels warm. Suddenly he has a bout of coughing, and greenish-yellow sputum trickles out of his mouth.

Logic The fever, cough, and purulent sputum suggest pneumonia. Dyspnea and cyanosis tell the intern that the infection is very severe or that it is superimposed on a pre-existing pulmonary disorder. Semi-stupor may arise from the severity of the illness, spread of the infectious process to the central nervous system, anoxia, CO_2 retention, or an as yet unidentified factor.

Data Additional information is obtained from the ambulance attendant and a neighbor who says that the patient is a virtual recluse, keeps pretty much to himself, and is rarely seen outside his one-room flat. Through the thin walls separating their apartments, she has heard the patient

having severe coughing spells over the years. Recently she noticed mail and newspapers piling up at his door, so she called the police, who entered and found the patient on the floor.

No further history was obtainable at that time. However, a quick physical examination revealed temperature, 102.4°F; pulse, 120; respirations, 30 and labored, with prolonged expiration; BP, 130/90; dehydration of the skin and mucus membranes; deep cyanosis of the lips and nail beds; heavy tobacco stains on the first three fingers of his right hand; distended neck veins; and expiratory wheezes all over the chest, with inspiratory rales and dullness at the right base. Heart sounds were muffled, and there were no gallops, murmurs, or rubs, although these findings may have been obscured by the noises in his chest. The point of maximal impulse was at the lower left sternal border, the liver was enlarged (15 cm) and tender, and there was 2+ presacral and ankle edema.

Logic Much information has been added. Pneumonia seems fairly certain, perhaps at the right base. Wheezes, chronic cough, and smoking suggest the patient may have underlying chronic obstructive pulmonary disease (COPD). Distended neck veins, right ventricular lift, enlarged liver, and edema point to right ventricular failure, secondary to pulmonary hypertension and COPD. With this background, the cyanosis and stupor probably represent severe anoxemia and hypercarbia. Acute respiratory failure may quickly occur when a pulmonary infection is superimposed upon COPD. The patient is critically ill and needs emergency care to tide him over the acute episode and restore him to his chronic state of poor health.

Data The intern arranges for the patient's admission to an inpatient facility on the other side of town, but only after first seeking and then getting the approval of the person designated as the "secretary to the authorization for admissions officer" at the other end of the telephone line.

Before the transfer, baseline studies are obtained and emergency measures for acute respiratory failure (ARF) are initiated. The chest radiograph shows moderate cardiac enlargement, increased bronchovascular markings, and an area of consolidation in the right lower lobe. The ECG shows sinus tachycardia, tall peaked P waves in leads II, III, and aVF, and right axis deviation. There are 18,000 white blood cells per mm^3 with 88% PMNs, and the hematocrit is 56. Arterial blood gases are pH, 7.30; PO$_2$, 38 mm Hg; PCO$_2$, 64 mm Hg.

Logic The radiograph confirms the clinical impression of pneumonia. The ECG offers evidence of right ventricular strain and right atrial hypertrophy as seen in cor pulmonale. The blood count reflects the acute suppurative process, as well as the erythrocytosis that may result from long-standing hypoxia.

The chronic hypoxemia of COPD is caused by a severe ventilation-perfusion mismatch in which perfused tissue is inadequately ventilated because of infection, secretions, mucus plugs, and spasm of bronchi. The hypoxemia results in pulmonary artery vasoconstriction, pulmonary hypertension, cor pulmonale, and eventual right ventricular failure. Chronic hypercarbia is not too well explained by the known pathophysiology, but it does exist, and it worsens markedly when another illness such as pneumonia supervenes. The CO$_2$ retention results in respiratory acidosis; the pH in this patient is only modestly low because renal compensating mechanisms retain bicarbonate.

Data Emergency measures included intratracheal and oral suction, intravenous aminophylline, and oxygen delivered by nasal prongs at 1 to 2 L/min.

Logic Suction removes purulent secretions, aminophylline aims to relieve bronchospasm, and low-flow oxygen is administered so as to gradually raise the PO$_2$ without depressing respiration. Patients with chronic CO$_2$ retention experience blunting of their CO$_2$-dependent drive to breathe and the respiratory center becomes driven mainly by the low PO$_2$. Unrestrained oxygen administration may cause respirations to stop and/or further elevate the PCO$_2$.

Data Additional treatment is deferred pending hospitalization, more studies, and observation. It will include an appropriate antibiotic for infection, a β-agonist for bronchospasm, a diuretic for sodium retention, hypotonic fluids for dehydration, and very careful monitoring of blood gases and respirations.

The patient, already slightly improved and less stuporous, is admitted to the intensive care unit, under the care of an intern who serendipitously happens to be the wife of the intern in the emergency department. Transfer of information is readily achieved, and the husband and wife team are able to conjoin their efforts and exchange progress reports from time to time. In addition, because both feel a little insecure about the management of acute respiratory failure, they decide to use this case as a basis for problem-based learning. Both will read about COPD, its complications and its management, and will pose questions to one another when they are off-duty.

Shortly after admission, ampicillin is begun, and gradually increasing concentrations of oxygen are delivered via a Venturi mask. By Day 3, the patient is markedly improved, oriented, afebrile, less dyspneic, no longer cyanotic, and blood gases are pH, 7.36; PO$_2$, 54 mm Hg; and PCO$_2$, 50 mm Hg. Cough and expectoration continue, although the sputum color has changed from yellow to white. Chest radiograph shows partial resolution of the pneumonic process.

He is now able to elaborate on the history: He has been coughing and expectorating for at least 10 years, smoked 1 to 2 packs of cigarettes daily until approximately 1 week ago, and recently he has developed shortness of breath on even mild exertion.

On the night of Day 5, the patient now being much improved, the husband and wife physicians, both having the same night off, ask each other questions while indulging in a bottle of their favorite wine:

1. **What roles do chronic bronchitis and emphysema play in the production of COPD?**

   Chronic bronchitis is said to exist when documented cough and expectoration have been present for 3 months per year for 2 consecutive years. It is characterized by cough and expectoration, and results from inflamed, infected, and spastic bronchi and bronchioles.

   Emphysema results from a loss of normal alveolar elasticity. Alveoli stretch and tear as the lung becomes hyperinflated and loses tissue.

   These two distinct processes usually coexist in various degrees to produce COPD, one sometimes more dominant than the other. Both are associated with airways obstruction: bronchitis because of structural pathologic changes in the bronchioles, and emphysema because of loss of elastic recoil, resulting in the loss of radial traction that normally occurs with inspiration. Alterations in the clinical picture of COPD depend on which of the two processes is dominant. Table 15.5 tabulates the important differences between them.

2. What are their causes?

Bronchitis results from bronchial infections, cigarette smoking, and air pollution. Heavy smokers have an average decline of 40 to 45 mL of 1-second forced expiratory volume per year—twice as much as in nonsmokers. There are various toxins in cigarette smoke, in addition to nicotine, which cause ineffective ciliary motion, alteration of mucus, and affect alveolar macrophage function. In industrialized areas, air pollution consists of organic and inorganic dusts, other particulate matter, and noxious gases such as sulfur dioxide. Exhaust fumes from internal combustion engines also play a role.

In emphysema, the alveolar walls lose their elasticity as a result of deficiency of antiproteases. In all likelihood, these deficiencies are genetically determined. Many patients with emphysema have been shown to have deficient or absent α_1 antitrypsin. In this situation, proteases such as elastase are in a position to damage alveolar walls. Cigarette smoking is also a factor in causing emphysema; smoke inhibits antiproteases and causes polymorphonuclear leukocytes to release proteolytic enzymes.

3. What is a "blue bloater" and a "pink puffer?"

The former term addresses the patient with COPD who predominately has chronic bronchitis. This patient is cyanotic as a result of anoxemia and erythrocytosis and has edema because of cor pulmonale. A "pink puffer" refers to the patient with COPD whose picture is predominantly that of emphysema. That patient is not cyanotic and has good color because anoxemia is mild, although he or she is markedly short of breath.

4. What is acute respiratory failure (ARF)?

This term refers to the situation wherein the patient's PO_2 drops by 10 to 15 mm Hg or more, or where any level of hypercapnia is associated with an arterial pH that is less than 7.30. Patients with COPD may develop ARF when an acute infection occurs in the tracheobronchial tree, when air pollution suddenly worsens as in the case of an inversion, as a result of excessive sedation or narcotics, or when a complication such as thromboembolism, pneumothorax, or pneumonia occurs.

5. Describe the chest radiograph in patients who have COPD.

In COPD patients with predominant bronchitis, the radiographic findings early on may be normal. But later, the heart is enlarged because of right ventricular hypertrophy and associated left ventricular anoxia; there are increased bronchovascular markings, especially at the bases.

In COPD patients who have predominant emphysema, the lungs are hyperinflated, bullae may be present, the diaphragm is flat and low, and the heart

TABLE 15.5. Distinguishing Features: Bronchitis and Emphysema

CHARACTERISTICS	CHRONIC BRONCHITIS	EMPHYSEMA
Pathology	Inflamed spastic bronchi	Loss of elasticity
Pathophysiology	Airways obstruction	Airways obstruction
	V:P mismatch	V:P mismatch
Dyspnea	Mild	Severe
Cyanosis	Yes	No
Cough	Early and severe	Late
Sputum	Copious	Scant
Bronchial infections	Yes	No
PaO$_2$	Decreased	Small decrease
PaCO$_2$	Increased	Normal
Hematocrit	Increased	Normal
Pulmonary hypertension	Severe	Mild
Cor pulmonale	Common	Rare
Edema	Yes	No

PaO$_2$ = arterial oxygen partial pressure; PaCO$_2$ = arterial carbon dioxide partial pressure; V:P = ventilation-perfusion.

shadow appears small and vertical (Fig. 15.17). Features of both conditions often coexist in the same patient.

6. What is the general clinical course of the patient with COPD?

There is progressive worsening of underlying pulmonary function that is primarily involved with CO_2-O_2 exchange. Intermittent exacerbations result from infection or worsening pollution. There is little pulmonary reserve, and rapid deterioration occurs if heart failure, pneumonia, spontaneous pneumothorax, or thromboembolism supervenes.

Data On Day 7, the patient appears much better. Vital signs are normal, although he still gets short of breath on only minimal exertion. Pulmonary function tests show a low FEV_1; residual volume (RV) and total lung capacity (TLC) are above normal, as expected. He is given detailed instructions regarding smoking, diet, and avoidance of infections, and is advised to have a flu injection each year.

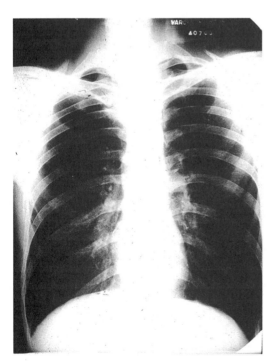

▶ **Figure 15.17.** Severe emphysema: lungs hyper-aerated, low diaphragm, and long narrow cardiac silhouette (not this patient).

Questions

1. A 42-year-old woman with known α_1-antitrypsin deficiency suddenly develops sharp left chest pain and shortness of breath. Examination discloses tympany, absent breath sounds, and absent fremitus in the left chest. The trachea appears to be shifted to the right. She has a:
   (a) left pleural effusion.
   (b) right pleural effusion.
   (c) left pneumothorax.
   (d) pneumonia.

2. All but which one of the following physical signs are commonly seen in severe COPD?
   (a) Cyanosis
   (b) Clubbing
   (c) Pursed lips
   (d) Wheezes

3. A patient with known COPD wakes up with shortness of breath and wheezing. Examination does not differ from her usual findings except for the presence of loud wheezes heard predominantly in the left hemithorax. Which is the most likely cause of her acute symptoms?
   (a) Left ventricular failure
   (b) Bronchial asthma
   (c) Left bronchial obstruction
   (d) Pneumonia
   (e) Cancer left main stem bronchus

Answers

1. **(c) is correct.** One must postulate she has emphysema with blebs and that one perforated. The tracheal shift to the right suggests a high tension pneumothorax. Urgent treatment is indicated. The physical signs are characteristically those of free air in the left hemithorax.

2. **(b)** clubbing is unusual unless bronchiectasis coexists. Pursed lips facilitate effective exhalation. Cyanosis and wheezes are common.

3. **(c) is correct.** Unilateral wheezes suggest left bronchial obstruction by tumor, foreign body, or mucus plug, most likely the latter. Although (e) is possible, the symptoms would not occur so suddenly; choices (a) and (d) would have associated symptoms and signs; choice (b) is possible, but not so suddenly, and not unilateral. Aspiration and measures to loosen secretions are indicated.

COMMENT This was a relatively straightforward case of COPD complicated by pneumonia and right ventricular failure who then developed acute respiratory failure. The patient bordered on the need for intubation and mechanical support.

COPD is a very common disease; its incidence is on the increase, and it currently affects approximately 20% of all adult men, in various degrees of severity, but mostly mild. There are still many gaps in our understanding of the pathophysiology of this group of diseases, such as exactly how α_1-antitrypsin deficiency results in alveolar wall destruction and what is the precise mechanism for airways obstruction in emphysema.

The diagnosis is fairly easy, but the physician must be aware of the various complications that may occur. Judicious administration of oxygen and ventilatory support are keystones of treatment. For this disease, preventive medicine is of paramount importance. *(P.C.)*

Suggested Readings

Angstman GL. Diagnosing COPD. How to identify patients with irreversible obstruction of the airways. Postgrad Med 1992;91(1):61–62, 65–67.

Anonymous. Standards for the diagnosis and care of patients with chronic obstructive pulmonary disease. Am J Respir Crit Care Med 1995;152(5, pt 2):S77-S121.

Chapman KR. Diagnostic dilemmas in obstructive airway disease. Hosp Pract (Off Ed) 1993;28(2A): 71–78, 81–88, 91.

Dennie C, Coblentz CL, LeBlanc P. Evaluation of the emphysematous patient. Chest Surg Clin N Am 1995;5(4):635–657.

Kronenberg RS, Geriffith DE. Chronic bronchitis. Key points in evaluation. Postgrad Med 1993;94(8): 84–90.

MacNee W. Pathophysiology of cor pulmonale in chronic obstructive pulmonary disease. Part one. Am J Respir Crit Care Med 1994;150(3):833–852.

MacNee W. Pathophysiology of cor pulmonale in chronic obstructive pulmonary disease. Part two. Am J Respir Crit Care Med 1994;150(4):1158–1168.

Gastrointestinal Problems

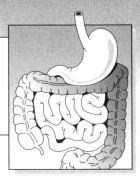

A consideration of gastrointestinal (GI) diseases must also include the diseases of this tract's appendages: the liver, gallbladder, and pancreas. You are therefore looking at a very large number of organs and diseases, from the mouth to the anus. The symptoms and signs are abundant, and ancillary studies are of great value.

Principal symptoms are dysphagia, anorexia, nausea, vomiting, "indigestion," pain, bleeding, perception of a mass, diarrhea, constipation, distention, and jaundice. Each symptom in itself may be a patient's chief complaint, although combinations are common.

In addition to the finding of a palpable mass, tenderness, distention, jaundice, hepatomegaly, or the various stigmata of cirrhosis, much help can be obtained from the physical examination.

However, many diagnostic studies must often be done before the final solution is reached. These include studies of the stool and urine, blood chemistry determinations, liver and pancreatic function tests, contrast radiographs, radionuclide studies, ultrasonography, endoscopy, biopsies, computed tomographic (CT) scans, magnetic resonance imaging (MRI), arteriography, percutaneous transhepatic cholangiography (PTC), and endoscopic retrograde cholangiopancreatography (ERCP)—an armory of diagnostic weapons. The exact roles, indications, benefits, risks, and preferential order of these studies are yet to be delineated in the various cases that follow.

The most frequent GI problems are usually not serious. The 1- or 2-day episode of nausea, vomiting, and diarrhea—acute gastroenteritis—is the single most common disorder; it clears spontaneously and needs little problem solving. Also frequent are acute gastric insults, indigestion, dyspepsia, psychogenic GI symptoms, and constipation; the latter two must be regarded with caution. The following conditions, although

less common (but still not uncommon), need more thought and resolution: ulcer, hepatitis, ileitis, ulcerative colitis, acute and chronic pancreatitis, acute cholecystitis, cholelithiasis, appendicitis, intestinal obstruction, and bleeding. Cirrhosis of the liver is in a class by itself because it is so very common in special subsets of the population. And at the tail end of this list are hemorrhoids—very common and easily diagnosed, yet often the scapegoat for symptoms originating in a more serious proximal lesion.

Lurking in the background, waiting to be mistaken for almost every disease just mentioned, is carcinoma occurring anywhere in the GI tract. It must not be overlooked.

Diverticulosis, gallstones, and hiatal hernia are common radiographic or autopsy findings (15 to 35% of adults have one or more of these three); therefore, the patient's symptoms are not necessarily attributable to these usually asymptomatic situations. The fact that a hiatal hernia can be demonstrated does not mean the patient's symptoms are due to the hernia; the same can be said for the other two radiographic findings.

To be remembered is the fact that many GI symptoms originate from diseases other than in the GI tract. Nausea, anorexia, and vomiting are commonly seen in uremia, Addison's disease, and congestive heart failure. Diarrhea or constipation may result from disease of the thyroid, parathyroid, or adrenal gland.

Medications taken for coexisting medical disorders may cause GI symptoms as well as more serious complications. One has but to leaf through the *Physicians' Desk Reference* to see the high incidence of nausea, vomiting, diarrhea, jaundice, and GI bleeding that may result from the use of nonsteroidal anti-inflammatory drugs (NSAIDs), other analgesics, and antibiotics.

Perhaps nowhere in medical practice must

there be a closer liaison between the primary care physician, the surgeon, and the radiologist than in GI tract disease. For obvious reasons, the distinction between medically and surgically treated disease must be made. The dividing line is often not clear, overlap may occur, and continuing consultation is often needed. Medically treated diseases develop surgical complications, and vice versa. A bleeding ulcer should be treated concurrently by the surgeon and primary care physician; the surgeon should not be hurriedly consulted at the last minute.

Two more points should be made. First, the reader should have an idea of the relative incidence of GI diseases. Expect to see a Zollinger-Ellison syndrome or Whipple's disease once in a lifetime, cancer of the stomach once every few years, cancer of the colon once every few months, a new peptic ulcer once a month, and a simple GI upset or psychogenic GI reaction daily.

Second, the reader must appreciate the fact that some GI diseases have many faces and presentations to the physician. Peptic ulcer can first be seen with classic symptoms, nondescript indigestion, perforation, hemorrhage, or obstruction. Regional enteritis can have a presentation of fever of unknown origin, right lower quadrant pain, intestinal obstruction, or an anal fistula. Cirrhosis can first be noted by asymptomatic hepatomegaly, a swollen abdomen, massive hemorrhage, acute alcoholic hepatitis with jaundice, or liver failure and impending coma. *(P.C.)*

DIFFICULTY IN SWALLOWING

Paul Cutler and Leonard Bentch

Data A 60-year-old woman visits your office with an 8-month history of difficulty in swallowing. The patient first noticed the problem when she was unable to eat a steak while dining in a restaurant. Since then she has had intermittent difficulty swallowing both liquids and solids and has lost 10 lb.

Logic Dysphagia must always be taken seriously. A few critical questions will determine the order of statistical likelihoods and the urgency with which tests must be done.

First—what is the location of the dysphagia?

Difficulty in the neck may be functional, neurologic, obstructive, or referred from a lower lesion. Although the sensation of dysphagia from lower lesions may be referred upward, the reverse is not true. The classic teaching that the patient can point to the site of the obstruction is only partially correct. If the symptom is high in the chest, you cannot be sure of its origin; but if it is lower in the chest, it may indeed indicate the location of the obstructing process.

Second—what kind of dysphagia is it? If only solids are involved, a mechanical obstruction that calibrates the food passing through it is suspect. This allows liquids and small particles to pass freely, but obstructs foodstuffs that approach the diameter of the opening. The normal esophagus is 20 mm in diameter; only some persons will have significant dysphagia if the diameter still exceeds 15 mm, but every one will have dysphagia if the diameter is narrowed to 11 mm (area decreased to one fourth of normal). On the other hand, if the patient has difficulty with both solids and liquids, then the passageway is pinhole in size (unlikely), or the problem is due to a motility disorder of the esophagus. Such disorders may include hypopharyngeal dysfunction due to neurologic disease, diffuse esophageal spasm, connective tissue disorders such as scleroderma, and distal esophageal sphincter dysfunction (achalasia).

Third—is the dysphagia continuous or intermittent? Progressive continuous worsening, first involving solids and later liquids too, suggests organic obstruction by cancer or stricture. Intermittency makes you think of a spastic lesion that waxes and wanes, or an organic lesion like a diverticulum which empties itself, thus temporarily relieving symptoms. Achalasia can be either continuous or intermittent, although not so progressively relentless as cancer.

Data On asking these questions, you learn that the discomfort on swallowing is in both the xiphoid area and the base of the neck. The dysphagia involves both liquids and solids, although the severity of the obstruction varies from time to time.

Logic Because of the intermittency of symptoms, you think mainly in terms of a disturbance of esophageal motility and/or a spastic, hypertensive lower esophageal sphincter (LES). But because many other serious diseases of the esophagus exist, you recall the various problems that can cause dysphagia and wish to rule them out.

Cervical dysphagia (difficulty arising in the neck) can be caused by globus hystericus; this is a feeling of a lump in the throat that occurs between meals and causes no real dysphagia. It is a manifestation of anxiety. Various neurologic diseases involving the brain stem or bilateral corticobulbar tracts cause difficulty in initiating the act of swallowing. In this instance, the patient chokes, coughs, and regurgitates through the nose, especially when trying to swallow liquids. Zenker's diverticulum in the hypopharynx can fill with food and obstruct swallowing until the pouch empties itself by regurgitation; this allows a brief symptom-free interval. Myasthenia gravis creates difficulty because of weakness of voluntary muscles that initiate swallowing. The Plummer-Vinson syndrome causes upper dysphagia because of high esophageal webs.

Medication-induced stricture is a more common cause of dysphagia. This may be seen in older patients taking quinidine-like drugs and large potassium tablets, and in any patient taking tetracycline compounds.

Data With this foreboding list in mind, you inquire about and note no other neurologic abnormalities, no difficulty with eye movements, no drooping eyelids, no feeling of a constant "lump in the throat," no history of regurgitation of undigested identifiable food, and no regurgitation of liquids through the nose. There is no evidence of anemia, the nails are not spoon-shaped, and the tongue is not smooth. Reflexes and cranial nerves are normal. No mass is felt in the side of the neck. The patient is a nonsmoker; examination of the chest reveals normal findings, and there are no enlarged lymph nodes.

Logic This quick subset of the history and physical examination has ruled out all the conditions associated with cervical dysphagia. A neurologic disease would not selectively affect only swallowing, nor would myasthenia gravis. There are no clues to speak on behalf of Plummer-Vinson syndrome or Zenker's diverticulum.

You now concern yourself with the rest of the esophagus, and the list of possibilities is equally formidable. Mainly you consider cancer, achalasia, and peptic esophagitis with stricture. Diffuse esophageal spasm and scleroderma are less common. Caustic stricture is easily eliminated by the lack of a history of swallowing a caustic. Diverticula in the middle and lower

esophagus occur, but they rarely if ever cause symptoms. She takes no medications that can cause stricture.

Diffuse esophageal spasm, like achalasia, is a disease of the visceral afferent nerves of the esophagus resulting in uncoordinated spasms demonstrable by motility studies. It is less common than achalasia and its pathophysiology is poorly understood.

Data There is no history of heartburn, indigestion, regurgitation of undigested nonacid material, choking and coughing that awaken the patient during sleep, anorexia, or weakness. Also, there are no symptoms or signs of arthritis, Raynaud's phenomenon, or tightening of the skin.

Logic Absence of heartburn weighs against peptic esophagitis. Although there is no evidence of scleroderma, dysphagia can be its first manifestation. This disease affects the smooth muscle and results in aperistalsis and secondary acid-peptic reflux due to a weakened lower esophageal sphincter. Progressive acid reflux will cause a lower esophageal stricture to form, just as in peptic esophagitis.

You suddenly remember that diseases outside the esophagus can also cause dysphagia, so a quick search is made for such possible causes.

Data The thyroid gland is not enlarged or hard; there is no auscultatory hint of mitral stenosis, nor can you feel, hear, or see evidence of an aortic aneurysm or a mediastinal mass. A normal chest radiographic finding rules out the latter three possibilities. While waiting for this radiograph, you complete the physical and neurologic examinations. All findings are normal there, too.

Logic The diagnostic field has been narrowed to either cancer of the esophagus or a motility disorder. The latter seems most likely.

Data Further discussion with the patient discloses that she has always considered herself to be "a slow eater," and over the past 10 years she has habitually "washed down" her food with liquids. The dysphagia is worse when she is out in company, but better when she can eat at her own pace at home. She tells of dysphagia that at times "hurts my heart."

Logic This history is becoming classic for achalasia. In this disease there is degeneration of the myenteric plexus in the esophageal submucosa. Nerve transmission is severed and the signal for peristalsis or lower esophageal sphincter relaxation cannot be transmitted. Large quantities of food and liquid create enough pressure, especially when the patient is erect, to intermittently force material into the stomach by overcoming the intrinsic pressure of the lower esophageal sphincter. Often, during sleep, liquid and food regurgitate from a distended esophagus, causing the patient to choke, cough, and sometimes even develop aspiration pneumonia. Patients often notice foul breath. However, these symptoms are not present in this case.

On the basis of history, you may not be absolutely certain of the cause of dysphagia, although you can determine likelihoods and guide those who will do further diagnostic procedures. The investigation of dysphagia is stereotyped. It includes an esophagram, upper GI series, and esophagogastroduodenoscopy in all cases. A blood count for anemia, a stool examination for occult blood to detect an ulcerating gastroesophageal lesion, and a chest radiograph complete the work-up. Because of similar visceral innervation, esophageal pain can sometimes mimic cardiac pain, so an electrocardiogram (ECG) and exercise tolerance test may be necessary. However, because the prominent symptom in this case is dysphagia, chest pain that is only reminiscent of cardiac pain would not warrant such study.

An esophagram is the safest of the first three studies mentioned, but it misses a significant number of carcinomas and other esophageal abnormalities, especially in the upper third. GI radiographs may detect carcinoma of the cardia. Fiberoptic esophagogastroduodenoscopy is most reliable but has more risk. It should generally follow an esophagram so that areas of potential hazard and sites of biopsies can be identified beforehand. The esophagram allows the fluoroscopist to watch peristalsis and the movement of the barium bolus—not generally possible with endoscopy.

A chest radiograph may demonstrate a dilated esophagus or a large hiatal hernia. Cervical dysphagia should always be initially evaluated with a barium or water-soluble contrast study because endoscopy may lead to inadvertent perforation of a Zenker's diverticulum or a proximal high-grade esophageal obstruction.

Data An esophagram demonstrated a dilated esophagus, with narrowing at the esophagogas-tric junction (Fig. 16.1). Endoscopy revealed a macerated esophagus with retained food and a

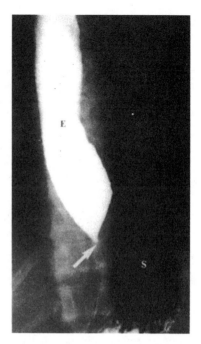

▶ **Figure 16.1.** Esophageal achalasia. Arrow points to the level of the gastroesophageal junction where a beak is formed by the column of barium. E = esophagus; S = stomach.

sharp narrowing at the LES. However, with gentle pressure the endoscopist was able to guide the endoscope through this narrowing with a definite "pop" as the instrument was advanced under direct vision. The endoscopist noted a classic "rosette" formation of the distal esophagus. On withdrawing the scope, no evidence of a mucosal lesion was seen. Especially important is a retroflex view of the proximal stomach to exclude a neoplasm arising in the cardia that might lead to "pseudo-achalasia."

An esophageal motility study was then done. It found aperistalsis in the body of the esophagus and a hypertensive LES that relaxed only 50% (from 60 to 30 mm Hg) after both dry and wet swallows (complete relaxation is normal). Complete blood count and urinalysis yielded normal results, and the stool tested negative for occult blood.

Logic A functional abnormality of the esophagus was suspected and proved. Achalasia is now established. Diffuse esophageal spasm was ruled out by radiographic and motility studies. Specific treatment may begin. The therapeutic modalities available include pneumatic dilation, surgical my-otomy, and the (experimental) injection of botulism toxin into the LES.

Questions

1. Given a patient with solid food dysphagia and a history of severe "heartburn" for many years, the most likely cause is:
   (a) carcinoma of the distal esophageal segment.
   (b) reflux esophagitis with secondary stricture formation.
   (c) Schatzki's ring.
   (d) scleroderma with secondary stricture.

2. If the patient's complaint had been cervical dysphagia, which of the following diagnoses could have been excluded with absolute certainty?
   (a) Globus hystericus
   (b) Pseudobulbar palsy
   (c) Carcinoma of the lower esophageal segment
   (d) None of the aforementioned

3. Anginoid pain is sometimes seen in patients with achalasia, diffuse esophageal spasm, or reflux esophagitis. This pain closely simulates angina because:
   (a) food lodging in the esophagus presses on the heart and causes cardiac pain.
   (b) visceral afferent fibers from the lower esophagus and the heart enter the spinal cord at the same level.
   (c) both pains are relieved by nitroglycerin.
   (d) patients with thoracic pain often fear the worst and imagine their chest pain to be cardiac in origin.

4. In which of the following esophageal diseases would a motility study be least likely to help?
   (a) Scleroderma
   (b) Carcinoma of the esophagus
   (c) Peptic stricture
   (d) Achalasia

Answers

1. **(b) is correct.** The presence of solid dysphagia indicates a structural abnormality that blocks the passage of food. Heartburn leads you to believe that reflux esophagitis has been present, and therefore the most logical diagnosis would be a peptic stricture. Carcinoma must always be excluded; biopsy of the lesion at endoscopy is a necessity. Schatzki's ring, an indentation at the squamocolumnar junction, is also possible, but is not

usually associated with heartburn and is almost always asymptomatic. Scleroderma with reflux and peptic stricture is rare.

2. **(d) is correct.** Cervical dysphagia generally points the clinician toward disease of the upper esophagus. However, it is a well-established clinical observation that obstruction of the lower esophageal segment can be perceived by the patient as cervical dysphagia. Therefore, the history alone cannot absolutely exclude carcinoma of the lower esophageal segment. Choices (a) and (b) cause symptoms in the neck, although, strictly speaking, globus does not cause true dysphagia. Pseudobulbar palsy is caused by bilateral partially resolved strokes; phonation and deglutition are disturbed because the lower cranial nerves on both sides are affected.

3. **(b) is correct.** The angina-like pain that sometimes accompanies dysphagia is due to stretching and stimulation of the visceral afferent fibers of the esophagus. These pain fibers enter the spinal cord at the same level as pain fibers from the heart, and they are often perceived as a squeezing chest pain that is at times virtually indistinguishable from angina. Therefore, the older patient may have coexistent angina, or only angina rather than esophageal disease. An ECG or exercise tolerance test may be indicated. Choices (c) and (d) are both true; however, neither explains the similar nature of the pains. Choice (a) has no pathophysiologic basis.

4. **(b) is correct.** A study of esophageal motility is expected to help uncover motor disturbances. Scleroderma is characterized by aperistalsis and hypotension of the lower esophageal sphincter. Peptic stricture in general demonstrates normal peristalsis, but shows a hypotensive sphincter that allows reflux of gastric contents. Achalasia has the combination of aperistalsis and a hypertensive lower esophageal sphincter. There are usually no characteristic abnormalities in carcinoma of the esophagus.

COMMENT This case study confronts us with a single key clue that may have multiple causes. Therefore the problem solver forms initial hypotheses—in this case a long differential diagnosis. On the basis of three historical points—location, type, and discontinuity of dysphagia—the list is rapidly narrowed. Other bits of pertinent negative information exclude additional diagnostic possibilities.

Two hypotheses remain plausible—cancer and achalasia. The diagnostic protocol is routine and a diagnosis is clearly made on a preconceived diagnostic sequence of esophagram, fiberoptic endoscopy, and motility-pressure studies. The patient has achalasia.

But in recent years it has become increasingly clear that peptic esophagitis with resulting spasm and stricture is very common. Careful studies of the lower esophageal sphincter have shown a causal relationship between a patent lower esophageal sphincter and gastroesophageal reflux. This results in frequent heartburn, eventual peptic esophagitis, and even stricture with dysphagia. The link to hiatal hernia is unproved, but reflux is abetted by the delayed gastric emptying seen in unrelated disease states such as diabetes. Furthermore, the patient with frequent heartburn due to reflux knows that caffeine, nicotine, alcohol, and chocolate exacerbate the reflux and the heartburn. To prove the existence of gastroesophageal reflux, manometry is impractical, endoscopy is widely used, a standard acid reflux test using a pH electrode is helpful, and barium radiography may give information in more advance states. Radionuclide scintiscanning may be useful; the stomach is loaded with a nonabsorbable isotope, and a gamma ray camera records the reflux over the lower end of the esophagus. *(P.C.)*

PROBLEM-BASED LEARNING Dysphagia leads to a study of many diseases both inside and outside the esophagus. Begin with a standard textbook for general orientation. There you learn a little about all conditions associated with difficulty in swallowing. Then progress to a textbook of gastroenterology for further details about the individual diseases. A complete study requires that you read recent literature where you will find that there is much ongoing research in the area of the lower esophageal sphincter. When finished, you should know all about:

- The causes of dysphagia
- Neuromuscular diseases such as pseudobulbar palsy, amyotrophic lateral sclerosis, multiple sclerosis, myasthenia gravis, and myotonia dystrophica—each of which may cause dysphagia
- How collagen disorders such as scleroderma and dermatomyositis cause dysphagia
- Disorders of esophageal motility—diffuse esophageal spasm and achalasia

- Dysfunction of the lower esophageal sphincter, gastroesophageal reflux, and peptic esophagitis
- Strictures caused by acid or lye or drugs
- The possible role of hiatal hernia
- Esophageal diverticuli (including Zenker's)
- Carcinoma of the esophagus
- Schatzki's ring
- Globus hystericus
- Plummer-Vinson syndrome and esophageal webs
- Extraesophageal diseases, such as thyroid cancer, lung cancer, substernal thyroid, aortic aneurysm, and mitral stenosis—each of which may cause dysphagia
- How esophageal disease causes chest pain
- The various diagnostic procedures needed to assess dysphagia—manometry, barium radiography, endoscopy, and scintiscanning: their uses, limitations, operating characteristics, and interpretation

And that's a lot to swallow!

Suggested Readings

Hendrix TR. Art and science of history taking in the patient with difficulty swallowing. Dysphagia 1993; 8(2):69–73.

Kadakia SC. Coping with achalasia. Postgrad Med 1993;93(5):249–250, 253–258, 260.

Lorenz R, Jorysz G, Tornieporth N, et al. The gastroenterologist's approach to dysphagia. Dysphagia 1993;8(2):79–82.

CASE 43

INDIGESTION

Suzanne Rose and Ernest Urban

Data Intermittent episodes of "indigestion" for 5 years bring a 45-year-old Mexican-American mother of three children to your office. She describes the indigestion as an upper abdominal fullness associated with gurgling noises and gas. This discomfort comes 1 to several hours after meals, lasts for a variable number of hours, then gradually disappears. There is no pain or heartburn. Over the last few months these symptoms became more frequent, occurred several times per week, and lasted for longer periods of time.

Logic The symptom complex of patients with indigestion can be vague and nonspecific, or it may be clear-cut and suggest a specific disorder. For example, duodenal ulcer may cause heartburn and epigastric pain several hours after eating; this is relieved by food or alkali. Gastroparesis may have a presentation of early satiety, bloating and distention, and postprandial nausea and vomiting. Peptic esophagitis causes symptoms like those of peptic ulcer; dysphagia may also be present. But atypical symptoms may include chest pain, hoarseness, asthma, and sore throat. Stomach cancer causes anorexia and early satiety. Gallbladder disease was thought to cause indigestion after ingestion of fried or fatty foods, but this is probably not so. Right upper quadrant pain is characteristic of gallstones, although stones do not cause indigestion. Gastrointestinal symptoms of anxiety states are vague, variable, and often nondescript.

Descriptions of indigestion vary. They include complaints such as gas, belching, heartburn, dyspepsia, bloating, discomfort, pain, gurgling noises, fullness, distention, and cramps. Typical syndromes are uncommon. Usually there is an overlap of symptoms from one digestive disease to another, and it is difficult to be certain of a diagnosis without studies.

The term non-ulcer dyspepsia (NUD) is used to describe unexplained gastrointestinal symptoms that suggest an upper GI tract problem. There are three major criteria associated with this diagnosis: the patient complains of a wide range of symptoms; symptoms are chronic and have existed for at least 3 months; and the symptoms remain unexplained after appropriate evaluation. Such criteria may be fulfilled by motility disorders such as gastroesophageal reflux disease (GERD), gastroparesis, enterogastric reflux gastritis, small intestinal dysmotility, and biliary dyskinesia. Such disorders are difficult to diagnose with certainty. Also possibly included in NUD are non-motility problems such as gastroduodenitis related to *Helicobacter pylori* or *Giardia lamblia* infection, and perhaps even to augmented visceral pain perception.

Data Further history does not elicit much additional significant information. The patient has experimented by avoiding spicy and fried foods, broiling meat, and omitting various vegetables and desserts. She has the impression that fatty and fried foods could be responsible for her symptoms. Antacids are of no help. Her appetite is good, and her weight has remained constant at 170 to 175 lb for at least 10 years. Occasional headaches are relieved by salicylates; she does not smoke and rarely drinks alcohol.

Her first child was delivered by cesarean section 22 years ago because of severe toxemia of pregnancy; the other two children are twins, 2½ years younger. Menses have been normal both before and since the pregnancies. A few weeks after the birth of her last two children she had several episodes of severe colicky upper abdominal pain that woke her at night. She felt distended each time, but the pains rapidly abated and she sought no medical advice.

Otherwise, the medical history is negative. She has three healthy younger sisters and a healthy 70-year-old mother. Her father died of a myocardial infarction at 62. The patient is a homemaker who left paid employment when she married.

Logic The fact that the patient is fat, female, fecund, and fortyish suggests gallstones. Several episodes of pain years ago could represent gallstone pain or the passage of stones or gravel. Incomplete intestinal obstruction from postoperative adhesions was possible. The constancy of weight and duration of symptoms weigh against cancer. Her dietary experimentation led nowhere. There is no pattern of periodicity, symptom relationship to meals, or relief by alkali. The picture remains unclear.

Data Physical examination disclosed a healthy-appearing but overweight woman. All findings were normal or negative, including the rectum, pelvis, stool for occult blood, and sigmoidoscopy. A low midline scar was noted. There was no epigastric tenderness, and no abdominal masses or organs were palpated.

Logic Again no help! A stool without occult blood and the absence of pallor preclude a bleeding gastrointestinal lesion but do not rule out intermittent bleeding. No masses or organs were palpable, but her obesity makes this negative finding unreliable. The absence of tenderness is fairly reliable and would eliminate an active ulcer, and certainly an acutely inflamed gallbladder.

You must now distinguish between *functional* and *organic* disease. This is a vital distinction. There is much information to show that "functional disorders" result from alterations in motility or dyskinesias of the gastrointestinal tract. Psychologic disturbance *may* play a role. But future clinical studies and new disease concepts may disprove the nervous or functional aspects of some subsets of this hodgepodge of gastrointestinal disorders. Organic diseases, on the other hand, have identifiable pathologic or structural lesions. Those disorders resulting from known hormonal or enzyme deficiencies are either considered to be organic or belong in a gray zone.

Approximately 50% of patients with "indigestion" have no organic disease. Middle-aged women predominate. The onus on the physician is great. A label of "functional gastrointestinal disorder" or "nervous stomach" is difficult to erase once established. This label must often be revised if symptoms change or new symptoms develop. Remember that patients with functional disorders develop organic disease with the same frequency as the general population.

With these thoughts in mind, you list the traditional causes of indigestion for further consideration. These include:

1. Peptic esophagitis and GERD
2. Peptic ulcer
3. Cancer of the stomach
4. Chronic cholecystitis with cholelithiasis
5. Aerophagia and other functional disorders
6. Malabsorption
7. Chronic pancreatitis
8. Pancreatic pseudocyst
9. Right ventricular failure with visceral congestion
10. Anginal equivalent
11. Abdominal epilepsy or migraine
12. Lack of proper dentures

A number of listed entities can be rapidly screened by history and examination. The absence of diarrhea, no abdominal pain, no history of acute pancreatitis, no evidence for heart failure, no relationship of symptoms to exertion, and the presence of teeth easily rule out most of diagnoses 6 to 12. The first five diagnoses are the most common and merit the most consideration. **Data** You decide to go fishing in the upper abdomen for an additional lead and order a blood count, urinalysis, ECG, chest radiograph, plain radiograph of the abdomen, sedimentation rate, and 18-test blood chemistry profile (including bilirubin, transferases, alkaline phosphatase, and proteins). All test results are normal. The plain radiograph of the abdomen shows normal renal size, no radiopaque calculi in the gallbladder or urinary tract, and no abnormal gas patterns.

Logic Again, no help from the tests so far. She is scheduled for an ultrasound study of the gallbladder the next day. Although 80% of kidney stones are radiopaque, only 20% of gallbladder stones are; the remaining 80% are radiolucent cholesterol stones.

Data The patient cancels her tests and postpones them 2 weeks hence because her eldest daughter will be visiting with the new grandchild. In the meantime she is told to keep a diary of her symptoms in relation to meals, type of food, and time of day.

Ten days later, she returns with a story of two episodes of colicky right upper quadrant pain radiating to the shoulder. The pain waxed and waned over several hours, then abated, leaving her sore and tender. The first episode occurred in the middle of the night after her last appointment, and the second episode was 2 days ago, approximately 2 hours after lunch. She said that she felt restless with the pain and could not find a comfortable position. The character of the pain was similar to labor pain and similar to the episodes she had had years ago.

The examination reults are normal except for slight right upper quadrant tenderness.

Ultrasound shows a normal liver; there are multiple stones in the gallbladder, but the common bile duct does not appear dilated (Fig. 16.2).

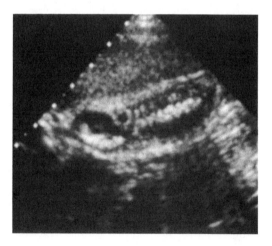

▶ **Figure 16.2.** Ultrasound reveals thickened gallbladder wall. Acoustic shadows indicate many stones in the lumen.

The results of an upper GI series are normal; there is no evidence of gastroesophageal reflux, ulcer, or cancer.

Logic Ultrasound is relatively inexpensive, safe, generally available, and highly reliable. Its 95% sensitivity for biliary calculi makes it a first-line diagnostic procedure when stones are suspected. You are not surprised to find stones. There is an increased incidence of cholelithiasis in Mexican-Americans; it is most likely a reflection of the increased incidence of cholelithiasis seen in the American Indian. Also, approximately 10 to 20 million Americans of all ethnic backgrounds have gallstones—that is, 5 to 10% of the population.

But are the stones related to her symptoms? To the episodes of pain, probably yes! To the long-standing indigestion, probably not! The association of symptoms other than pain with gallbladder disease is chancy. In fact, the relationship of fatty food intolerance and gallstones is purely fortuitous. It has been nicely demonstrated that fatty food intolerance is more frequent in patients with normal than with abnormal cholecystograms. So much for a popular but mistaken concept introduced as far back as 1908 and still not expunged.

Patients who have gallstones and atypical symptoms have a 50% chance of having their usual symptoms persist after cholecystectomy.

Data After careful consideration, consultation, and discussion with the patient, surgery was advised. A laparoscopic cholecystectomy was performed. The gallbladder wall showed evidence of acute and chronic inflammation. There were many stones of varying size within the gallbladder (Fig 16.3); the common duct was of normal caliber. Recovery was uneventful.

Logic Even though the symptoms and diagnosis could not be definitely related, surgery was indicated. An elective procedure in a healthy patient bears little risk. One third to one half of patients with gallstones will develop severe symptoms or serious complications. At that point, the surgical risk is much higher. Furthermore, cancer of the gallbladder can result from stones. And, because ursodeoxycholic acid for dissolution of biliary calculi is slow, only partially effective, and does not prevent stone recurrence, surgery is still the best treatment.

Data Six months later the patient consults you again. For a few weeks after the cholecystectomy she seemed to be relieved of her symptoms, but

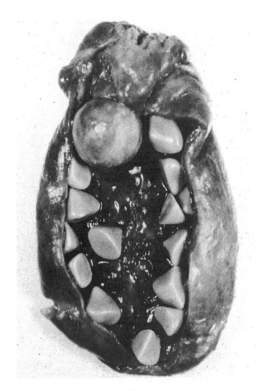

▶ **Figure 16.3.** Multiple gallstones within resected gallbladder.

over the past few months her indigestion returned and now seems to be getting worse. She noticed an increasing amount of bloating and gas, and there have also been several bouts of diarrhea. She has not been out of the country and no family members have had similar symptoms. Examination results are completely normal. The cholecystectomy scar is well healed and not tender.

Logic This situation is not rare. Was the diseased gallbladder unrelated to the symptoms? Was her original disease not uncovered? Does she have a new disease? Is she psychoneurotic? Diarrhea has been added to the cluster of symptoms, but it does not seem to be of infectious origin.

Data Further inquiries are made. Her home situation does not seem to be stressful despite having three children. She does not seem disturbed, anxious, tense, or depressed. The stools are watery but contain formed solid material. Borborygmi frequently precede a sudden need to go to the toilet. The solid part of the stool is of normal caliber, and there is no blood, mucus, or pus.

Logic Again the matter of organicity arises. At least on the surface, no psychologic problems are present. You know that irritable bowel syndrome is the most common chronic gastrointestinal disorder seen in clinical practice. Although it causes much distress, it has no serious consequences. It is characterized by chronic crampy abdominal pains and constipation, or chronic intermittent watery diarrhea, or a combination of both. The stools may contain much mucus and are sometimes pencil-like; or the stool may be passed frequently in small amounts, yet there is no increase in the total amount of stool. A fact that must always be considered when seeing patients with such complaints is that these symptoms mimic more serious or curable diseases.

Mistakes in this area are common. The absence of blood, pus, and mucus in the stool makes infectious or ulcerative colitis less likely but does not exclude them. And be aware that the common denominator for all forms of irritable bowel syndrome is alteration in intestinal motility for which psychologic disturbances may or may not be responsible.

Data Sigmoidoscopy results are normal. Stool culture shows only normal flora, and no ova or parasites are seen on careful microscopic examination. Barium enema reveals no abnormality. You are perplexed and ready to label the symptoms functional despite the absence of environmental stress. The patient tells you again that she has explored dietary manipulations without success.

Logic Suddenly an idea flashes through your mind. Lactose intolerance of *varying degrees* occurs in 50% of adult Mexican-Americans, 70% of black Americans, and almost 100% of Asians and American Indians, but in less than 15% of whites of northern European ancestry. The symptoms are wholly consistent with lactose intolerance. Milk products containing lactose are widely present in foods, often being added as fillers or extenders. They are present in such items as cream of chicken soup, some breads, and many cookies, as well as the more obvious dairy products.

Data You inquire in detail about the use of milk and dairy products. She drinks several cups of coffee with milk or cream each day, eats ice cream, and has milk with cereal for breakfast. She has not liked the taste of milk since her late teens but never thought much about it and never related her indigestion to milk or milk products.

An oral lactose tolerance test is done. After 50 g of oral lactose, the blood glucose levels are 86, 89, 94, and 96 mg/dL at fasting, 30, 60, and 90 minutes after ingestion. The patient complained of considerable bloating, gas, and several loose, watery bowel movements during and for several hours after the test.

A hydrogen breath test was simultaneously performed. Expired air samples were collected at intervals after lactose ingestion and analyzed for hydrogen content by gas chromatography. The test results were positive for lactose intolerance.

Logic Lactose intolerance is now proved. The amount of lactose used is equivalent to that found in approximately 1 liter of milk. The blood glucose results indicate a flat curve (a rise of less than 20 mg/dL). These values plus the exacerbation of symptoms are excellent evidence that the patient is lactase deficient and therefore lactose intolerant. Recall that lactose is split by the mucosal enzyme lactase into glucose and galactose before absorption. Unsplit lactose remains in the intestinal lumen where it exerts an osmotic effect. When the lactose and greater amount of water drawn with it reach the colon, enteric bacteria flourish and some even split lactose. Thus, gas, bloating, and diarrhea result. This is a specific malabsorption, and absorption of all other nutriments by the small intestine remains unimpaired.

The lactose tolerance test has a 20% false-positive and a 20% false-negative rate. The breath test is much more sensitive and specific. Intestinal bacteria act upon undigested and unabsorbed lactose to form hydrogen, which is excreted in the breath.

A lactose-free diet or the use of lactase supplements are excellent diagnostic and therapeutic tests.

Data The patient is given detailed instructions about a low-lactose diet and calcium supplementation because elimination of a wide range of foods containing lactose may lead to calcium deficiency and osteopenia. She is informed of the need to read labels in order to learn the composition of the packaged foods she buys. You consider prescribing a new commercial lactase preparation which, when added to milk, hydrolyzes the lactose and makes it drinkable; but you decide to try diet alone.

Two months later she reports back to you—free of symptoms.

COMMENT Two organic problems existed in this patient. Each caused symptoms—cholelithiasis and lactose intolerance. This combination is not so unusual. Chance alone dictates that two common conditions will occur together in a smaller but definite number of persons—(product of the probabilities). Fortunately, a psychoneurotic label was avoided.

Beginning with a broad range of disorders that might cause "indigestion," the list was whittled down by the absence of numerous highly sensitive clues until only two or three possible diagnoses remained. Discussion often centered on the operating characteristics (sensitivity and specificity) of various clues, and of the lactose tolerance and hydrogen breath tests, until reasonable certainty was established by a therapeutic trial.

Other carbohydrate malabsorption syndromes have been described. More recently, fructose and sorbitol malabsorption have been implicated as causes of similar symptoms. One entity known as "chewing gum disorder" has been described in patients chewing large amounts of dietetic gum, with sorbitol as the sugar, which acts as an osmotic agent and may cause urgent diarrhea. *(P.C.)*

Suggested Readings

Fisher RS. Non-ulcer dyspepsia: Candidate disorders. Gastroenterol Endosc News 1993;18–21.

Montes RG, Perman JA. Lactose intolerance: Pinpointing the source of nonspecific gastrointestinal symptoms. Postgrad Med 1991;89:175–184.

Saavedra JM, Perman JA. Current concepts in lactose malabsorption and intolerance. Ann Rev Nutr 1989; 9:475–502.

Tally NJ, Phillips SF. Non-ulcer dyspepsia: Potential causes and pathophysiology. Ann Intern Med 1988; 108:865–879.

CASE 44

DIARRHEA AND WEIGHT LOSS

Glenn W.W. Gross and Elliot Weser

Data Watery, nonbloody, non-mucus-producing diarrhea brings a 48-year-old man to your office. Although these symptoms have been intermittently present for 12 years, they have gotten worse, especially over the past 2 years. He now has several stools daily and gets up at night to go to the toilet. The diarrhea is accompanied by abdominal cramps, excessive flatulence, and loud noises in the abdomen. During the past 2 years he has lost 20 lb. Several physicians told him he had a "nervous colon," and one of these physicians ordered a barium enema performed that had normal results. Otherwise, he has always been well.

Logic You react with surprise and disbelief that such severe symptoms could possibly be considered functional, especially with weight loss. Many organic diseases characterized by chronic diarrhea come out of your memory tape: (1) parasitic diseases, such as amebiasis, giardiasis, strongyloidiasis; (2) primary small or large bowel disease, such as regional enteritis, ulcerative colitis, and tuberculosis; and (3) endocrine-induced diarrhea caused by hyperthyroidism, gastrinoma, carcinoid, or diabetes (Table 16.1).

The absence of gross blood in the stool makes a mucosal ulcerating disease such as ulcerative colitis unlikely, and the chronicity argues against a bacterial dysentery. Cancer is unlikely in view of the 12-year illness. It is important to consider a malabsorption disorder because there has been recent documented weight loss. The cramping and borborygmi indicate increased peristalsis and therefore disease of the small intestine.

Data The stools are bulky, frothy, float, and smell foul. Despite his symptoms, the patient's appetite is excellent and food intake remains normal. He drinks no coffee or alcohol and takes no laxatives. He has no risk factors for human

TABLE 16.1. Major Causes of Chronic Diarrhea

1. Infections—viral, protozoal, fungal, bacterial
2. Inflammatory bowel disease
   (a) Regional enteritis (Crohn's)
   (b) Ulcerative colitis
3. Malabsorption syndromes
4. Endocrine causes—hyperthyroidism, Addison's disease, carcinoid, gastrinoma, VIP–secreting adenoma
5. Colon cancer or lymphoma
6. Tuberculous enterocolitis
7. Drugs

VIP = vasoactive intestinal peptide.

immunodeficiency virus (HIV) infection and takes no medications.

Examination shows normal vital signs, evidence of weight loss, scattered ecchymoses of the skin, cracking at the corners of the mouth (cheilosis), a smooth red tongue, and a protuberant abdomen with increased bowel sounds. There is no tenderness, surgical scars, or organ enlargement in the abdomen. Moderate pretibial and ankle edema are present. All other findings, including those of flexible sigmoidoscopy, are normal.

Logic Normal sigmoidoscopy results make ulcerative colitis and amebiasis unlikely because these diseases usually involve the rectum and sigmoid. However, the rectum may be spared in Crohn's disease of the colon or elsewhere in the gastrointestinal tract because skip areas are common.

The character of the stools almost certainly indicates that the patient has steatorrhea and malabsorption. Fat and fermentation gas entrapped in the stool give it the observed appearance with a density less than water—hence it floats.

Weight loss in the face of an excellent appetite suggests that ingested calories are not being used and further points to impaired absorption. A hypermetabolic state, such as hyperthyroidism, may also produce weight loss and diarrhea with preservation of appetite and food intake, but this is unlikely in the absence of the usually present physical findings of tachycardia, tremor, and thyromegaly.

Ecchymoses suggest a clotting defect such as hypoprothrombinemia resulting from fat-soluble vitamin K deficiency. The cheilosis and smooth tongue indicate vitamin B complex deficiency, and the edema is compatible with hypoproteinemia.

Malabsorption seems likely. The causes include intestinal lymphoma, regional enteritis (Crohn's), celiac sprue, severe liver disease, bacterial overgrowth in the small intestine (blind loop syndrome), Whipple's disease, intestinal lymphangiectasia, and chronic pancreatic exocrine insufficiency. The absence of fever, abdominal mass, or specific tenderness reduces the likelihood of regional enteritis and lymphoma. There are no stigmata of liver disease. Tests are needed to corroborate malnutrition and malabsorption. As we proceed, it is important to distinguish between digestion and absorption, because an increased loss of nutrients in the stool can reflect a disorder of either process. The tests commonly used in the clinical evaluation of suspected malabsorption are listed in Table 16.2.

TABLE 16.2. Tests Commonly Used in the Clinical Evaluation of Suspected Malabsorption

Complete blood count, serum chemistries, prothrombin time

Thyroid function studies

Specific nutrient levels (iron, folate, vitamin B_{12}, fat-soluble vitamins)

72-hour fecal fat collection

Small bowel biopsy

Breath hydrogen test(s)

D-xylose absorption test

Secretin test

Plain abdominal radiograph, small bowel series

Endoscopic retrograde pancreatography

Schilling's test (multiple phases)

Digestion begins in the mouth and stomach (pepsin), but occurs mainly in the upper small intestine (SI) under the influence of the pancreas (lipase, amylase, trypsin) and small intestinal cells (disaccharidases). The sites where various nutrients are absorbed are: iron, calcium, water-soluble vitamins, and fats in the proximal SI; hexose sugars in the proximal and mid-SI; amino acids all over the SI, but mainly in the mid-SI; bile salts and vitamin B_{12} mostly in the SI; and water and electrolytes in the proximal colon.

Data Blood count shows a mild anemia (hematocrit 35%, hemoglobin 10 g/dL) with a nondiagnostic blood smear. Serum potassium is low (2.8 mEq/L); thyroid function (T_4 and T_3 resin uptake) is normal; serum calcium is low (7.8 mg/dL); total protein is low (5.1 g/dL) with a low albumin (2.2 g/dL); liver function test results are normal except for the prothrombin time (22 seconds: control 12 seconds); serum cholesterol is reduced (96 mg/dL), as are the carotene (18 μg/dL) and triglycerides (42 mg/dL). Blood glucose, 5-hydroxyindoleacetic acid in the urine, and serum gastrin levels are normal.

The chest radiographic finding is normal. Upper gastrointestinal and small bowel radiograph series show moderate diffuse dilatation of the small bowel and thickened scalloped folds, compatible with a malabsorption pattern; pancreatic calcifications and narrowing of the ileum are not present.

The barium enema finding is normal. An intermediate strength purified protein derivative (PPD) skin test result is negative. The stool tests are negative for ova, parasites, and blood (Hemoccult test).

Logic These tests substantiate *malnutrition* and suggest but do not absolutely document *malabsorption* or indicate its cause. Diabetic autonomic neuropathy, carcinoid, and gastrinoma are now unlikely. Low potassium may result from chronic diarrheal loss. The other low blood chemistry values are related to depleted lipid and nitrogen stores caused by poor fat and protein absorption. Protein may also be lost by "weeping" of albumin into the intestinal lumen through a damaged mucosa. The low total serum calcium may be caused by decreased binding to reduced serum albumin and a decrease in ionized serum calcium from reduced absorption. Calcium malabsorption is the result of two factors: binding of calcium to malabsorbed fatty acids, and vitamin D deficiency caused by this vitamin's fat solubility and subsequent poor absorption. Tetany may result.

Fat-soluble vitamins (A, D, E, and K) are poorly absorbed and cause the low carotene and low prothrombin levels. Vitamin B complex deficiency accounts for the tongue and cheilosis, although vitamin B_{12} malabsorption can smooth the tongue, too. Anemia can result from poor absorption of iron, vitamin B_{12}, or folic acid, and its cause needs clarification with more studies.

The radiographs do not show changes characteristic of regional enteritis (Crohn's), ulcerative colitis, or any abnormality of the gastrointestinal tract that might indicate bowel stasis and bacterial overgrowth (multiple diverticula, fistulas, or blind loop). There are no pancreatic calcifications, epigastric pain, history of alcoholism, or episodes of acute pancreatitis to suggest chronic pancreatitis and pancreatic insufficiency. The normal chest radiograph and negative purified protein derivative skin test make intestinal tuberculosis unlikely. Intestinal parasites are excluded by the stool study.

It is important to exclude cirrhosis and chronic pancreatitis even though they are uncommon causes of maldigestion and consequent malabsorption.

If, contrary to the stated data, the patient drank too much alcohol and had epigastric pains, diabetes, severe steatorrhea, and pancreatic calcifications, marked deficiency of exocrine pancreatic function would be your first diagnostic consideration. Such an obvious instance needs no further tests. But in doubtful, on-the-fence cases, you might wish confirmation. The *secretin* test measures duodenal fluid and bicarbonate after intravenous (IV) secretin administration. The *combined secretin-cholecystokinin* test measures intraluminal duodenal amylase, lipase, trypsin, and chymotrypsin after an intravenous infusion of the secretagogue. Or you can simply measure the *fecal chymotrypsin* content.

If the liver size and feel are normal, and there are no stigmata of chronic severe liver disease, the liver may be virtually eliminated as the cause of malabsorption. When severe liver disease is clearly evident by history and physical examination, another cause for malabsorption may still be present and must be sought.

Data A D-xylose absorption test (25 g oral dose) reveals a low urinary excretion of 2.3 g (9.2%). The 3-day fecal fat excretion test is increased and averages 16 g/d (16% of daily fat intake).

A lactose breath hydrogen test shows a significant rise in breath hydrogen (increase of > 20 parts per million) at 3 hours after lactose ingestion. Endoscopic retrograde pancreatography and a secretin stimulation test reveal normal pancreatic duct morphology and normal exocrine pancreatic function, respectively.

Finally, a small bowel (distal duodenal) biopsy was done at upper endoscopy. Histologic examination revealed total atrophy of the intestinal villi, with a dense infiltrate of lymphocytes and plasma cells in the lamina propria (Fig. 16.4). The patient was diagnosed as having *celiac sprue* (gluten enteropathy), and a strict gluten-free diet was initiated. Within 2 weeks his diarrhea gradually subsided, and he gained 20 lb in weight over the next 6 months. A repeat small bowel biopsy 1 year later was normal.

Logic The specific absorption tests clearly demonstrated a generalized malabsorptive state. Not only was steatorrhea present, but there also was impaired D-xylose and lactose absorption. Steatorrhea may be caused by diseases that impair the normal digestion of fat (such as pancreatic insufficiency with decreased lipase activity) or disease that impair the absorption/transport of otherwise normally digested fat (such as primary small bowel diseases, or conditions that deplete or alter the bile acid pool and lead to defective micelle formation in the gut lumen).

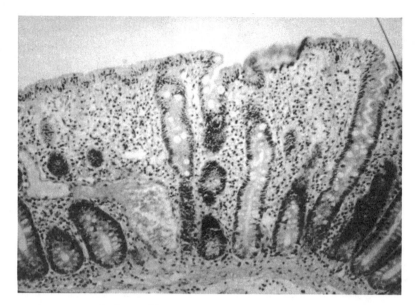

▶ **Figure 16.4.** Photomicrograph of a small bowel biopsy specimen from a patient who has celiac sprue displaying the characteristic villous atrophy, crypt hyperplasia, intraepithelial lymphocytes, and lymphocytic infiltration of the lamina propria. The exact mechanism for gluten's effect on the mucosa is not clear.

The abnormal D-xylose and lactose absorption point to a primary mucosal disease most likely involving the proximal small bowel, which is the major site of absorption of these sugars. The villous atrophy is associated with not only reduced carbohydrate absorption but also with decreased activity of intestinal disaccharidases, particularly lactase. Thus impaired lactose hydrolysis is largely responsible for malabsorption of this sugar. Intraluminal maldigestion of lactose (lactase deficiency), rather than mucosal malabsorption (impaired transport) of its constituent sugars, could alternately account for the late rise in breath hydrogen after lactose ingestion.

The small bowel biopsy has characteristic histologic changes in some mucosal malabsorptive diseases, including celiac sprue, Whipple's disease, lymphangiectasia, and abetalipoproteinemia (acanthocytosis). Gluten is a protein found in wheat, rye, oats and barley—but *not* in rice and potatoes.

In this patient the typical histologic changes of celiac sprue and the definite improvement on a gluten-free diet established the diagnosis.

The diagnosis of generalized malabsorption is first suggested by a history of chronic diarrhea and weight loss, usually accompanied by physical findings associated with malnutrition. It is possible, however, to have a disorder in which there

is selective malabsorption of a single nutrient, such as lactose in primary lactase deficiency, vitamin B_{12} in isolated ileal Crohn's disease, and glucose or galactose in monosaccharide transport carrier deficiency. The diagnosis of generalized malabsorption depends on demonstration of absorptive defects involving more than one nutrient, usually including an abnormal fecal excretion of fat. The specific disease causing the malabsorption is determined by additional physical findings (i.e., abdominal mass, localized tenderness), characteristic radiograph changes, intestinal biopsy, breath hydrogen testing, structural and/or functional studies of the pancreas, and in some cases surgical exploration.

Questions

1. Steatorrhea may occur in all but which one of the following?
   (a) Isolated lactase deficiency
   (b) Small intestinal bacterial overgrowth
   (c) Insufficient lipase secretion
   (d) Intestinal lymphoma
2. Increased fecal fat excretion with a normal D-xylose test result most likely suggests:

(a) Celiac sprue

(b) Ulcerative colitis

(c) Diffuse intestinal lymphoma

(d) Pancreatic insufficiency

3. Steatorrhea caused by insufficient digestion of fat would be likely if the gastrointestinal radiograph shows:

(a) a blind loop.

(b) regional ileitis.

(c) pancreatic calcifications.

(d) dilated scalloped small bowel loops suggestive of celiac sprue.

4. Intestinal biopsy is particularly helpful in the diagnosis of:

(a) Crohn's disease.

(b) pancreatic insufficiency.

(c) intestinal lymphoma.

(d) celiac sprue.

Answers

1. **(a) is correct.** Isolated lactase deficiency is a very common, specific defect that impairs only the digestion (hydrolysis) of lactose and is not accompanied by steatorrhea. Bacterial overgrowth in the small intestine leads to deconjugation of bile acids, which results in poor micelle formation and impaired fat absorption. Insufficient lipase secretion, as seen in exocrine pancreatic insufficiency, results in inadequate fat hydrolysis before absorption. Intestinal lymphoma may directly impair the mucosal transport of fat.

2. **(d) is correct.** Pancreatic insufficiency results in lipase deficiency, which impairs the hydrolysis of fat and thus reduces its overall absorption. Intestinal mucosal function is usually normal, and thus a D-xylose absorption test should be normal. Celiac sprue and intestinal lymphoma are likely to have impaired mucosal transport, and thus the D-xylose absorption test result would be abnormal. Being a disease of the colon, ulcerative colitis should impair the absorption of neither fat nor D-xylose.

3. **(c) is correct.** The presence of pancreatic calcifications on radiograph would point to chronic pancreatitis and reduced lipase secretion. Fat *digestion* (hydrolysis) would likely be impaired. Bacterial overgrowth in the blind loop syndrome and decreased absorption of bile salts from the ileum in regional enteritis would result in poor micelle formation and decrease the *absorption* of fat. A diffusely dilated small bowel ("malabsorption pattern") on radiograph would more likely suggest that a primary intestinal disease such as celiac sprue is decreasing the absorption.

4. **(d) is correct.** There are specific mucosal diseases that can be diagnosed by histologic examination. Celiac sprue is the most common one, and a patient with malabsorption and the typical histologic changes detected at small bowel biopsy most likely has this disease. Detection of circulating anti-gliadin or anti-endomysial antibodies supports the presence of celiac disease, and clinical improvement on a gluten-free diet confirms the diagnosis. Exocrine pancreatic insufficiency does not alter the intestinal mucosa. In Crohn's disease and intestinal lymphoma, histologic findings are not sufficiently specific to support a precise diagnosis by biopsy, and additionally the patchy distribution of these diseases often leads to biopsies that miss the area of pathology.

COMMENT There are numerous tests and procedures that may help solve problems such as this one. But the clues offered by the history and physical examination go far in establishing the diagnosis. One might question the need for many of the tests that were done.

Diarrhea, weight loss, good appetite, and the nature of the stool add up to malabsorption. The absence of alcoholism, abdominal pain, and stigmata of cirrhosis virtually eliminate diseases of the pancreas and liver as causes for malabsorption. This points to the small intestine as the site of disease.

The small intestinal biopsy and the response to specific treatment offered a degree of diagnostic certainty that left no room for false positivity. *(P.C.)*

Suggested Readings

Craig RM, Atkinson AJ Jr. D-xylose testing: A review. Gastroenterology 1988;95:223–231.

Perman JA. Clinical application of breath hydrogen measurements. Can J Physiol Pharmacol 1991;69:111–115.

Romano TJ, Dobbins JW. Evaluation of the patient with suspected malabsorption. Gastroenterol Clin No Am 1989;18:467–483.

Trier JS. Celiac sprue. N Engl J Med 1991;325:1709–1719.

CASE 45

SUDDEN UPPER ABDOMINAL PAIN

Carlos Pestana

Data A 43-year-old man arrives at the emergency department at 6 am complaining of severe abdominal pain that he has had all night. He is accompanied by his wife. As you start your evaluation of the problem, you notice that he is lying on the stretcher on his back with his knees drawn up, and he is retching and vomiting a very small amount of greenish fluid. While you are asking your first few questions he changes position twice, lying on his side but still with the knees drawn up. It is obvious that he is in great pain.

Logic Your initial observation and the complaint with which he registered have already given you several clues. The problem is acute, has lasted approximately 12 hours, and is a problem of abdominal pain. His appearance and the fact that he sought help at a rather inconvenient hour suggest that the pain is severe. Furthermore, even though you were trained to take a history first and then do a physical examination, you cannot help but notice his position and the fact that he moves around seeking relief. The fetal position is frequently assumed with pancreatic pain.

Acute abdominal pain brings to mind perforated ulcer, acute pancreatitis, mesenteric thrombosis, biliary colic, ureteral colic, and a host of other disorders. It is unusual to thrash around seeking relief if there is an irritating fluid loose in the belly, so that perforated ulcer, bile peritonitis, free perforation of a diverticulum, or other examples of visceral perforation are less likely. Let us go on and get the details about the pain.

Data The patient relates that he was in his usual state of good health until last night. He began to experience epigastric pain at approximately 8 pm, shortly after he returned home from a party at which he ate and drank heavily. The pain began gradually, and built up to full intensity in approximately 1/2 hour. It was constant in nature, very severe, radiating straight through to the back, and was accompanied by nausea and vomiting shortly after its onset. He vomited one or two cupfuls of greenish material, but later he simply retched without bringing much up. The pain has remained constant in nature, location, and intensity. He has taken no medications for it.

Logic An experienced clinician would already have a tentative diagnosis based on pattern recognition. The description is classical for acute pancreatitis. You would not easily elicit such a concise summary from a patient or his wife, but you could achieve it only by careful questioning. We start by setting the time of onset: he says last night. You press on: does he really mean last

night, or has he been sick for 2 or 3 days and things got worse last night? No, he was fine until last night. OK, how did it begin? What was he doing at the time? It makes a big difference if he got the pain right after being run over by a truck, as opposed to lying quietly in bed. It turns out that he had just returned home after an unusual meal—a heavy one, with lots of drinking.

This pattern fits pancreatitis, but also would fit acute alcoholic gastritis, a flare-up of an otherwise tame duodenal ulcer, food poisoning, or plain old upset stomach of the television commercial variety. The latter is unlikely, in view of the duration and severity of the pain. In food poisoning, we would expect vomiting and diarrhea, and the pain would be of a colicky nature (intermittent pain with a crescendo-decrescendo pattern). An angry duodenal ulcer can give much pain, particularly one that penetrates into the pancreas or, even more so, one that perforates. The fact that he is moving around is a small clue against the latter, but does not rule it out. Acute alcoholic gastritis should have been somewhat relieved with vomiting, and would have produced bleeding—it sounds unlikely.

We press on with the details. Just how sudden was the onset? If he had been calmly reading the paper, and suddenly, on line 10 of column 2, he was struck by a bolt out of the blue, you would think of a perforation, most commonly a perforated ulcer (but it could also be a diverticulum). If it were almost as sudden, but then took on a colicky pattern, you would think of a stone suddenly moving—biliary or ureteral. On the other hand, the slow buildup suggests an inflammatory condition: pancreatitis, diverticulitis, appendicitis, and so forth. But he has already located his pain in the epigastrium, and the pain has not moved from there, so lower abdominal conditions are less likely.

He next told us that the pain was constant in nature, again what you expect from inflammation of a solid organ or from irritating fluid loose in the belly. The radiation straight through to the back is typical for pancreatic pain. Nausea and vomiting may accompany many acute abdominal conditions, including pancreatitis. If vomiting had preceded the pain, one would have seriously considered a perforation of the lower esophagus, but it was the other way around.

We have been building a clinical picture that we recognize as pancreatitis. But we must rule out other possibilities. The anatomic approach is a good way to make a list. Persistent epigastric pain suggests disease of organs in that vicinity: stomach, pancreas, duodenum, biliary tree, liver, lower esophagus, colon on the abdominal side; and heart and lungs just above the diaphragm. We quickly consider possibilities: gastritis, gastric or duodenal ulcer perforation, acute cholecystitis, biliary colic, acute hepatitis, esophageal perforation, colonic perforation, lower lobe pneumonia, pulmonary embolus, or myocardial infarct. We have already cast doubt upon some of these; the others are still possible. Further information will help.

Data A review of systems is quickly done. There are no other symptoms referable to the gastrointestinal tract. Specifically, there is no bleeding, no diarrhea, and no dysphagia. The respiratory system offers no additional clues. There is no cough, shortness of breath, or sputum, and the epigastric pain has no relationship to respiratory movements. Cardiovascular symptoms are also absent. The pain does not radiate to the left arm, is not perceived as tightness in the chest, and is not accompanied by palpitations. The urinary system is also noncontributory. There is no dysuria and no radiation of the pain to the inner thigh or scrotum. Other systems are equally negative. He has never had an episode like this before, and "has never been sick."

Logic The negative information gleaned from the review of systems makes us doubt that there is pulmonary or cardiac disease. The urinary tract, never seriously in our thoughts, recedes even further into the background. The upper gastrointestinal tract and its adjacent organs (liver, biliary tree, and pancreas) are the most likely sources. Let us proceed with the physical examination.

Data Vital signs were taken before you arrived: temperature is 37.2°C, blood pressure is 70/50, pulse rate is 140, and respirations are 36 per minute. You recheck them yourself, and he is indeed that hypotensive. You also note that the pulse is feeble and fast but regular. The patient is clearly dehydrated. Head, neck, and chest are not remarkable, but the abdomen is. There is generalized distention, tenderness to deep palpation in the epigastrium, muscle guarding, and rebound tenderness. The lower abdomen is somewhat tender also, but not so much as the epigastrium; there is no rebound or muscle guarding in the lower abdomen. Percussion does not help much;

it does not sound like a drum, but it is not dull either. You cannot quite decide whether there is ascites or gaseous distention. The pain on deep palpation discourages further investigation. Bowel sounds are present but very sporadic. Rectal examination is unremarkable.

Logic "Pattern recognition" again: shock, signs of an acute upper abdomen, and relatively subdued abdominal findings are what you expect from pancreatitis. A perforated ulcer should give you a boardlike abdomen throughout, with rebound everywhere, and probably no bowel sounds at all. Shock would be expected also. Another devastating catastrophe, mesenteric occlusion, might lead to shock but would give more alarming generalized findings, except in the very old. Mesenteric occlusion would be more likely in an older person or in someone with an irregular pulse or a recent myocardial infarct, suggesting an embolus. Acute hepatitis or acute cholecystitis would have localized the findings to the right upper quadrant and would ordinarily not lead to shock. Lower thoracic pathology, although unlikely on the basis of the review of systems, is still a faint possibility.

Data You start a central venous line where you read a central venous pressure of zero, and then proceed to infuse Ringer's lactate rapidly until plasma arrives from the blood bank. A Foley catheter goes in to monitor hourly urinary output. You draw blood for the laboratory and order a hemoglobin, white blood cell count, serum amylase, and serum calcium. Your hospital offers an automated collection of tests for the same price, so you get all the electrolytes, as well as several liver enzymes. A nasogastric (NG) tube is placed, and various staff members arrive to do an ECG, a chest radiograph, and an upright radiograph of the abdomen that you have ordered. Urine has not yet begun flowing.

Shortly thereafter, results begin to pour in: the hemoglobin is 20 g/dL, white blood cell count is 8200/mm³, serum amylase level is 1250 units/L, and serum calcium level is 5 mg/dL (normal is 10). The other electrolyte studies are unremarkable, as are those for liver enzymes. Blood glucose level is normal. Bilirubin, however, is 4 mg/dL with 2.5 mg direct. The ECG and chest radiographic findings are normal.

The radiograph of the abdomen shows several distended loops of small and large bowel, no air-fluids levels, and no free air under the diaphragm. You do not quite see it, but the radiology resident points out a loop of small bowel in the mid-abdomen and the fact that there is no gas beyond the mid-transverse colon; he calls these a "sentinel loop" and a "colon cutoff sign."

Logic Things have fallen into place. The crucial finding is the elevated serum amylase level. The upper level of normal is 125 units/L. His value, at 1250, is unequivocally high. That number alone, with a different clinical picture, would not diagnose pancreatitis, because other diseases can elevate the amylase level; but in this instance it does. Do we need pictures to confirm the diagnosis? Should we add a sonogram or CT scan? For diagnosis alone, we probably do not. If we want to monitor the development of complications, or determine the genesis of the pancreatitis, the CT scan and the sonogram would have a role to play.

One of the findings is worrisome: the low serum calcium level. In Ranson's criteria, that is one of the elements that may add up to a bad prognosis. But so far, none of the others are there. He is younger than age 55 and has no elevation of the white blood cells (WBC), no hyperglycemia, and no abnormalities in liver enzymes.

His evolution within the next couple of days will add valuable prognostic signs. The resolution of the clinical picture with appropriate medical management (essentially putting the pancreas at rest) would be the most reassuring course of events, and the one that most patients will demonstrate.

Worsening, on the other hand, will signify progression to hemorrhagic disease and the possible development of the dreaded complication of a pancreatic abscess. The hematocrit would drop, the blood urea nitrogen (BUN) rise, blood gases would show a low PO_2 and metabolic acidosis. Fluid deficit would be manifest by large IV fluid requirements to maintain good hemodynamics. Failure of the serum calcium to respond to calcium administration would be particularly ominous.

Were any of the aforementioned to develop, we would certainly want to get a CT scan. A contrast-enhanced study is the method of choice to delineate the pancreas. A normal picture would indicate that the disease, if present, is mild. More frequently, the edema and distortion by the inflammatory process will be visible, and more important, the complication that if overlooked would be quite lethal—pancreatic necrosis and subsequent abscess—should be clearly shown (Fig. 16.5).

A cheaper sonogram might also show an edematous pancreas if the distended loops of paralytic bowel do not get in the way. Because of that potential limitation, sonogram is not the best way to look at the gland, but on the other hand with the sonogram you might get a free confirmation of the diagnosis while you are looking for the cause of the problem.

This brings us to a consideration of etiology. Does he have pancreatitis secondary to biliary tract disease (unusual in the male), or is it due to alcohol abuse? You will eventually visualize the gallbladder, but it is not essential that you do so right now. The initial treatment is identical for either type of pancreatitis. To rule out biliary tract disease a sonogram is the procedure of choice; it is at least 95% sensitive for stones in the gallbladder. But even before doing this simple, noninvasive, cheap, and highly reliable test, you rethink the history. As you ponder the question of when to get the sonogram, you realize that you did not ask about alcohol intake.

Data The patient says that he drinks only socially and usually in moderation. You wonder if he indeed has biliary tract disease, but at that point his wife calls you aside. "Doctor," she says, "he drinks at least two fifths of whiskey every week. I wish you would get him to stop." "Madam, I will try," you respond.

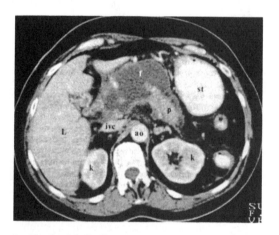

▶ **Figure 16.5.** Severe acute pancreatitis (not the patient in Case 45). Computed tomography with contrast demonstrates enhancement of only the distal body of the pancreas (p). The rest of the pancreas does not enhance and is lost in the fluid (f) extending from the pancreatic bed. Other organs are labeled.

Questions

1. Several pathologic entities are listed in the numbered column. In the lettered column, descriptions of different types of pain are listed. Match the pain descriptions with the diagnoses.

   (1) Acute myocardial infarct
   (2) Pulmonary embolus to a lower lobe
   (3) Perforated peptic ulcer
   (4) Penetrated peptic ulcer
   (5) Acute pancreatitis
   (6) Mesenteric artery occlusion
   (7) Biliary colic
   (8) Acute rupture of the lower esophagus

   (a) Colicky pain in the right upper quadrant of the abdomen, nausea, and vomiting
   (b) Cyclic epigastric pain relieved by meals that changes to constant pain radiating to the back, unrelieved by meals
   (c) Crushing type epigastric pain radiating to the left arm
   (d) Sudden severe epigastric pain following repeated vomiting
   (e) Epigastric pain of sudden onset, aggravated by deep breathing, in a patient immobilized in bed for a hip fracture
   (f) Generalized constant abdominal pain in a 78-year-old man 5 days after a myocardial infarction
   (g) Constant epigastric pain radiating to the back in an alcoholic patient who just had a heavy meal
   (h) Generalized abdominal pain of sudden onset in a patient who has chronic indigestion

2. Assume we have the same patient as the one discussed in this case presentation. The history and physical findings are the same, except that he has had pain for only 6 hours, and his blood pressure is normal. The laboratory values are: hemoglobin, 16 g/dL; WBC, 8200/mm³; serum amylase level, 180 U/L; serum calcium level, 8 mg/dL; bilirubin level, 1.2 mg/dL. These values in such a patient:
   (a) rule out pancreatitis.
   (b) are nondiagnostic, thus suggesting the need for exploratory laparotomy.
   (c) are nondiagnostic, thus suggesting the need for further observation and additional tests.
   (d) confirm the presence of early pancreatitis.

3. Given a history and physical findings identical to those described in the case presentation, but of 48 hours' duration instead of 12 hours, what would be the significance of a serum amylase level of 180 U/L?
   (a) It would rule out pancreatitis.
   (b) It would be nondiagnostic, indicating the need for exploratory laparotomy.
   (c) It would be nondiagnostic, indicating the need for an additional test.
   (d) It would confirm the diagnosis of acute pancreatitis.

4. A 43-year-old man has severe, constant, generalized abdominal pain of sudden onset and of 6 hours' duration. He lies quietly in the supine position, perspiring profusely. He is in shock and has a rigid silent ab-

domen. There is free air under the diaphragm as revealed by an upright radiograph of the abdomen. What significance does a serum amylase of 1250 U/L have in this case?
   (a) It confirms a diagnosis of acute pancreatitis.
   (b) It suggests that a duodenal ulcer has penetrated into the pancreas.
   (c) It suggests that gas-forming organisms have produced acute suppurative pancreatitis.
   (d) None of the aforementioned

5. A 56-year-old obese woman sees you for acute severe epigastric pain and vomiting that has been occurring on and off for 24 hours. She does not drink alcohol, but smokes one pack daily and has diabetes mellitus. Over the past 2 years she has had similar although much milder episodes. Examination shows tenderness and mild rigidity in the epigastrium and right upper quadrant. The temperature is 38.3°C, and no jaundice is visible. Which of the following is correct?
   (a) The negative alcohol history rules out pancreatitis.
   (b) Perforated peptic ulcer is likely, and a gastrointestinal radiographic series is indicated.
   (c) Acute cholecystitis is likely, and a sonogram or DISIDA isotope scan might clinch the diagnosis.
   (d) Acute cholecystitis is unlikely because there is no jaundice.
   (e) An ultrasound study that shows gallstones makes the diagnosis of acute cholecystitis certain.

Answers

1. (1-c), (2-e), (3-h), (4-b), (5-g), (6-f), (7-a), (8-d).

2. **(c) is correct.** The clinical picture is very suggestive of pancreatitis, even if limited to a duration of 6 hours. A normal serum amylase early in the course of the disease does not rule out its presence; it may take several more hours for the values to go up. Because of the relatively localized and mild degree of signs of peritoneal irritation, it would be safe to initiate conservative medical management (fluid replacement, nasogastric suction) and repeat the tests several hours later. This short period of observation would also allow collection of urine for a 2-hour urinary amylase level—another valuable test to diagnose or rule out pancreatitis. Faced with an unclear picture, most physicians would get a CT scan of the abdomen. If the latter does not clarify the issue, and certainly if the clinical picture deteriorates, an exploratory laparotomy would be indicated.

3. **(c) is correct.** Elevation of the serum amylase occurs early in the disease, although it can be missed in the first few hours. It also disappears early—in approximately 1 or 2 days. This patient could have had elevated values before he was seen and tested. If he had been under observation for 48 hours and multiple tests had persistently shown normal values, the diagnosis would be ruled out. But if first seen at 48 hours, your best test would be the urine amylase level. It rises a bit more slowly than the serum amylase level, but it stays elevated for a longer time. Some physicians would recommend a serum lipase in these circumstances. A CT scan would be in order and exploratory laparotomy might be needed.

4. **(d) is correct.** The description is classical for a perforated hollow viscus, and a perforated ulcer would be the most likely possibility. An elevated serum amylase level is not pathognomonic of acute pancreatitis; it can occur in other acute abdominal conditions, including a perforated duodenal ulcer. A penetrated ulcer does not produce the acute abdomen described in this question. There is no need to invoke the pancreas to explain the high serum amylase. This case is one where the clinical picture vastly outranks other findings in making a correct diagnosis.

5. **(c) is correct.** Pancreatitis can occur in teetotalers. Barium radiographs are certainly not indicated for possible perforation of an ulcer; an upright radiograph for free subphrenic air should be obtained. Jaundice is present if the common bile duct is obstructed or if there is extensive inflammation, but its absence certainly does not exclude cholecystitis. Both (c) and (e) are correct, but (c) is more correct. The presence of gallstones does not guarantee that the acute episode is related because stones are so common in obese middle-aged diabetic women. However, sonograms nowadays can not only show stones, but can also demonstrate the presence of pericholecystic fluid and a thick, inflamed gallbladder wall. If the test is not helpful, a DISIDA scan might resolve the issue; if no radioactivity is promptly detectable over the gallbladder, the cystic duct must be obstructed by stone, inflammation, or both. In doubtful cases, (c) and (e) might be considered equally correct. If a patient has repeated episodes of right upper quadrant pain, and you are seeing her between episodes or when the picture is not acute, ultrasound imaging is the procedure of choice.

COMMENT An upper abdominal catastrophe requires a quick direct approach. You cannot spend the time required for a complete data base. Anatomically we are dealing with the upper abdomen and its contents. A cluster of pain, vomiting, and shock makes a recognizable pattern of fairly typical acute pancreatitis. The other possibilities quickly pass through your mind and you rule them out, proving pancreatitis most likely by a series of well-chosen questions and a brief localized examination. The conclusive studies are the markedly elevated serum amylase level, low calcium level, and absence of air under the diaphragm. Probability theory may be invoked to predict the presence of pancreatitis in an alcoholic. Sequence of events (pain preceding emesis) was considered to rule out a perforated esophagus. The reliability, specificity, and sensitivity of the serum amylase were detailed in several examination questions.

The author has taken you into the inner recesses of his mind and told you the multitude of thoughts he experienced in seconds. He would have no doubt solved this problem in the time it took you to read the first paragraph. An acute upper abdomen plus shock in a boozer would mean acute pancreatitis—"nine times out of ten"; then a few tests to confirm the hypothesis. (P.C.)

Suggested Readings

Gupta PK, Al-Kawas FH. Acute pancreatitis: Diagnosis and management. Am Fam Physician 1995;52(2): 435–443.

Clinical policy for the initial approach to patients presenting with a chief complaint of non-traumatic acute abdominal pain. Ann Emer Med 1994;23(4): 906–922. [Patients do not show up in an emergency department with a label that says "acute pancreatitis." They show up with acute abdominal pain. This policy paper, written by a committee, details how emergency medicine physicians are expected to work up such patients. Maybe a foretaste of the "cookbook" medicine that older physicians fear so much, or conversely a much-needed set of guidelines for younger professionals who will practice in the era of managed care.]

Steinberg W, Tenner S. Review article: Acute pancreatitis. New Engl J Med 1994;330(17):1198–1210.

 C A S E 46

PAINLESS JAUNDICE

Raymond A. Rubin

Data Painless jaundice brings a 23-year-old man to your office. He tells you that he has had moderately severe pruritus, mostly on the legs and feet for the past few months, and that he had consulted a dermatologist several times with only minimal relief. But over the past few weeks he noted that his eyes and skin turned yellow, his stools became the color of clay, and his urine the color of strong tea. Except for some mild fatigue, he has felt well, has had a good appetite, and has lost no weight. In particular, he has had no pain or abdominal discomfort.

Logic The approach to the patient with painless jaundice is tempered by the clinical context. For example, the most common cause of painless jaundice in a previously healthy patient his age is viral hepatitis. In a 75-year-old, the focus would be on malignant disease of the bile ducts or pancreas.

The causes for jaundice are legion. They can be divided into three general categories—*hemolytic, hepatocellular,* and *obstructive* jaundice. Hemolytic jaundice is caused by the excessive destruction of red blood cells (RBCs); it results in moderate elevations of indirect-reacting bilirubin (up to 4 or 5 mg/dL) that is bound to albumin and does not spill over into and discolor the urine. Hepatocellular jaundice can be caused by hepatitis A, B, C, D, or E, various drugs, alcohol, and cirrhosis, and results from the inability of the damaged hepatocyte to extract, conjugate, or excrete bilirubin. Obstructive jaundice is caused by stone, stricture, or cancer obstructing the common bile duct.

Considerable overlap in these categories may exist and mixed pictures may be seen. For example, although hemolytic jaundice does not usually damage hepatocytes and cause liver enzyme elevations, excessive hemolysis may sometimes result in gallstones or anoxic damage to liver cells. The liver cell disease of cirrhosis may be associated with autoimmune hemolytic anemia. Long-term bile duct obstruction may damage liver cells.

Information regarding color changes of the stool and urine is not always so forthcoming as in this case. Usually patients notice yellow sclerae first and the rest of the obstructive jaundice tableau is elicited by specific questions. This combination of color changes points to a pathophysiologic state known as "cholestatic jaundice"—a condition characterized by obstruction to the flow of bile from the liver into the duodenum. Causes for cholestasis (Table 16.3) can be

TABLE 16.3. Causes of Cholestatic Jaundice (Jaundice, Dark Urine, Light Stool)[a]

Hepatitis—some severe cases
Stone in common bile duct
Cancer
(a) Metastatic in porta hepatis
(b) Gallbladder with metastases
(c) Cholangiocarcinoma
(d) Ampulla of Vater
(e) Pancreas
Pancreatitis (with narrowing of common bile duct)
Certain drugs
Rare causes
(a) Choledochal cyst
(b) Stricture, common bile duct
(c) Primary sclerosing cholangitis
(d) Primary biliary cirrhosis

[a]Diagnoses 1, 3(a), and 5 are intrahepatic; the rest are extrahepatic.

intrahepatic—in some cases of hepatitis, swollen hepatocytes block the flow of bile through the canaliculi—and *extrahepatic*—in which stricture, stone, or cancer chokes off the common bile duct (Fig. 16.6).

The normal serum bilirubin level is 0.3 to 1.0 mg/dL. It is derived mostly from the breakdown of old red blood cells in the spleen and exists in the blood as indirect-reacting bilirubin. The liver cells conjugate it to bilirubin glucuronide (direct-reacting bilirubin) that is excreted in the bile. If there is an impedance to excretion—either intra-hepatic or extrahepatic—the direct-reacting bilirubin, in an as yet unexplained manner, reen-ters the general circulation, elevates the serum bilirubin level, and spills over into and darkens the urine.

The fact that pruritus preceded the onset of jaundice is interesting and suggests that the prob-lem lies more with obstruction to flow of bile than with a predominantly inflammatory disease of the liver. The reason for pruritus has never been clearly identified; there is no correlation between the severity of pruritus and the concen-tration of bile salts in either the serum or skin.

Data More history! The patient has never been jaundiced before and has not had contact with anyone he has recognized as being jaundiced. He has not had any fevers, chills, nausea, vomiting, diarrhea, melena, hematochezia, or change in bowel habit. When again questioned, he reaf-firms that he has had no pain, no weight loss, and no anorexia. He denies any heterosexual or ho-mosexual activity, intravenous drug use, or tat-toos. Occasionally he drinks a modest amount of alcohol, mostly beer and wine.

With the exception of severe and recurrent si-nusitis, he has been in good health. He was treated with various suppressive antibiotics in the past, and for several months he has been taking daily trimethoprim-sulfamethoxazole. He takes no other medications or herbal preparations. There is no family history of liver disease; he is a graduate music student who lives at home with his parents and younger sister.

Logic Many pertinent negatives in the history tend to exclude some diagnostic contenders. The presence or absence of pain, and its characteris-tics if present, is a key feature in the jaundiced patient. A stone in the common bile duct often causes colicky right upper quadrant pain, though

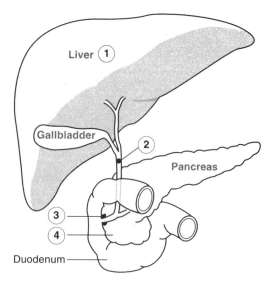

▶ **Figure 16.6.** Sites for causes of cholestatic jaun-dice. 1 = liver; 2 = common bile duct: stone, stric-ture, cholangiocarcinoma, primary sclerosing cholangitis; 3 = carcinoma: ampulla of Vater; 4 = carcinoma: head of pancreas.

there are instances where the stone may remain silent for years and obstruct with little or no dis-comfort. Gallbladder stones cause pain but do not obstruct the common bile duct. Malignan-cies usually cause no pain, though there are in-stances where cancers of the gallbladder or pan-creas are associated with pain or discomfort.

Although cancer is not a credible hypothesis because of the patient's age, the good appetite and stable weight are also reassuring. The ab-sence of gastrointestinal symptoms weighs against the possibility of primary sclerosing cholangitis (PSC), an unusual cause of jaundice in which 70% of cases occur in association with inflamma-tory bowel disease (IBD)—either ulcerative col-itis or regional ileitis (Crohn's disease).

There are no risk factors for viral hepatitis, or alcohol-related, or heritable diseases. Stricture of the common bile duct is unlikely without previ-ous surgery or a history of pancreatitis. The treat-ment with antibiotics warrants another look. Sul-fonamides have been associated with both hepatocellular and cholestatic forms of hepatic in-jury. Although many drugs are hepatotoxic, no-table ones include anabolic steroids, chlorpro-mazine, isoniazid, and acetaminophen.

Data The physical examination is remarkable for

the obvious severe jaundice and longitudinal scratch marks on the legs. Everything else is normal. There is no right upper quadrant tenderness, no masses are palpable, the liver is neither enlarged nor tender, the spleen is not palpable, and there are no stigmata of chronic liver disease such as palmar erythema, spider telangiectasias, testicular atrophy, gynecomastia, or distended abdominal wall veins. The stool is grayish-tan and it contains no blood.

Logic There is no physical evidence for hepatitis, cirrhosis, portal hypertension, gallbladder disease, wasting, or malignancy. Suspicion narrows in the direction of the common bile duct and obstruction somewhere in its course.

Data The blood count is normal, there is no eosinophilia, and serologic tests for hepatitis A, B, and C viruses have negative results.

Blood chemistry levels are as follows: bilirubin, 22.5 mg/dL (normal 0.3 to 1.0); alkaline phosphatase, 1900 IU/L (normal, 35 to 115); aspartate aminotransferase (AST), 100 IU/L (normal 1 to 36); alanine aminotransferase (ALT), 138 IU/L (normal 1 to 45); albumin, 3.5 g/dL (normal 3.2 to 5.2); and prothrombin time, 19.5 seconds (normal 11 to 13.4).

Logic Viral hepatitis is excluded. Weighing heavily against the possibility of sulfonamide-induced hepatotoxicity are the absence of eosinophilia, the rarity of its occurrence with this drug, and the length of time it has been taken. Still, it might be wise to discontinue its use.

The marked elevation of the alkaline phosphatase level and only modest elevations of levels of hepatocellular enzymes strongly suggest substantial cholestasis resulting from obstruction in the biliary system rather than from liver cell damage (Table 16.4). Imaging studies will be required to detect intrahepatic or extrahepatic ductal dilatation.

Although the normal serum albumin indicates intact hepatic synthesis function, the prolonged prothrombin time suggests otherwise. The liver manufactures prothrombin from vitamin K, which is absorbed from the intestine. Insufficient prothrombin and a resultant prolonged prothrombin time may result from either inadequate absorption of vitamin K or defective synthesis of prothrombin in the liver. Absorption depends in part upon the presence of bile within the intestine, and if there is obstruction to the flow of bile, vitamin K is not absorbed. Parenteral vitamin K restores the prothrombin time to normal if liver function is intact.

Data The prothrombin time normalizes within 36 hours after two doses of parenteral vitamin K. Ultrasound study of the abdomen shows normal size liver and spleen, no stones visible in the gallbladder or in the common bile duct, and no cysts or tumors of the bile ducts or pancreas. Minimal intrahepatic ductal dilatation is noted, and although the common bile duct, especially in its distal portion, could not be clearly visualized, there appeared to be echogenic material within it.

Logic The response to vitamin K is reassuring of hepatic functional integrity. Even though ultrasound is highly sensitive for dilated extrahepatic ducts, gallbladder stones, and hepatic and pancreatic masses, it fails to detect 40% of stones in the common bile duct and often incompletely visualize its distal portion. It is most unlikely that this young, healthy male patient with no risk factors would have a stone, let alone have a stone that is silent.

The findings are inconclusive, and further study is indicated. Computed tomography offers no advantage over ultrasound in such cases. Percutaneous transhepatic cholangiography is good for visualizing the ducts, but it is technically achievable only if intrahepatic ducts are substantially dilated. Endoscopic

TABLE 16.4. Related Chemistry in Three Basic Types of Jaundice

TYPES	SB DIRECT	SB INDIRECT	AST–ALT	AP
Hemolytic	nc	↑↑	nc	nc
Hepatocellular	↑↑↑	↑	↑↑↑	↑
Obstructive[a]	↑↑↑	↑	↑	↑↑↑

[a]This case.
SB = serum bilirubin; AST–ALT = aspartate aminotransferase–alanine aminotransferase; AP = alkaline phosphatase; nc = no change; ↑ = small increase; ↑↑ = moderate increase; ↑↑↑ = marked increase.

retrograde cholangiopancreatography is an excellent tool for visualizing (and performing biopsy, if indicated) the ampulla of Vater and the entire biliary and pancreatic ductal systems—where the pathology in this case is apt to be found.

Data ERCP demonstrates mild narrowing of the common bile duct and common hepatic ducts. There are multiple short bandlike strictures alternating with beadlike areas of dilatation in the common bile duct, the hepatic ducts, and some intrahepatic ducts (Fig. 16.7). Arborization of peripheral intrahepatic bile ducts is decreased. A cytologic specimen obtained from the distal end of a dominant stricture tests negative for malignant cells.

A liver biopsy shows disruption of the normal architecture by bridging fibrosis. The portal tracts display a chronic inflammatory infiltrate, intense bile duct proliferation, and cholestasis with duct plugging and occasional areas of extravasated bile.

Logic Both the ERCP and the liver biopsy are strongly supportive of a diagnosis of *primary sclerosing cholangitis* (PSC), even though intense periductal fibrosis or "onion-skinning" was not noted. This unusual and strange disease is immunologically mediated and has no known cause. It is often associated with IBD, is characterized by thickened bile ducts with narrow beaded lumina, and cholestatic jaundice with pruritus. Sometimes it is seen in patients who also display evidence of retroperitoneal fibrosis. It seems that this patient belongs to the 30% subset of patients with PSC who do not have IBD.

More recently, a related (secondary) variant has been seen as a result of infections associated with and as a result of acquired immunodeficiency syndrome (AIDS)—*Cryptosporidium, Microsporidia,* and cytomegalovirus (CMV).

PSC has a chronic indolent course and results in late hepatic failure. Treatment is unsatisfactory. It may consist of pharmacologic agents (ursodiol, methotrexate, and other immunomodulatory agents); endoscopically guided balloon dilatation of strictures; and liver transplantation.

Questions

1. If the ultrasound study in the case just presented had shown dilated intrahepatic ducts, the next best test or action would have been:
   (a) CT scan
   (b) Stop trimethoprim-sulfamethoxazole administration and observe
   (c) Percutaneous transhepatic cholangiography (PTC)
   (d) ERCP

2. A 56-year-old man, who is known from a previous study to have stones in the gallbladder, develops right upper quadrant pain, vomiting, and fever. Examination discloses a temperature of 101°F, right upper quadrant tenderness, and mild jaundice. He has:
   (a) acute cholecystitis.
   (b) stone in the cystic duct.
   (c) stone in the common bile duct.
   (d) hepatitis.

3. A 65-year-old woman complains of anorexia, weight loss, and weakness. She is both pale and jaundiced. Which of the following clues best directs you to the correct diagnosis?
   (a) Stool positive for occult blood
   (b) Hard left supraclavicular node
   (c) Enlarged nodular liver
   (d) Blood glucose 190 mg/dL

Answers

1. **(c) is correct.** With dilated ducts, some physicians would go directly to PTC, because detailed visualization of the biliary tree would be easy to achieve from above. Others would prefer ERCP at once because it offers better views of the lower biliary duct system. A CT scan offers no more than ultrasound. The presence of dilated ducts eliminates drug-induced hepatitis, so (b) would be fruitless.

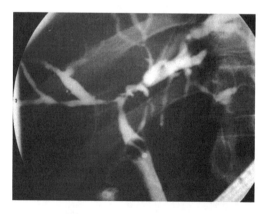

▶ **Figure 16.7.** Primary sclerosing cholangitis. Endoscopic cholangiogram with balloon catheter in place shows multiple areas of stenosis involving right and left and common hepatic ducts.

2. **(a),** acute cholecystitis, is clearly present, but it alone would not cause jaundice unless in addition the common bile duct is obstructed by a stone or contiguous inflammation. Choices (a) and (b) or (a) and (c) may be correct. Infectious hepatitis may present similarly, in which event the stones would be coincidental.

3. **All are helpful.** Choice (a) may direct you to a gastrointestinal carcinoma, but this finding is highly nonspecific. Choice (c) tells you that metastases exist in the liver but does not reveal the source. Choice (d) informs you of diabetes; this is a hint for carcinoma of the pancreas, but ordinary diabetes is common in this age group, and the finding may be coincidental. Choice (b), a hard left supraclavicular node (Virchow's), speaks for a cancer whose primary site may be in the breast, lung, or pancreas. The matter of which clue is best is debatable.

COMMENT The onset of jaundice is always a diagnostic challenge. Much significance is usually attached to the presence or absence of associated abdominal pain, but as this case demonstrates, exceptions to generally accepted concepts are common. It is notable that the three categories of disease associated with jaundice—hemolytic, hepatocellular, obstructive—may be distinguished by their clinical features and in great measure by the blood chemistries. However, because one category often causes or is accompanied by another, the overall picture may become fuzzy.

Diseases in the right upper quadrant offer huge amounts of relevant data and pertinent negatives in the history and physical examination, and their understanding requires familiarity with the vast number of pathophysiologic processes that are at work—digestion, absorption, synthesis, detoxification, and excretion.

Although the patient's age played a critical role in the evaluation of data, in the present era of high-technology tests, the key to solving this patient's problem lay in whether or not the bile ducts were dilated and determining which imaging procedure to use.

Although this patient turned out to have an unusual disease, the problem solver must carefully note that the jaundiced patient is most apt to have one of the three most common causes—hepatitis, stone, and cancer. *(P.C.)*

Suggested Readings

Aldersley MA, O'Grady JG. Hepatic disorders. Features and appropriate management. Drugs 1995; 49(1):83–102.

Banerjee B. Extrahepatic biliary tract obstruction. Modern methods of management. Postgrad Med 1993;93(4):113–117.

Buckley SE, DiPalma JA. Recognizing primary biliary cirrhosis and primary sclerosing cholangitis. Am Fam Physician 1996;53(1):195–200.

Fennerty MB. Primary sclerosing cholangitis and primary biliary cirrhosis. How effective is medical therapy? Postgrad Med 1993;94(6):81–88.

Krell H, Enderle GJ. Cholestasis: Pathophysiology and pathobiochemistry. J Gastroenterol 1993;31(suppl)2: 11–15.

C A S E   47

JAUNDICE AND PAIN

Paul Cutler

Note: Two cases of jaundice (Cases 46 and 47) are intentionally presented because they illustrate the diagnostic logic of two different clinicians who approach the problem of jaundice in two distinctly different settings.

Data A 70-year-old woman who retired to Mexico 6 months ago returns to the United States because of nausea, vomiting, jaundice, and right upper quadrant pain for 1 week. Her illness began with the gradual onset of anorexia and right upper quadrant discomfort, followed the next day by nausea and vomiting. By the third day her husband noted that her skin and eyes were slightly yellow, and she observed the urine getting dark and the stools becoming light. The pain got much worse and became a dull steady ache that seemed to wax and wane and did not radiate to the back or to anywhere else in the abdomen. On admission to the hospital she was still vomiting, could not eat, and was complaining of pain.

Logic The diagnostic possibilities in an elderly woman with jaundice and pain are many, but principal concern centers around whether this problem needs medical or surgical treatment.

The combination of jaundice, dark urine, and light stools tells you that obstruction to the flow of bile (*cholestasis*) exists. Your job is to determine whether the cause is *intrahepatic* (hepatocellular disease) or *extrahepatic* (stone, stricture, sclerosing cholangitis, cancer of the bile ducts, ampulla of Vater, or pancreas; or metastatic cancer to the porta hepatis from many possible primary sites). The mode of treatment depends on this important distinction; for if the patient has hepatitis or metastatic cancer to the liver, treatment is medical. If there is a removable or bypassable obstruction, the treatment is ultimately surgical (Table 16.5).

The tenet that painless jaundice means cancer and painful jaundice means biliary tract stone is no longer reliable, because pain may be present or absent in either condition. Furthermore, hepatitis may be present with pain of variable degree and varying types. In general, though, colicky pain suggests bile duct obstruction by a stone, whereas a constant dull ache points more in the direction of hepatitis, cholecystitis, pancreatitis, or pancreatic carcinoma. In this case the pain is not clearly colicky nor is it constant, so that cancer, stone, and hepatitis all merit concern.

Even with the minimal history obtained so far, additional judgments can be made. Viral hepatitis is extremely common in Mexico and deserves strong consideration. Miliary tuberculosis and amebic abscess, although also frequent in Mexico, are less likely to cause prominent jaundice and severe pain. Gallbladder disease (acute cholecystitis with cholelithiasis) is common in this age group, regardless of the geography. Think of bile duct stricture if there has been previous surgery in the area.

Drug- or alcohol-induced hepatitis are additional considerations. Almost any drug may rarely cause hepatitis. But notorious in this regard are anesthetics (halothane, chloroform); tranquilizers (phenothiazines, haloperidol, diazepam, chlordiazepoxide); antidepressants (iproniazid, tricyclics); anticonvulsants (phenytoin, carbamazepine); antiarthritics (gold, allopurinol, probenecid, nonsteroidal

anti-inflammatory drugs); all the hypoglycemics; antithyroidal drugs; some antimicrobials (clindamycin, isoniazid, rifampin, sulfonamides); cardiac drugs (methyldopa, quinidine); and most cancer chemotherapeutic agents.

Cancer always hovers in the background at this age. But a sudden onset of symptoms, the absence of weakness, weight loss, and anorexia, plus the absence of symptoms indicating a primary site would weigh against it.

Data Additional history reveals that the patient felt perfectly well until this episode. She ate well, slept well, and never had similar symptoms before. There were no prodromes of arthritis, arthralgia, pruritus, or urticaria (to suggest hepatitis) nor had there been any change in bowel habit except for 2 weeks of nonbloody diarrhea shortly after arriving in Mexico. She had had no cough, sputum, hemoptysis, fever, or weight loss. The rest of the systems review was equally devoid of positive symptoms.

History indicated no previous surgery. She has had mild diabetes mellitus for 12 years, controlled by diet alone, and recent hypertension treated with hydrochlorothiazide; no other drugs have ever been taken. She smoked one pack of cigarettes daily until 10 years ago but gave up the habit as a result of widespread anti-smoking publicity, and she has been drinking one to two glasses of wine with supper nightly for the past 20 years. Otherwise she consumes no alcohol. Family history is negative for gallbladder disease, stone, or cancer, and nobody in her home or family was recently jaundiced. She eats no raw seafood and has had no injections or transfusions in the recent past. The patient is a successful artist, and her husband is an author.

Logic The additional history is helpful in eliminating or discounting certain possibilities. Previous good health weighs against cancer. Drug hepatitis is unlikely because hydrochlorothiazide only rarely causes hepatitis. Alcohol consumption is very modest and chronic liver disease is unlikely. Viral hepatitis is rendered less likely by the absence of common prodromes and by the absence of factors such as eating raw shellfish, contact with jaundiced persons, or a history of injections. The episode of severe diarrhea 6 months ago was probably infectious, though we do not know the cause, and amebiasis is always possible. There are no symptoms to suggest active pulmonary tuberculosis.

TABLE 16.5. Causes of Jaundice

Hemolysis
Hepatitis—A, B, C, D, E   Alcohol, drugs
Stone, stricture, stenosis of common bile duct
Cancer—liver, bile duct, ampulla, pancreas

It is important to note that infectious hepatitis only sometimes has prodromal symptoms. More often its onset is marked by nausea, anorexia, and subsequent dark urine and jaundice. At times, the disease may present with high fever, at others, with only jaundice.

Data Physical examination disclosed a somewhat anxious, obese, obviously jaundiced woman complaining of persistent abdominal discomfort. Vital signs were: temperature, 38.5°C; pulse, 90; respirations, 18; blood pressure (BP), 160/90; and head, neck, and chest findings were normal. The liver was enlarged (15 cm by percussion in the right midclavicular line, and palpated 4 cm below the rib cage) and exquisitely tender on palpation and percussion, but the spleen was not palpable, the abdomen was not distended, and there was no evidence of ascites. In addition, there were no stigmata of chronic liver disease. Pelvirectal examination was negative and the stool was light tan and negative for occult blood. There was no asterixis, and Babinski's signs were absent.

Logic A tender, enlarged liver speaks strongly for infectious hepatitis. The absence of stigmata of chronic liver disease (spider nevi, palmar erythema, distended abdominal veins) weighs against a long-standing or decompensated liver disorder such as cirrhosis. Fever and tenderness are consistent with acute cholecystitis, hepatitis, or liver abscess. The blood pressure seems well-controlled. Cholestasis is confirmed by the light stool and dark urine, though you cannot yet decide if the obstruction is intrahepatic or extrahepatic. There is no evidence of hepatic encephalopathy.

More studies are urgently needed. It is necessary to decide if and when surgery should be performed, and medical therapy may be urgent if you are dealing with an abscess or cholangitis. Surgery in the face of acute hepatitis might be disastrous (10% mortality), and biliary tract obstruction and subsequent infection together with diabetes have an even higher mortality.

Data Except for 4+ bilirubin, the urinalysis is normal; urobilinogen is absent. The complete blood count shows no anemia, and there are 10,000 white blood cells per cubic millimeter, with 50% lymphocytes and 50% polymorphonuclear leukocytes (5% of the lymphocytes are atypical). Electrolytes, creatinine, and amylase are normal. Blood glucose is 240 mg/dL. Prothrombin time is 3 seconds longer than the control. Total bilirubin is 12.0 mg/dL (direct 7.0, indirect 5.0 mg); AST (formerly SGOT) is 1100; ALT (formerly SGPT) is 800 IU/L (normal is less than 40); and alkaline phosphatase is 200 IU/L.

The hepatitis A virus (HAV) antibody of the IgM type (IgM anti-HAV) is absent; the hepatitis B surface antigen (HBsAg) is absent; and the hepatitis C virus (HCV) antibody (anti-HCV) is absent. The serologic test for amebiasis also has negative results.

Twenty-four hours after intravascular vitamin K, the prothrombin time falls to equal the control. Chest radiograph, ECG, and plain abdominal radiograph findings are normal. In particular, there are no radiopaque calculi, no air in the biliary tree, and no ileus.

Logic Acute infectious hepatitis with considerable liver cell necrosis seems likely, even though there is as yet no immunologic confirmation. Although this is somewhat disturbing, it must be remembered that it may take 10 to12 days before serologic evidence is present in some patients.

There are currently at least five known types of hepatitis virus—A, B, C, D, and E—all having immunologic serum markers that are antigens in some cases, antibodies in others. If all tests are negative, consideration may be given to other causes—cytomegalovirus, Epstein-Barr virus, mononucleosis, and Coxsackie virus.

Hepatitis A virus is an RNA virus, is transmitted enterically by food, water and raw shellfish, and has a low mortality. Hepatitis B virus is a DNA virion, is transmitted parenterally by blood or needle, and may result in chronic hepatitis. Hepatitis C (formerly non-A, non-B) is caused by an RNA virion, and it too is transmitted parenterally by blood or needle, and may result in chronic hepatitis. Hepatitis D is caused by a defective RNA virus and it requires the presence of HBsAg for its expression. Hepatitis E is seen mainly in East Asia.

The absence of polymorphonuclear leukocytosis weighs against abscess and cholecystitis, whereas the lymphocytosis is consistent with hepatitis. Urobilinogen is absent from the urine because no bile is entering the gut (Table 16.6). Precluding hemolytic jaundice are the absence of anemia, the relatively low indirect bilirubin, the

TABLE 16.6. The Urobilinogen Story

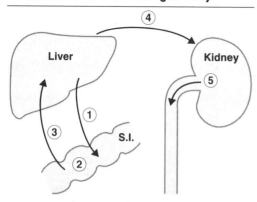

1. Liver excretes conjugated bilirubin
2. Bilirubin and gut bacteria → urobilinogen
3. Urobilinogen to liver via portal vein
4. Spills over to kidney
5. Excreted by kidney

Clinical Application

1. Obstruction of common bile duct and/or antibiotics that alter gut flora result in absent urine urobilinogen.
2. Urobilinogen reappears in urine when obstruction begins to abate.

TABLE 16.7. Pathophysiologic Differences Between Major Types of Cholestatic Jaundice

Features	CAUSES OF CHOLESTASIS (JAUNDICE, DARK URINE, LIGHT STOOL)	
	Hepatitis	Stone/Cancer
AST, ALT	↑↑↑↑	↑
AP	↑	↑↑↑↑
Hepatocytes	swollen	normal
Intrahepatic ducts	narrow	wide
Obstruction[a]	intrahepatic	extrahepatic
Schematic		Stone or tumor

[a]How conjugated bilirubin re-enters the circulation is not clearly understood in either type of obstruction.
AST = aspartate aminotransferase; ALT = alanine aminotransferase; AP = alkaline phosphatase.

high total bilirubin, and the marked bilirubinuria. Diabetes is confirmed by the high glucose, but it is difficult to evaluate control in the presence of an acute process. The slight prothrombin time prolongation responded well to vitamin K, suggesting that liver function in this regard must be adequate, and that a relative lack of bile salts in the gut may have accounted for this abnormality. More important, the normal prothrombin will permit invasive procedures.

The levels of enzymes are quite high, whereas the alkaline phosphatase level is only two or three times normal. This suggests acute liver disease rather than bile duct obstruction, where the reverse would be true (Table 16.7). Less than 25% of gallstones in the United States are radiopaque, and biliary tract sepsis can occur in the absence of biliary tract air, so these negative findings are of limited usefulness.

More sophisticated diagnostic techniques are necessary. There is a wide variety of noninvasive and invasive procedures available. When the serum bilirubin exceeds 4 mg/dL, ordinary cholecystographic techniques do not visualize the gallbladder or ducts. Other available procedures include liver-spleen isotope scan, ultrasound (US), computed tomography, magnetic resonance imaging, thin-needle percutaneous transhepatic cholangiography, liver biopsy, and endoscopic retrograde cholangiopancreatography—each of which has its specific indications, values, and limitations. How to decide which to do? The least invasive test with the highest yield is best. But these two criteria may not coincide. Under certain circumstances you might be forced to do the most invasive procedure first, because it has the highest yield, and time may be a cogent factor.

Data An abdominal sonogram (US) was unfortunately of poor quality and dilated intrahepatic ducts could not be excluded. CT was not available as the equipment was being repaired. A liver-spleen isotopic scan demonstrated uneven uptake in an enlarged liver that was without discrete filling defects and without significantly increased uptake in the spleen and marrow.

Logic The isotope scan is consistent with a diffuse liver disease; the absence of a "cold area" weighs against amebic or bacterial abscess or large metastatic modules, and the lack of increased uptake by the spleen weighs against portal hypertension.

Because the isotope scan seldom gives valuable information in cases of obstructive jaundice, it has largely been replaced by CT and US. It seems that in this case, it may have been wiser to repeat the US or wait for the CT.

Sonography in experienced hands may detect stones in the gallbladder, but even if they are present they may not necessarily explain the patient's jaundice because stones are so common in this age group. On the other hand, sonographic or CT demonstration of dilated intrahepatic ducts would strongly imply biliary tract obstruction and laparotomy might be justified. The sonogram should also detect an abscess.

So far, then, the cholestatic jaundice appears to arise from acute diffuse liver disease. A diagnosis requiring surgery seems less likely, but the persistence of severe pain is worrisome. If you were certain of hepatitis, you might wait and watch. But the picture is neither black nor white, and you decide that, because greater certainty is needed, invasive procedures that visualize the biliary tree should be done.

Data All the previously mentioned studies had been obtained during the first 48 hours after admission. During this time, the patient received analgesics for pain and intravenous fluids with insulin coverage. The pain abated somewhat, but persisted.

On Day 3, thin-needle PTC was performed and failed to visualize the biliary tree. Before terminating the procedure, a Menghini needle biopsy was done and yielded a 3-cm core of brown tissue.

Logic When properly done, thin-needle cholangiography successfully visualizes *dilated* bile ducts in 100% of patients and demonstrates normal ducts in 60 to 70%, so that failure to visualize the biliary tree made extrahepatic obstruction highly unlikely. Needle biopsy of the liver was therefore unlikely to enter a dilated duct and could be considered a safe procedure. Its purpose was to confirm a diagnosis of hepatocellular disease and to further justify a conservative course of close observation.

Data The biopsy was followed by hypotension, tachycardia, right upper quadrant rebound tenderness, and a decrease in hematocrit. She was given 2 units of packed red blood cells. On the following day the biopsy revealed acute viral hepatitis with cholestatic features but was without bridging necrosis or fatty infiltration. By this time she had recovered from her biopsy complication of probable liver tear with hemoperitoneum.

Over the next 5 days the patient improved clinically. Pain and tenderness subsided and at the time of discharge she was feeling and eating well. Repeated viral studies returned on the day of discharge. Both the IgM anti-HAV and the immunoglobulin G (IgG) anti-HAV had become strongly positive, which indicated both a diagnosis of hepatitis A and a good prognosis. The levels of bilirubin and hepatic enzymes returned to normal in the ensuing 6 weeks.

Logic Most cases of hepatitis do not require hospitalization. But, today's strict guidelines for admission notwithstanding, hospital care is indicated in patients who have a marked increase in the prothrombin time, low serum albumin, hypoglycemia, very high serum bilirubin, or who may have severe vomiting and dehydration, and/or are suffering much pain.

One might justifiably question the wisdom of doing invasive risky procedures when the diagnosis of acute hepatitis was already reasonably certain. But the primary care physician and collaborating surgeon did not wish to overlook a surgical lesion in a patient exhibiting some atypical features. In their judgment this was the wisest course to follow. Perhaps they were wrong.

Questions

1. Assume that the patient just presented had a prothrombin time of 25 seconds that was not correctable by vitamin K. Needling the liver would have been precluded. The sonogram was of no help, and the patient continued to be sick with pain, jaundice, and fever. Your next step would be:
   (a) exploratory laparotomy.
   (b) give antibiotics.
   (c) ERCP.
   (d) wait and watch.

2. If this patient had no palpable liver, a very high alkaline phosphatase level, only slightly elevated levels of liver enzymes, normal prothrombin time, colicky pains, and leukocytosis, and no invasive procedures had yet been done, you would:
   (a) perform surgery.
   (b) give antibiotics.
   (c) order ERCP.
   (d) order "skinny" needle PTC.

3. A 60-year-old man becomes jaundiced after a 2-month period of anorexia and weight loss. Serum bilirubin is 10 mg/dL, ALT is twice normal, alkaline phosphatase is 10 times normal, and serum glucose is 220 mg/dL. Which of the following could explain the entire picture?
   (a) Carcinoma of the pancreas
   (b) Carcinoma of the stomach with liver metastases
   (c) Diabetes mellitus
   (d) Choices (b) plus (c)

4. Return to the patient in the case. Suppose the radiograph of the abdomen had revealed radiopaque stones in the general area of the gallbladder, and the CT liver scan showed a 6-cm single round posterior filling defect near the porta hepatis. Also suppose that ultrasound of the liver found that the defect was cystic. No invasive studies had yet been done, and the blood count showed a marked polymorphonuclear leukocytosis. The probabilities are that the disease causing the patient's acute problem is:
   (a) acute cholecystitis with cholelithiasis.
   (b) hepatitis.
   (c) cancer with metastases.
   (d) amebic liver abscess.

Answers

1. **(c) is correct.** Provided an expert endoscopist is available, this procedure should tell if there is common bile duct obstruction. If (c) were unavailable, (b) and (d) would be the best choices because surgery in the face of severe hepatocellular disease carries enormous risks. If there were no improvement, a therapeutic dilemma would be present, and the surgeon's hand might be forced.

2. **(c) or (d)** still remain the best choices because even typical cases of seeming extrahepatic obstruction occasionally turn out to have intrahepatic cholestasis and surgery may be dangerous under such circumstances. The techniques that distinguish *extrahepatic* (surgical) from *intrahepatic* (nonsurgical) forms of jaundice are among the most significant advances in hepatology. They should be used when available because they are reasonably safe and are far more accurate than clinical judgment alone. In their absence, you would initiate antibiotic therapy, and you would probably perform surgery at a time that would be determined by the clinical course.

   Legitimate differences of opinion may exist in this instance. Some clinicians might go directly to surgery because the clinical picture seems so characteristic of common duct obstruction.

3. **(a) and (d) are correct.** Cancer of the pancreas may cause obstructive jaundice, and diabetes may develop if the neoplasm extensively replaces the body and tail. Common genetic diabetes mellitus may also occur, but it does not account for the other symptoms. Stomach cancer with metastases may be present, but it does not explain the diabetes. Choice (d) represents a concurrence of diseases that explains the whole picture.

4. **(d) is correct.** The "hole" in the liver, fever, leukocytosis type of pain and tenderness, and her residency in Mexico all point to an amebic abscess that can cause jaundice if adjacent to the common duct. Although the patient also has stones, it is less likely that this is causing her illness; it does not account for the large single filling defect, although it could cause multiple abscesses by ascending suppurative cholangitis. Hepatitis could not account for a large filling defect either. Cancer with metastases is unlikely in view of previous good health; furthermore, the filling defects are more apt to be multiple, and cancer is not so apt to cause an acute picture such as is seen here.

COMMENT Papers that propose to solve the common riddle of cholestatic jaundice still flood the journals. These attest to the fact that this issue is not yet solved, and diagnostic procedures and sequences are variable. No single strategy is optimal for all patients, for, as always, there are many individual variables, and each case must be handled differently.

Yet some facts are well established and a few protocols are strongly advocated for the patient who has cholestatic jaundice. But do we need *diagnostic road maps* or can we get to the same destination by simply following the *road signs*? Must we rely on the preconceived plans of others, or do we have sufficient gray matter to think our own way through the morass of procedurists who beckon this way or that?

The diagnostic accuracy of the combined history, physical examination, and laboratory tests should approach 90%. For example, given a 22-year-old healthy patient with the recent onset of nausea, anorexia, cholestatic jaundice, and an enlarged tender liver, the diagnosis is infectious hepatitis—almost for certain. Given a 56-year-old reasonably healthy woman with repeated episodes of right upper quadrant pain who now has colic, fever, and cholestatic jaundice, the diagnosis is stone in the common bile duct with retrograde infection—almost for certain. And given a 65-year-old man with a 3-month downhill course, recurrent diffuse abdominal pains, an enlarged nodular liver, and cholestatic jaundice, the diagnosis is metastatic cancer to the liver—almost for certain.

But there are great numbers of patients who cannot be so neatly categorized. For them you must perform diagnostic procedures. And even for those whose diagnosis is reasonably certain, some procedures may be necessary too. The question is, which procedure for whom, when, and in what order? Today's consensus may change as diagnostic techniques become more refined and their operating characteristics become firmly established.

The procedures of greatest use are (a) ultrasound, (b) CT scan, (c) PTC, (d) ERCP, and (e) liver biopsy. Ultrasound is good for detecting gallbladder stones, liver abscesses or metastases, and intrahepatic biliary duct dilatation; it has no risks and is not costly. The CT scan is of equal value but is more costly and may involve the injection of intravenous dye. PTC and ERCP are both good for visualizing the biliary tree and detecting extrahepatic obstruction with radiopaque contrast dye. The former has a respectable morbidity and is best for upper biliary obstructions. The latter has less risk but requires great skill; however, it is especially good for detecting pancreatic and ampullary lesions, and obstructions closer to the lower part of the biliary tree. Both are costly. Liver biopsy has its risks, especially if ducts are dilated.

The disease spectrum with which we deal has already been presented in the case discussion. If you are not satisfied with the degree of probability established by the clinical picture, further procedures must be done. The sensitivity, specificity, success rate, complications, and cost of each procedure is well established in good institutions with expert procedure performers. Because the figures for the operating characteristics of each test are in the 75 to 90% range, the tests have high accuracy and reliability. But the results are not that good everywhere. This must be borne in mind when the report is "equivocal," "compati-ble with," "of poor quality," "suggestive of," "unobtainable," or "suboptimal reading."

If the patient almost certainly has hepatitis, do nothing. But if the clinical estimate of hepatitis likelihood is .80 or less, then the $P(D)$ for extrahepatic cholestasis is .20 or more. In that event, do an ultrasound study.

The sonogram has a 90% sensitivity for dilated intrahepatic ducts and a 10% false-negative rate. Therefore, if the ducts are not visibly dilated, observe the patient. If the patient gets well, hepatitis is almost certain and nothing further needs to be done. But if the patient continues to exhibit unremitting cholestatic jaundice, a liver biopsy should be obtained. A biopsy showing hepatitis warrants continued observation; but if such is not the case, and especially if the biopsy shows bile duct dilatation, then opacification of the biliary system is indicated. You may have encountered one of the 10% of patients whose ultrasound study is falsely negative. Do a PTC or ERCP.

Go back to the original setting, but suppose the sonogram shows dilated intrahepatic ducts. Proceed directly to PTC or ERCP, or both if necessary, and be prepared to request arteriography, guided needle biopsy, and whatever is required on your voyage of discovery.

In this case, and especially in other cases where the probability of extrahepatic biliary obstruction is even greater, you must establish the cause of obstruction. Some form of surgery may be necessary, and surgeons generally prefer to know in advance what they will encounter. *(P.C.)*

Suggested Readings

Borsch G, et al. Clinical evaluation, ultrasound, cholescintigraphy, and endoscopic retrograde cholangiography in cholestasis: A prospective clinical study. J Clin Gastroenterol 1988;10:185.

Dusheiko GM. Rolling review—the pathogenesis, diagnosis and management of viral hepatitis. Aliment Pharmacol Ther 1994;8:229.

Frank BB, et al. Clinical evaluation of jaundice: A guideline of the patient care committee of the American Gastroenterological Association. JAMA 1989;262:3031.

Hoofnagle JH, DiBisceglie AM. Serologic diagnosis of acute and chronic viral hepatitis. Semin Liver Dis 1991;11(2):73.

LOWER ABDOMINAL PAIN

Arthur S. McFee

Data Brought to the emergency department by his father, a 5-year-old boy complains of abdominal pain that has been present for several days. The pain started in the middle of his abdomen and was like a "cramp." It settled in both lower quadrants and became steady and sharp but hard to localize; his right side seemed more uncomfortable.

More history reveals anorexia and nausea but no vomiting, and he has not felt like taking any food or water for 2 or 3 days. He has not had a bowel movement for 24 hours. Several of his brothers and sisters have recently been sick with gastrointestinal "flu," which they presumably contracted at school. Each has been ill for 2 to 3 days. Their illnesses were associated with nausea, vomiting, diarrhea, and transient cramping pain relieved by bowel movements.

This is the patient's third visit to the emergency department in 4 days. After brief examinations, he was discharged at the first two visits with a diagnosis of viral gastroenteritis.

Logic With this history, and in this age group, you must think primarily of acute appendicitis. Other possibilities merit some consideration too. A few very simple initial thoughts pertain. The character of the pain changed. In the first few hours it was colicky and periumbilical, indicating a source of obstruction within the nerve distribution of the appendix and small bowel. As time passed, it became sharp and constant, but poorly localized. The mechanisms causing the two types of pain are different; local irritation of the peritoneum followed obstruction of an organ. Tenderness should be demonstrable in the area of suspected inflammation, because it promptly follows the development of local peritoneal irritation. Presumably, no such changes occurred with the siblings who were ill and recovered.

Poor localization of the new sharp pain tends to steer you away from an immediate diagnosis of classical appendicitis. In addition, the fact that considerable acute bowel disease has been present among the siblings distracts you.

The history gives two important additional clues regarding acute inflammatory disease of the gastrointestinal tract—nausea and anorexia. Each is a nonspecific symptom and is present in many diseases. Anorexia is, however, the single most common symptom seen in acute appendicitis. Its presence does not confirm the diagnosis, but its absence casts doubt. The fact that the patient has not had a bowel movement in 24 hours is highly significant and does not support a diagnosis of common gastrointestinal infectious disorders which, as a group, cause mucosal irritation and diarrhea.

The length of the history is important. Acute appendicitis is a short-lived process. Ordinarily, if untreated, rupture occurs 18 to 24 hours after its onset. Accordingly, after some days, one must seek signs consistent with a complicated or ruptured appendicitis.

The fact that the patient had been discharged twice from the emergency department before this visit underlines a very important consideration. After the first 24 hours, the clinical picture of right lower quadrant inflammatory disease, especially appendicitis, is usually not clear. It very frequently is not clear in the *pediatric* patient. In this case, admission to the hospital for observation *by one doctor* would have been appropriate at either visit and would have led to a much more expeditious diagnosis. Observation over a period of time *by a single individual* is invaluable in defining the existence and nature of many inflammatory intra-abdominal problems.

Data A physical examination is done. The young boy is lying very quietly in bed and does not move much. He appears ill and has poor skin turgor and a dry mouth; rectal temperature is 39°C, pulse is 120, and respirations are 18. Moderate tenderness is present in both lower abdominal quadrants. Bowel sounds are present. Point tenderness cannot be elicited at the junction of the lateral and middle thirds of a line joining the right anterior superior iliac spine and the umbilicus (McBurney's point). Neither forced hyperextension (psoas sign) nor forced external rotation (obturator sign) of the right thigh causes pain. No masses can be defined in the groin or femoral canals.

A rectal examination reveals an area of exquisite tenderness at the tip of the examining finger on the right side. A mass is felt in this area, and the central portion is distinctly soft. No stool is present in the rectal vault.

Logic The physical examination is most significant. Fever and tachycardia are present. The patient with peritonitis tends to lie quietly in bed. Motion and occasionally breathing hurt. The demonstration of localized point tenderness within the pelvis on the right side indicates an inflammatory lesions in this area. The presence of a mass with a softened center suggests a fluctuant abscess. In a young male patient with such a history for more than 24 hours, a diagnosis of appendicitis must be strongly considered.

Constipation and the absence of stool in the rectum tend to confirm an acute perirectal inflammation. Bowel sounds are present and indicate that the inflammatory process has been quite efficiently walled away in the pelvis and has not caused diffuse peritonitis and ileus. Dehydration accounts for the general appearance of the patient because he has neither eaten not drunk well for 2 or 3 days.

The examination is most helpful in ruling out alternate considerations. The patient with ureteral colic ordinarily does not have peritoneal irritation; he or she may seek a comfortable position and thrash about in bed in so doing. Furthermore, such pain is persistently colicky, does not localize, tends to radiate downward often to the external genitalia, and is often accompanied by urinary frequency and hematuria.

A tender palpable mass in the groin would indicate an inguinal or femoral hernia with obstruction and strangulation as the source of the problem. In either case, obstructive symptoms of nausea, vomiting, and cramps would precede the development of sharply localized peritoneal signs in the hernia sac.

For this patient to have "classical" appendicitis, one would expect to find well localized right lower quadrant tenderness in keeping with the peritoneal irritation in that area. The localized point tenderness is now in the pelvis. Nevertheless, it must be regarded, as in other areas, as the single most important sign confirming the presence of intra-abdominal acute inflammation. In simple uncomplicated acute appendicitis in the right lower quadrant, tenderness is most often localized at McBurney's point. After rupture, it overlies the abscess that has formed. This sign may be difficult to demonstrate, depending on the location of the abscess, but its importance as an indicator of intra-abdominal inflammation cannot be minimized.

Data Final studies are done. A chest radiograph has normal findings; flat and upright abdominal radiographs reveal a 6- to 8-cm air-filled loop of ileum in the right lower quadrant; hemoglobin is 16.5 g/100 mL; hematocrit, 49%; WBCs, 20,000/mm^3 with 79% polymorphonuclear leukocytes are noted; and a urinalysis with 15 RBCs and 10 WBCs per high-powered field is recorded. The temperature is 38.8°C.

Logic The additional information confirms an acute inflammatory process in the right lower quadrant (elevated WBC count, fever, and sentinel ileal loop). The term "sentinel loop" refers to a single area of small or large bowel distended with gas. It signifies that peristalsis is deficient or absent at that point and gas, which normally does not collect sufficiently to cause distention, is delayed in its passage. It signals the presence of an adjacent inflammatory process.

Pyuria and hematuria suggest a urinary tract disorder, but do not exclude appendicitis. These urine abnormalities may result from inflammation adjacent to the bladder or ureter, and may indeed be seen as a result of appendicitis itself. The elevated hemoglobin level and hematocrit indicate hemoconcentration and dehydration.

Because this patient is a young man, one need not consider sources of inflammation associated with the female pelvic genitalia. These problems would include ectopic pregnancy, pelvic inflammatory disease, tubo-ovarian abscess, and ovarian cysts with their complications of rupture or twisting.

One should not overlook other more obscure problems such as muscle strain in an active young man. A strain, although producing severe abdominal wall signs, is rarely associated with colic. A mass may even be present if an intramuscular or rectus sheath hematoma exists.

Acute appendicitis can produce a number of variations of the basic clinical signs. The appendix is a mobile mesenteric organ, and can reside in a 360-degree circle of rotation in several planes. Accordingly, right upper quadrant pain and tenderness simulating cholecystitis, absence of right lower quadrant tenderness (retrocecal appendix), or the picture described here, can be seen. In each, a sequence of colicky pain followed by peritoneal signs *referable to the location of the appendix* is present. You must seek to demonstrate the local tenderness in the area where the appendix might lie.

Some diseases of the ileum and right colon mimic appendicitis and are often indistinguishable except at the operating table. Right colon diverticulitis, Crohn's disease of the ileum, cecal ulceration, perforating cecal carcinoma, and appendiceal carcinoid tumors are examples. In the foregoing diseases, with the exception of those that initially cause appendiceal obstruction, the element of periumbilical cramping may not be seen and right lower quadrant pain is predominant. Almost all are associated with varying degrees of nausea and anorexia.

In the patient who seeks medical care late in the course of the disease, both a computed tomographic scan of the abdomen and ultrasound may be helpful. The computed tomographic scan may reveal an area of significantly decreased density that displaces adjacent structures and is suggestive of an abscess. The sonographic study may indicate a right lower quadrant or pelvic cystic structure that is also consistent with an abscess (Fig. 16.8). *Neither study is used in the primary diagnosis of acute appendicitis.* Both studies may produce much information in the long-standing, neglected, or complicated patient. There are a variety of isotopic scans that may serve to locate occult abscesses that accompany long-standing appendiceal disease.

In the last few years, some attention has been given in the literature to considering the predictive value of serum markers such as C-reactive protein levels, or a combination derived from the gross white blood cell count, the percentage of white blood cells as polymorphonuclear leukocytes, and the actual count per cubic millimeter of polymorphonuclear leukocytes. Although these studies may serve to confirm the diagnosis of appendicitis in questionable cases, their specificity is not such as to render them useful primary diagnostic techniques.

Before committing a patient to an operation, laparoscopy is sometimes advocated when the diagnosis is uncertain. This technique can also be employed for the final surgical treatment. However, it is not a primary diagnostic tool in the management of standard acute appendicitis.

At the extremes of age—in the very young and the very old—appendicitis is a very difficult diagnosis to make because it is not suspected and demonstrates few localizing signs. In the pediatric patient, fever is common early in the course of the disease, and the history is that of an "upset

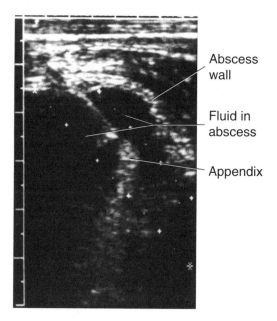

▶ **Figure 16.8.** Ultrasound study demonstrates periappendiceal abscess (not deemed necessary for the patient in Case 48).

stomach," possibly diarrhea, and poor feeding. In the older patient, fever is rarely seen unless rupture has taken place. The physical examination in the pediatric patient may be very revealing, must be carefully and gently done, and may be the only means of securing a diagnosis. In the elderly patient, physical signs and complaints may be few until a well-established abscess is present, and sepsis has occurred. It must therefore be a diagnosis of suspicion in everyone without clear findings who has not had an appendectomy.

A history of multiple visits to the emergency department with the innocuous diagnosis of viral gastroenteritis should raise the suspicion of some other inflammatory disease. Ordinarily, the diagnosis of gastroenteritis in these instances is supported by the presence of diarrhea along with cramping, nausea, and vomiting.

More important, this type of problem is usually limited to 2 or 3 days; the more severe inflammatory diseases are not.

The value of examinations *by a single individual* for the patient in whom the diagnosis is initially uncertain cannot be overemphasized. Admission to the hospital or emergency department observation ward is easily effected and a diagnosis is ordinarily clear within 8 to 12 hours. In our patient, by all odds, the best consideration is a ruptured pelvic appendicitis with abscess formation.

Data This was confirmed at the operating table.

Questions

1. A 38-year-old woman has had severe, crampy right lower quadrant pains for several days that are getting progressively worse. There was no preceding epigastric or periumbilical pain, significant fever, or anorexia. She has had a similar episode in the past. Each of the following is possible except which one?
   (a) Temperature 38.8°C, tender right lower quadrant, diarrhea, and anal fistula
   (b) Physical examination results normal, 20 red blood cells per high-powered field in urine
   (c) Acute appendicitis, even if there is no anorexia, and the temperature is normal
   (d) A small tender mass in the right inguinal area

2. You elicit a history of severe left lower quadrant pain for 2 days in a 48-year-old woman. The pain is constant, there is marked tenderness, the temperature is 38.3°C, and the WBC count is 18,500/mm³ with 86% polymorphonuclear leukocytes. Rectal and pelvic examinations are refused. Which of the following is possible?
   (a) Acute diverticulitis
   (b) Acute appendicitis
   (c) Torsion of an ovarian cyst
   (d) Peridiverticular abscess

3. The most sensitive clue in the diagnosis of acute appendicitis is:
   (a) tenderness over McBurney's point.
   (b) leukocytosis.
   (c) right lower quadrant pain.
   (d) anorexia.

4. The most specific clue in the diagnosis of acute appendicitis is:
   (a) tenderness over McBurney's point.
   (b) leukocytosis.
   (c) right lower quadrant pain.
   (d) anorexia.

5. You see a 42-year-old woman who seems to have a classical case of acute appendicitis. She has been sick for 12 hours, leukocytosis is present, urinalysis is normal, the temperature is 37.7°C, and the rectal and pelvic examinations are normal. She has a 3-inch distorted right lower quadrant scar. An operation was performed at age 22, 2 years after her marriage. She does not know exactly what was done but thinks her appendix may

have been removed. Drainage and healing took 6 weeks. Her parents and relatives are dead or unavailable. She has been in excellent health. You should:
   (a) perform prompt appendiceal exploration.
   (b) observe for 24 to 48 hours.
   (c) obtain old hospital records.
   (d) do complete barium radiograph studies of upper and lower gastrointestinal tracts.

Answers

1. **(c) is correct.** Acute appendicitis is unlikely in the presence of crampy pain for several days; there was no preceding epigastric or periumbilical pain, and there is no fever or anorexia. By this time, fever would invariably be present. The others, however, are all distinct possibilities. Choice (a) describes a patient with regional enteritis. The type of pain and hematuria (b) suggest a ureteral calculus. A tender inguinal mass with crampy pain (d) points to an incarcerated, possibly strangulating, hernia.

2. **All are correct.** Diverticulitis is most likely present and presents in this manner. Appendicitis cannot be ruled out—the appendix may be on the left side (malrotation). Pelvic disease of various types can cause this picture. The inflamed diverticulum or, for that matter, the appendix, may have already ruptured and resulted in an abscess.

3. **(d) is correct.** Anorexia is almost universally present, although it is nonspecific. Leukocytosis may not be present in the event of poor host response. McBurney's point is tender only if the appendix is in the classic location. Right lower quadrant pain may not be present if the appendix is ectopic, in the case of infants who cannot give pain descriptions, or in the elderly who may overlook or fail to appreciate pain.

4. **(a) is correct.** The classically located inflamed appendix gives point tenderness at McBurney's point. Leukocytosis is very nonspecific. So is anorexia. Right lower quadrant pain can be caused by a host of illnesses. Questions 3 and 4 show the difference between clue specificity and clue sensitivity.

5. **(a) is correct.** This is a judgment decision. Were it not for the old scar, there would be no decision to make. But the scar could represent drainage of an appendiceal abscess or some other operation, and the appendix might have been left intact (not ordinarily done today). Twenty-year-old hospital records are not usually obtainable. Radiograph studies take time and offer little. Regional ileitis may be suspected by information revealed by upper gastrointestinal radiographs, but if surgery must be done anyway, this can be confirmed on the table

with very little added risk. Observation for 24 to 48 hours is risky and may result in perforation with abscess formation. But observation for 8 to 10 hours permits a more firm distinction between nonspecific abdominal pain and acute appendicitis, and therefore some physicians might prefer to observe the patient for several hours. The patient's health is good, and a surgical disease, probably appendicitis, is likely. The risk of surgery is small compared with the risk of doing nothing.

COMMENT This was *not* a textbook case of acute appendicitis, for typical cases hardly exist anymore. Many clues in the data base make you think of other possibilities—"flu" in the family, pain in *both* lower quadrants, earlier "viral gastroenteritis," absence of tenderness over McBurney's point, and an abnormal urinalysis.

Consideration was given to Crohn's disease, ureteral calculus, and viral gastroenteritis. In other age and gender subsets, such a presentation might include a consideration of colon cancer with perforation, urinary tract infection, diverticulitis, pelvic inflammatory disease, and so forth.

The author of this case led you gently from one bit of evidence to another and rendered a clear exposition of his logic as he reached a conclusion. Further expansion of the clinical reasoning process is found in the mini-cases (questions and answers). *(P.C.)*

Suggested Readings

Connors TJ, Garch IS, Ramshaw BJ, et al. Diagnostic laparoscopy for suspected appendicitis. Am Surg 1992;61(2):187–189.

Guidry SP, Poole GV. The anatomy of appendicitis. Am Surg 60 1994;(1):68–71.

Jeffrey RD, Jian KA, Nghiam HV. Sonographic diagnosis of acute appendicitis: Interpreted pitfalls. Am J Roentgen 1994;162(1):55–59.

CASE 49

SWELLING OF THE ABDOMEN

H. Leonard Bentch

Data Dr. Jones, an obstetrician, refers you a 32-year-old married woman who sought his advice because she missed two menstrual periods and noticed mild abdominal swelling. She thought she was pregnant. Dr. Jones thought she was not because the uterus was normal in size and the pregnancy test was negative. He further commented that she would not have noticeable abdominal swelling so early even if she were pregnant. But then he gave you a little more to worry about by saying, "the right adnexa was normal, but I could not feel the left; and the blood count was normal except for a hemoglobin of 10 g/dL and a hematocrit of 33%."

Logic It was appropriate for the patient to consult her obstetrician. Not only did she think she was pregnant, but she, like many women, looks to her obstetrician-gynecologist for primary care. During the childbearing years, secondary amenorrhea is most commonly due to pregnancy. However, there are many other causes including inflammatory, metabolic, endocrine, infectious, and psychogenic disorders.

Mild anemia is not unusual in menstruating women who lose 5 to 10 mg of iron with each period and do not quite replace it in their diet. However, in conjunction with a large abdomen and amenorrhea it causes you some concern.

Data The patient's comment that she has been unable to close her skirt for the past month plus a quick look convince you that her abdomen is enlarged.

Logic Before going further, you think of the many causes of abdominal distention. Localized enlargement can result from large cysts (ovary, pancreas, mesentery); tumors (uterus, ovary); or a huge liver or spleen. Diffuse abdominal swelling can be caused by one of the traditional five—fat, feces, flatus, fluid, and fetus. Occasionally an ovarian cyst will be so large as to give diffuse swelling. Also, two or more items may coexist, such as hepatosplenomegaly and ascites.

It is common for patients to complain of abdominal distention for simple reasons like recently acquired obesity, severe constipation, or the presence of much gastrointestinal gas. This may need little problem solving: a few questions, then feel and tap the abdomen. For obesity—a pinch! For constipation—a history! And for gas—tympany on percussion. If still in doubt, a radiograph of the abdomen will help distinguish between the five "fs," but a radiograph is ill-advised if pregnancy is suspected. Remember that gaseous distention plus abdominal cramps can augur intestinal obstruction.

Data The patient is the head nurse in the dialysis unit at your hospital. In addition to her two chief complaints, she noted mild fatigue, soreness of the wrist and hand joints, and a nonpruritic rash on her face and arms. These were attributed to a combination of overwork and the irritating scrub soap used in the unit. She had gained 15 lb despite dieting, and had taken a diuretic for the swelling. She had been depressed by the recent death of a favorite dialysis patient. Her appetite was good, and she had no abdominal pain or indigestion. She neither smokes nor drinks alcohol. History is negative except for an appendectomy and allergy to penicillin.

Vital signs are normal except for a temperature of 37.7°C. A large 1- × 2-cm dark nevus seems particularly stark on her back compared to her sallow complexion. No spider angiomas are seen, though there is a slightly scaling urticarial rash on the face and hands. The abdomen is generally protuberant and dull to percussion, except for tympany around the umbilicus. Shifting dullness, fluid wave, and the puddle sign cannot be elicited, and there is no bulging in the flanks. No masses are felt; the spleen is not palpable, although the liver has 14 cm of vertical height and reaches 3 cm below the costal margin in the midclavicular line. It is slightly enlarged and ballotable. The liver edge is firm and blunt. The lungs are clear, there is a grade 2/6 systolic ejection murmur at the base, and two-plus ankle edema is present. Dr. Jones' findings on pelvic examination are confirmed, and the rest of the examination findings are normal.

Logic The case is a complex one, has many ramifications, and you realize that many diagnostic studies will be needed. *Ascites* is the key clue about which your investigation will center. Fever, rash, heart murmur, and mild hepatomegaly are found on physical examination. Also, the mild anemia is significant in this setting.

Much related and unrelated information is now available and must be sorted out. As a dialysis unit nurse, your patient is exposed to hepatitis, tuberculosis, bacteria and viruses of all sorts, drug availability, and depression. Fever is worrisome and suggests infection, inflammation, or neoplasia. The nevus is probably a false clue, because most patients have several such lesions. But malignant melanoma with liver and peritoneal implants cannot be dismissed.

Slight liver enlargement and ascites suggest liver disease. The absence of spider angiomas does not rule out liver disease, especially in the nonalcoholic, but no other stigmata such as parotid swelling and palmar erythema are present. The textbook signs of fluid wave and shifting dullness have poor sensitivity and specificity except in severe cases. You are reasonably certain of ascites because ballottement of the liver is a more accurate sign. The firm blunt liver edge further suggests liver disease.

Another concern is for infective endocarditis superimposed upon perhaps another disease. The fever, anemia, and heart murmur suggest this possibility. Nor have you yet settled the issue of the impalpable left adnexa. A huge ovarian cyst can fill the abdomen and mimic ascites, yet not be felt in the pelvis.

Data A chest radiograph shows a normal-sized heart, no pulmonary infiltrates, and a small right pleural effusion. An abdominal radiograph shows normal air distribution and an overall groundglass hazy appearance characteristic of ascites.

Logic You review the common causes of ascites:

1. Cirrhosis of the liver
2. Congestive heart failure
3. Metastatic cancer—breast, colon, ovary

as well as some of the less common ones:

4. Tuberculous peritonitis
5. Nephrotic syndrome
6. Constrictive pericarditis
7. Inferior vena cava, hepatic vein, or portal vein thrombosis
8. Myxedema (hypothyroidism)
9. Pancreatic carcinoma, cyst, or inflammation
10. Malnutrition

The first three conditions cause more than 90% of cases of ascites. Age and geography are factors. Possibilities 2, 3, and 8 are unlikely at age 32. Diagnoses 4 and 10 are much more common in underdeveloped, primitive, or impoverished areas.

Data Abdominal paracentesis is performed and 50 mL of clear straw-colored fluid are removed. The blood and ascitic fluid studies return: hematocrit 31%; WBC 4200/mm^3, normal differential; platelets 80,000/mm^3; ALT level, 550 U/L (normal 5 to 41); alkaline phosphatase level, 200

U/L (normal 30 to 115); and bilirubin level, 1.7 mg/dL (normal 0.1 to 1.5). The urinalysis and the rest of the blood chemistry determinations are normal. The prothrombin time is 12 seconds. T_4 and thyroid-stimulating hormone levels are normal. Abdominal sonography confirms the presence of diffuse intraperitoneal fluid. The spleen is prominent, portal vein flow is noted toward the liver, and no other masses are found.

The ascitic fluid shows 20 cells per cubic millimeter, no red blood cells, 75 mg glucose, 1.5 g protein, and 4 U of amylase per deciliter. The Gram's stain exhibits no organisms, the culture reveals no growth, and no malignant cells are seen on cytologic study.

The results of two blood cultures are negative. Protein electrophoresis discloses only 2.5 g albumin, but 4.1 g globulin/dL; marked β-γ bridging is noted. A liver-spleen scan shows patchy hepatic uptake, no lucent areas, and an enlarged spleen and increased radioactive material in the spleen and bone marrow.

Logic The clinical problem is becoming clear. She has ascites and the fluid is a transudate. Infection, inflammation, and neoplasia appear most unlikely. Had you accidentally tapped a pancreatic or ovarian cyst, the glucose content would have been almost nil in both, and the amylase would be high in the former. Furthermore, these cysts would have been accompanied by an abnormal gas pattern seen in a plain radiograph of the abdomen because the gas-filled bowel would have been displaced. More important, the abdominal sonogram would have identified the cysts. Tuberculosis would have shown a lymphocytic exudate. The imaging study, her age, and the absence of tumor cells weigh against cancer.

Endocarditis is unlikely because blood cultures are negative, and no embolic phenomena are noted. Heart failure and constrictive pericarditis are ruled out by the normal (except for the murmur) heart examination, the absence of rales, and the absence of distended neck veins. Nephrotic syndrome is excluded by the normal urinalysis. Myxedema can be excluded by the normal thyroid function studies, as well as by a look at her face.

On the other hand, the physical examination, liver enzymes, protein electrophoresis, and liver-spleen scan point directly to a diffuse disease of the liver.

Some findings are now explained. Because a diseased liver cannot manufacture adequate albumin or detoxify aldosterone, hypoalbuminemia and secondary hyperaldosteronemia (with salt and water retention) result. Both act in concert to cause the ankle edema and pleural effusion seen in this patient.

Fever may be related to the disease process in the liver. Anemia occurs for many reasons in liver disease; these include hemolysis, gastrointestinal bleeding, and depressed marrow function. The heart murmur remains incompletely explained, although it may result from the anemia or fever, or it could be a normal finding. Low platelets, and anemia too, can be caused by hypersplenism secondary to portal hypertension. Amenorrhea probably results from an alteration in the metabolism of hormones upon which normal ovulation and menstruation depend.

Severe liver disease causes ascites in many ways: portal hypertension with weeping of fluid from the surface of the liver and throughout the portal bed; low serum protein; intrahepatic lymphatic obstruction; and the inability to metabolize aldosterone.

The type of diffuse liver disease remains to be determined (Table 16.8). Because she does not drink alcohol, it is not alcoholic cirrhosis. But at times it may be difficult to prove that alcoholism exists if there is a co-dependent relationship with other family members. Rare causes of chronic liver disease must be considered, especially if there is specific treatment. Alpha$_1$-antitrypsin deficiency is excluded by the presence of alpha$_1$-

TABLE 16.8. Types of Diffuse Chronic Liver Disease

Alcoholic cirrhosis (Laënnec's)

Biliary cirrhosis

  (a) Primary

  (b) Secondary

Primary sclerosing cholangitis

Chronic viral hepatitis—B, C, D

Chronic autoimmune hepatitis

Hemochromatosis

Wilson's disease

Alpha$_1$-antitrypsin deficiency

globulin on electrophoresis, but it is not currently treatable. However, other inborn errors such as hemochromatosis and Wilson's disease are treatable and they must be excluded by normal serum ferritin and ceruloplasmin levels.

Primary biliary cirrhosis is a rare disease, especially in women younger than age 50; it is notable for connective tissue and immunologic disorders associated with manifestations of liver disease, and is nearly always marked by an elevated antimitochondrial antibody (AMA) level. Secondary biliary cirrhosis is caused by extrahepatic biliary tract obstruction—usually the result of stone in or stricture of the common bile duct in a previously operated patient. It presents with the clinical features of obstructive jaundice and is usually associated with dilated intrahepatic bile ducts on sonography. Primary sclerosing cholangitis presents with obstructive jaundice and occurs more often in the presence of inflammatory bowel disease (ulcerative colitis or Crohn's disease).

Chronic active hepatitis, perhaps with subsequent cirrhosis, is probably present in this patient. This may be caused by either an autoimmune process or by previous infection with hepatitis B, C, or B and D viruses; hepatitis A does not cause chronic hepatitis. Although there is no history of hepatitis, this group of diseases must be eliminated by appropriate serologic tests. It is especially important to consider the hepatitis C antibody in a nurse who works in a dialysis unit.

Autoimmune chronic active hepatitis is a very likely explanation for this patient's condition. In the event that the antinuclear antibody (ANA) test will yield positive results in high titer; rare patients have normal ANA but elevated levels of anti-smooth muscle and anti-liver, anti-kidney, and anti-muscle antibodies.

Data The prothrombin time is normal, and the platelet count is diminished although adequate ($> 50,000/mm^3$). Directed needle biopsy of the liver is performed with the aid of laparoscopy. The classic histologic changes of autoimmune chronic active hepatitis are found (Fig. 16.9). Immunologic studies are as follows: hepatitis B core antibody and hepatitis B surface antigen are absent; hepatitis C antibody is absent; AMA is absent; and ANA is present at 1:1280 in a diffuse pattern.

Logic These results establish the exact diagnosis and explain all the findings. The patient has developed autoimmune chronic active hepatitis,

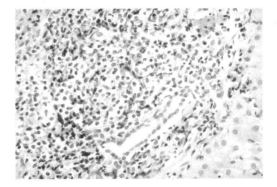

▶ **Figure 16.9.** Histologic changes in autoimmune chronic active hepatitis; disruption of architecture, degeneration of hepatocytes (lower right), and heavy infiltration of chronic inflammatory cells.

and her illness has nothing to do with occupational exposures. The rash and arthralgias represent immunologic manifestations of the disease. This diagnosis is likely in cases in which viruses, genetic derangements, and hepatotoxic drugs have been eliminated from consideration.

You can now offer the patient a thorough explanation of the disease as far as is now known, its natural history, the available medications, and their potential side effects. Treatment with corticosteroids and immunosuppressant drugs (azathioprine) should result in the prevention of cirrhosis.

COMMENT After considering the various causes of abdominal swelling in a young woman, *ascites* became the key clue from which an initial differential diagnosis was formed. Most causes of ascites were eliminated by the absence of accompanying clues in the history and examination. An enlarged ballotable liver having a firm blunt edge offered strong evidence that ascites was due to chronic liver disease. Consideration was then given to various types of chronic liver disease, and the final diagnosis was reached by eliminating all causes except one, and that one was decisively proved by serologic studies and liver biopsy.

Misleading features such as depression, overwork, occupation, possible alcoholism, use of scrub soap, and a large nevus clouded the picture and had to be suppressed. Fever, anemia, and heart murmur clustered to falsely suggest the presence of an additional disease. The sensitivity and specificity of classical clues for ascites entered into the diagnostic logic, and the importance of abdominal paracentesis in weeding out the causes of ascites was evident.

The various clinical features of chronic liver disease were clearly correlated with the underlying pathophysiology all along the way. *(P.C.)*

Suggested Readings

Desmet VJ, Gerber M, Hoofnagle JH, et al. Classification of chronic hepatitis: Diagnosis, grading and staging. Hepatology 1994;19(6):1513–1520.

Maddrey WC. Chronic hepatitis. Dis Mon 1993;39(2): 53–125.

Vierling JM. Immune disorders of the liver and bile duct. Gastroenterol Clin N Am 1992;21(2):427–449.

 CASE 50

BLACK STOOLS

Suzanne Rose and Ernest Urban

Data A 68-year-old retired police officer is brought to the hospital several hours after fainting while on the commode. He had passed two to three black, tarry, malodorous stools each day for the past 2 days; he attributed these to something he "must have eaten." He did feel a little lightheaded from time to time, and on the day of admission he actually passed out after passing considerable black stool. The color was noted and verified by his son, who drove him to the emergency department.

On arrival, he felt weak and looked pale but had no other complaints. Nothing like this had ever happened before. The patient reported that he was in excellent health and had no other symptoms or previous serious illnesses. His only prior surgery was at age 11 for an appendectomy. He was taking no medications regularly. He did take an occasional aspirin for rare headaches and last took two aspirins 3 months ago. He denied alcohol abuse but admitted to an occasional beer, and he smokes a half-pack of cigarettes a day.

Logic Before delving into the specific cause for such a presentation, you must concern yourself with two issues. First, how severe is the blood loss and how urgently is treatment needed? Second, is the bleeding from the upper or lower gastrointestinal tract?

Stabilization of the patient is critical. You must assess the patient's volume status and re-plenish it with fluids and blood products if necessary. Once this is done, you may address the cause of the bleeding. Although it is possible he may have had a vagal episode during a bowel movement, it is more likely he fainted from blood volume depletion subsequent to acute blood loss.

Data The vital signs are: temperature, 37°C; respirations, 16; BP, 130/80; and pulse, 96 while lying down. On sitting up, the pulse rises to 120 and the BP falls to 100/60. A large bore IV is placed and the patient is given normal saline. A second large bore IV is placed for additional access. Blood studies are drawn for complete blood count (CBC), platelets, prothrombin time (PT), partial thromboplastin time (PTT), and electrolyte and liver tests. A specimen is sent for type and cross-match, and a normal ECG is obtained. A nasogastric tube is gently passed into the stomach, and the aspirate shows coffee-ground material without fresh blood that clears with a liter of lavage. The stat hematocrit is 28%.

Logic The vital signs are consistent with orthostatic hypotension and support the theory of volume loss. The "tilt test" for orthostatic hypotension yields a positive result if the pulse rate increases more than 20 beats per minute, or the systolic blood pressure drops more than 20 mm Hg when the patient moves from the supine to the sitting position. It indicates significant acute blood volume loss, usually greater than 1000 mL in adults. The actual volume loss required for a positive tilt test result will also depend on the ability of the patient's vascular system to respond with peripheral vasoconstriction.

The hematocrit of 28% is low but it may not accurately tell you how much blood has actually been lost. It may take 6 hours to fully re-equilibrate the blood volume, and a hematocrit after fluid repletion and hemodilution may be significantly lower.

It is important to assess accurately the aspirate from the nasogastric lavage. The presence of coffee-ground material is highly suggestive of old blood in the upper GI tract. If the specimen is clear and contains bile, this indicates that the bleeding is unlikely to have originated proximal to the ligament of Treitz—from the esophagus, stomach, or duodenum. If clear and with no bile, only the esophagus and stomach may be excluded. You may be misled, however, if bleeding took place several hours ago and has now stopped. Because tube trauma may cause blood in the gastric aspirate, the tube must be passed gently.

The major diagnostic considerations at this time are: (1) duodenal ulcer; (2) acute gastritis; (3) esophageal varices. Other possibilities are far less common.

Data Further history is not contributory. There is no family history of gastrointestinal cancer. There are no known toxic exposures. The patient denies any change in bowel habits before this and there has been no diarrhea, constipation, indigestion, dysphagia, nausea, anorexia, weight loss, or abdominal pain. He has not been evaluated regularly and has never had health care maintenance evaluation with a flexible sigmoidoscopy.

Physical examination reveals normal heart and lungs. The abdomen is soft and nontender, and there is no hepatosplenomegaly. There are no skin stigmata of liver disease. On rectal examination there is black stool that is guaiac positive (dark blue-green as revealed by the Hemoccult test)—a finding consistent with melena. After a fluid bolus and hydration, the pulse slows to 86 beats per minute, and the patient appears to have improved.

Logic It is always important to test the stool for blood. In this case, however, you are fairly certain that the black color was caused by blood because of the syncope, pallor, and the appearance and odor of the stool. In other cases, black stools may be caused by the ingestion of iron and bismuth medications and large quantities of spinach, licorice, green beets, and certain berries. It takes at least 5 to 10 mL of blood per day to make the stool test positive 50% of the time with the Hemoccult test, and 30 mL of blood per day results in 93% positive reactions. At least 60 mL, and more likely more than 100 mL, result in the stool turning black (melena).

The source of blood in the stool cannot always be determined by the color. Generally speaking, bleeding from the midtransverse colon down is red, and more proximal bleeding is black. But this varies with the amount of bleeding and the transit time of the blood. Massive upper GI bleeding can be black, maroon, or red, depending on how long it takes the blood to reach the rectum, and whether there is enough time to permit bacterial action on the hemoglobin. Bright red rectal bleeding originating in the lower GI tract may come from polyps, cancer,

diverticula, angiodysplasias, or hemorrhoids. The latter three conditions are very common in older persons and the presence of any one does not guarantee that it is the source of bleeding. A direct relationship must be established. The presence of only black stool usually excludes blood loss from the descending colon down.

A physical examination in cases of this sort must note the presence or, as in this case, the absence of stigmata of liver disease. You look for things like jaundice, palmar erythema, spider angiomata, and telangiectasias. Their absence, plus the normal-sized liver, virtually exclude portal hypertension and variceal bleeding that may result from cirrhosis of the liver.

Data The repeat hematocrit is 23%. The red blood cells are hypochromic and microcytic on blood smear and by determination of the indices. Platelets are adequate, and the PT and PTT are normal. The patient is admitted to the intensive care (ICU) unit for further management. Two units of packed RBCs are given. A gastrointestinal consultant is asked to evaluate the patient with esophagogastroduodenoscopy (EGD).

Logic The drop in the hematocrit represents further hemodilution as fluid moves from the tissues into the vascular system. The platelet count, PT, and PTT disclose no evidence of a bleeding disorder. Hypochromic microcytic anemia suggests that chronic blood loss may have antedated the acute hemorrhage. This indicates that the bleeding lesion may have been oozing over some time and recently bled heavily, or that another cause may exist.

EGD is the initial test of choice for two purposes. First of all, it affords a direct visualization of the lining of the esophagus, stomach, duodenal bulb, and second portion of the duodenum. Second, there are therapeutic maneuvers that may be performed via the endoscope that may reduce the risk of rebleeding, may result in less blood product requirements, and may avoid the need to refer the patient to surgery. There is no role for an upper GI barium study in this particular situation. Barium will coat the upper GI lining and make any further therapeutic intervention more difficult to perform.

Data Once the blood has been transfused and the vital signs are stable, EGD is performed with conscious sedation in the intensive care unit. The esophagus has normal mucosa without any evidence of varices. In the stomach there are linear erosions in the proximal stomach consistent with NG tube trauma. Antral gastritis is seen with a few erosions. The retroflex view of the stomach is normal and shows no evidence of varices. As the duodenal bulb is entered, a 2- × 2-cm ulcer is seen. There is oozing at the edges of the ulcer, and a small protuberance consistent with a visible vessel with nearby clot is noted. The descending duodenum is evaluated before any intervention and appears normal. The scope is withdrawn back into the bulb, and the lesion is treated with cautery and excellent hemostasis. The endoscope is removed, and the patient tolerated the procedure quite well. An H_2 receptor blocker drip had already been started upon admission to the ICU, and orders are written for empiric treatment for *Helicobacter pylori* (Fig. 16.10).

Logic Endoscopy identified the bleeding lesion. The visible vessel indicated a high risk of rebleeding; accordingly the lesion was cauterized.

The H_2 receptor blocker therapy was initiated to reduce the acid environment. Upper GI tract ulcers are most commonly related to either NSAID medication or to the presence of *Helicobacter pylori*. Because there was no recent history of NSAID or aspirin use, it was not unreasonable to treat this patient empirically for *H. pylori*. Such treatment has been shown to reduce the recurrence of peptic ulcer disease.

Data The patient was observed in the ICU for 36 hours with no evidence of further bleeding. He was transferred to a regular medical bed. The iron studies were consistent with an iron deficiency anemia. An elective colonoscopy was scheduled before the patient's hospital discharge.

Logic Although the patient may have had upper GI tract mucosal disease with inflammation and oozing over time, the evidence of iron deficiency in the RBCs requires the evaluation of the lower GI tract in order to rule out an additional, possibly neoplastic, lesion.

The diagnostic options include: (1) flexible sigmoidoscopy; (2) barium enema (thick, thin, or with air contrast); and (3) fiberoptic colonoscopy. The former may miss the 30% of colonic lesions beyond the sigmoid. Contrast studies may coat the lesion making it less accessible to biopsy and/or removal. The latter is considered the procedure of choice by most clinicians in these circumstances.

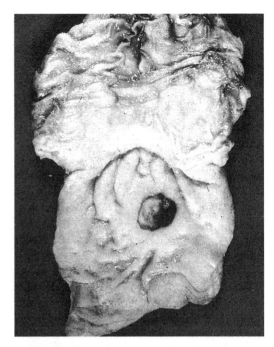

▶ **Figure 16.10.** Bleeding duodenal ulcer just beyond pylorus. This specimen is from another patient who required surgical treatment. Note clot within the ulcer.

Colonoscopy is a relatively safe test that can evaluate the colonic mucosa with direct visualization. Lesions can also be addressed during the procedure. Polyps can be removed by biopsy or snare technique. The risk of colonoscopy is approximately 1 in 1000 for an adverse event, which could include infection, reaction to the conscious sedation medications, bleeding, or perforation. This latter complication may be serious and almost always requires surgical repair, but the chance of a perforation is low. You must always view any situation in terms of risks and benefits. There are risks to not doing the procedure, which in this case could mean not identifying and removing a lesion that could otherwise prove life-limiting.

Data The colonoscopy was performed in the GI laboratory. The external and digital examination results were normal. The colonoscope was advanced to the cecum. The terminal ileum was entered and was visualized to be normal. The preparation was good. The findings included diverticulosis of the left colon and two polyps were seen and removed. One polyp was located at 50 cm in the left colon and was pedunculated (on a stalk). It was 1.5 cm in size. The stalk was snared; electrocoagulation was applied, and the polyp was removed and retrieved and sent to pathology. The second polyp was an 8-mm polyp seen in the proximal transverse colon; it was also removed by cold snare. This was sent to pathology. The retroflex view of the rectum showed internal hemorrhoids. The polypectomy sites were evaluated and showed good hemostasis. The patient tolerated the procedure without any difficulty (Fig. 16.11).

Pathologic study revealed that the polyps were tubular adenomas. There was no evidence of carcinoma.

Logic The colonoscopic findings included diverticulosis. This is a very common finding in our society and may be attributable to our western low-fiber diet that results in weakness in the colon wall. Most persons suffer no consequences of these lesions. Diverticula may become infected and result in diverticulitis. They rarely may bleed. When bleeding occurs, it usually signifies the erosion of a feeding vessel. However, a guaiac-positive stool should never be attributed to diverticulosis alone.

Data The patient was discharged from the hospital with the following medications: antibiotics to treat the *H. pylori infection,* omeprazole, and iron supplements; he was to be followed up as an outpatient.

Logic In this case, the prime bleeding site was identified as a bleeding duodenal ulcer. A second bleeding site was sought because of evidence of hypochromic anemia and chronic blood loss. Although colonic polyps were discovered and removed, they were not deemed to be bleeding, and it was reasonably assumed that the patient had bled small amounts from the duodenal ulcer before the major bleed.

In other cases, if the site of GI bleeding cannot be readily identified by endoscopic procedures, the problem solver may resort to isotopes or arteriography.

A tagged RBC scan after the intravenous injection of technetium 99m-labeled autologous RBCs may detect small pockets of radioactivity from blood loss as slow as 0.1 mL/min. This technique locates the general area of bleeding but does not identify the lesion; it is generally not useful in upper GI bleeding where liver and spleen scintillation dominate the field. Selective

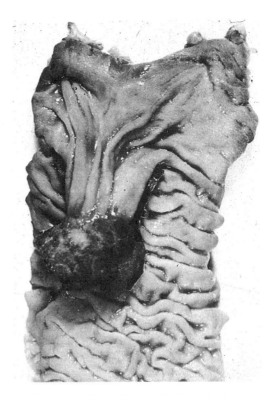

▶ **Figure 16.11.** Pedunculated colon polyp (not the patient in Case 50).

arteriography may locate and define a lesion or at least demonstrate an intraluminal collection of dye. Blood loss of at least 0.5 mL/min is necessary to visualize the bleeding site by angiography. Sometimes an arteriovenous malformation may be visualized. Angiography, if done, must be performed before barium studies. The various diagnostic procedures that may help you locate the cause of gastrointestinal bleeding are listed in Table 16.9.

COMMENT The patient with black stools and syncope has a medical emergency. Your first job is to stabilize the patient with fluids and blood. As in this case, the rest of the history and examination follow at a slower pace.

The next job is to determine if bleeding is from the upper or lower gastrointestinal tract. Early gastric aspiration and EGD are indicated, and if negative, attention must be given to the colon. But in this case the bleeding was from an ulcer—perhaps the commonest cause of such a clinical situation. Nevertheless, after appropriate

TABLE 16.9. Evaluation of Gastrointestinal Bleeding

TEST	INDICATION
EGD	Evaluation of UGI bleeding; allows for diagnosis as well as therapy
Colonoscopy	Evaluation of LGI bleeding; may identify lesions such as AVMs, polyps, cancers, ischemia, colitis
Flexible sigmoidoscopy	Only evaluates left colon; may be used with air-contrast barium enema to evaluate guaiac-positive stool
UGI series	No role in the evaluation of acute bleeding; may be diagnostic for other problems—e.g., gastric outlet obstruction
Barium enema	Air-contrast study may be used to evaluate guaiac-positive stool; no role in brisk bleeding; does not allow for therapy
Enteroclysis	Barium evaluation of small bowel to rule out tumors, strictures, Crohn's
Enteroscopy	Endoscopic view of small intestine to jejunum to evaluate obscure bleeding
Tagged RBC scan	Used to locate general area of bleeding, but does not identify etiology of bleeding source
Angiography	Used in rapid, brisk bleeding to identify source; there may be a therapeutic option of embolizing the source of bleeding

EGD = esophagogastroduodenoscopy; UGI = upper gastrointestinal; LGI = lower gastrointestinal; AVM = arteriovenous malformation.

treatment, an additional lesion causing chronic blood loss was sought but not definitely found.

The author is mindful that the initial clinical manifestation of duodenal ulcer may be hemorrhage or perforation, and that there may be, as in this case, no history of either typical or atypical indigestion and heartburn. Of particular note are the discussions regarding the reliability and operating characteristics of data obtained from the color of the stool, tests for occult blood, gastric aspiration, and the various imaging procedures used here. *(P.C.)*

Suggested Readings

Freeman ML. The current endoscopic diagnosis and intensive care unit management of severe ulcer and other non-variceal upper gastrointestinal hemorrhage. Gastrointest Endosc Clin N Am 1991;209–239.

Laine L, Peterson WL. Bleeding peptic ulcer. N Engl J Med 1994;331:717–727.

NIH Consensus Conference. Therapeutic endoscopy and bleeding ulcers. JAMA 1989;262:1369–1372.

CASE 51

VOMITING OF BLOOD AND DYSPNEA

Raymond A. Rubin

Data The ambulance arrives at the emergency department with a 62-year-old man who just vomited large quantities of bright red blood and is complaining of weakness, dizziness, and shortness of breath. His supine blood pressure is 70/50, pulse 120, respirations 24, and he is pale, cold, and clammy.

Logic This patient requires immediate resuscitation. Being hypotensive in the supine position suggests loss of at least 30 to 40% of his intravascular blood volume. The dyspnea may indicate that, in addition to the gastrointestinal bleeding, he may have cardiac ischemia and congestive heart failure, or that he may have aspirated blood. The ABCs of basic cardiac life support dictate instant attendance to airway, breathing, and circulation before configuring the differential diagnosis for an upper gastrointestinal hemorrhage.

Data He is brought into the treatment area at once. Nasal oxygen is administered, dual large bore intravenous lines are inserted, and normal saline is rapidly infused. Blood is drawn and sent for CBC, biochemistry profile, coagulation studies, and type and cross-match for 4 units of blood. A pulse oximeter registers a saturation of 91% on 4 liters of oxygen per minute.

The repeat supine BP and pulse are 90/60 and 110. The patient says he is less dyspneic and denies chest pain. A 12-lead ECG shows a 2-mm ST depression in leads II, III, and aVF. A urinary catheter is inserted. The patient adamantly refuses placement of a nasogastric tube.

Logic He appears to be stabilizing. The ECG is consistent with inferior wall myocardial ischemia, and, rather than a primary cardiac event, it appears more likely that the hypotension caused by acute blood loss has compromised coronary perfusion.

While instituting emergency measures, you think of what may be wrong. Primary considerations are duodenal or gastric ulcer, cirrhosis with varices, and acute erosive or hemorrhagic gastritis. Less common possibilities include Mallory-Weiss (M-W) tear, peptic esophagitis, and stomach cancer. More unusual causes include vascular malformations, leiomyoma of the stomach, hereditary hemorrhagic telangiectasia, Dieulafoy's lesion, and aortoduodenal fistula (Table 16.10).

Inquiry into the cause of the problem proceeds side by side with treatment. Because of the delicate situation, it must be done with the least number of questions and examining techniques. Fiberoptic gastroduodenoscopy will be done as soon as hemodynamic stabilization is attained. You seek answers to the following questions:

- Is there a previous history of heartburn or indigestion?
- Is the patient an alcoholic, or has he had hepatitis?
- Does he take aspirin, steroids, NSAIDs, or other drugs?
- Does he have anorexia, weight loss, and early satiety?
- Did he vomit several times before blood comes up?
- Does he have stigmata of cirrhosis (large liver, palmar erythema, spider angiomata)?
- Are there telangiectasias in the skin or mucous membranes?
- Is there a mass, tenderness, or pulsation in the epigastrium?

The answer to each question helps to eliminate diagnostic possibilities if they are negative or absent and helps to confirm them if they are positive or present.

Data The patient appears more comfortable. His BP is 100/60 and pulse 96. There were no previous episodes of hematemesis. He had been feeling quite well until 5 days ago when he felt lightheaded and nauseated. Subsequently he noticed that his stools turned black and tarry and that he felt fatigued, but this did not stop him

TABLE 16.10. Causes of Upper Gastrointestinal Bleeding[a]

Acute gastritis—drugs, NSAIDs, aspirin, alcohol
Gastric or duodenal ulcer
Mallory-Weiss tears
Varices (cirrhosis of liver)
Neoplasms (stomach)
Arteriovenous malformation
Peptic esophagitis
Dieulafoy's lesion
Hemobilia
Aorto-enteric fistula

[a]Listed from most common to least common.

from doing his work at the post office. He relates having dyspnea on exertion for the past year and describes a "transient ischemic attack"(TIA) that occurred 6 months ago. In the remote past he had been diagnosed as having a peptic ulcer that was treated with buttermilk and bicarbonate. He takes two aspirins each day "to protect his heart" and occasionally uses ibuprofen for "rheumatism." There has been no weight loss, and his appetite is good.

Typically, he drinks two or three beers nightly and will frequently share a bottle of wine with his wife at dinner. While speaking with him, you convince him of the necessity of placing a nasogastric tube. The gastric contents resemble coffee grounds admixed with some red blood, and the drainage clears with only 500 cc of iced saline lavage.

A focused physical examination reveals anicteric sclera, pallor, a right carotid bruit, no neck vein distention, no adenopathy, an S_4, basilar rales, apex beat in the left 6th intercostal space 11 cm from the midsternal line, a midline vertical abdominal scar, no tenderness, a liver spanning 10 cm in the midclavicular line, and no palpable splenic tip. Rectal examination finds tarry stools streaked with fresh blood. There are no cutaneous stigmata of liver disease such as palmar erythema and spider angiomata.

Logic Cardiac enlargement and basilar rales indicate mild left ventricular failure. This was caused by the superimposition of acute hypoxemia upon preexisting coronary disease. In view of the ECG abnormality, the history of a TIA, and the carotid bruit, it is not unreasonable to presume that he has coronary atherosclerosis.

Perhaps more germane to the acute issue, there is no evidence for chronic liver disease with bleeding varices, and no previous symptoms to suggest cancer, esophagitis, or recent ulcer. The so-called classic description of ulcer symptoms is more often absent than present, and although a history of retching and bilious vomiting followed by hematemesis is classic for M-W tears at the esophagogastric function, this history is forth-coming in only half of documented cases. The taking of aspirin and NSAIDs causes concern for acute hemorrhagic gastritis or ulcer disease.

Data The patient explains that the abdominal scar is from the surgical repair of an abdominal aortic aneurysm 7 years ago.

Logic The aneurysm and its repair raises the specter of an unusual cause of acute upper GI bleeding—aortoduodenal fistula. Other causes yet to be considered are angiodysplasias, neo-plasms, esophageal ulcer, rupture of an aberrant proximal stomach artery (Dieulafoy's lesion), and hemobilia (bleeding into the biliary tree). Until the advent of flexible endoscopy, the true preva-lence of angiodysplasias was underestimated; they are relatively common in the elderly and in pa-tients with hereditary hemorrhagic telangiecta-sia. But the discovery of an arteriovenous mal-formation does not guarantee that a patient's bleed is from that source.

Hematobilia is often secondary to biliary tree trauma but may also result from malignancies, ruptured aneurysms, and gallstones. No specific cause for GI bleeding is found in 5 to 10% of pa-tients who have acute upper GI bleeding.

Data Laboratory work returns. The initial he-moglobin is 10g/l and the hematocrit is 29%. The mean corpuscular volume (MCV), random distribution width (RDW) of the red blood cells, platelet count, and coagulation studies are within normal limits. Notable in the chemistry profile is a BUN of 64 mg/dL and a creatinine that is 1.6 mg/dL.

After blood transfusions are begun, the pa-tient is transferred to the medical intensive care unit. Upper endoscopy is performed to the sec-ond portion of the duodenum. Mild antral gas-tritis and a 3-mm duodenal ulcer with a bland yellow exudate is noted.

Logic Once a patient with upper GI bleeding is hemodynamically stabilized, urgent endoscopy must be performed. The patient's mild cardiac is-chemia does not contraindicate this procedure; prevention of further bleeding will stabilize the cardiopulmonary status. Even in the setting of ongoing bleeding, endoscopy successfully identi-fies the offending lesion with greater than 90% accuracy. It is especially good for finding small tears or erosions and for identifying features that predict a high risk of rebleeding, such as visible vessels in an ulcer bed or active arterial spurting.

The expeditious determination of the specific cause of the bleeding may be used to guide im-mediate therapy, such as the use of an intravenous H_2 receptor antagonist for ulcer or gastritis, and vasoconstrictive therapy for esophageal varices. Moreover, therapeutic instruments can be passed down the channel of the endoscope to arrest the bleeding. For example, thermal probes can coag-ulate a bleeding ulcer or angiodysplasia, local in-filtration of epinephrine can stop bleeding from an M-W tear, and direct injection of irritating chemicals can stop variceal hemorrhage.

In this patient, the cause of the massive GI bleed has not yet been identified. The mild gas-tritis and bland ulcer do not explain the clinical presentation. Although it is possible that a small M-W tear or Dieulafoy's lesion could have been missed at endoscopy, the diagnostic possibility of greatest concern—and beyond the reach of an endoscope—is an aortoduodenal fistula.

As for the initial blood count, the hematocrit first obtained in a patient with acute blood loss does not accurately reflect the volume of blood lost. Because the hematocrit is expressed as the percentage of the total blood volume comprised by red blood cells, it does not decrease until blood volume has been restored by fluids. The normal MCV and RDW argue against substan-tial *chronic* blood loss. The elevated BUN level and relatively normal creatinine level reflect both the absorption of digested blood and prerenal azotemia.

Data A CT scan of the abdomen is obtained that same afternoon. It demonstrates loss of the fat plane between the aorta and the third portion of the duodenum and a small retroperitoneal fluid collection. The patient underwent emergent sur-gical excision of the aortic graft, over-sewing of the aorta, and extra-anatomic bypass grafting.

Logic Aortoduodenal fistulas may result from atherosclerotic disease or infections, but the vast majority are related to a prior prosthetic aortic graft. The third or fourth portion of the duodenum is involved in 80% of patients. As in this case, most patients experience a self-limited herald bleed several days before the massive hemorrhage. The mortality of this condition is high; the patients are elderly, and the hemorrhage may be accompanied by endovascular infection. A high index of suspicion is required to make this important and life-saving diagnosis because the fistula is often difficult to detect with endoscopy, cross-sectional imaging, and aortography.

The mortality rate of patients with upper GI hemorrhage depends on the age of the patient and the cause of the hemorrhage. A higher mortality rate for older patients reflects the effect of co-morbid illnesses such as atherosclerotic, pulmonary, and renal diseases. Bleeding varices have a high mortality. Patients who have acute gastritis and bleeding ulcer fare generally well. Survival is best following a M-W tear and for those in whom, after a thorough search, a specific diagnosis cannot be made.

Questions

1. If the patient had been an alcoholic and had shown all the stigmata of cirrhosis including severe portal hypertension, then the cause of the bleeding would have been:
   (a) varices.
   (b) ulcer.
   (c) gastritis.
   (d) any of the aforementioned.
2. Mallory-Weiss syndrome is more common than was originally thought. It occurs in a patient who is vomiting or retching violently and then starts to vomit blood. The cause is:
   (a) alcohol-induced gastritis.
   (b) steroid-induced ulcer.
   (c) tear of gastric mucosa near esophagogastric junction.
   (d) tear of gastric mucosa near gastroduodenal junction.
3. In reference to determining the site of GI bleeding, which of the following clinical deductions is incorrect?
   (a) The patient vomits blood, is not alcoholic, and has no clinical evidence of cirrhosis. Varices are a highly unlikely cause.
   (b) The patient vomits blood, and stools are tarry black. Carcinoma of the colon is not the cause.
   (c) The patient has black tarry stools. Duodenal ulcer may be the cause.
   (d) The patient has black tarry stools, and the gastric aspirate is clear. Bleeding from the duodenum is ruled out.

Answers

1 **(d) is correct.** Patients with alcoholic cirrhosis commonly bleed from any of the three causes. Although varices are common, bleeding may occur from ulcer or gastritis even if varices are present. In fact, gastritis may be more common than varices as a cause of bleeding in the cirrhotic patient.
2. **(c) is correct.** The tear occurs because a sudden increase in intragastric and intra-abdominal pressure results in forceful traction through the hiatus against the fixed crux of the diaphragm. This causes a tear of the gastric mucosa at or just below the gastroesophageal junction. Bleeding can be minor or very severe. This usually occurs in alcoholics or in patients who have a hiatal hernia.
3. **(d) is correct** because it is incorrect. The patient may have stopped bleeding. Choices (a), (b), and (c) are correct possibilities. In circumstance (a), there is usually evidence of portal hypertension to imply varices. In (b), hematemesis tells you that the lesion must be proximal to the ligament of Treitz. Bleeding from a duodenal ulcer in (c) may alter the stool, yet not cause hematemesis if bleeding is not very rapid.

COMMENT The urgency of this case clearly demonstrated that treatment must at times precede the establishment of a precise diagnosis. The differential diagnosis for the causes of hematemesis was divided into common, less common, and rare possibilities. Although most causes on this list were easily eliminated by selected subsections of the history and examination, there were many distractions such as possible alcoholism, the use of NSAIDs and aspirin, and the presence of concomitant left ventricular failure.

The need for, practical uses of, and limitations of prompt endoscopy were noted in that, although endoscopy eliminated many contenders, it uncovered a small nonbleeding duodenal ulcer—in this case, a false-positive clue. For, had it not been for the abdominal scar and the belated history of an aneurysm repair, the correct diagnosis might not have been made premortem. CT, of course, provided the final sensitive and specific clue for the diagnosis of an aortoduodenal fistula. *(P.C.)*

Suggested Readings

Katz PO, Salas L. Less frequent causes of upper gastrointestinal bleeding. Gastroenterol Clin N Am 1993;22(4):875–879.

Lieberman D. Gastrointestinal bleeding: Initial management. Gastroenterol Clin N Am 1993;22(4):723–736.

Nagy SW, Marshall JB. Aortoenteric fistulas. Recognizing a potentially catastrophic cause of gastrointestinal bleeding. Postgrad Med 1993;93(8):211–212, 215–226, 219–222.

CASE 52

CRAMPS AND NAUSEA

Arthur S. McFee

Data A 45-year-old woman comes to the emergency department complaining that she has had "intestinal flu" for the past 3 days. It began with cramping, periumbilical pain, anorexia, and nausea. The episodes of cramping were severe and frequent at first, but then they came less often and had almost disappeared by the second day, at which time she felt that she was better. She not only denies diarrhea, but notes that she has had no stool nor has she passed gas for 2 days.

However, toward the end of the second day she began to feel uncomfortably full, and her clothes felt tight. That night she vomited and continued to do so until admission to the hospital on Day 3. Her last vomitus was particularly foul-tasting and consisted of dark greenish-brown liquid material (feculent vomiting). Several hours before admission she noted a different type of abdominal pain that was steady, sharp, and localized to the left lower quadrant (LLQ).

Logic This history is characteristic of distal small bowel obstruction. The patient thought she had "intestinal flu" because of the cramping. If that were so, she would have had diarrhea too. Occasionally, as in this case, the patient assumes improvement as the cramping pain diminishes. Actually, she is much worse.

Vomiting can be a late sign with distal obstruction. Nausea and anorexia are common symptoms that give no clues to the specificity of the diagnosis. Often the patient with a distal lesion may not seek help for several days until distention and feculent vomiting occur. Feculent vomitus originates in the small bowel. It indicates distal small or large bowel obstruction and is noted only after prolonged incessant vomiting has emptied the proximal gastrointestinal tract.

The advent of a new, more steady pain indicates peritoneal irritation and a different pain mechanism. It is a very significant symptom that tells you something else is happening.

The concurrent onset of vomiting and cramps usually indicates a more proximal obstruction and causes the patient to seek aid much earlier in the course of the disease. Proximal obstructions are those that take place at the gastric outlet, the duodenum, or the first two or three feet of jejunum.

Data History reveals good health with no major diseases. She has three children, all delivered by cesarean section; the youngest is 14 years old. Ten years ago she underwent an abdominal hysterectomy for fibroids. The systems review, family history, and patient profile reveal negative or normal findings.

Logic Fibrous adhesions within the coelom are the preponderant cause (80%) of bowel obstruction in the patient who has undergone an abdominal operative procedure. Although most develop this obstruction within 1 or 2 years of surgery, it can occur much later. In the patient who develops a similar picture in the absence of prior surgery, the most common cause of obstruction is an internal or external hernia. Other causes of distal bowel obstruction include colon cancer, volvulus, intussusception, foreign body, gallstone, regional ileitis, and diverticulitis (Table 16.11).

Data Physical examination discloses a very sick patient who is lying quietly in bed. The vital signs are: temperature, 38.7°C; pulse, 105; respirations, 24; and BP, 90/70. Skin turgor is poor, mucous membranes are dry, and the eyes are sunken. Although the heart and lungs are normal, the diaphragm moves poorly. There is marked abdominal distention and bowel sounds are absent. Point tenderness and rigidity can be defined in the LLQ at the site of her present pain. The abdomen is tympanitic, and a succussion splash is elicited, but

TABLE 16.11 Causes of Distal Intestinal Obstruction

Hernia
Adhesions
Colon cancer
Volvulus
Intussusception
Gallstone
Foreign body
Regional ileitis
Diverticulitis

no masses can be palpated. Pelvirectal examination reveals marked left adnexal tenderness and an empty rectal ampulla. No inguinal, femoral, or umbilical herniae are noted. There are midline and transverse lower abdominal incisions; each is well healed, firm, and without hernia.

Logic The prime impression is that you have a very ill patient who exhibits many signs of dehydration and has an acute surgical abdomen. By itself, it means nothing that the patient is lying quietly in bed. Together with the LLQ pain, point tenderness, and rigidity, it indicates the presence of peritoneal irritation and confirms the historical report of a different type of pain starting hours before admission.

Other significant physical findings are present in the abdomen: First, there is marked distention due to dilated air and fluid-filled loops of intestine; this situation is indicated by tympanites and a succussion splash and is characteristic of distal bowel obstruction. If the obstruction were proximal, abdominal distention would not be noted because the upper bowel empties itself quite well by vomiting, and the process is largely concealed beneath the costal margin.

Second, lack of bowel sounds can result from several causes. In the absence of peritonitis, a distended edematous bowel gradually loses its ability to sustain effective peristalsis. Bowel sounds and cramps diminish as peristalsis decreases, and they may indeed vanish altogether. In the presence of peritonitis from any cause, a reflex paralysis or ileus of the bowel occurs; it may be localized to the area adjacent to the inflammation, or be generalized if the peritonitis is widespread or

severe. Extra-coelomic processes, such as pelvic or spinal fractures or abscesses and pneumonia, can also cause reflex ileus with absent bowel sounds.

Left adnexal tenderness can result from acute tubo-ovarian inflammation causing secondary bowel obstruction, or it may simply mean that inflamed tender bowel is being felt in this area. Hysterectomy does not necessarily include removal of the adnexae. The fact that no masses were palpable in the abdomen may merely reflect the difficulties of examination in the presence of tenderness and distention. An empty rectum is compatible with obstruction.

The physical examination buttresses the historical impression of distal mechanical bowel obstruction followed by an inflammatory process. This can only mean that obstruction with strangulation or perforation has occurred. A rapid work-up and treatment are mandatory.

Data Chest and abdominal radiographs show a normal chest with an elevated diaphragm, and a marked layering "stepladder" pattern of air-filled small bowel with air-fluid levels apparent in the upright position (Fig. 16.12). It is impossible to

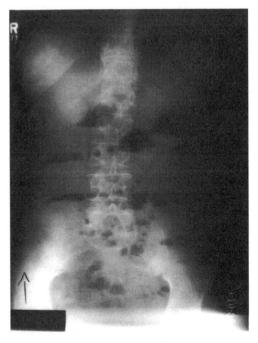

▶ **Figure 16.12.** Small bowel obstruction. Note air-fluid levels in small intestine giving characteristic 'stepladder' pattern.

define a normal colon pattern of gas, and no air is seen in the distal large bowel.

Complete blood count shows: hemoglobin, 16.5 g/dL; hematocrit, 47%; white blood cell count, 21,800/mm^3; 91% polymorphonuclear leukocytes. Only 30 mL of urine are obtained: specific gravity is 1.034, and the urine is ketone positive, but all other findings are normal or negative. Serum sodium is 136; potassium, 3.2; bicarbonate, 15 mEg/L; blood urea nitrogen, 46; glucose, 100; and creatinine, 1.6 mg/dL.

Proctosigmoidoscopy is normal to 25 cm, although some difficulty is encountered due to tenderness. After some discussion on the appropriateness of radiologic contrast studies, a barium enema is performed; its results are normal.

Logic The radiographs confirm obstruction; the site is not apparent, but it is certainly not in the colon. Blood and urine studies indicate dehydration, hemoconcentration, electrolyte depletion, ketosis, acidosis, and decreased renal blood flow with prerenal azotemia and scant concentrated urine. The marked leukocytosis suggests an acute inflammatory process.

In this setting, contrast radiographs are not generally productive of more information than can be adduced by history and physical examination. However, a carefully done barium enema is reasonably innocuous and rules out obstruction in the colon. In very suspicious instances, a water-soluble contrast agent can be substituted for barium. Most carcinomas of the colon (60 to 70%) causing obstruction should be visible by a proctosigmoidoscopy, or certainly by flexible sigmoidoscopy; colon malignancy causing obstruction can be effectively ruled out by these studies. Furthermore, the absence of anemia and no history of rectal bleeding weigh against colon or rectal cancer.

In general, an upper gastrointestinal series of radiographs is contraindicated in this type of patient for several reasons. It is doubtful that the contrast material in many instances will pass out of the stomach; retained food and fluid will render good visualization difficult; and if obstructed, the contrast material will only reveal the point of obstruction without identifying the cause—not a helpful item of information. Lately, however, water-soluble agents, *not* barium, have been employed in timed studies to demonstrate individuals with partial obstruction for whom observation may be appropriate.

CT scan and ultrasonography are both compromised by the presence of multiple loops of distended air- and fluid-filled bowel; however, each has been used in numerous studies to help define strangulation or identify masses. Each may be very effective in diagnosis, especially when combined with water-soluble contrast media. MRI studies are not used in the diagnosis of bowel obstruction. Diagnostic laparoscopy may be a great help if one is dealing with obstruction based on adhesions, carcinomatosis, or a single identifiable lesion; it may also be therapeutic. Basically, obstruction remains a diagnosis that depends mainly on clinical evidence (history and physical examination). All other techniques are used as confirmatory studies.

Data Over the next 4 hours, the patient is intensively prepared for surgery with intravenous fluids, appropriate electrolytes, gastrointestinal suction, and antibiotics. The blood pressure rises, the pulse falls, and urinary output rises to 30 to 50 mL/h. Ketosis, acidosis, and electrolyte disorders are ameliorated.

Exploratory laparotomy reveals an area of extensive fibrous adhesions surrounding a left cystic ovary. Approximately 1.5 feet of distal ileum are entrapped within this cystic mass and are strangulated. The adhesions are lysed, the ovary and tube are removed, gangrenous small bowel is resected, and an anastomosis is performed. The patient makes an uneventful recovery and is discharged well in 8 days.

Logic Several important lessons are to be learned. The exact cause for obstruction need not necessarily be known, but an operation is mandatory to relieve both the effects of the obstruction and the obstructing mechanism itself.

In most cases of simple mechanical intestinal obstruction, preoperative treatment can proceed on a planned basis, unless the obstruction is high. Proximal high obstruction, in addition to causing a rapid depletion of body fluid and electrolytes, poses the further danger of aspirated vomitus, pneumonia, or asphyxiation. If an obstruction results in intestinal strangulation, signs of peritoneal irritation are additionally present (fever, tenderness, abdominal wall rigidity). Therefore, in a case of high obstruction or peritoneal irritation, treatment before surgery must proceed rapidly. A dead or perforated viscus cannot be long tolerated, because systemic sepsis and shock may cause the patient's death.

Questions

1. Assume the same clinical presentation: cramping pain followed by increasing distention and vomiting. The patient is 62 years old and has had no previous surgery. Although the bowels had always been normal, large amounts of laxatives were taken over the previous 3 months for increasingly more severe constipation. Physical examination results are normal. The most likely diagnosis is:
   (a) cancer of the sigmoid colon.
   (b) acute diverticulitis.
   (c) obstruction in a femoral hernia.
   (d) Crohn's disease of the colon.

2. A 23-year-old woman has the acute onset of cramping abdominal pain, distention, and vomiting. She had an appendectomy at age 8. Distention and very active borborygmi are present. Bilateral inguinal adenopathy is believed to be the result of fungal infection of the feet. A tender mass, 1 cm in diameter, is noted near one lymph node just inferior to Poupart's ligament on the left side. The most likely diagnosis is:
   (a) acute inguinal lymphadenitis.
   (b) Richter's femoral hernia.
   (c) inguinal hernia.
   (d) fibrous adhesions in the abdomen.

3. A 14-year-old male is hit by an automobile and sustains a severely fractured pelvis and a pulmonary contusion. No intra-abdominal bleeding is demonstrated on peritoneal lavage. Four days later he develops pneumococcal pneumonia. Six days after the accident, abdominal distention is still present, bowel sounds are absent, and he has passed no stool or gas. He has never complained of colicky pain. The abdomen is soft and not tender. He has:
   (a) fibrous adhesions as a result of lavage.
   (b) obstruction from an internal hernia.
   (c) reflex paralytic ileus without obstruction.
   (d) need for urgent surgery.

4. A 58-year-old man with a clear-cut picture of intestinal obstruction had an operation for the repair of two inguinal hernias 1 year ago and an appendectomy for a ruptured appendix 2 years ago. For the past 6 months he has had bright red rectal bleeding with most bowel movements, but no change in bowel habit. Examination shows distention but no tenderness, a large, easily reducible, right recurrent inguinal hernia, and internal hemorrhoids that are not bleeding at that moment. After reduction of the hernia, evidence of obstruction continues. The obstruction is most likely caused by:
   (a) carcinoma of the left hemicolon.
   (b) recurrent right inguinal hernia.
   (c) adhesions from previous surgery.
   (d) carcinoma of the cecum.

Answers

1. **(a) is correct.** Diverticulitis is associated with tenderness and guarding. A femoral hernia is not present. Choice (d) does not have this type of presentation. A distal bowel obstruction in this age group, under these circumstances, is most likely caused by cancer. The left colon is narrow, and cancers there are usually of the "napkin-ring" constricting type, so obstruction occurs early.

2. **(b) is correct.** A small tender mass in the femoral canal, associated with the picture of intestinal obstruction, indicates an obstructed femoral hernia. Because this canal is small, it is common for the obstruction to be caused by only a knuckle of bowel rather than an entire loop; this is called a Richter's hernia. Although (a) could account for a tender mass, it could not cause obstruction. Postappendectomy adhesions could cause obstruction but would not cause a tender femoral mass. The location of the mass weighs against an inguinal hernia; besides, femoral hernias are more common than inguinal hernias in women.

3. **(c) is correct.** Both a retroperitoneal hematoma resulting from fractured pelvis and pneumonia can cause reflex paralytic ileus. The clinical picture of obstruction (colic and borborygmi) is not present, and there are no findings of peritoneal irritation (tenderness and guarding). Adhesions from lavage are rare. Surgery is not indicated, and bowel activity will return with appropriate nonsurgical measures.

4. **(c) is correct.** Admittedly, there is an overlap of findings and possibilities here. With rectal bleeding, cancer of the left colon is a distinct possibility at this age, even though hemorrhoids are present; the absence of change of bowel habit weighs against this impression. The larger recurrent hernia is probably not the cause of obstruction because of its size, easy reducibility, and lack of improvement after it was reduced. Cancer of the right colon rarely causes obstruction unless it is at the site of the ileocecal valve; this is because the right colon is wide, and lesions there tend to be fungating rather than constricting. Thus, they present with anemia, occult bleeding, and unexplained fatigue. This leaves us with adhesions, the most common cause of obstruction in a patient with previous surgery. Of course, proctosigmoidoscopy and barium enema before surgery are especially indicated in this patient.

COMMENT The author meticulously analyzed each of the symptoms and signs in this patient, and although he took the reader through each diagnostic procedure currently used in cases like this, he pointed out that diagnosis rests almost entirely upon the basic history and physical examination.

The triad of anorexia, nausea, and cramps is not specific, but when combined with obstipation, distention, and vomiting, obstruction becomes very likely. In a 45-year-old woman with intestinal obstruction who has always been in good health, yet has had four abdominal operations and has no observable hernia, the likelihood that the obstruction is caused by adhesions is between .80 and .95. (P.C.)

Suggested Readings

Joyce WP, Delaney PV, Gorey TF, et al. The value of water-soluble contrast radiology in the management of acute small bowel obstruction. Ann R Coll Surg Engl 1992;74(6):422–425.

Keating J, Hill A, Schroeder D, et al. Laparoscopy in the diagnosis and treatment of acute small bowel obstruction. J Laporosc Surg 1992;2(5):239–244.

Maginte DD, Gage SN, Harmon BH, et al. Obstruction of the small intestine: accuracy and role of CT in diagnosis. Radiology 1992;188(1):64.

Ogata M, Imai S, Hosotani R, et al. Abdominal ultrasonography for the diagnosis of strangulation in small bowel obstruction. Br J Surg 1994;81(3):421–424.

CASE 53

FEVER, CONFUSION, ALCOHOL

Paul Cutler

Data A 50-year-old man, in whom Laënnec's cirrhosis was proved by biopsy 2 years ago, was brought to the emergency department by his family because of fever and confusion for 24 hours. Even since this diagnosis was made, he continued to drink 1 pint of 86-proof whiskey daily as he had done for 30 years before. He never had a gastrointestinal hemorrhage, and his ascites had been treated with attempted salt restriction and 100 mg of hydrochlorothiazide daily.

Logic Altered mentation in an alcoholic patient with known liver disease requires three sets of considerations. First, you think of hepatic or portal-systemic encephalopathy (PSE) as a likely explanation.

But second, you must also consider other central nervous system disturbances in a patient with this background. These include acute alcoholic intoxication; other drug intoxication; acute hallucinosis; delirium tremens; Wernicke-Korsakoff encephalopathy; hypoglycemia; acute infections (meningitis, pneumonia, sepsis); and subdural hematoma from the head trauma that heavy drinkers often incur. And third, alcoholism does not exempt him from the cerebrovascular accidents that nondrinkers get. Each of these many diseases can present with similar behavior disorders, although the fever favors some more than others.

Data Additional history obtained from the patient and his family confirmed that he had been drinking his usual amounts up to and including the very day of admission to the emergency department. He never experienced "the shakes," hallucinations, or delusions, and he had suffered no recent head trauma. Although he ate poorly, he had no nausea, vomiting, hematemesis, or known melena and has taken no other drugs.

Logic Because he has not stopped drinking and has not had the usual manifestations of delirium tremens, alcohol withdrawal syndromes can probably be excluded. Similarly, the absence of a recent history of hematemesis, melena, and other drug ingestions make GI bleeding and drug intoxication unlikely.

Data Physical examination disclosed an unkempt, poorly nourished man who looked much older than his age. The vital signs were: temperature, 39°C; pulse, 106; BP, 128/70; respirations, 20; and no orthostatic changes were present. He was slightly lethargic and disoriented to time and place, but he had no gross tremor, perseveration, confabulation, or ideas of reference. There were no signs of head trauma such as ecchymoses, hematomas, or lacerations; the sclerae were slightly icteric, ocular movements were normal, pupils reacted well, and the fundi were normal.

Muscular tone was somewhat increased so that neck stiffness and tests for Kernig's and Brudzinski's signs were uninterpretable. There was temporal muscle wasting, parotid enlargement, numerous spider angiomas, and palmar erythema, but no gynecomastia. His breath had a musty odor suggestive of fetor hepaticus. The heart and lungs were normal; but the abdomen was moderately distended and the umbilicus was effaced. Chest hair was present. There was no caput medusae, although some distended abdominal veins were present. The liver was ballotable 3 cm below the costal margin, and its vertical percussion span was 15 cm in the midclavicular line; the splenic tip was palpable. No abdominal tenderness was noted, and bowel sounds were present although faint. The testes were normal in size, rectal examination was normal, and the stool was brown and tested negative for occult blood. The extremities showed palmar erythema and white fingernails, but no clubbing or Dupuytren's contractures.

On neurologic examination, there were no lateralizing signs, and deep tendon reflexes were 3+ and symmetric. Bilateral "hand flap" (asterixis) was present, and Babinski's signs were absent. His signature was shaky, and his performance of a number-connecting test was very slow.

Logic The history and physical examination were directed at trying to distinguish between the cited diagnostic possibilities. Based upon the presence of asterixis and fetor hepaticus in a patient with severe chronic liver disease (portal hypertension, ascites, and other stigmata), PSE is by far the most likely explanation for the patient's altered mental status. Although asterixis is a nonspecific sign that may be present in other forms of organic encephalopathy, fetor hepaticus appears to be specific for PSE when it is detected.

Note the presence of many physical signs that are characteristic of cirrhosis but the absence of some that are often present (testicular atrophy, gynecomastia, loss of chest hair). Also, in PSE, Babinski's sign is often present.

Subdural hematoma is less likely without neurologic signs, but it is certainly not ruled out even in the absence of a clear-cut trauma history. Wernicke-Korsakoff psychosis is unlikely in the absence of ophthalmoplegia, confabulation, and polyneuritis, and there is no focalizing neurologic evidence of a stroke.

Although PSE may occur in the course of decompensated liver disease, especially in the presence of portal hypertension with shunting, it is often precipitated by GI bleeding, other sources of increased enteric protein load, infection, hypokalemic metabolic alkalosis, or sedative/narcotic administration. This patient's fever is of special concern. Further studies are therefore directed at determining which of the precipitating factors may be present, and at finding the cause of the fever itself (Table 16.12).

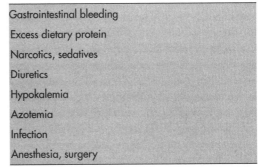

TABLE 16.12. Causes of Portal-Systemic Encephalopathy

Gastrointestinal bleeding
Excess dietary protein
Narcotics, sedatives
Diuretics
Hypokalemia
Azotemia
Infection
Anesthesia, surgery

Data Chest radiograph and ECG findings were normal. Abdominal radiograph showed diffuse haziness compatible with ascites; the liver and spleen were not clearly visualized. The nasogastric aspirate was clear and negative for occult blood. Except for 1+ bilirubin, the urinalysis results were normal. Other emergency laboratory data included a hemoglobin/hematocrit of 8.6/30, which was unchanged from tests done 2 months ago. There were 20,000 WBC per mm^3, of which 75% were polymorphonuclear and 15% were band cells; the blood smear showed poikilocytosis and anisocytosis with a normal number of platelets. Blood chemistry determinations were: urea nitrogen, 36 mg/dL; bilirubin, 5 mg/dL; sodium, 130 mEq/L; potassium, 2.5 mEq/L; chloride, 99 mEq/L; and bicarbonate 34 mEq/L. Serum and urine amylase levels were normal. Prothrombin time was 16 seconds (control 12), which was unchanged since last measured 2 months ago. Minimal intoxication was indicated by a blood alcohol level of 50 mg/dL. The results of a toxicology screen for sedatives and tranquilizers in the blood and urine were negative.

Logic GI bleeding is highly unlikely on the basis of a negative history of hematemesis or melena, the absence of detectable blood in the stool and gastric aspirate, and the stable though abnormal hematocrit. The cause of the anemia remains to be determined, but in patients with cirrhosis the usual cause is previously undetected episodes of GI bleeding from varices, ulcer, or gastritis. The low level of blood alcohol and the negative toxicology screening results make drug encephalopathy unlikely.

Mild azotemia may have resulted from diuretic-induced fluid losses. The elevated blood urea level may contribute to encephalopathy by diffusing across the gut mucosa, where bacterial ureases reduce it to absorbable ammonia.

Hypokalemia and an elevated serum bicarbonate level suggest a metabolic alkalosis. This may be caused by thiazide diuretics, lack of potassium supplementation, volume contraction, and the secondary hyperaldosteronism that sometimes occurs in patients with cirrhosis and ascites. Alkalosis also aggravates PSE by increasing the diffusion of ammonia into (central nervous system) cells where it may be trapped as ammonium ion, resulting in disturbed oxidative metabolism.

Although the EEG, arterial blood gases, arterial ammonia, and spinal fluid ammonia or glutamine determinations may help to confirm PSE, the clinical picture is reasonably complete and such additional studies are not likely to change your approach. Furthermore, the exact biochemical disturbance responsible for PSE has not yet been verified.

Recent reports incriminate false neurotransmitters and enhanced GABA neurotransmitters as causes of the mental aberrations. However, the serum ammonium level has approximately a 90% correlation with the existence of PSE, and is said to come about because the diseased liver is unable to convert gut-derived ammonium into urea.

Data Rehydration with 5% dextrose in water was guided by a central venous pressure monitor, and potassium chloride was carefully supplemented to correct possible excessive water loss and metabolic alkalosis. Dietary protein was withheld, tap water enemas were given, and oral lactulose was started—all counter-encephalopathy measures—while the evaluation proceeded.

Logic You should be especially concerned about the unexplained fever and leukocytosis. Alcoholic cirrhotic patients are predisposed to tuberculosis (pulmonary, meningeal, peritoneal, and miliary), bacterial meningitis, pneumonia (aspiration), spontaneous bacterial peritonitis in the presence of ascites, and other sources of sepsis. Each can precipitate PSE but may also threaten life by the nature of the infection itself. Although alcoholic hepatitis may cause fever and leukocytosis all by itself, there is nothing in the data so far obtained to suggest a marked worsening of liver function or sudden increase in hepatic cell necrosis.

Pneumonia is excluded by the normal chest examination and negative chest radiograph, and urinary tract infection is unlikely with a normal urinalysis. However, the examination and culture of the cerebrospinal and peritoneal fluids are the most important tests, and these should be performed as emergency studies on the day of admission.

Data A lumbar puncture yielded clear colorless fluid under normal pressure. The proteins, glucose, and cell count were normal. Fluorochrome stain, Gram's stain, and India ink preparation were all negative. Cultures for various pathogens were begun.

Midline paracentesis below the umbilicus obtained 20 mL of straw-colored, slightly cloudy fluid: specific gravity, 1.020; proteins, 3.7 g/dL; glucose level, 40 mg/dL; and the amylase level was undetectable. There were 1800 WBC/mm³, of which 90% were polymorphonuclear leukocytes. Gram's stain showed gram-negative rods, and fluorochrome stain results were negative.

Logic The picture is now clear. Meningitis, septicemia, and tuberculosis are excluded. Most important, there is strong evidence that the patient has peritonitis that is no doubt the cause of his acute deterioration. The paracentesis fluid has the characteristics of an exudate; numerous polymorphonuclear leukocytes are counted, and bacteria are present. This disorder may occur spontaneously in the complete absence of physical signs of peritonitis and in the absence of any obvious focus of intra-abdominal suppuration. Gram-negative organisms, especially *Escherichia coli,* are the usual offenders.

Data Ticarcillin and tobramycin were added to the intravenous fluids in an effort to treat this frequently catastrophic complication of cirrhosis and ascites. Other tests of liver function were sent to the laboratory. Skin tests for tuberculosis and fungi were also applied. Blood cultures were drawn.

Over the next 48 hours, evidence of PSE abated, urine output rose, the blood urea nitrogen level fell to normal, the temperature dropped, and general improvement was noted. Culture of the blood and ascitic fluid yielded a heavy growth of *E. coli* sensitive to the antibiotics in use.

While the course of treatment continued, studies were done to seek out a focal infection. Abdominal plain radiographs and repeated physical examinations failed to detect any suggestion of intra-abdominal suppuration such as biliary, pancreatic, periappendiceal, or diverticular disease. Intermediate strength purified protein derivative and fungal test results were negative; mumps antigen was present; total serum bilirubin was 4.6 mg/dL (3.0 mg direct); alkaline phosphatase was 280 IU/L; AST, 120 IU/L; serum proteins, 5 g/dL; and albumin, 2.5 g/dL.

Logic Tuberculosis is ruled out by the skin test and lack of lymphocytes in the exudate. The liver tests are what you would expect with chronic liver disease, and the modest AST level is not in keeping with severe acute necrosis. There is no apparent source for the infected peritoneal fluid, so it is assumed to be spontaneous. A gallium isotope scan for intra-abdominal suppuration was deemed unnecessary.

Data The patient was discharged after completion of antibiotic treatment. In the meantime, his diuretic was changed to spironolactone given in doses adjusted to remove 1/2 lb of ascitic fluid per day. Attempts to have him curtail alcohol were considered hopeless. Arrangements were made to follow him at frequent intervals.

Logic When a patient with Laënnec's cirrhosis takes a sudden downhill course, you must think of hepatoma, portal vein or hepatic vein thrombosis, peritonitis or other forms of infection, acute alcoholic hepatitis, marked electrolyte disturbances, and the hepatorenal syndrome, as well as PSE and some of its causes (Table 16.13).

Although this patient clearly had alcoholic cirrhosis, it is wise to remember that cirrhosis may be caused by other disorders, and some of these, such as Wilson's disease, hemochromatosis, secondary biliary cirrhosis, and cirrhosis due to chronic active hepatitis, may respond to treatment and should be sought.

TABLE 16.13. Complications of Cirrhosis

Portal hypertension
Bleeding esophageal varix
Ascites
Spontaneous bacterial peritonitis
Portal-systemic encephalopathy
Hepatorenal syndrome
Coagulopathy
Hepatoma
Portal vein thrombosis

Cirrhosis has many faces. Liver disease of itself has few symptoms. A large liver may be discovered in a patient who sees a physician for an unrelated problem. Other common presentations are those related to the associated alcoholism: acute alcoholic hepatitis, acute alcoholic intoxication, and delirium tremens. Last, the patient may not see a physician until he or she has noticed jaundice, has PSE, GI hemorrhage, ascites, or an infectious complication.

Data Problem list:

1. Alcoholism
2. Portal cirrhosis
3. Acute bacterial peritonitis
4. Portal-systemic encephalopathy

COMMENT Disorientation in a patient who has cirrhosis and alcoholism suggests many possibilities. But the presence of fever suggests a small cluster that rapidly limits the diagnostic hypotheses, unless there are two independent processes going on. At any rate, pertinent negative clues helped rule out many possibilities, and highly specific decisive clues such as fetor hepaticus and the nature of the ascitic fluid confirmed the two new diagnoses that were present.

This patient presented with many complications of cirrhosis—ascites, portal hypertension, hypokalemic alkalosis, peritonitis, and encephalopathy—each having adversely compounding effects on the others. Cause-and-effect relationships were multiple and complex. For example, cirrhosis, portal hypertension, and ascites laid the background for peritonitis. Portal hypertension with shunting, hypokalemic alkalosis, and peritonitis combined to precipitate PSE.

Given a patient with PSE and fever, the experienced clinician would have quickly sought out the main problem with a paracentesis, because that is where the answer is most apt to lie. (P.C.)

Suggested Readings

Aldersley MA, O'Grady JG. Hepatic disorders. Features and appropriate management. Drugs 1995; 49(1):83–102.

Butterworth RF. Pathogenesis and treatment of portal-systemic encephalopathy: An update. Dig Dis Sci 1992;37:321

Chung RT, Jaffe DL, Friedman LS. Complications of

chronic liver disease. Crit Care Clin 1995;11(2): 431–463.

Mousseau DA, Butterworth RF. Current theories on the pathogenesis of hepatic encephalopathy. Proc Soc Exp Biol Med 1994;206(4):329–344.

DIARRHEA AND FEVER

Jamie A. Selingo

Data Several days after returning from a trip to Cancun, Mexico, a 36-year-old woman began passing five to six large volume, liquid, brown stools daily. Her bowel habits had previously always been regular—one formed movement daily. None of the friends who traveled with her developed similar symptoms. The diarrhea continued off and on for 6 months, during which time she saw several physicians who prescribed medication for a "nervous colon" that gave no permanent relief. Occasionally the diarrhea was accompanied by diffuse crampy abdominal pain, and more recently she had documented fevers to 101°F.

Logic Traveler's diarrhea often affects U.S. residents who visit Mexico within the first week of travel; the diarrhea can occur during the visit or after returning home. The illness may begin abruptly with cramps and diarrhea. Accompanying symptoms such as fatigue, nausea, anorexia, headache, arthralgias, and fever are common.

Bacterial pathogens account for at least 80% of cases, thus accounting for the efficacy of preventive antibacterial medications. *Escherichia coli* is the most common causative agent of traveler's diarrhea throughout the world, although *Campylobacter jejuni, Shigella, Aeromonas, Salmonella, Entamoeba histolytica,* and *Rotavirus* are important causes, too.

Although the association of this patient's travel history with the onset of diarrhea is compelling, it should be remembered that traveler's diarrhea is usually short-lived, with symptoms lasting fewer than 3 days in 90% of patients. Infection with *Shigella* and *Salmonella* and amebiasis may cause symptoms for several months. At times their symptoms may be so severe as to resemble inflammatory bowel disease (IBD)—ulcerative colitis or Crohn's disease. Because none of her companions got sick, and because symptoms have lasted for 6 months, other possible causes of diarrhea and fever need to be explored.

Data The patient states that the diarrhea appears to be worse in the morning. Avoiding lactose in the diet has not altered the stool pattern, nor has fasting. The stools are without an unusual color and are not greasy. The fevers are intermittent and sometimes accompanied by chills. Over the past 6 months she has noted increasing fatigue, mild anorexia, and a 10-pound weight loss. She has not had any of the following: cough, shortness of breath, dysuria, rash, eructations, easy satiety, nausea, vomiting, postprandial bloating, right upper quadrant pain, tenesmus, hematochezia, or mucus in the stool.

The only medication she takes is an oral contraceptive. She lives with her boyfriend, and they have been monogamous for 3 years. She has not been married, has no children, denies alcohol or drug use, and drinks only a glass of wine with dinner. A maternal uncle and cousin have been diagnosed as having "colitis."

Logic The addition of fever, weight loss, and fatigue to the clinical picture points in the direction of a few chronic intestinal infections (amebiasis, salmonellosis) as well as toward the possibility of IBD. You must be sure to ask about related extraintestinal manifestations of IBD in the eyes, mouth, joints, and skin—such as aphthous ulcers, iritis, migratory arthritis, and rashes (pyoderma gangrenosum or erythema multiforme). Although unlikely in a young patient, malignancies, including lymphoma and endocrine neoplasias—carcinoid, vasoactive peptide-secreting pancreatic adenomas, and gastrinoma—are rare and unusual possible causes for chronic diarrhea.

Data Other than for mild diffuse arthralgias, further questioning reveals no evidence of any extraintestinal manifestation of IBD.

On examination, she is a thin, pale woman who appears chronically ill but is in no acute distress. The vital signs are: BP, 120/80; pulse, 90; respirations, 20; temperature, 100.6°F; and weight, 99 lb. Her conjunctiva and nail beds are pale, and small, mobile, nontender lymph nodes are palpable in the neck. Bowel sounds are somewhat hyperactive, and the abdomen is soft, with mild tenderness to deep palpation in both lower quadrants.

The liver and spleen are not palpable, and there are no abdominal masses, joint effusions, or rashes. Digital rectal examination reveals brown stool that tests positive for occult blood; no anal fissures or perineal fistulae were evident.

Logic Physical examination suggests a chronic illness, probable anemia, and gastrointestinal blood loss. The differential diagnosis has not changed; it includes chronic infectious diarrhea, IBD, and much less likely, a malignancy.

Data A CBC shows hematocrit 28%; 2500 WBC/mm³, 69% neutrophils, 10% lymphocytes, 18% monocytes, 2% eosinophils, 1% basophils, and normal platelets. Biochemistry profile is entirely normal. Three stool specimens for ova and parasites test negative; stool culture tests negative for pathogens. *Clostridium difficile* toxin is not detected in a stool specimen, and the serum *E. histolytica* titer is normal.

Logic Although it may be difficult to diagnose chronic bowel infections merely with stool specimens, the negative results of various studies in this case do not support an infectious etiology for the diarrhea and fever. The unexpected leukopenia with a low lymphocyte count raises the specter of HIV-related diarrhea—the most frequent gastrointestinal complaint in patients who have AIDS. The onset of diarrhea in such patients is a harbinger of deteriorating immune function, and it is sometimes the initial clinical manifestation. Depending on the methods used to isolate the opportunistic organism, the offender is identified in more than half the cases.

Data The patient appears quite frightened when confronted with the possible implications of her low white blood cell count. She again denies intravenous drug use and relates that she has had six sexual partners in her lifetime. She and her current partner have engaged in unprotected vaginal intercourse for years. He has no known risk factors for acquiring AIDS and appears healthy. Neither the patient nor her partner has ever been tested for antibody to HIV-1. Despite strong urging, she refuses testing at the current time.

Logic Although there is strong suspicion of HIV-related disease, it cannot be confirmed. To exclude or confirm IBD, colonoscopy is the next logical step in a patient with chronic diarrhea, abdominal pain, fever, and anemia.

Data A colonoscope is advanced to the terminal ileum. Mucosal changes are noted from the rectum to the splenic flexure and again in the cecum. The findings include edema, erythema, friability, granularity, a mucopurulent exudate, and aphthoid erosions. The intervening colon and terminal ileum are normal. Biopsies from the involved areas show cryptitis and microabscess formation. No granulomas are seen, but there are occasional eosinophils within the lamina propria. Viral cultures for cytomegalovirus have negative findings. Stool for acid-fast staining tests negative for mycobacteria and *Cryptosporidium*.

Logic These endoscopic and pathologic findings are consistent with IBD. Because of the discontinuous involvement and aphthoid erosions, Crohn's colitis is considered more likely than ulcerative colitis. Granulomas seen in the biopsies would be strongly suggestive of Crohn's disease, although their absence does not exclude this diagnosis. Infectious colitis is still a possibility, but no offending pathogens have as yet been identified. It seems reasonable to treat the patient for Crohn's disease.

Initial anti-inflammatory treatment for Crohn's colitis typically includes oral aminosalicylates and/or corticosteroids. For patients who have inflammatory bowel disease restricted to the left colon, enemas may be used to administer these medications locally, while sparing systemic adverse effects.

Data After a negative PPD test result is documented, the patient is started on oral prednisone 40 mg/d, sulfasalazine 500 mg po qid, and a low-residue diet. Over the next several weeks, her appetite improves, and her fevers abate. The diarrhea, however, is unchanged. The complete blood count remains essentially unchanged.

Logic The patient has not improved on standard initial therapy for Crohn's colitis. Although this might reflect refractory disease, in light of the leukopenia, this lack of response again raises suspicion about HIV-1-related infections. In particular, infection with cytomegalovirus can closely mimic the clinical presentation of IBD, even producing perineal disease, fistulae, and bowel perforations. Infection with CMV can be very difficult to diagnose, and usually relies on blood cultures, documentation of virally mediated cytopathic effect on tissue specimens, and more recently, analysis of serum by polymerase chain reaction for viremia. You must convince her of the need for further tests.

Data The serum HIV-1 antibody test finding is positive; the CD4 count is 120/mm³ (normal, 550 to 1190/mm³). The patient now relates that a man with whom she had frequent unprotected vaginal intercourse 4 years ago had recently died of complications related to AIDS. The patient is counseled regarding the need for safe sexual practices and testing of her current sexual partner. She is started on anti-retroviral therapy and prophylaxis against infection by *Pneumocystis carinii*.

Regarding her "colitis," although blood cultures are negative for CMV, a repeat rectal biopsy demonstrates inclusion bodies consistent with this infection (Fig. 16.13). The azulfidine is discontinued, and the prednisone is tapered off. Specific antiviral therapy improves her symptoms to the point where she remains afebrile and passes one to two soft bowel movements daily.

The numerous possible causes of diarrhea in patients with AIDS are outlined in Table 16.14. **Logic** One wonders whether the search for HIV should have been more diligent before steroids were started. The leukopenia is distinctly atypical for patients with IBD. The use of corticosteroids

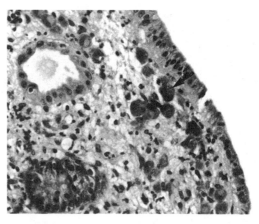

▶ **Figure 16.13.** Biopsy of rectal mucosa. Inclusion bodies (arrow) are consistent with cytomegalovirus infection.

TABLE 16.14 Differential Diagnosis of Diarrhea in AIDS

Protozoal Infections	Bacterial Infections
Cryptosporidium[a]	*Salmonella*[a]
Isospora belli[a]	*Shigella, Campylobacter*[a]
Microsporidia[a]	*Mycobacterium avium—intracellulare*[a]
Giardia lamblia	*Mycobacterium tuberculosis*
Entamoeba histolytica	Small bowel overgrowth
Leishmania donovani	**Fungal Infections**
Blastocystis hominis	Histoplasmosis
Viral Infections	Coccidioidomycosis
Cytomegalovirus[a]	**Idiopathic**
Herpes simplex	'AIDS enteropathy'
Adenovirus	
HIV?	
Gut Neoplasms	
Lymphoma	
Kaposi's sarcoma	
Pancreatic Insufficiency	
Infectious pancreatitis (CMV, MAI)	
Drug-induced pancreatitis (pentamidine)	
Tumor invasion (lymphoma, Kaposi's sarcoma)	

[a]More frequent.
AIDS = acquired immunodeficiency syndrome; HIV = human immunodeficiency virus; CMV = cytomegalovirus.

in patients with HIV disease increases the risk for the development of opportunistic infections.

Detection of the HIV antibody by enzyme-linked immunosorbent assay (ELISA) is currently the most widely used screening test for HIV infection. The sensitivity and specificity of this assay is approximately 99%, but false-positive results do occur, especially in low-risk populations. A positive test by ELISA is typically confirmed by a Western blot assay.

Final problem list:

1. AIDS
2. AIDS colitis
3. Opportunistic cytomegalovirus infection

COMMENT One- or two-day episodes of diarrhea and cramps are among the two or three most common disorders of humankind. They do not prompt visits to the doctor's office. Those episodes that extend beyond a week are cause for concern, especially if accompanied by fever and other symptoms. This prompted the construction of a long differential list, each member of which had to be eliminated by the absence of clinical features, mainly in the history and physical examination, but also as a result of laboratory tests.

HIV-associated enteropathy, as well as HIV-related diseases in other organ systems, is a diagnosis of exclusion that can be made only after other forms of usually treatable diarrheal disease have been excluded—and the test results for HIV are positive.

Another important lesson! The place where a person gets sick may not necessarily be related to the cause of the illness. *(P.C.)*

Suggested Readings

Barlett JG, Belitsos PC. AIDS enteropathy. Clin Infect Dis 1992;15:726.

DuPont HL, Ericsson CD. Prevention and treatment of traveler's diarrhea. New Engl J Med 1993;328:1821–1827.

Gazzard BG. Diarrhea in human immunodeficiency virus antibody-positive patients. Semin Liver Dis 1992;12:154.

Simon D, Brandt LJ. Diarrhea in patients with the acquired immunodeficiency syndrome. Gastroenterol 1993;105:1238.

Renal and Electrolyte Problems
A: Renal Problems

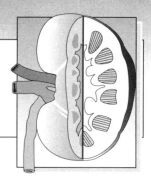

"What is the kidney but an infinitely artful device for turning the sweet wines of Shiraz into urine?" It is natural that the filtrate of such a process should reflect so much of what goes on in the kidney itself. Not surprisingly, urinalysis often delivers the key clue in a patient who has kidney disease. The presence of white blood cell (WBC) casts, red blood cell (RBC) casts, doubly refractile fat bodies, coarse granular casts, or bacteria tells us much of what is wrong. Significant bacteriuria denotes infection; WBC casts tell us that the infection is in the tubule where casts are forming; and RBC casts indicate that the RBCs that originate in the glomerulus are incorporated into casts that are forming in the tubule. Whether or not all the wine is being turned into urine is measured by the blood urea nitrogen (BUN) or serum creatinine level—determinants of kidney function.

These simple laboratory examinations are essential in kidney disease and give much valuable information. Other than in the patient who has chronic uremia, or in the patient who has large palpable kidneys, the physical examination rarely offers key clues. The history, however, is another story. A few symptoms may put us directly on the diagnostic trail.

Bloody urine often augurs serious disease, but it does not locate or denote the pathologic process. Colicky pain usually indicates ureteral obstruction by a stone. Frequency and burning on urination suggest infection somewhere in the lower urinary tract. A downhill course including nausea, weight loss, anorexia, and gastrointestinal and neurologic symptoms may indicate chronic renal failure, although other nonrenal diagnostic possibilities exist. Acute renal failure has no characteristic symptoms except perhaps for nausea, vomiting, and lack of urine formation; but this cluster usually occurs in the course of a disease whose severe nature (shock,

sepsis) may obscure its renal effects. A progressively downhill course suggests cancer, too; the kidney and prostate are frequent primary sites, and additional symptoms need not be present. Other common presentations of patients with renal disease are: peripheral edema in the nephrotic syndrome; flank pain and fever in acute pyelonephritis; and albuminuria found on routine examination.

Frequently a patient is not aware of kidney disease until renal failure, hypertension, and their complications occur—visual defects, stroke, heart failure, coronary thrombosis, or electrolyte disturbances.

Prostatic hypertrophy, prostatic cancer, and bladder cancer, although not kidney diseases, are mentioned in this chapter because they are so prevalent and often cause urinary tract symptoms similar to some of the renal disease presentations just described.

As has been noted for other disease systems, there are very many kidney diseases, but only a handful of commonly seen diseases. These include urinary tract infection, calculi, obstructive uropathy, acute and chronic renal failure, neoplasms, and the nephrotic syndrome. Know these, and you know a substantial core.

It is important to note that kidney disease is often found coincidentally in the course of work-up for another illness, or may exist as part of a generalized disease. The patient who has marginally compensated renal function may decompensate under the stress of pneumonia or congestive heart failure. Sometimes abnormal urinalysis results or an elevated blood urea nitrogen level is found during a routine insurance, military, or employment-related examination. Then, too, there are a large number of multisystem diseases that also affect the kidneys—myeloma, systemic lupus erythematosus, infective endocarditis, diabetes mellitus (DM), and hepatic failure.

As for diagnostic clues derived from further studies, the past three decades have seen a host of new and valuable invasive and noninvasive techniques evolve for diagnosing kidney disease, as well as for other organ systems. This armamentarium includes ultrasound, computed tomography (CT), magnetic resonance imaging and angiography, digital subtraction, arteriography, and biopsy. The exact role of each and the benefits of one over the other remain for current and future research to delineate as we aim for specificity, sensitivity, economy, and safety.

The matter of bilateral renal vein thrombosis and the nephrotic syndrome (Which comes first?) has not been clarified in the past few years. Their frequent coexistence seems to be more than coincidence. Doubt no longer exists about the relationship of analgesic abuse to chronic tubulo-interstitial nephritis and subsequent papillary necrosis; the villains are phenacetin (no longer available) and possibly acetaminophen.

The common use of dialysis and renal transplantation, perhaps more than anything else, has added understanding to the pathophysiology of renal failure and has advanced and broadened the field of nephrology. These therapeutic modalities have been springboards for quantum leaps into many other fields—organ transplantation, immunology, and, unfortunately, infectious disease. By creating a large population of immunocompromised hosts, we have unwillingly given birth to numerous nosocomial infections. There is an ever-escalating conflict between new drugs and "funny bugs," and between new-generation antibiotics and transformed microorganisms. Patients on dialysis and those with surrogate kidneys are good subjects for the investigation and demonstration of altered hormonal, electrolyte, and mineral disturbances, as well as drug-chemical interactions. A *textbook* of new problems exists in this subset of patients. (P.C.)

BLOODY URINE

Meyer D. Lifschitz

Data A 57-year-old man's urine has been intermittently red over the past few weeks. He has had no flank pain, abdominal pain, or pain referred to the groin or testis. But he has had a narrowed stream, increasing hesitancy, worsening urgency and frequency of urination, and nocturia two to three times nightly for the previous 6 months.

Logic Red urine usually means blood in the urine—hematuria. But red urine cannot be absolutely equated with blood nor does blood always make the urine red. Hemoglobin (excessive hemolysis), myoglobin (acute muscle necrosis), porphyrins, laxatives containing danthron or phenolphthalein, foods like red cabbage or beets, and drugs like rifampin and phenazopyridine hydrochloride can also make the urine red.

On the other hand, some of the aforementioned conditions can make the urine smoky gray, dark brown, or even orange. "Cola-colored" urine usually refers to bilirubin. Blood may become dark gray or brown as the hemoglobin becomes oxidized.

Note too that the patient has symptoms that suggest lower urinary tract obstruction. Benign prostatic hypertrophy (BPH), stricture, bladder neck obstruction, and cancer of the prostate are all possible. The red urine and the obstructive symptoms could be causally related. Because you want to know what the chief complaint signifies, a urinalysis is done first.

Data A freshly voided urine specimen is diffusely pink and cloudy and shows innumerable RBCs and a trace of albumin. The last portion of the voiding was just as pink as the first. The specific gravity is 1.024, pH 6, and there is no glucose. Careful microscopic examination finds one white blood cell and a few hyaline casts per high-powered field. No bacteria, crystals, or abnormal casts are seen.

Logic Much information is immediately available. The patient indeed has hematuria. The absence of much protein and RBC casts tends to rule out the glomerulus as the source of the RBCs. Lack of crystals make a stone less likely but does not rule it out; crystals can appear in showers. Infection is rendered unlikely by the absence of WBCs, WBC casts, and bacteria. A urine culture is not deemed necessary. The high specific gravity implies reasonably good kidney function.

Gross or microscopic hematuria must always be investigated except in women with symptoms of obvious severe cystitis. Always make sure the blood is not vaginal in origin.

If considerable albumin and especially RBC casts are present in the urine too, the source of bleeding lies in the nephron, and a medical kidney disease is present. Depending on the patient's age and history, the cause may be analgesic nephropathy, immunoglobulin A nephropathy, acute post-streptococcal glomerulonephritis, membranoproliferative glomerulonephritis, Henoch-Schönlein purpura, or other immune complex glomerulopathies. If such were the case, a renal biopsy might be needed because treatment differs for the various types.

Had no RBCs been found, either the patient had temporarily stopped bleeding (a common occurrence) or the discoloration was due to a cause other than hematuria. A further search would have been indicated. Note that there is no hurry to investigate hematuria. It takes very little blood to make the urine red. Exsanguination via the urinary tract is virtually impossible.

Data There have been no previous episodes of hematuria or history of stone disease. The patient has felt well, the systems review and medical history are negative, and the family history is negative for kidney disease. He does not ingest large quantities of milk or alkali, takes no vitamin supplements, and has no gastrointestinal symptoms or known bone diseases.

Logic The causes of hematuria are many and can be listed in anatomic sequence from the kidney down to the urethra. By and large, we are dealing mainly with *cancer, stone,* or *infection.* Starting with the kidney, there can be trauma, tumor, stone, polycystic disease, tuberculosis, infarct, pyelonephritis, or glomerulonephritis. Trauma is evident by history, stones are painful, and an infarct must postulate a source; the latter two can be ruled out by the absence of associated symptoms. The history gives no evidence for any of the causes of hypercalcemia and stones (milk–alkali syndrome, excessive vitamin D, and so forth).

Proceeding downward, there may be carcinoma or a stone in the ureter. The bladder may be affected by cancer, stone, or inflammation. Cancer is often asymptomatic, stone is usually painful if it is too large to pass, and inflammation is apparent if associated acute severe frequency, urgency, burning, and dysuria exist.

The prostate and urethra can be the source of hematuria too. BPH causes bleeding from venous distortions and varices, and prostatic cancer causes it by direct bladder wall invasion. Urethral malignancies are uncommon but do bleed too.

Do not forget the hemorrhagic disorders (overanticoagulation and thrombocytopenia) that may be manifested by hematuria or may unmask underlying silent neoplasms. Geography, sex, and age influence our logic. If the patient lives in Egypt, the most common cause of hematuria is schistosomiasis of the bladder (Egyptian hematuria). Bladder stones are very common across North Africa and central Asia. Men everywhere are prone to prostate problems, whereas women have a much higher incidence of hemorrhagic cystitis. Children are afflicted with acute glomerulonephritis, but cancer is more common in adults.

Many of the aforementioned diagnostic possibilities have already been ruled out. The most serious problem is still to be considered. Cancer (bladder or kidney) accounts for 25% of patients with hematuria. Stones account for almost 25%, too, but the absence of any type of pain, crystals, and an underlying cause refutes this possibility.

Another clue can help localize the source. If only the first portion of the urine sample is bloody, the bleeding is urethral. If the urine is diffusely bloody, the source is from the vesical neck up. Large clots or drops of blood at the end of urination suggest bleeding from the bladder. Wormy clots indicate bleeding from the ureter above the bladder.

Data Physical examination reveals a well-developed slim man who is in no acute distress and does not look sick. Two abnormalities are noted. The lower abdomen is full and tenderness, dullness, and urgency are noted on percussion. Rectal examination discloses a 3+ enlarged smooth, firm, nontender prostate; it contains no hard nodules. The stool is guaiac negative. There are no masses in the abdomen, no band keratopathy, and no tenderness over the kidneys.

Logic Absence of band keratopathy weighs against prolonged severe hypercalcemia. Kidney cancer is not ruled out by the absence of palpable masses; kidneys themselves are rarely palpable and a mass would have to be quite large and in the lower pole to be felt. He does seem to have an enlarged prostate that is causing obstructive symptoms and urinary retention. Its effect on kidney function must be determined. Examination of the prostate gland is vital in cases such as this.

Data Laboratory tests show a normal blood count. The urinalysis is repeated and the findings are the same as before. An 18-test blood chemistry profile is completely normal except for BUN, 50 mg/dL; creatinine, 1.8 mg/dL; and calcium, 11.1 mg/dL. The latter three are repeated and found to be correct. Alkaline and acid phosphatase and prostatic specific antigen are normal.

Logic Cancer of the kidney (hypernephroma) can secrete a parathormone-like substance that elevates the calcium level, as well as erythropoietin, which causes polycythemia. Hypercalcemia is present; polycythemia is not. The absence of band keratopathy suggests that the modest hypercalcemia is not longstanding. Renal malfunction with a disproportionately elevated BUN level suggests pre- or postrenal azotemia. Prerenal azotemia is not likely because the physical examination findings are normal, and there is no evidence for gastrointestinal bleeding (stool negative). The large prostate and bladder suggest that the azotemia is most likely the result of prostatic obstruction. A normal acid phosphatase and prostatic specific antigen are against prostatic cancer.

Data The chest radiograph, abdominal radiograph and electrocardiogram (ECG) are normal except for apparent bladder distention. In particular, no metastatic lesions are noted in the lung (a favorite site for hypernephroma), the renal contours are not well visualized, and the ECG shows no evidence of hypercalcemia.

Logic So far, we have eliminated many possibilities but have not pinpointed the cause for the hematuria. Further studies are needed. First do an intravenous pyelogram (IVP), but only after determining lack of allergy to iodine and to any previously done IVP. The mild azotemia does not preclude doing an IVP because intrinsic renal disease and dysfunction are considered unlikely.

Data An IVP was performed the next day. It demonstrated a normally functioning left kidney. The right kidney was somewhat enlarged, and the upper pole, which was functioning poorly, appeared to have a distorted, thinned-out calyx and protruded beyond the rest of the renal contour. Both ureters visualized adequately and the ureters and collecting systems were moderately dilated. The bladder was enlarged, and there was a postvoid residual volume of 200 to 300 mL. Intrusion of a large prostate into the bladder base was visible. No stones were seen in this study.

Logic A right upper pole carcinoma is strongly suspected; 90% of stones are radiopaque, so this entity is virtually ruled out. The bilateral hydroureter, mild hydronephroses, and large residual volume are diagnostic of bladder outlet obstruction and are most likely due to the patient's enlarged prostate. Diminishing renal function no doubt results from the obstruction. The small loss of functioning renal tissue in the right upper pole could not possibly account for the elevated BUN level. Prompt relief of the obstruction with an indwelling catheter is indicated.

Data After the insertion of a Foley catheter, 3000 mL of urine were excreted in the first 24 hours. Three days later, the BUN and creatinine levels approached normal. Obstructive symptoms vanished.

Logic Were this the only problem, a prostatectomy would have been done. But the right upper pole lesion is the critical situation and must be diagnosed before prostate surgery is attempted.

The lesion in the upper pole is either a benign cyst or a malignant tumor and a distinction must be made by an ultrasound study or a computed tomographic (CT) scan. Both give essentially the same information, but the former is less costly, less invasive, easier to do, and may have greater capacity for making the crucial differentiation between cyst and tumor.

Data The next day an ultrasound study showed a lesion with irregular echogenicity, which suggested a solid rather than a cystic lesion (Fig. 17.1). On the following day, a renal arteriogram was performed via the right femoral artery. This revealed a highly vascular tumor in the upper pole of the right kidney, a typical tumor blush and abnormal vessels, but no aberrant or anomalous arteries. Radiographs taken in the late venous filling phase showed no evidence of tumor infiltrating the renal vein.

Logic The diagnosis is now reasonably certain. The IVP distortion was not caused by a cyst. The patient has a carcinoma of the right kidney (hypernephroma), and there is no evidence of spread beyond the kidney. It is probably resectable and surgery is indicated. Careful attention must be given to adequate hydration so that the hypercalcemia gives no problems while it lasts. A catheter may be needed for a brief time to main-

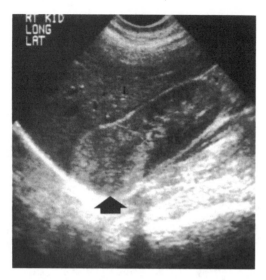

▶ **Figure 17.1.** Renal cell carcinoma. Ultrasound image in the long axis of the right kidney (RK) reveals a solid mildly hyperechoic mass (arrow) at the upper pole. L = liver.

tain normal renal function. Prostatectomy will be done at a future date if the kidney lesion is resectable, and there are no evident metastases.

If the initial ultrasound study had shown a *purely cystic* lesion, you might then have performed a guided needle aspiration with cytologic study, or perhaps done nothing referable to the cyst. Had the renal lesion been only partially cystic, aspiration first, followed by surgery if the fluid were bloody or contained neoplastic cells, would be the route for some, direct surgery for others.

Most physicians obtain a renal arteriogram before surgery in order to (a) define the renal vascular anatomy, (b) determine renal vein invasion, and (c) confirm the diagnosis.

Consider another scenario in this patient. The IVP is normal or shows a lesion that proves to be a benign cyst. In these circumstances you must hunt further for a hematuria-causing lesion. Cystoscopy is indicated. This procedure will detect a bladder neoplasm and note the degree of prostatic hypertrophy. In older people the search may end at this point even if nothing is found. If blood is seen coming from a ureteral orifice, retrograde pyelography may be done to find a rare ureteral tumor. Prostatic hypertrophy as a cause for hematuria is a diagnosis made by exclusion; renal and bladder cancer *must* be ruled out. In

younger persons arteriography may detect an arteriovenous malformation.

If there is a suspicion of coexisting prostatic cancer, as in this case, it may be diagnosed by newer more sensitive techniques for measuring the prostate specific antigen and the acid phosphatase, isotope bone scans for metastases, and aspiration biopsy. But because this patient will shortly need prostatic surgery too, further studies were deferred until then.

You might justifiably debate the necessity for all the diagnostic procedures done for this patient. Before recent years, the IVP was enough; but this resulted in the removal of too many benign cysts and normal kidneys. Here, the IVP and sonogram were probably sufficient. But if the IVP and sonogram were equivocal, nobody would argue against doing a CT scan, a needle aspiration, and/or an arteriogram. Where the diagnosis of tumor is reasonably certain, many would question the need for a risky invasive arteriogram to guide the surgeon, and the need for a sometimes-performed inferior vena cavagram to detect direct tumor invasion.

In a child with hematuria, suspect infection, immune-complex glomerulonephritis, sickle cell anemia, Wilms' tumor, or a congenital anomaly. This differential necessitates a careful urinalysis, urine culture, hemoglobin electrophoresis, an IVP, and a voiding cystourethrogram.

Questions

1. If this patient had shown a normal IVP, the next diagnostic maneuver would have been cystoscopy. Given the same clinical picture, what would have been the most likely finding?
   (a) Cancer of the bladder
   (b) Hemorrhagic cystitis
   (c) Bladder stone
   (d) Cancer of the urethra
2. In a patient with obstructive uropathy, all of the following would be expected except?
   (a) BUN-to-creatinine ratio greater than 20
   (b) No urine production for 24 hours
   (c) Urine osmolality equal to plasma osmolality
   (d) Urine pH 6.0
3. A 56-year-old man has 5 to 10 RBCs per high-powered

field in his urine on a routine insurance examination. Otherwise nothing abnormal was found. Which statement is correct?

   (a) It is only mild microscopic hematuria and can be ignored.

   (b) Even though mild, it should be rechecked in a month.

   (c) If no albumin or RBC casts are noted, it is not significant.

   (d) It should be immediately investigated.

4. Hypernephromas are slow-growing, retroperitoneal, and rarely present as masses in the abdomen. However, they can present in a variety of ways other than hematuria. These include all but which one of the following?

   (a) Fever of unknown origin

   (b) Pulmonary embolus

   (c) Bilateral leg edema

   (d) Pathologic fracture of the femur

5. Draw an algorithm that starts with gross hematuria; uses three diagnostic procedures (IVP, CT scan, and cystoscopy); and has four possible endpoints ([1] renal cancer, [2] renal cysts, [3] bladder cancer, and [4] no diagnosis).

Answers

1. **(a) is correct.** Cancer of the bladder is the most likely of the four. It usually gives no symptoms—just bleeding. Cystitis, on the other hand, whether caused by infection or drugs (cyclophosphamide), is associated with severe symptoms, which are not present in this patient. Bladder stones cause bleeding, but an IVP would have detected this. In cancer of the urethra, blood would have been primarily in the initially voided portion of the specimen; the urine would not have been uniformly pink.

2. **(b) is correct.** Obstructive uropathy can be present for months to years and renal function may deteriorate, yet urine formation continues. A ratio of BUN to creatinine greater than 20 is common in obstructive uropathy, presumably because of decreased tubular fluid flow rate that leads to increased urea resorption, and thus a higher BUN. A defect in renal concentrating ability and an inability to maximally acidify urine are common in obstructive uropathy, so that (c) and (d) result.

3. **(d) is correct.** Microscopic hematuria can have the same serious causes as gross hematuria. The presence of 5 to 10 RBCs, confirmed by immediate recheck, is definitely abnormal. Choices (a) and (b) are therefore obviously wrong courses to follow. The absence of albu-

min and RBC casts tends to rule out a glomerular source of the blood, but by no means rules out other serious diseases like cancer.

4. **(d) is correct.** Hypernephromas do not metastasize like other tumors. They do not spread to long bones, so a pathologic fracture of the femur would be quite uncommon. However, they do grow into the renal vein and up the vena cava; tumor emboli to the lungs or partial vena cava obstruction with bilateral leg edema can result. Because the tumor often contains necrotic tissue, fever of unknown origin may be a mode of presentation. Remember that polycythemia and hypercalcemia detected on a routine blood screen can also be initial presentations. These result from the production of hormone-like materials—erythropoietin-like substance and parathyroid hormone-like substance (or even 1,25-dihydroxycholecalciferol, which is the active form of vitamin D).

5. First, perform an IVP. If mass is revealed, perform a CT scan; this distinguishes between cyst and tumor. If no renal mass is found, perform cystoscopy; this results in bladder cancer or no diagnosis.

COMMENT After a careful consideration of the distinction between red urine and bloody urine, hematuria was established as the key clue and a list of diagnostic possibilities was formed. A urinalysis was the initially obtained portion of the data base—not the usual order.

Numerous possibilities were ruled out with pertinent negative clues. Bayes' probability theory was properly respected because only common possibilities were seriously considered; geography, age, and sex created various subsets of population in whom the probabilities differed. The presence of two genitourinary diseases, each of which can cause hematuria, established another Boolean overlap. Although both BPH and cancer of the kidney can cause bloody urine, there were other features present that related to only one or the other (renal mass, urea retention, urine retention). Indeed, the cause for the hematuria was never clearly attributed to one or the other condition, but treatment for cancer took precedence.

A dendrogram approach to the solution would have been simple. Answer a series of questions: (1) Is it blood? (2) Is there any pain? (3) Are there symptoms of infection? (4) Is the prostate or bladder enlarged? (5) Is a renal mass palpable? And so forth. *(P.C.)*

PROBLEM-BASED LEARNING   You have just learned a few things about a patient with hematuria. In order to have a well-rounded knowledge of the subject, you should read and know all about:

- The causes of hematuria
- What else may make the urine red
- The concomitant urine abnormalities that guide you
- The significance of microscopic vs. gross hematuria
- Hemorrhagic cystitis
- Carcinoma of the kidney, its pathologic types, varied clinical presentations, the role of excessive "erythropoietin," and the use of the IVP, CT, MRI, MRA, ultrasound, and arteriography in defining the lesion
- How to distinguish renal cancer from renal cyst
- Polycystic kidneys
- How hematologic disorders cause hematuria
- Benign prostatic hypertrophy and carcinoma of the prostate, their clinical pictures, how each may cause hematuria, the value of the acid and alkaline phosphatase and prostatic specific antigen tests and of ultrasound
- The role of aspiration for renal cysts and biopsy for prostatic cancer
- How kidney stones may cause hematuria, yet no pain
- Obstructive uropathy
- Carcinoma of the bladder and the role of cystoscopy and ultrasound in its diagnosis

Learn this, and you have added another 5% to your medical information base.

Suggested Readings

Curry NS. Small renal masses (lesions smaller than 3 cm): Imaging evaluation and management. Am J Roentgenol 1995;164(2):355–362.

Levine E. Renal cell carcinoma: Cinical aspects, imaging diagnosis, and staging. Sem Roentgenol 1995; 30(2):128–148.

Novick AC. Management of the incidentally detected solid renal mass. Sem Nephrol 1994;14(6):510–522.

FREQUENT AND PAINFUL URINATION

Marvin Forland

Data   A 23-year-old woman sees you because of frequent and painful urination for 2 days. This had never happened before her marriage 6 months ago, but since then she has had four similar episodes. She has the impression they are related to sexual intercourse, although she cannot be sure. Fever, chills, gross hematuria, or back pain are never present. Twice she was treated with 1-week courses of nitrofurantoin and promptly got better. On the other occasions she got well without treatment.

There is a 19-year history of juvenile-onset diabetes mellitus (DM) that has been regulated with NPH insulin before breakfast and dinner. Blood sugars are checked approximately twice daily and approach normal range. She has been remarkably free of problems and symptoms related to her diabetes.

Logic   The history is typical of recurrent lower urinary tract infections—urethritis-cystitis.

Among the most common problems seen in primary care are urinary tract infections. They occur in infants, children, men, and women; but the spectra of causes differ. It is notable that after age 60, 5 to 15% of men and women experience such infections.

The patient's diabetes seems well controlled according to blood tests and lack of polyuria and thirst. However, there are a number of factors that require more careful evaluation before merely instituting another brief course of antibacterial therapy.

First, the organism causing these infections has never been identified. When bacteria are found, 95% are gram-negative bacilli (mostly *Es-*

cherichia coli, some *Aerobacter-Klebsiella*); the remainder consists of gram-positive cocci, *Proteus, Pseudomonas,* and fungi. This may be related to the anal-urethral-bladder route of bacterial spread. Specific local infections around the genitalia can also cause dysuria and frequency. These include gonorrhea, herpes progenitalis, *Monilia,* and *Trichomonas vaginalis*. The gold standard of growth of ≥ 100,000 colonies of a urinary pathogen per milliliter of urine to establish urinary infection has been modified for symptomatic patients. The predictive value of the criterion of ≥ 100 per milliliter of coliform organisms is high and considered to provide optimal sensitivity and specificity for clinical decision making. When similar symptoms occur in the absence of bacterial growth, considerations include infection with an organism not isolated on routine culture preparations, such as *Chlamydia trachomatis,* or a functional disorder of the bladder.

Second, these episodes have recurred over a brief period of time. They may be marriage related, and may be of benign origin. However, recurrent urinary tract infection (UTI) under any circumstances is an indication for careful evaluation. You must look for congenital, anatomic, functional, or obstructive factors that can be the predisposing cause for infection. Obstruction to urine flow is a principal concern and it may be either functional or anatomic. Such abnormalities can exist at any level of the collecting system from the urethral meatus to the renal pelvis.

Here, sex and age are important clues. Youngsters with UTIs frequently have structural abnormalities and congenital defects such as ureterovesical reflux, bladder neck obstruction, ureteropelvic obstruction, horseshoe kidney, and so forth. These predispose to infection. For, as in other systems of the body, obstruction often leads to infection.

A 28-year-old sexually promiscuous man may have gonorrhea with a urethral stricture. Young and middle-aged men develop acute prostatitis with a typical picture of severe urinary symptoms, fever, and marked prostatic tenderness. They also commonly have chronic prostatitis, which is often asymptomatic but causes recurrent episodes of cystitis. Whereas the efficacy of three-day therapy for uncomplicated lower urinary tract infection is well established, her treatment was prolonged because of the concurrent, long-standing diabetes mellitus.

In an older multigravida woman, think of a poorly emptying bladder caused by a large cystocele. And in the 65-year-old man, remember prostatic hypertrophy. It commonly causes retrograde infection.

A third important consideration here is diabetes. Increasing data suggest that UTIs are more frequent in women with DM than in nondiabetic women, with a high prevalence of upper tract involvement in the former. Why this is not so in males remains speculative. But it is well established that serious complications like papillary necrosis and perinephric abscess are more common in DM. Another point to remember is that long-standing DM can cause neurogenic impairment of bladder emptying, thus predisposing to infection.

Data More facts are obtained. The family history, review of systems, and previous medical history give no helpful information. Vital signs are normal, and the patient does not look sick. There are scattered microaneurysms and a few hard yellowish exudates in the fundi. No tenderness is noted over the kidneys or bladder, and Murphy's sign is absent. Other than decreased proprioception in the legs and absent Achilles tendon reflexes, the examination is normal. There is no discharge and the urethral meatus is normal in situation and appearance. A clean-catch midstream urine specimen is collected while the patient is in the lithotomy position.

Logic Several important bits of information are revealed. There is no evidence of a local specific infection such as moniliasis, frequent in poorly controlled diabetes. In addition, the absence of kidney tenderness and fever is important in separating upper UTI from lower UTI. Fever is the most valuable clue in the differentiation of the two. Note that the urine specimen was easily collected without adding the risk of introducing infection by catheterization. The fundi show specific evidence of diabetic retinopathy, and the neurologic abnormalities support the impression of early diabetic neuropathy.

Data Preliminary data are available. The complete blood count is normal. The sterilely collected urine specimen was divided into two aliquots. One was used for immediate study, the second for routine culture and sensitivity. Routine urinalysis shows pH 5.5, protein 2+, glucose trace, 20 to 30 white blood cells with clumps per high-powered field, and one to two hyaline casts with an occasional granular cast per low-powered field. There are no WBC casts. Many bacteria are seen in the unspun specimen. A Gram's stain of a dried smear shows gram-negative rods.

Logic Bacteria and WBCs in an unspun clean-catch specimen confirm a UTI of bacterial origin. The presence of bacteria correlates well with a culture growth of at least 100,000 colonies per milliliter and provides a useful screening method. In fact, more than 10 WBCs per high-powered field of centrifuged urine suggest that infection is present. More than one bacterium/oil-immersion field from a stained unspun specimen is predictive of 100,000 or more colonies/mL of urine and indicates an infectious process. Gram's stain helps identify the organism. Pyuria without bacteriuria might hint at tuberculosis. The proteinuria and casts suggest possible concomitant diabetic glomerulosclerosis in keeping with other evidences of microangiopathy noted. The absence of WBC casts and a normal peripheral WBC count are further evidence against kidney involvement by infection.

Data Pending the results of culture, trimethoprim-sulfamethoxazol is given. The patient returns in 48 hours and the symptoms had cleared. Culture grew more than 100,000 colonies of *E. coli*, sensitive to all agents, but resistant to nitrofurantoin. Repeat urinalysis showed persistent 2+ proteinuria and casts, but a rare WBC and no bacteria. Continuation of trimethoprim-sulfamethoxazol for a full 7-day course is recommended, and the patient is asked to collect a 24-hour urine sample for protein and creatinine. Blood is drawn for an 18-test blood chemistry determination.

Logic Response to treatment was excellent. *E. coli, Pseudomonas* species and *enterococci* are the most common pathogens. Radiograph studies were deferred pending evaluation of renal function. The greater risk of renal function complications associated with intravenous pyelography in diabetics is well known.

Data Further studies return. Serum creatinine is 1.0 mg/dL, and creatinine clearance is 85 mL/minute—both normal. Blood glucose is 128 mg/dL; other blood chemistry tests are normal. When she sees her physician the next week, renal ultrasonography and voiding cystourethrogram are ordered. Both are normal, and there is no residual urine or evidence of obstruction. The radiologist comments that the kidneys look slightly larger than normal for the patient's stature.

Logic Although the patient may well have diabetic nephropathy based on the urine findings and the slightly enlarged kidneys, function is still normal. Radiographic studies rule out anatomic, congenital, and obstructive abnormalities that could be responsible for the recurrent UTIs. Diabetic neuropathy with incomplete bladder emptying is excluded, and there is no evidence of reflux or undiagnosed papillary necrosis.

Data A repeat urine culture is negative, and the urinalysis stays the same. The patient is apprised of her diabetic status and reassured that the infections are not serious. Postcoital voiding and cleansing of the urethral meatus with a mild soap solution are recommended. She is to return promptly if symptoms recur.

Logic You realize that recurrence is common. But you are aware that the diagnosis of UTI is often plagued by silence. Chronic cystitis has a high prevalence, yet may be asymptomatic. Chronic pyelonephritis may silently destroy the kidneys and cause renal failure in the presence of an anatomic abnormality.

On the other hand, acute infections speak out with signs and symptoms. Acute pyelonephritis usually presents a classic picture that subsides in several days. It did so even before the antibiotic era. Yet sometimes this infection may progress to renal abscess, perinephric abscess, necrotizing papillitis, or gram-negative sepsis. These serious and often life-threatening complications may be detected by computed tomographic scan and blood culture.

Should your patient's next infection involve her kidneys too, you must be well aware of such complications because some are more apt to occur if DM is present.

Questions

1. The features most strongly suggesting renal parenchymal involvement in an acute UTI are:
   (a) suprapubic tenderness
   (b) clumps of WBCs in the urine
   (c) fever
   (d) WBC casts

2. Acute pyelonephritis with flank pain, fever, chills, and pyuria can be seen in which of the following clinical settings?
   (a) Colicky pain radiating to testis associated with hematuria
   (b) 6 months of pregnancy
   (c) Cystoscopy with ureteral catheterization for diagnostic purposes
   (d) Previous IVP showed marked hydronephrosis of one kidney

3. Obstruction predisposes to infection. The site of obstruction may determine the clinical picture. Which of the following is untrue?
   (a) Large obstructing prostate glands may cause repeated episodes of cystitis or epididymo-orchitis.
   (b) Obstructing prostate glands can cause bladder hypertrophy, many symptoms, hydronephroses, and renal failure.
   (c) Urethral strictures in younger men, and congenital valves at the vesicourethral junction in male children, can cause the same picture as in (b).
   (d) Bilateral ureteral obstruction can cause silent deteriorating renal function.

Answers

1. **(c) and (d) are correct.** Fever is not seen with simple urethritis-cystitis. It indicates renal and sometimes prostatic involvement. WBC casts tell us the WBCs are in the tubules where casts form. Suprapubic tenderness goes with bladder inflammation. Clumps of WBCs are seen no matter where the UTI is.

2. **All are correct.** Situation (a) suggests a stone obstructing the ureter, and obstruction often leads to infection. Pregnant women are susceptible to kidney infection because pregnancy causes hydroureters and poor drainage. Instrumentation always carries a risk of introducing infection. The previous IVP in (d) suggests the presence of ureteropelvic obstruction by an anomalous renal artery.

3. **No answers are untrue.** This question is designed to demonstrate the various levels and types of obstructive uropathy and how obstruction at each level can cause serious problems. (d) can result from stones, strictures, cervical cancer, and retroperitoneal fibrosis.

COMMENT Diagnosis was no problem here. Diabetes was prominent in the author's thinking,

both from the standpoint of overlapping complications (neuropathy, retinopathy, nephropathy) and because of its relationship to UTIs through a variety of known and unknown mechanisms.

Many complex cause-and-effect relationships were present. For example, diabetes can cause infection in three ways. The first is direct and unknown; the second is via autonomic neuropathy; the third is by the presence of associated moniliasis. Diabetes, sexual intercourse, pregnancy, obstruction, congenital anomaly, poor drainage, and instrumentation can combine in various ways to cause infection.

Sex and age alter the statistical likelihoods of the underlying causes for UTI. So do the presence of other genitourinary diseases and the taking of certain immunity-altering drugs.

Upper and lower UTI were differentiated by a number of clues. Fever and WBC casts are highly specific and sensitive in this regard. That is to say—fever is reliable in distinguishing between upper and lower UTI, but not in distinguishing UTI from infection in another area. However, if both clues are present, then the evidence for an upper UTI becomes overwhelming. *(P.C)*

Suggested Readings

Kunin CM, Van Arsdale White L, et al. A reassessment of the importance of "low-count" bacteriuria in young women with acute urinary symptoms. Ann Intern Med 1993;119:454–460.

Patterson JE, Andriole VT. Bacterial urinary tract infections in diabetes. Infect Dis Clin N Am 1995; 9:25–51.

Stamm WE, Hooton TM. Management of urinary tract infections in adults. N Engl J Med 1993;329: 328–334.

 CASE 57

SHARP FLANK PAIN

Meyer D. Lifschitz

Data Excruciating waves of sharp left-sided abdominal pain radiating to the left groin bring a 38-year-old man to the emergency department. Over the past 10 years, he had three similar episodes and passed three kidney stones; once the pain was on the right side. There is no burning, urgency, or frequency of urination. The diagnosis seems clear, so you inject 75 mg of meperidine hydrochloride, start intravenous fluids, and hospitalize the patient because of persistent and unrelieved pain. He does not know the cause for his stones and never had a work-up. A urinalysis done in the emergency department shows 20 to 30 RBCs per high-powered field and nothing else.

Logic   Treatment takes temporary precedence over the complete study. But already there is evidence that the patient has recurrent stones involving both sides of the urinary tract, so a unilateral obstructive anomaly is unlikely. Also, there are no symptoms to suggest concurrent infection.

Data   The colicky pains subside after several hours. A plain radiograph of the abdomen shows an 8-mm irregular radiopaque calculus lodged in what seems to be the upper third of the left ureter. The patient is instructed to void all urine specimens through a strainer, to save any debris, and to call the nurse if pain recurs. He goes to sleep, but not before blood samples are drawn and another urine specimen is obtained for analysis and culture.

Logic   Now you begin to consider the various causes of stones. Many have a clear-cut pathophysiologic explanation; some do not. It is important to realize that most renal stones are single episodes and do not recur; their cause is unclear and little if any work-up is needed. Concern exists mainly when the stones are recurrent and you suspect an underlying potentially curable or preventable disorder. The etiology and chemical composition of stones are often easily related (Table 17.1).

Triple phosphate stones occur in the presence of chronic urinary tract infection, usually with *Proteus* species, although sometimes with other gram-negative bacilli. This organism is a urea-splitter, creates an alkaline pH, and liberates much NH4+—an ideal situation for the precipitation of such stones.

Uric acid stones occur from hyperuricemia and excessive uric acid excretion due to gout, chemotherapy for malignancies, and myeloproliferative disorders. They also occur when the serum uric acid is normal and the urine pH is persistently low, as in chronic diarrheal states and ileostomies.

Cystine stones result from an inherited disorder, begin to form in early childhood, and exist in other members of the family. Such patients usually die of renal failure at a young age.

TABLE 17.1. Chemical Composition of Renal Stones

COMPOSITION	PERCENTAGE
Calcium oxalate, phosphate, or both	67
Triple phosphate or $MgNH_4$ phosphate	15
Uric acid	8
Cystine	4
Miscellaneous	6

$MgNH_4 =$

TABLE 17.2. Causes of Kidney Stones

Hypercalciuria
Hyperparathyroidism
Hypervitaminosis D
Milk-alkali syndrome
Prolonged immobilization
Gout
Sarcoid
Unknown

Calcium stones are by far the most common, are radiopaque, and consist of oxalate, phosphate, or both. They have many causes. Twenty-five to forty percent of calcium stone formers excrete excessive calcium in the urine, which in men is > 300 mg/24 h, and in women is > 250 mg/24 h. Of these, hyperparathyroidism causes 5%; sarcoidosis, milk-alkali syndrome, hypervitaminosis D, and prolonged immobilization cause a few more. But most are the result of *idiopathic hypercalciuria* whose cause is not definitely known but may be related to increased absorption from the gut or increased excretion by a "leak" through the kidney. The latter group has a strong family history. In 20% of those with idiopathic hypercalciuria there is associated hyperuricemia, which results in mixed stones.

In a large percentage of stone formers (20 to 60%) no metabolic defect is ever found. Some have slightly high excretion of calcium and oxalate, but the levels are still within upper-normal limits. Further research and clarification are needed as to the causes of kidney stones. (Table 17.2).

Data Your patient has awakened, so you take his history. He does not ingest large quantities of milk and cheese or take absorbable alkali, vitamins, or drugs. There is no indigestion or heartburn, although he has recently been constipated; and he has had no joint pains or stiffness. Systems review is negative for additional data, and the family history is not significant for stones.

Logic The milk-alkali syndrome (excessive calcium intake) is excluded; so is vitamin D intoxication. He has no upper gastrointestinal symptoms to suggest hyperparathyroidism, although constipation is often seen with this disease. The lack of symptoms of urinary tract infection weighs against stone formation from that cause, although smouldering chronic renal infection can exist without symptoms. There are none of the joint complaints often seen in sarcoidosis. The negative family history rebuts inheritable stone-forming diseases such as cystinuria and xanthinuria.

Other items in the history may guide your judgment in evaluating renal stone disease. *Age* is one such factor. Hyperparathyroidism and idiopathic hypercalciuria are uncommon before puberty, whereas metabolic disorders that cause stones (cystinosis, primary hyperoxaluria, and renal tubular acidosis) start early in childhood. *Gender* is important too; the stones of idiopathic hypercalciuria are five times more frequent in males, whereas hyperparathyroid stones are twice as common in females. *Diet and drug* history may reveal vitamin D fads, excessive milk and/or alkali, or large oxalate intake (rhubarb). *Geography* is a factor in that stones are far more common in the southeast United States, North Africa, and all across central Asia.

Data Physical examination discloses a well-nourished healthy-looking man who now looks comfortable. The vital signs are normal. Except for the heart, there are no positive findings. In particular, there are no masses in the neck, no band keratopathy, no lymph node enlargement, and no renal tenderness. The apex beat is in the fifth left intercostal space, 12 cm from the midline; there is a grade 3/6 high-pitched pansystolic murmur at the apex radiating to the left axilla. Otherwise the heart is normal and the lungs are clear.

Logic There is no physical evidence of hyperparathyroidism, although parathyroid adenomas are only rarely palpable. The lack of renal ten-derness is difficult to interpret. Cardiac findings are typical for an enlarged heart secondary to mitral regurgitation. This is most likely a result of rheumatic heart disease, although there is no history of an acute episode of rheumatic fever or a previously heard heart murmur. At any rate, it is not related to his stone disease, and clear lungs indicate that he is not in left ventricular failure.

Data He has two more brief episodes of pain not requiring a narcotic. Laboratory results return the next day. The urine is normal except for 20 to 30 RBCs per high-powered field and some crystals of calcium oxalate. The result of a nitroprusside test of the urine is negative for cystine, and the Sulkowitch test shows 4+ calciuria. The serum calcium, phosphorus, alkaline phosphatase, creatinine, and uric acid levels are normal, as are the rest of the blood chemical tests. Urine culture is negative, and the complete blood count is normal.

Logic The RBCs are expected. Calcium oxalate crystals in the urine are not diagnostic because they are omnipresent; large quantities might have some significance. The strongly positive Sulkowitch test indicates hypercalciuria, yet the serum calcium is normal. This suggests the entity of idiopathic hypercalciuria. Renal function is normal and gout is unlikely in the absence of joint symptoms, tophi, and hyperuricemia. Hyperparathyroidism is now even more remote in the presence of normal calcium and phosphorus levels. With a negative culture and the absence of leukocytes in the urine, the likelihood of chronic renal infection is also remote.

Data Chest radiograph shows a moderately enlarged left ventricle, but the lungs are clear, and there are no enlarged nodes. The ECG indicates left ventricular hypertrophy. An intravenous pyelogram demonstrates a normal right kidney and ureter; the left renal pelvis and left ureter are slightly dilated above the calculus, which is clearly within the ureter and is now in the lower third. There is no postvoid residual, and no other stones are seen (Fig. 17.2).

Logic The fact that the stone has moved down and is less than 10 to 12 mm in size suggests it will pass by itself. Sarcoidosis can be excluded by the negative chest radiograph, absence of lymph nodes, normal proteins, and normal calcium. The heart studies corroborate the physical findings; for now and the immediate future no car-

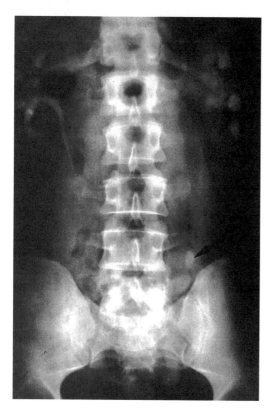

▶ **Figure 17.2.** Intravenous pyelogram demonstrates small stone in distal left ureter and dilated calyces.

diac treatment is needed, although investigation for valve replacement may be in order later.

That evening you reprogram your fading memory by reading about nephrolithiasis because you have not encountered the problem for many months. You are reminded that the clinical pictures and presentations by patients with renal stones may vary. Stones may be silent, may cause only microscopic or gross hematuria, may give pain, may aggregate in the renal pelvis to form a staghorn calculus, may destroy kidney function, may predispose to infection, or may precipitate primarily in the distal nephron resulting in nephrocalcinosis. Staghorn stones have varying radiopacity, are usually made of struvite ($MgNH_4PO_4$) and are associated with chronic infections caused by *Proteus* organisms. Multiple papillary calcifications are notable in distal renal tubular acidosis; the malfunction in the distal nephron results in hyperchloremic acidosis and excessive calcium excretion, causing nephrocalcinosis and eventual renal failure.

Stones cause pain only when they obstruct or are migrating. As they pass down to the lower third of the ureter, the pain that was in the flank radiates to the groin, thigh, or testicle. When the stone lodges in the intramural portion of the ureter at its junction with the bladder, frequency and urgency are added to the picture, thus simulating infection. Because the ureter is 10- to 12-mm wide, stones larger than 1 cm have difficulty passing and may cause great pain. Once the stone drops into the bladder it is easily passed because the urethra has a larger caliber. A clinking sound in the toilet bowl tells you that all is over—until the next episode that may be months or years away. At other times it may silently cause obstructive changes in the ureter, pelvis, and calyces above it.

Data Next morning, the stone is passed and collected in a strainer. Analysis shows pure calcium oxalate. A 24-hour urine collection while the patient is on a low-calcium diet shows: creatinine clearance 120 mL/minute; phosphate tubular reabsorption, 90%; uric acid, 300 mg/24 h; and calcium, 450 mg/24 h. All laboratory findings are normal, except the calcium excretion, which is markedly elevated. Repeat serum calcium and phosphorus levels are normal.

Logic These findings are helpful. The stone composition tells you that this is the most common type of stone; it is not basically uric acid that has precipitated a coat of calcium oxalate around it. Chemical studies of the urine offer further evidence against hyperparathyroidism and hyperuricosuria. The high amount of urinary calcium, even on a restricted calcium intake, suggests either hyperabsorption of calcium from the gut, or a renal leak of calcium. In either event, hypercalciuria is the cause of the patient's stones.

Because most hospitals are not equipped to distinguish between the two possible mechanisms of idiopathic hypercalciuria, the patient is started on hydrochlorothiazide 50 mg twice daily. This reduces urine calcium excretion and should diminish or eliminate renal calcium stone formation; serial urine and serum calcium determinations will be made. He is also advised to drink liberal amounts of fluid. Recent treatment strategies that either diminish calcium absorption from the gut or decrease its excretion in the urine have their drawbacks. For the moment, the use of thiazides to decrease calcium excretion seems to offer less deleterious effects.

It might be well to mention that the aforementioned mechanisms of stone formation do not tell the entire story. Solubility products, matrix nucleation, saturation and supersaturation indices, precipitation, crystallization, and stone inhibition factors in the urine are more and more being recognized as playing important roles.

Overriding many of these mechanisms is the balance between solute and solvent as well as the urine pH. A decrease in available solvent (water) or an increase in solute (calcium, oxalate, and so forth) may work separately or together to form stones. And last, the acidity or alkalinity of the urine is a potent force in determining which if any crystals may deposit.

The importance of capturing and analyzing the stone, and of performing a detailed urologic and metabolic work-up at least once in the life of a stone-former, cannot be overemphasized. Most have remediable metabolic disorders. Moreover, you must also be aware of the interrelationship and interactions between *stone, obstruction,* and *infection,* because often one causes the other.

But the entire story is still untold.

Questions

1. In reference to uric acid stones, which of the following statements is incorrect?
   (a) They are usually radiolucent.
   (b) They are often found in overexcreters of uric acid (> 600 mg/24 h).
   (c) They are often found in patients with persistently alkaline urine.
   (d) They are often found in association with tophaceous deposits in the ear cartilage and recurrent episodes of acute monarticular arthritis.
2. Approximately 90% of stones are radiopaque. The rest are not visualized by ordinary radiographs; contrast methods or chemical tests must be used if stone is suspected yet not visible. Which of the following are radiopaque?
   (a) Triple phosphates
   (b) Cystine
   (c) Oxalates
   (d) Xanthines
3. Whereas calcium oxalate stones are common, and the cause is usually an excess of calcium, in a small percentage of cases hyperoxaluria is the basic defect. This can occur in which of the following circumstances?
   (a) Malabsorption syndrome
   (b) An inherited deficiency of D-glyceric dehydrogenase
   (c) Pyridoxine deficiency
   (d) Excessive rhubarb ingestion
4. The clinical picture in a 48-year-old male diabetic patient suggests that he is passing a stone. Plain radiograph of the abdomen shows a 1.5-cm calcification in the left midabdomen. Which of the following statements may be true?
   (a) Intravenous urography visualizes both ureters, and the calcified area is outside the ureter.
   (b) Intravenous urography reveals a radiolucent area in the left midureter; there is dye above it, and the calcification is outside the ureter.
   (c) The pain continues, and the patient develops fever and chills.
   (d) The serum uric acid is 10.4 mg/dL.

Answers

1. **(c) is correct** because it is wrong. Uric acid stones tend to form in persistently acid urine because of their insolubility at a low pH; thus, this type of stone may be caused by a defect in ammonia production so that the kidneys must excrete their net acid production each day in the form of titratable acid. In this way uric acid stones can form in the absence of hyperuricemia and hyperuricosuria. Choice (a) is a true statement, but at times uric acid serves as a nidus for calcium deposition, and the stone becomes partially radiopaque. Excessive uric acid excretion is the principal cause of this type of stone; it occurs in most cases of gout; hematoproliferative disorders, especially with the beginning of treatment; and the Lesch-Nyhan syndrome (an inborn error of metabolism characterized by an overproduction of uric acid). Choice (d) is a classic clinical description of gout.
2. **(a), (b), and (c) are correct.** Triple phosphates contain calcium. Cystine is radiopaque because of its sulfur content. Oxalates are combined with calcium. Xanthine is radiolucent, as are uric acid stones and some small but not dense calcium-containing stones. Newer imaging techniques show versatility in detecting stones that were formerly not demonstrable by the usual methods.
3. **All are correct** and can cause stones because of excessive oxalate excretion in the urine. In the malabsorption syndrome, which is associated with a variety of diseases, calcium is bound to fatty acid in the gut,

thereby leaving oxalate free for absorption. Normally much oxalate is bound to calcium and excreted in the stool. Enteric disease is the most common cause of hyperoxaluria. Choice (b) is a description of primary oxaluria, in which a deficiency of the stated enzyme interferes with normal metabolic pathways and results in hyperoxaluria. These children develop stones and calcifications early and usually die of uremia by age 20. Rarely, pyridoxine deficiency interferes with similar metabolic pathways, resulting in oxalate stones. Rhubarb contains much oxalate and can also cause stones by hyperoxaluria.

4. **All may be true.** The calcified area is probably a calcified mesenteric node and the stone, if present, may be radiolucent. The radiolucent area delineated by contrast in answer (b) may be a uric acid stone, a blood clot, a tumor, or a sloughed renal papilla. Diabetic patients are prone to severe infections of the kidney with renal papillary necrosis and sloughing. Anything that causes bleeding may cause the clot. An impacted stone may cause retrograde infection of the kidney (c). And, of course, the patient may also have hyperuricemia, a condition that occurs more commonly in diabetics than in the rest of the population—much more often than a simple concurrence.

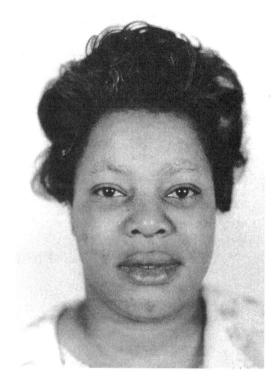

▶ **Figure 17.3.** Note facial puffiness, especially in periorbital areas.

Suggested Readings

Halabe A, Sperling O. Uric acid nephrolithiasis. Mineral Electro Metab 1994;20(6):424–431.

Klugman V, Favus MJ. Diagnosis and treatment of calcium kidney stones. Advances Endocrinol Metab 1995;6:117–142.

LeRoy AJ. Diagnosis and treatment of nephrolithiasis. Am J Roentgenol 1994;163(6):1309–1313.

CASE 58

SWELLING OF FACE AND LEGS

Marvin Forland

Data A 32-year-old woman consults her physician because of intermittent swelling of the face, hands, and legs for one month. Although she felt well, she became increasingly aware of periorbital puffiness on awakening, tightening of her rings, and ankle swelling toward the end of the day. More recently, her legs were also swollen on awakening. Despite no change in her normally good appetite or in her usual food intake, she noted a gradual 10-lb weight gain (Fig. 17.3).

Logic This woman has generalized edema as noted by gain in weight and swelling of the face, legs, and hands. When fluid retention and edema occur (expansion of the interstitial component of the extracellular fluid volume), three possibilities immediately come to mind: *congestive heart failure* (CHF), *cirrhosis of the liver,* and the *nephrotic syndrome.* Less likely considerations are idiopathic cyclic edema, often characterized by abrupt weight changes correlating with the menstrual cycle, and hypothyroidism where brawny swelling can be mistaken for pitting edema. Venous or lymphatic obstruction in the legs can be ruled out by the presence of facial and hand edema, too.

Constrictive pericarditis is an unusual and dramatic cause of edema although curable if discovered. Protein-losing enteropathy is another rare cause; suspect it if edema occurs in the absence of heart, liver, or kidney disease, and the serum protein is low. Localized edema of the face and eyelids may be caused by trichinosis, and edema may occur on the paralyzed side in hemiplegia. In children, acute post-streptococcal glomerulonephritis may cause edema, but this disease has other obvious hallmarks—hypertension, hematuria, rising antistreptolysin titer, and so forth.

In each of the three main considerations, decreased renal blood flow (RBF) invokes the renin-angiotensin-aldosterone system. This results in sodium and water retention in an effort to preserve effective arterial blood volume. But other mechanisms are at work too. In CHF, edema is caused by increased capillovenous pressure as well as by decreased cardiac output and diminished RBF. Cirrhosis causes edema in many ways; hypoalbuminemia, portal hypertension, intrahepatic lymphatic obstruction, and inability to destroy antidiuretic hormone and aldosterone contribute to sequestration of fluid in the abdomen and elsewhere. Then, a decreased RBF initiates the renal mechanism for salt and water retention. The sequence of events in nephrotic syndrome is: glomerular defect, massive proteinuria, hypoalbuminemia, edema, decreased RBF, renal retention of salt and water, and more edema. Adding to this sequence is an increased fractional catabolism of the decreased serum albumin pool, which is related to increased destruction of filtered proteins by the renal tubular cells (Fig. 17.4).

Data Further history reveals excellent previous health and two uneventful full-term pregnancies 8 and 5 years ago. She takes no medication, does not smoke, and averages one alcoholic drink each week. There is no history of hepatitis or jaundice. She tolerates activity and exercise quite well, does not get dyspneic or fatigued on exertion, is comfortable in cold weather wearing no more clothes than others, and has normal bowel habits and an unchanged menstrual pattern. Recently she has had nocturia once or twice nightly, and has noticed some "foaminess" in the toilet bowl after completing urination. The edema is unrelated to her menstrual cycle.

Logic Good exercise tolerance and lack of dyspnea or fatigue on exertion tend to exclude CHF. Furthermore, there is no history of congenital heart disease, acute rheumatic fever, hypertension, or murmurs, which might be expected in a young woman with CHF. Absence of drug or alcohol abuse and no history of jaundice make severe liver disease unlikely. Tolerance to cold, normal bowel habits, and absence of other related

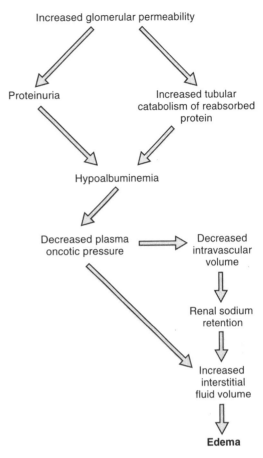

▶ **Figure 17.4.** A model for the pathophysiology of edema in the nephrotic syndrome predicated on the primacy of hypoalbuminemia.

symptoms refute thyroid hypofunction; cyclic premenstrual edema is denied by the history. Nocturia is a common manifestation of edema from any cause and relates to more effective renal perfusion in the reclining position. Foamy urine occurs in patients with massive proteinuria. So far, then, the evidence points to the kidney as the source of her illness.

Data Physical examination reveals a well-nourished patient. Vital signs are blood pressure (BP), 110/70; pulse, 80 and regular; respirations, 12; and temperature, 36.6°C. No jaundice or pallor is noted. The neck veins are not distended and the examination of the heart and lungs is normal. There are no rales, flatness, dullness, or altered fremitus, and breath sounds are normal (no evidence for congestion or effusion). The apex beat is normally located, heart sounds are normal, and there are no S_3, S_4, or murmurs noted. Spleen and liver are not palpable, and ascites cannot be detected. None of the stigmata of cirrhosis are present. No definite facial edema is noted at this time, although the legs show 2+ pitting edema to the midcalf. Several fingernails display whitish arcuate bands parallel to the lunulae. The remainder of the examination is normal.

Logic Cirrhosis can now be ruled out by the absence of historical or physical evidence. CHF is also excluded by the normal cardiac and pulmonary findings. Myxedema, only a remote consideration, is virtually eliminated by the absence of its facial features, the type of edema, and normal reflexes. Constrictive pericarditis can be excluded by the absence of cardiac abnormalities, distended neck veins, Kussmaul's sign, prominent y descents in the jugular veins, and by the presence of leg edema without hepatomegaly and ascites.

The only abnormal findings are edema of the legs and some clues to its cause. The whitish bands in the nailbeds are called Muehrcke's lines; they develop during periods of severe hypoalbuminemia (less than 2.0 g/dL). The nephrotic syndrome is strongly suspected. There is clinical evidence of *edema, hypoalbuminemia,* and *severe proteinuria* (foamy urine)—a highly suggestive cluster.

Data Initial laboratory tests have now returned: the hemoglobin and hematocrit levels and white blood cell count are normal. Urinalysis shows: pH 6.0, trace of glucose, urobilinogen and bilirubin absent, protein 4+ (by sulfosalicylic acid method); one white blood cell and one red blood cell per high-powered field; and two to four hyaline casts with occasional fatty inclusions, and one oval fat body per low-powered field.

Logic The heavy proteinuria, casts with fatty inclusions, and fat bodies add further strength to the diagnosis of a nephrotic syndrome. Advanced renal insufficiency is probably not present if the hemoglobin level is normal. The few red blood cells and white blood cells on urine examination suggest we are not dealing with a typical glomerular inflammatory process. A trace of glucose in the urine may suggest diabetes mellitus, a possible cause for the nephrotic syndrome, but mild glycosuria is often present with massive albuminuria as an apparent consequence of impaired proximal tubular function.

In general, the proteinuria of renal-caused nephrotic syndromes consists mainly of albumin

because it is the smallest of the major protein molecules. A loss of more than 3.5 g/1.73 m²/24 h is considered a prerequisite for the diagnosis. But κ and λ chains slip through in multiple myeloma. Other proteins may be lost too. A low thyroxine (T_4) and increased triiodothyronine (T_3) resin uptake may result from leakage of thyroid-binding globulin, loss of transferrin can cause hypochromic microcytic anemia, and loss of antithrombin III can result in a hypercoagulable state (iliofemoral or renal vein thrombosis).

In the nephrotic syndrome, hepatic synthesis of lipoproteins is increased and catabolism is often decreased. This results in hyperlipidemia, an increase in low-density lipoproteins and cholesterol, and the presence of lipid bodies in the urine (fatty casts, oval fat bodies, and doubly refractile maltese crosses). The lipid abnormalities are not always present in the nephrotic syndrome.

The physician now orders a series of laboratory studies that fall into four major categories:

1. To exclude hypothyroidism, T_3 and thyroid-stimulating hormone (TSH) are ordered.
2. To confirm the diagnosis of nephrotic syndrome, she orders a serum protein electrophoresis, total serum proteins, serum cholesterol, and 24-hour urinary protein.
3. To evaluate the status of renal function, she orders a serum creatinine and requests a urine creatinine level on the 24-hour collection.
4. To seek a cause for the nephrotic syndrome, she orders a 2-hour postprandial blood glucose, antinuclear antibody (ANA) test, and serum C'3 complement level.

This laboratory series may only initiate the search.
Data The T_3 and TSH are normal. Serum protein electrophoresis shows a decrease in albumin and $α_1$- and $γ$-globulins, with a mild increase in $α_2$- and $β_1$-globulins; total proteins are 5.1 g/dL (albumin 2.1 g and globulin 3.0 g). Twenty-four-hour urine protein excretion is 6.4 g. Serum cholesterol is 390 mg/dL. Serum creatinine is 0.9 mg/dL and creatinine clearance is 94 mL/minute. The 2-hour postprandial blood glucose is 98 mg/dL; ANA is absent, and serum complement is normal. The rest of the findings from the 18-test chemistry profile (including liver function tests) and the Venereal Disease Research Laboratory test are normal or negative.

Logic The cluster needed to establish the existence of the nephrotic syndrome is clearly present: (1) edema, (2) proteinuria (usually but not necessarily more than 3 to 5 g/24 h), and (3) hypoalbuminemia (less than 3 g/dL). Increased blood cholesterol is often although not necessarily found. Liver disease is excluded. Kidney function is normal, and there is no evidence for diabetes or systemic lupus erythematosus (SLE)—two common causes for the syndrome under discussion.

Pause a moment and again consider the sequence of events resulting in the nephrotic syndrome before searching further for a cause. Whatever the etiology—streptococcal infection, diabetes, or blood vessel disease—the common denominator is glomerular injury. This allows for protein leakage and increased urinary protein. Loss of protein in the urine (plus other factors, such as increased fractional catabolism) leads to decreased serum protein, decreased colloid osmotic pressure, and edema. This in turn causes decreased blood volume and then decreased RBF, which activates the renin-angiotensin-aldosterone sequence as well as other renal mechanisms. Thus, salt and water are retained and edema is compounded.

Diabetic glomerulosclerosis is ruled out by the absence of diabetes. SLE can be dismissed by the absence of cardinal clinical features (rash, arthritis, pleuritis, and so forth) and the absence of immunologic abnormalities (ANA and complement testing). But a list of all the other causes of the nephrotic syndrome could fill a page. Included are various types of idiopathic glomerulonephritis, amyloidosis, multiple myeloma, other connective tissue diseases, allergens, drugs, and acute infections. Bilateral renal vein thrombosis, once thought to be a cause of the nephrotic syndrome, now appears to be its consequence. Thrombosis of one or both renal veins is seen especially in membranous nephropathy, membranoproliferative glomerulonephritis, and amyloidosis (Table 17.3).

As the physician considers the extensive list of disease processes that may result in altered glomerular permeability and massive proteinuria, he or she must carefully regard age, sex, and geography. In some still developing areas, amyloidosis related to tuberculosis may be the leading cause. In the tropics, quartan malaria provides the antigen for an immune complex form of nephrotic syndrome. Lipoid nephrosis (minimal change lesion)

TABLE 17.3. Major Causes of the Nephrotic Syndrome

Diabetes mellitus
Systemic lupus erythematosus
Glomerulonephritis (immune complex disease)
Certain drugs (see text)
Multiple myeloma
Amyloidosis
Lipoid nephrosis
Neoplastic disease

is responsible for 80% of all cases in children. SLE and other collagen diseases would be prominent considerations in our patient—a young woman—although from the evidence acquired so far, these diseases are not present. If the patient were older, primary amyloidosis, multiple myeloma, or underlying malignancy might deserve more attention.

Exposure to penicillamine, tridione, paramethadione, probenecid, captopril, gold, mercury, and bismuth is easily ruled out, as are bee stings, poison oak, and poison ivy—all possible causes of the nephrotic syndrome.

It is interesting to note how many other primarily extrarenal diseases may affect the kidneys and produce a nephrotic syndrome by known and unknown mechanisms. These include infections such as endocarditis and secondary syphilis; neoplastic diseases like lymphomas, Hodgkin's disease, leukemia, and carcinomas; and some general disorders such as sarcoidosis, diffuse vasculitis, sickle cell anemia, and others that have already been mentioned.

We have considered and excluded the many generalized diseases that affect the kidney and thus cause the nephrotic syndrome. At this point, one of the varieties of glomerulonephritis must be highly suspect, because this group is indeed the most common cause for the nephrotic syndrome in adults. What was called "Bright's disease" or chronic glomerulonephritis is now known to consist of many different entities. All are associated with glomerular disease, usually postulated to be of immune mediation; but the histopathologic changes may be proliferative, membranous, or both—focal or diffuse. And so we inherit a host of long-named diseases that differ mostly in their microscopic appearance. But the histologic type must be identified, for it helps determine the natural course of the disease, the prognosis, and the treatment.

Therefore, a renal biopsy must be done. *Minimal change disease* (nil lesion, lipoid nephrosis, foot process disease) is the predominant cause of nephrotic syndrome in children but it also occurs in adults. Its names derive from the fact that ordinary light microscopy reveals nothing abnormal; electron microscopy shows effacement of the epithelial foot processes. In most other instances, the histologic findings provide us with diagnoses of mesangial proliferative glomerulonephritis, focal and segmental glomerulosclerosis, membranous glomerulopathy, membranoproliferative glomerulonephritis, and other unclassified lesions.

The various renal diseases just mentioned may for the most part eventually lead to what was and still is known as chronic glomerulonephritis with its associated hypertension, symmetrically contracted kidneys, and renal failure.

Data After consultation with the patient and her husband, the patient is admitted to the hospital for a renal biopsy. Preliminary intravenous pyelography demonstrates normal kidney size, function, and location; no tumors, cysts, or hydronephrosis are seen. A urine culture shows no growth. A bleeding disorder is ruled out by a normal platelet count, prothrombin time, and partial thromboplastin time and bleeding time. Percutaneous renal biopsy is obtained, and the specimen is sectioned for light, electron, and immunofluorescence microscopy. There are no complications. Characteristic lesions of membranous glomerulopathy, an immune complex form of glomerulonephritis, are found on the three forms of microscopy.

Finding the cause was easy. The difficult problem is treatment.

Questions

1. The same patient is seen 3 years later. She has been treated intermittently with steroids, immunosuppressives, and diuretics without beneficial effect. Massive edema is now present. You would not be surprised to find any of the following except:
   (a) hypertension.
   (b) serum creatinine, 4.0 mg/dL.

   (c) ascites and pleural effusion.
   (d) urine 24-hour albumin = 0.5 g.
2. The nephrotic syndrome could be related to each of the following clinical circumstances except:
   (a) patient receiving phenytoin for epilepsy.
   (b) patient with recently diagnosed carcinoembryonic antigen-positive colon adenocarcinoma.
   (c) patient with large tongue, malabsorption, orthostatic hypotension, and cardiac hypertrophy without apparent cause.
   (d) patient under treatment for rheumatoid arthritis.
3. You see a 62-year-old woman with the recent onset of severe edema of the legs. There is no edema apparent elsewhere. Examination is otherwise completely normal. The urinalysis shows +3 glucose and a trace of albumin. Serum albumin is 3.5 g/dL. Which of the following statements is/are true?
   (a) She may have diabetes, which is causing a nephrotic syndrome.
   (b) CHF may be causing her swollen legs.
   (c) She may have diabetes, but it is not causing her swollen legs.
   (d) Her edema may be caused by venous or lymphatic obstruction in the legs or pelvis; a pelvic examination may supply the answer.

Answers

1. **(d) is correct,** because a marked decrease in albuminuria would not be expected. However, progressive renal failure with an elevated creatinine level, and worsening fluid retention with ascites and pleural effusion, occur in the natural course of the disease, often despite treatment. Hypertension is common in renal failure for most cases.
2. **(a) is correct.** Tridione and pardione used for petit mal can cause nephrosis. Phenytoin does not. Patient (b) probably has an immune complex nephropathy. Patient (c) has manifestations of primary amyloidosis, and patient (d) might have renal amyloidosis secondary to rheumatoid arthritis, or a nephrotic syndrome from treatment with gold injections or penicillamine. Therefore (b), (c), and (d) can definitely be associated with a nephrotic syndrome.
3. **(c) and (d) are correct.** Heavy glycosuria suggests diabetes mellitus, but she has no nephrotic syndrome for diabetes to cause. Nephrotic syndrome is negated by the urine and serum protein values. A large pelvic mass or neoplasm could cause swollen legs by obstruction of veins or lymphatics. Bilateral thrombophlebitis could exist too. Choice (a) is wrong for the same reason that (c) is correct. Choice (b) is impossible in the presence of an otherwise normal physical examination.

COMMENT The time-conscious physician would immediately consider the few major causes of generalized edema and use a stepwise approach. Liver disease and CHF are ruled out with a few questions, a look at the patient, and a listen to the heart and lungs. Serum proteins and urinalysis would prove the cluster to be caused by kidney disease—the nephrotic syndrome. The specific etiology would be suspected by considering probabilities as they relate to commonness, age, sex, and geography. History or associated physical findings might offer the decisive clue, although renal biopsy is often the ultimate diagnostic study, with the highest specificity and sensitivity in this arena. *(P.C.)*

Suggested Readings

Humphreys MH. Nephrology forum: Mechanisms and management of nephrotic edema. Kidney Int 1994;45:266–281.

Lewis EJ. Idiopathic membranous nephropathy—to treat or not to treat? N Engl J Med 1993;329:127–129.

Madaio MP. Nephrology forum: Renal biopsy. Kidney Int 1990;38:529–543.

Ponticelli C, Passerini P. Treatment of the nephrotic syndrome associated with primary glomerulonephritis. Kidney Int 1994;46:595–604.

 C A S E 59

COMA AND OLIGURIA

Paul Cutler

Data A 64-year-old man was brought to the emergency department after having been found comatose in his room. He was seen by a neurologist and a neurosurgeon who diagnosed a cerebrovascular accident after a computed tomographic scan demonstrated infarction of a large area supplied by the left middle cerebral artery. A lumbar puncture disclosed no cellular elements. He was then admitted to the medical intensive care unit.

On the evening of his admission, routine blood chemistry tests done earlier in the day revealed: BUN, 60 mg/dL; creatinine, 7.2 mg/dL; glucose, 85 mg/dL; Na^+, 142 mEq/L; K^+, 6.0 mEq/L; CI^-, 92 mEq/L; CO_2, 17 mEq/L; Ca^{++}, 8.0 mg/dL, phosphate, 5.0 mg/dL; uric acid, 19.3 mg/dL; hemoglobin and hematocrit,

17.3 g/dL and 52%, respectively; WBC count, 11,400/mm³; and platelets, 420,000/mm³.

Logic At this point, the only certainties are that the patient has renal insufficiency and has suffered a cerebrovascular accident. Although most of our thoughts and efforts center around his stroke, we are curious about the azotemia. First, determine whether the renal failure is acute or chronic in nature. The history may be helpful in making this decision.

Data The patient was brought to the hospital by his landlady who discovered him unresponsive after not having seen him for 2 days. She knew little of his medical problems except that he was on a low-salt diet because of high blood pressure and had suffered a stroke 2 years previously, but he had no apparent residual neurologic impairment.

Logic You wonder whether the elevations of the BUN and creatinine levels are new or old. Did renal failure precede the stroke, or was it the result of the stroke? Previous laboratory reports would be helpful if available. Although the history does not document any chronic renal disease, the prior history of high blood pressure is consistent with underlying renal disease. A closer look at the laboratory values may be informative.

The absence of anemia strongly suggests that the renal insufficiency is an acute problem. The high hemoglobin reflects a certain degree of dehydration and hemoconcentration. Whereas the electrolytes are typical of those found with chronic renal failure of this degree, the $K+$ is usually not this high. Patients with chronic renal failure are able to increase tubular secretion of $K+$ to compensate for their diminished renal mass. The $Ca++$ and phosphates are not helpful as the former will fall and the latter rise within 48 hours of the onset of acute renal failure (ARF). They are similarly altered in chronic renal failure (CRF). The markedly abnormal uric acid level is strongly suggestive of acute renal disease, because this compound is only mildly elevated in the chronic setting (9 to 12 mg/dL).

Thus, these data, especially the lack of anemia and the severe hyperuricemia, are indications that the renal failure is not only acute but new.

A sudden severe decrease in renal function in association with a decreased glomerular filtration rate, rapidly rising azotemia, and oliguria indicates the presence of ARF. Less than 400 mL of urine per 24 hours is insufficient for elimination of the normal load of waste products; this condition is called "oliguria." *Anuria* refers to 100 mL of urine or less/24 h.

Although the patient's stroke is of principal concern, ARF is close behind because it may cause complications and death. The common causes of such renal deterioration quickly confront you. Immediately you discard the 60% of cases that are due to surgery or trauma and consider the 40% that arise from other causes—*renal ischemia, renal damage,* or *renal obstruction.*

A radiograph of the abdomen to determine renal size may be helpful.

Data A flat radiograph of the abdomen is obtained, and the vertical renal size is 14 cm bilaterally—normal. (A sonogram was not considered necessary at this point).

Logic Small kidneys suggest a chronic process like chronic glomerulonephritis or pyelonephritis. Patients with polycystic disease and obstructive urologic disorders have enlarged kidneys. Those with amyloidosis and diabetic glomerulosclerosis who are in chronic renal failure usually have enlarged kidneys. The normal size in this case points to an acute renal process.

The next question to confront is the cause of the acute renal failure. In general, you should first consider the possibilities in the broadest terms, that is, prerenal azotemia, parenchymal renal disease, and postrenal (or obstructive) uropathy.

Prerenal azotemia results from decreased effective renal blood flow and decreased renal perfusion resulting in a lowered glomerular filtration rate. Aside from the shock and blood loss of surgery, anesthesia, or trauma, it may be caused by extracellular volume depletion, septic shock, cardiogenic shock, or "third space" loss (bowel obstruction, peritonitis, and so forth).

Postrenal defects are caused mainly by obstructive uropathy from an enlarged prostate; uncommonly, bilateral ureteral obstruction from retroperitoneal fibrosis occurs. Whether crystal, heme, or myeloma deposits in the tubules represent a renal or a postrenal problem is a moot point.

There are many renal parenchymal problems that can cause ARF. Essentially they result from a prolonged period of renal hypoperfusion, severe kidney infection, or acute tubular necrosis from drugs or chemical compounds such as nonsteroidal anti-inflammatory agents (NSAIDs), contrast media, heme pigments and aminoglycosides.

It is important to remember that often multiple causes are operative at the same time.

The physical examination and, again, the laboratory are helpful in these differentiations.

Data Physical examination reveals: BP, 140/80 supine, and 110/50 when tilted to 40 degrees; pulse, 100 and regular when supine, and 140 when tilted. Skin turgor is poor; there is tenting; and the mucous membranes are dry. Ophthalmoscopy reveals only moderate arteriolar narrowing. There is no jugular venous distention at 45 degrees. His right lower extremity is cool, discolored, and markedly swollen; because of the edema, pulses could not be verified as absent or present. There is no edema elsewhere, and pulses are palpable in the left leg.

Logic The etiology of the abnormal swollen leg is not certain. His landlady reported that when he was found in his room, his right knee was flexed and the leg positioned under his trunk and thigh.

The BP and pulse findings are consistent with a decreased effective extracellular fluid volume, possibly due to sequestration of fluid in the markedly edematous right leg and to lack of access to oral fluids. Thus, prerenal azotemia is a real possibility. However, parenchymal renal disease and obstructive uropathy are not excluded.

Data Further physical findings pertinent to his renal failure include a moderately enlarged smooth prostate but no suprapubic distention. The rest of the examination is normal except for evidence of a complete right hemiplegia.

Logic In this age group, the most likely cause of obstructive uropathy is benign prostatic hypertrophy. In a stroke victim, however, urinary retention due to an atonic bladder can also occur. At any rate, the bladder is not enlarged, so marked retention is not likely.

Data A Foley catheter is inserted into the bladder and only 30 mL of dark brown urine are obtained. The laboratory reports a urine Na^+ concentration of 60 mEq/L and an osmolality of 320 mOsm/kg of H_2O.

Logic The small urine volume rules out urinary retention with obstructive uropathy at the level of the prostate gland and is in keeping with ARF.

When in doubt it is sometimes necessary to do other procedures to exclude obstruction higher up. Techniques to visualize the calices, renal pelvis, and ureters include visualization by computed tomographic scan, ultrasound, or retrograde pyelography. But it is important to remember that the urine collecting system may not be visibly stretched until 48 hours after acute obstruction occurs.

If prerenal events (e.g., dehydration) were the cause of the azotemia, one would predict a urine sodium concentration of less than 10 mEq/L and a urine osmolality of greater than 500 mOsm/kg of H_2O. In that event, renal flow is altered but kidney function is still reasonably intact, and the kidney can still reabsorb sodium and concentrate urine (specific gravity 1.020 to 1.030). If the oliguria results from intrinsic renal disease, the urine sodium content will be high (>15 mEq/L) and the urine osmolality will be low (< 400 mOsm/kg).

Additionally, you will recall that the BUN is 60 mg/dL, and creatinine is 7.2 mg/dL. The normal ratio of BUN to creatinine is approximately 15:1. With azotemia due to either prerenal or postrenal causes, one expects the BUN level to be elevated out of proportion to the elevation in the creatinine level. This is due to the flow-dependent nature of urea reabsorption along the nephron; that is, at low flow rates seen with prerenal and postrenal azotemia, urea reabsorption is enhanced. Thus, the high urinary Na^+ concentration, the low urine osmolality, the relatively low ratio of BUN to creatinine, and the absence of obstructive findings have virtually excluded both prerenal and postrenal causes of renal insufficiency (Table 17.4). The differential diagnosis has therefore narrowed to those causes of ARF associated with renal parenchymal disease, as listed in Table 17.5.

TABLE 17.4. Laboratory Distinction between Prerenal and Renal Acute Renal Failure

	PRERENAL	RENAL
Urine	Benign	Casts, cells, albumin
BUN: creatinine	20:1	10–15:1
Urine Na conc	< 15 mEq/L	> 15 mEq/L
Osmolality	> 500 mOsm/L	< 400 mOsm/L
Urine sp g	1.020	1.010
FEna[a]	< 1%	> 2%

[a]The fractional excretion of sodium (FEna) is another standard for distinguishing prerenal and renal causes of acute renal failure. The numerator of this fraction is equal to the urine÷blood concentrations of sodium; the denominator is equal to the urine÷blood concentrations of creatinine. This ratio multiplied by 100 equals the FEna.
BUN = blood urea nitrogen; sp g = specific gravity.

TABLE 17.5. Causes of Acute Renal Failure Associated with Renal Parenchymal Disease

Glomerular disease—acute
  Glomerulonephritis
Vascular disease
  Vascular
  Arterial or venous obstruction
  Malignant nephrosclerosis
Tubulointerstitial disease
  Tubular precipitation
    Urates
    "Myeloma kidney"
  Papillary necrosis
  Acute interstitial nephritis
  "Acute tubular necrosis"
    Postischemia
      Hypotension
      Sepsis
    Nephrotoxins
    Heme pigments

Data Urinalysis: color, dark brown; specific gravity 1.012; pH 6; glucose absent; protein 2+; occult blood 3+; microscopic: many coarse granular pigmented casts; one to four renal tubular epithelial cells per high-powered field; an occasional WBC; and no RBCs or RBC casts.

Logic The urinalysis is extremely helpful in confirming that the problem is renal and not prerenal or postrenal. Furthermore, it helps narrow the list of parenchymal diseases that cause ARF.

In prerenal and postrenal uremia, the kidneys, at least in the acute stage, are reasonably intact, and there may be only minor albuminuria and few casts. Renal diseases, however, present with more albumin and abnormalities in the urine sediment, such as casts of all kinds, RBCs, and WBCs.

As for the renal diseases listed in the table, *acute glomerulonephritis* is effectively excluded by the absence of RBCs and RBC casts. Because avid salt retention and a urine sodium concentration of < 10 mEq/L is characteristic of this disease, the previously noted urine sodium concentration of 60 mEq/L argues against its presence.

Microscopic or gross hematuria is usually seen

in patients whose ARF is secondary to *vascular disease* or *arterial emboli*. Additionally, vasculitic diseases such as systemic lupus or polyarteritis nodosa are usually manifested by a skin rash, arthritis, and cytoid bodies on ophthalmoscopy. The normal blood pressure and relatively benign fundi weigh heavily against malignant nephrosclerosis.

This patient was noted to have severe hyperuricemia, and *tubular precipitation* of uric acid may be a cause of oliguric ARF. However, this situation is limited almost exclusively to patients with myelo- or lymphoproliferative diseases, especially after undergoing either radiation or chemotherapy. With treatment of these diseases, cell lysis releases into the circulation a large quantity of purine nucleotides that are metabolized to uric acid. We have no evidence, however, that this patient has such a disease or that he is undergoing such treatment. Finally, in such cases the urine sediment contains large amounts of precipitated uric acid; none was observed in this patient.

Papillary necrosis, when bilateral, may cause ARF. This disease is often associated with infection, the urinalysis usually reveals heavy pyuria, and it occurs mostly in patients with diabetes mellitus, sickle cell anemia, obstructive uropathy, or analgesic abuse. There is no evidence of any of these entities in this patient, although you cannot exclude the latter possibility.

Acute interstitial nephritis is generally related to a drug reaction (e.g., penicillin and its analogues) and is often accompanied by eosinophilia. In addition, acute inflammatory cells are frequently found in the urine sediment. There is no evidence for this diagnosis.

Acute tubular necrosis is the most common cause of ARF. A partial list of nephrotoxins includes various antibiotics (especially aminoglycosides), non-steroidal anti-inflammatory drugs, heavy metals, chlorinated hydrocarbons, and anesthetic agents. We have no knowledge of exposure to any known nephrotoxic agent; however, we cannot exclude this possibility. ARF is often observed in association with renal ischemia or vasoconstriction secondary to an acute myocardial infarction, burn, hemorrhage, or sepsis. The patient presented here did not have a documented episode of hypotension, but it should be emphasized that acute tubular necrosis can occur due to renal ischemia without *overt* hypotension

or shock. Yet burns, myocardial infarction, hemorrhage, and sepsis can be virtually excluded by inspection, ECG, normal blood count, and negative blood cultures.

Data An ECG showed only nonspecific ST-T changes; the chest radiograph was normal. Blood cultures drawn the day before were negative. No evidence or cause for sepsis can be found. As for the stroke, nursing and supportive care were given; the patient became more lucid. The cause of the ARF and right leg findings remained obscure. Marked oliguria persisted.

Logic However, the patient was noted to have one additional significant finding: dark brown urine. *Pigments,* specifically *hemoglobin* and *myoglobin,* are well-recognized causes of oliguric ARF. Recall that the urinalysis was positive for "occult blood," but no RBCs were noted. The "dipsticks" commonly used for occult blood use orthotoluidine, which yields a positive reaction with both hemoglobin and myoglobin. Thus, in the absence of RBCs this finding suggests either hemoglobinuria or myoglobinuria. In view of the normal complete blood count (that is, no evidence for hemolysis), it appears that myoglobinuria is present.

As pointed out, the patient was noted to have a discolored, markedly swollen right extremity. It is likely that as a result of his cerebrovascular accident the patient fell, and his position caused compression and ischemia of this lower extremity, resulting in muscle necrosis (rhabdomyolysis), myoglobinuria, and finally ARF (Fig. 17.5).

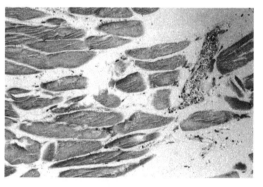

▶ **Figure 17.5.** Striated muscle necrosis is evidenced by the loss of nuclei, degeneration of cytoplasm, and interstitial edema, which result in the release of nephrotoxic substances (biopsy not done for the patient in this case).

Muscle necrosis as a cause of ARF has become more widely recognized. Prolonged pressure from coma caused by stroke or drug overdose, crush injuries, and sudden vascular occlusion to large muscles may cause muscle necrosis, along with the release of myoglobin and measurable large quantities of aldolase and creatine phosphokinase. The mechanism by which myoglobin damages the kidney is unknown. Indeed, myoglobin is probably not the offending agent and may only be a marker for the true toxin that accompanies it.

It should be noted that the stroke, rather than the uremia, was the probable cause of the patient's unconsciousness. But if not for the stroke, there would have been nausea, vomiting, somnolence, and stupor—the usual symptoms of ARF. **Data** After several days, consciousness returned, but the hemiplegia and aphasia persisted. Azotemia and oliguria continued for several weeks and then gradually improved. Special care was given to prevent problems such as thrombophlebitis, water and salt overload, hyperkalemia, infection, and other complications explained in question 2, which follows.

Questions

1. Necrosis of muscle tissue occurs under many circumstances. It is common in comatose patients who compress muscles for long periods of time. Rhabdomyolysis and myoglobinuria with ARF are associated with all the following except:
   (a) BUN-to-creatinine ratio < 10.
   (b) hypophosphatemia.
   (c) hypercalcemia.
   (d) hyperuricemia.
2. The chief cause of death in patients who have ARF is:
   (a) hyperkalemia.
   (b) severe acidosis.
   (c) infection.
   (d) pericarditis.
3. Following ARF, the kidney may secrete large quantities of dilute urine, yet azotemia may persist. Which of the following statements concerning this diuretic phase of ARF is true?
   (a) The risk of pericarditis is low.
   (b) The likelihood of hyperkalemia is reduced.
   (c) Sodium restriction should be continued.
   (d) Dialysis is never necessary.

Answers

1. **(b) is correct.** Hypophosphatemia does not occur with rhabdomyolysis. The soft-tissue necrosis may release large amounts of phosphate into the extracellular fluid space. This endogenous phosphate load coupled with renal failure causes marked and rapid hyperphosphatemia. Contrary to the general rule, a low BUN-to-creatinine ratio (a) may be seen with rhabdomyolysis due to the release of the muscle enzyme creatine, which is metabolized to creatinine. Although an increase in serum phosphate generally causes the serum calcium to decrease, hypercalcemia (c) may occur late in the course of ARF in this setting. This is thought to be caused by the release of deposited calcium from damaged muscle tissue. Finally, hyperuricemia (d) in the 20 to 30 mg/dL range may occur in this entity and is probably due to the release of purines from damaged muscle.

2. **(c) is correct.** Infection with resultant sepsis remains the primary cause of death in ARF. Catheters and intravenous tubes serve as sources of infection in the unconscious patient. The remaining choices are life-threatening complications of ARF, but these can be avoided or promptly treated as they occur.

3. **(b) is correct.** Because potassium excretion is at least in part flow-dependent, urinary potassium excretion increases with an increase in urine output. Pericarditis (a) may occur at any time during the course of ARF, and dialysis (d) may continue to be necessary because the glomerular filtration rate often remains severely compromised even during the diuretic phase of the illness. It may be necessary to liberalize sodium intake (c) because the urinary sodium concentration may remain elevated, and thus extracellular fluid volume depletion may occur if sodium restriction is continued.

COMMENT This case presents the reader with a treasure trove of pathophysiologic correlations. As the logic unfolded, several critical decision points had to be crossed: (1) Is the renal failure acute or chronic? (2) If acute, is it prerenal, parenchymal or postrenal? (3) If parenchymal, what are the possible causes?

The various categories of disease causing parenchymal ARF were considered and eliminated one by one mostly on the basis of the absence of highly sensitive clues in the history, physical examination, and laboratory features.

Dark scant urine that was positive for blood in the absence of RBCs, and a swollen leg in an unconscious patient were crucial clues in the solution of this problem. *(P.C.)*

Suggested Readings

Sillix DH, McDonald FD. Acute renal failure. Crit Care Clin 1987;3(4):909–925.

Wagener OE, Lieske JC, Toback FG. Molecular and cell biology of acute renal failure: New therapeutic strategies. New Horiz 1995;3(4):634–649.

Woodrow G, Brownjohn AM, Turney JH. The clinical and biochemical features of acute renal failure due to rhabdomyolysis. Ren Fail 1995;17(4):467–474.

CASE 60

NAUSEA, WEAKNESS, CONFUSION

Paul Cutler

Data The patient is a 58-year-old woman who has not felt well for more than a year, but has refused to see a physician. She was brought to the emergency department in a semi-stuporous confused state. A close friend provided the history. The patient has had progressive lassitude, weakness, confusion, depression, and torpor for many months.

Logic At this point many possibilities enter your mind. A progressive downhill course in a person this age suggests uremia, brain tumor, carcinomatosis, cirrhosis, chronic brain syndrome, drug abuse, alcoholism, or diabetic ketoacidosis.

Data In the past month she had anorexia, nausea, vomiting, and weight loss. More recently, itching and scratching of the skin, twitching motions around the face, and deep rapid breathing were noted. No further history is available.

Logic The possibilities are narrowing. In carcinoma, you would expect the gastrointestinal symptoms to precede or coincide with the downhill course; the reverse occurred here. The absence of both excessive thirst and frequent urination would refute diabetic ketoacidosis, although those symptoms might have been present but unnoticed by the friend.

Itching of the skin could be caused by: jaundice, uremia, lymphoma, skin diseases, drug allergy, diabetes, and psychogenic disorders. Jaundice, if present, would be apparent and could be related to metastatic cancer or cirrhosis. The other causes would become evident as information is gathered.

Twitching facial movements sound like hypocalcemia, although a focal irritative brain lesion could cause them too. The heavy breathing is also not specific. It could result from uremic acidosis, diabetic ketoacidosis, superimposed pleural effusion, pneumonia, or congestive heart failure. Weight loss is no mystery when there is anorexia, nausea, and vomiting.

So far, we have a patient with a 1-year downhill course, whose seven symptoms have appeared in the following order: weakness, nausea and vomiting, weight loss, itching, twitching, confusion, and heavy breathing. Although uremia seems to be the most likely common denominator, other possibilities must be ruled out.

The basic problem in chronic renal failure and resultant uremia is *loss of nephrons.* Two million nephrons at birth diminish to 1 million by age 50 to 60. When kidney disease reduces nephron numbers to 400,000 or less, the glomerular filtration rate and creatinine clearance fall to approximately one fourth to one third of normal. At this point, the adaptive mechanisms of the kidney can no longer maintain homeostasis, and the clinical picture of uremia begins.

Simply put, the purpose of the kidneys is to (1) eliminate metabolic waste products (30 g of solute per day); (2) secrete hormones (erythropoietin, renin, vitamin D analogue, prostaglandins, kallikrein-kinins); (3) maintain blood osmolality and blood volume; (4) regulate the concentration of electrolytes; and (5) govern acid-base balance.

When these regulatory functions are compromised or lost, most body organs are affected and profound changes occur. First, there is retention of nitrogen wastes and toxins. Blood volume expands but is easily depletable. Sodium concentration can fall; potassium may decrease or terminally increase; phosphates and acids are retained; and metabolic acidosis with Kussmaul's breathing may ensue. As phosphates are retained, serum calcium decreases, resulting in excessive secretion of parathyroid hormone (secondary hyperparathyroidism) and renal osteodystrophy. This is abetted by decreased absorption of calcium from the gut resulting from the inability of the kidney to convert vitamin D to 1,25-dihydroxy vitamin D_3, its active analogue.

Other derangements occur. Anemia results from the toxic depression of bone marrow, diminished formation of erythropoietin, shortened red cell survival (hemolysis), and frequent gastrointestinal bleeding; the anemia is usually normochromic and normocytic. Platelet function is impaired.

Hypertension is almost invariably present. It results from volume overload, excessive secretion of renin (renin → angiotensin → aldosterone), and other yet postulated mechanisms. As kidney function becomes further impaired, sodium as well as water is retained, thus contributing to the edema of concomitant congestive heart failure—a very common complication. Acute fibrinous pericarditis is also frequently seen as a complication of uremia. It is interesting to note that long-standing essential hypertension is the commonest cause of renal failure and uremia by virtue of the resultant arteriolar nephrosclerosis; yet all forms of kidney disease that progress to renal failure and uremia are causes of secondary hypertension. Hypertension and kidney disease have a mutually reciprocal cause-and-effect relationship.

Carbohydrate tolerance diminishes, and the liver produces increased triglycerides. In the central nervous system you see lethargy, impaired mentation, asterixis, seizures, and coma. The skin demonstrates pallor, urochrome pigment deposition, uremic frost, pruritus, and ecchymoses (from a coagulopathy). Anorexia, nausea, vomiting, ulcers, and bleeding are manifestations of gastrointestinal tract affliction. The breath is ammoniacal. Peripheral neuropathies are common and the chest radiograph often shows "uremic lungs" (perihilar hazy congestion) and cardiac hypertrophy.

These are the origins of the symptoms, signs, and paraclinical findings in chronic renal failure. And as you proceed to gather more information about the patient, the entire gamut of metabolic derangements must be kept in mind.

Data Physical examination reveals a dehydrated, pale, cachectic, unresponsive woman. Longitudinal scratch marks are noted all over the skin of the arms, legs, and anterior trunk. There is no jaundice, but the skin has a slightly yellow waxy cast. The BP is 220/120; pulse is 88; respirations 24 and deep; and temperature 37°C.

Logic Dehydration would be expected in a patient with vomiting and stupor who has no access to fluids. The scratch marks are only on accessible areas. Severe hypertension is present. The deep, somewhat rapid breathing suggests Kussmaul's respirations seen in severe metabolic acidosis from any cause. Retained chromogens cause the yellowish skin. Uremia becomes more likely.

Data The breath has a strong ammoniacal odor and white powdery material is noted over the face and hair roots. Tapping of the facial nerve in front of the tragus causes twitching movements of the corner of the mouth and adjacent cheek. The conjunctiva and skin are very pale.

Logic The uremic syndrome now appears definite. Uremic frost is present; it represents excretion by the skin of those waste products that are normally eliminated by the kidneys. The odor of the breath is unmistakable. It results from the breakdown of urea in saliva to NH_3. A positive Chvostek's sign in this instance represents probable hypocalcemia, even though this sign can also be seen in alkalosis and occasionally in normal persons. But you would not expect alkalosis in this clinical situation. Furthermore, the pallor is also part of the picture of renal failure (Fig. 17.6).

It is important to note that tetany and a positive Chvostek's sign are *uncommon* in uremia even though the serum calcium is low. The critical factor for these signs is the amount of *ionized* calcium. Acidosis favors ionization and alkalosis

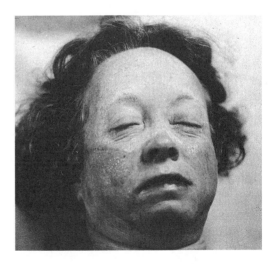

▶ **Figure 17.6.** Uremic patient. Note semistupor, pallor, and powdery uremic frost on face.

retards it. Thus, in other situations, you may see tetany with a normal serum calcium if alkalosis is present, and there may be no tetany, even in the presence of a low serum calcium level, if acidosis exists. Uremics develop tetany mainly if they are given large amounts of base to correct the acidosis.

Data Cervical veins are distended to the angles of the jaw with the patient lying at 45 degrees. Fine, moist end-inspiratory rales are heard at both bases. The apical impulse, strong and diffuse, is felt in the sixth intercostal space at the anterior axillary line. A grade 2/6 systolic ejection murmur is heard at the base of the heart, S_2 is loud, and a low-pitched sound is heard at the apex with the bell attachment approximately 0.15 second after S_2. Examination of the abdomen, rectum, genitalia, and extremities is normal.

Logic These findings indicate cardiac enlargement, left ventricular failure (loud S_2, S_3, and rales), and beginning right ventricular failure (distended neck veins). The failure results from hypertension that may be caused by the renal disease. Both cardiac and renal failure contribute to the deep rapid breathing. Valuable negative information is obtained. Liver disease is ruled out; the fact that the kidneys and prostate are not palpably enlarged will help to determine the cause for the patient's renal failure; the absence of hepatomegaly and leg edema tells you that right ventricular failure has only just begun. Note that congestive heart failure (CHF) can occur in the presence of dehydration.

Data Studies are as follows: hemoglobin, 8.5 g/dL; RBC count, 3 million per cubic millimeter; hematocrit, 25%; WBC count, 5800/mm^3; normal differential; urinalysis shows specific gravity 1.010, albumin +4, glucose and acetone absent, many fine and coarse granular casts, no RBCs, and no WBCs; urine culture negative; BUN, 230 mg/dL; creatinine, 16 mg/dL; glucose, 148 mg/dL; sodium, 128 mEq/L; potassium, 3.6 mEq/L; chloride, 85 mEq/L; bicarbonate, 12 mEq/L; pH, 7.2; calcium, 5.4 mg/dL; phosphorus, 5.6 mg/dL; ECG shows left ventricular hypertrophy with prolongation of the QT interval and ST segment; and chest radiograph shows cardiac enlargement and pulmonary congestion.

Logic The ECG and chest radiographic findings are what you would expect in a patient with uremia, hypertension, and CHF. The heart is enlarged and strained, the lungs are congested, and there is ECG evidence of hypocalcemia—prolonged QT interval and broad ST segment. Retention of phosphates by the kidneys plus decreased absorption of calcium from the gut cause the low serum calcium. Normochromic anemia results in part from the decreased production of erythropoietin. The blood urea nitrogen and creatinine are proportionately markedly elevated and confirm the existence of renal azotemia and uremia—the main problem.

It is thought that the acidemia of the uremic syndrome is the cause of nausea, anorexia, vomiting, and Kussmaul's respirations. However, the precise chemical, toxin, poison or poisons, that causes many other clinical manifestations (neuropathy, muscular disturbances, pericarditis, dermatologic changes, pruritus, and hematologic and immunologic disturbances) remains obscure.

Urine abnormalities indicate severe renal disease affecting the glomerulus and tubule. Low serum sodium stems from diminished intake, excessive vomiting, and defective tubular reabsorption. In other patients, injudicious salt restriction by the physician may be a contributing factor. Acidosis in chronic renal failure is caused by an impaired tubular mechanism for the excretion of acids, retention of sulfates and phosphates, loss of bicarbonate, and inability to form ammonia and conserve sodium. The elevated glucose level should be rechecked.

So far, there are four problems:

1. Chronic renal failure
2. Hypertension (secondary to 1)
3. CHF (secondary to 2)
4. Hyperglycemia

Uremia is well established by the symptoms, signs, and laboratory tests. Still to be determined is the specific renal disease causing renal failure. First, the hypertension and CHF need immediate treatment; digitalis, diuretics, and antihypertensive drugs must be especially carefully administered in the presence of uremia. Fluids and electrolytes need judicious juggling because the patient has dehydration and hyponatremia side by side with CHF; dialysis may be of great value.

Once treatment of CHF is begun, further thought can be given to the cause of chronic renal failure in this age group (Table 17.6).

TABLE 17.6. Common Causes of Chronic Renal Failure[a]

Essential hypertension and nephrosclerosis

Diabetes mellitus

Chronic glomerulonephritis

Chronic tubulo-interstitial nephritis

Chronic pyelonephritis

Obstructive uropathy with hydronephroses

Systemic lupus erythematosus

Polycystic kidneys

Analgesic abuse

[a]In approximate order of frequency.

Data Repeat studies confirm all the previous blood chemistry test results, except for several glucose determinations that are now normal. Plain radiograph of the abdomen shows easily defined kidney shadows that are much smaller than normal for this woman's size; no calculi are seen. So far as can be determined by history, discussion with friends, and checking the patient's apartment, there has been no analgesic abuse.

Logic The patient does not have diabetes, but it is interesting to note that mild glucose intolerance is commonly seen in advanced uremia. Conversely, if a known diabetic develops renal failure, the glucose tolerance may improve.

Kidney size serves to divide cases of chronic renal failure into those where kidneys are small because of tissue loss and fibrosis (arteriolar nephrosclerosis, glomerulonephritis, tubulo-interstitial nephritis, and chronic pyelonephritis), and those where kidneys are enlarged (hydronephrosis and polycystic disease). The small kidneys in this case point to the former and eliminate the latter.

The negative urine culture and the absence of WBCs and WBC casts in the urine rebut pyelonephritis. Systemic lupus erythematosus and diabetes are not considered causes for renal failure in this patient because tests disprove diabetes and other clinical features of systemic lupus erythematosus are not present.

Because the remaining diagnostic possibilities—glomerulonephritis and tubulo-interstitial nephritis—consist of a diverse group of diseases, some of which may benefit from steroids, a renal biopsy might be considered. But in the presence of markedly contracted kidneys, this degree of renal insufficiency with a chronic course, and the associated heart failure, a biopsy is not advisable in this case. Although arteriolar nephrosclerosis from long-standing hypertension is a viable diagnosis, a biopsy will not alter management. The possibility of finding a renal lesion that would respond to therapy is negligible in this setting and the microscopic appearance of an end-stage kidney may not permit etiologic definition.

Dialysis and eventual transplantation must be seriously considered.

Questions

1. Other physical findings commonly observed in end-stage kidney disease include all the following except one:
   (a) hyperactive reflexes.
   (b) ecchymoses.
   (c) abnormal fundi.
   (d) pericardial friction rub.
2. If the patient were male, and if the abdominal radiograph had shown large kidneys, all the following possibilities would have needed consideration except:
   (a) polycystic kidneys.
   (b) hydronephroses caused by prostatic obstruction.
   (c) hydronephroses caused by retroperitoneal fibrosis.
   (d) acute tubular necrosis.
3. The severe hypertension so often seen in patients with advanced bilateral kidney disease is:
   (a) caused by the kidney disease.
   (b) the cause of the kidney disease.
   (c) the result of hyperreninemia.
   (d) the result of abnormal sodium and water retention.

Answers

1. **(a) is not found.** Uremics may develop a peripheral neuropathy, first sensory and later motor; reflexes may be diminished. Choices (b), (c), and (d) could be expected because bleeding tendencies are common in uremia; the fundi usually show evidence of hypertension and renal disease (exudates, hemorrhages, arteriolar narrowing, and arteriovenous nicking); and a fibrinous pericarditis producing a friction rub is common.
2. **(d) is correct** because it does not fit the picture. Acute tubular necrosis is an acute disease characterized by nausea, vomiting, and oliguria or anuria. It has a recognizable cause (e.g., shock, sepsis, poison, or toxin); is rapid in onset; and does not cause large kidneys. The

other answers are all possible. Prostatic obstruction with big kidneys can exist in the presence of a large median lobe that may not be palpable on rectal examination, but the patient would also have symptoms of prostatic obstruction. Periureteral retroperitoneal fibrosis with hydronephroses usually has no demonstrable cause, although methysergide, used for vascular headaches, is a known offender.

3. **All are correct.** Long-standing severe hypertension can cause arteriolar nephrosclerosis. The reverse is also true; chronic kidney disease may cause hypertension. When it does, it is by either of two methods: 80% of patients who have end-stage renal disease have volume-dependent hypertension that is related to abnormal sodium and water retention; the remaining 20% have hyperreninemia.

COMMENT The presentation was not specific. It was necessary to cull the body systems for diseases that have a presentation of a downhill course plus cerebral and gastrointestinal manifestations. Pattern building established a cluster that indicated uremia, and thus the diseased organ was quickly pinpointed. The sequence whereby the downhill course preceded the other features tended to rule out primary brain or gastrointestinal disease.

The presence of CHF complicated the picture somewhat. A vicious circle of cause and effect was established whereby chronic renal failure (CRF) caused hypertension and then CHF, which in turn worsened the renal failure by decreasing renal blood flow. Furthermore, CRF caused nausea and vomiting, which further worsened the CRF by virtue of dehydration and decreased renal blood flow. Simpler cause-and-effect relationships were profusely used to explain the various findings in uremia.

The common causes for CRF in this age group were considered, and most were easily excluded on a clinical basis. Although a biopsy (essentially 100% sensitive and 100% specific) might define the precise histopathology, it was not considered necessary or valuable in this instance. Indeed, it might very well have revealed a multiplicity of pathologic processes going on at the same time.

Statistics for the causes of CRF vary, but for practical purposes the following estimates are acceptable. One fourth are caused by interstitial-tubular diseases (analgesics, pyelonephritis, polycystic disease, urate deposits, and obstructive uropathy); one fourth by vascular disease (nephrosclerosis); one fifth by systemic disease (diabetes, systemic lupus erythematosus, multiple myeloma, and so forth); one fifth by forms of glomerulonephritis; and the rest have unknown causes. Remember that in many instances a biopsy or autopsy in CRF shows mixed disease. For example, a diabetic patient with CRF may exhibit intercapillary glomerulosclerosis, arterial nephrosclerosis, arteriolar nephrosclerosis, and chronic pyelonephritis on microscopic examination. So too for other situations.

The mode of presentation for patients with CRF must be mentioned. Often evidence of diminished renal function is accidentally detected by routine screening of patients who have other primary problems. In some instances the patient sees the doctor for the early symptoms of CRF—for example, fatigue, weakness, pruritus, nausea and vomiting, hiccoughs, and so forth. On occasion the function of barely compensating kidneys is markedly worsened by an intercurrent event such as myocardial infarction. It is uncommon for patients to present with florid uremia as this patient did. *(P.C.)*

Suggested Readings

Friedman EA. Facing the reality: The world cannot afford uremia therapy at the start of the 21st century. Artif Organs 1995;19(5):481–485.

Harnett JD, Parfrey PS. Cardiac disease in uremia. Semin Nephrol 1994;14(3):245–252.

Ismail N, Becker BN. Treatment options and strategies in uremia: Current trends and future directions. Semin Nephrol 1994;14(3):282–299.

Price SR, Mitch WE. Metabolic acidosis and uremic toxicity: Protein and amino acid metabolism. Semin Nephrol 1994;14(3):232–237.

Renal and Electrolyte Problems
B: Electrolyte Problems

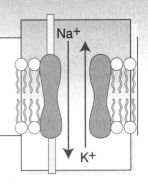

It is with reservation that a separate introduction is devoted to electrolyte disorder, because these are not diseases in themselves. They are syndromic manifestations of endocrine, renal, gastrointestinal, or brain diseases, or the result of injudicious treatment of cardiac, renal, or liver diseases.

Yet derangements of electrolytes cause profound clinical disturbances—even death. When an electrolyte disturbance occurs and is detected, finding its cause often requires careful investigation, and problem solving enters the picture.

These are usually complex situations, because an electrolyte disturbance depends on a balance between intake and output; the ratio of the total body electrolyte to total body water; numerous control mechanisms (antidiuretic hormone, renal function, aldosterone); iatrogenic factors (e.g., salt-restricted diets and potent diuretics); and so forth.

Water balance (dehydration and overhydration) and blood pH (acidosis and alkalosis) are integral parts of the subject of electrolyte disorders, because they often go hand in hand. Sodium and water disorders usually accompany each other; sodium depletion is always relative to the amount of water on board. Serum sodium concentration reflects the relative proportions of sodium and water in the serum, not the absolute amount of sodium in the body. The same can be said for potassium. Thus, either hyponatremia, hypernatremia, hypokalemia, or hyperkalemia can occur when the total body sodium or potassium content is decreased, normal, or increased.

Calcium, sodium, potassium, and magnesium are the principal cations, whereas phosphate, chloride, and bicarbonate are the principal anions associated with metabolic electrolyte disturbances. Of these, decreased or increased serum concentrations of calcium, sodium, and potassium give us the most concern.

You must bear in mind the fact that these disorders are frequently unnoticed; they occur in the course of other diseases and may be overshadowed by the prime problem. Furthermore, the manifestations of the electrolyte disturbance are often not very different from what you would expect in the natural course of the underlying disease. Hypopotassemia causes weakness, neuromuscular disturbances, cardiac arrhythmias, and death—what you might expect in a terminal cardiac patient who did not have a low serum potassium that was induced by potent diuresis. In addition, because the patient is taking digitalis, he or she is even more susceptible to arrhythmias that might be caused by the underlying heart disease.

Thus, the patient with severe advanced congestive heart failure may die seemingly from his heart disease unless severe hyponatremia can be distinguished and extracted from a backdrop of cardiac findings. Similarly, the patient with cancer of the kidney may die of uremia caused not by the malignancy but by an associated hypercalcemia. After all, would you not expect a cancer patient to die with nausea, vomiting, obtundation, and uremia?—all manifestations of hypercalcemia too!

Unless the physician is alert, an electrolyte disturbance may deliver the *coup de grace*—nobody being the wiser, even at the autopsy table! If you are aware of the possible derangements, then the electrocardiogram (ECG), serum and urine electrolyte concentrations, and serum and urine osmolality are accurate measuring tools. Even if you are not alert, the common use of batteries of chemical studies may call these problems to your attention—provided you carefully read the laboratory reports on the chart. *(P.C.)*

CASE 61

FATIGUE AND ABNORMAL ECG

Paul Cutler

Data You have been asked to cover another physician's practice for the weekend. Upon arriving at his office on a Saturday morning, the nurse gives you an ECG to evaluate. The patient from whom the ECG was obtained, a 24-year-old woman, had seen the doctor the day before, complaining of overwhelming fatigue and weakness so severe that she could hardly move. He felt that the complaint had a psychoneurotic basis, but in order to be sure he performed a complete examination and found nothing wrong other than what he thought were minor nonspecific ECG changes. The nurse further tells you that the patient is coming in shortly because she feels even worse than she did the day before.

As you review the ECG, you notice that it is unremarkable except for depression of the ST segments, lowering of the amplitude of the T waves, and a marked increase in the U waves, particularly in leads V_2 and V_3. The QT is markedly prolonged (0.68 second), and the heart rate is 72 beats per minute (Fig. 17.7).

Logic The amplitude of the U wave may be increased by certain drugs such as epinephrine or digitalis, or in patients with ventricular hypertrophy, bradycardia, or hyperthyroidism. But its association with hypokalemia is most noteworthy, especially in the absence of ECG evidence for the other conditions mentioned. The heart rate is neither abnormally fast nor slow. At this point, further historical information and data from the physical examination and plasma electrolytes must be obtained.

It is important to note the distinction between the ST-T changes caused by hypokalemia and hypocalcemia (Fig. 17.8).

Data The patient appears to be quite nervous and occasionally cries, and it is difficult to obtain a reliable history. She claims to have been in reasonably good health until 2 weeks before admission when she noted that she was tiring more easily than usual. In addition, she has had sleep disturbance and bouts of spontaneous weeping.

Logic At this point, inasmuch as you expect her to have hypokalemia, history regarding entities causing hypokalemia should be obtained. Table 17.7 classifies hypokalemic disorders and separates them into those caused by inadequate

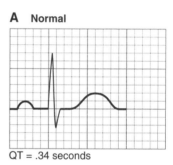

A   Normal

QT = .34 seconds

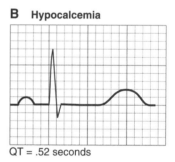

B   Hypocalcemia

QT = .52 seconds

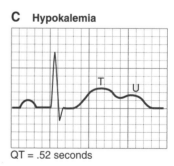

C   Hypokalemia

QT = .52 seconds

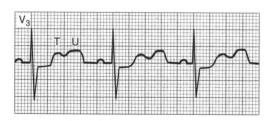

▶ **Figure 17.7.** Hypokalemia: depressed ST segments; prolonged QT interval (.68 seconds); and wide T-U complex, which are most notable in leads V_2 and V_3.

▶ **Figure 17.8.** Both B and C have a prolonged QT, but in B the prolongation is due to a wide ST segment, whereas in C the prolongation results from a U wave superimposed on the tail of the T wave.

TABLE 17.7. Classification of Hypokalemic Disorders

Inadequate dietary intake

Excessive renal loss

  Diuretics

  Mineralocorticoid excess

    Primary aldosteronism

      Adenoma

      Bilateral hyperplasia

    Cushing's syndrome or disease

      Primary adrenal disease

      Pituitary tumor

      Secondary to nonendocrine tumor

      Exogenous steroid administration

    Accelerated hypertension

    Renovascular hypertension

    Renin-producing tumor

    Adrenogenital syndrome

    Licorice excess

  Bartter's syndrome

  Liddle's syndrome

  Renal tubular acidosis

  Metabolic alkalosis

  Acute hyperventilation

  Starvation

  Ureterosigmoidostomy

  Antibiotics—carbenicillin, amphotericin, gentamicin

  Diabetic ketoacidosis

  Acute leukemia

Extrarenal loss

  Vomiting

  Diarrhea from various causes

  Chronic laxative abuse

  Villous adenoma

  Enterocutaneous fistulae

  Biliary fistulae

  Profuse sweating

Intracellular shift

  Alkalosis

  Periodic paralysis

  Barium poisoning

  Insulin administration

dietary intake, excessive renal loss, extrarenal loss, and intracellular shift.

Knowledge of these disorders cannot be completely obtained by history. Yet information about a number of them can be derived, particularly those relating to gastrointestinal losses of potassium and the use of diuretics. Some common causes of hypokalemia include gastrointestinal losses, vigorous diuretic treatment, and the presence of mineralocorticoid excess. The universal use of diuretics for hypertension and congestive heart failure probably represents by far the most common cause of this electrolyte disturbance.

Frequently the manifestations of an electrolyte disorder are not well defined, and you become aware of a disturbance only after obtaining routine electrolyte determinations. Yet certain clinical entities are so frequently the cause of electrolyte disturbances that you must constantly bear the possibility in mind when these clinical situations are encountered.

Data Further careful questioning of the patient was fruitless. She denied any gastrointestinal disturbances, drug usage, or hypertension. The remainder of the systems review was likewise negative. Her social history indicated that she had moved to the city from a small town in order to obtain a job, and she lived alone in a one-bedroom apartment. She neither drank nor smoked. Her family history was noncontributory.

The physical examination revealed an overweight young woman (60 inches tall, 154 lb) who, although not in acute distress, was crying intermittently. Vital signs were: Blood pressure, (BP) 110/70 without postural change; pulse, 70; respirations, 16; and temperature, 37°C. Examination of the head, eyes, ears, nose, throat, chest, heart, abdomen, rectum, and pelvis was normal or negative. Muscle strength was possibly diminished although there was some question as to her cooperation. The neurologic examination findings were normal. The patient was oriented to time, place, and person and has had no hallucinations or paranoid ideation.

Logic You are provided little positive information by the patient, but important negative data have been obtained. Her weight excludes starvation as a cause of the suspected hypokalemia. Likewise, she was not clinically hyperventilating and did not have hypertension. These negative clues are important because alkalosis causes potassium loss into the cells and out in the urine, and hypertensive diseases caused by corticoid excess have low potassium levels. Reflexes may be diminished or normal in hypokalemia.

While waiting for the blood electrolyte profile to return, you ponder the pathophysiology of hypokalemia. Potassium homeostatic mechanisms maintain a normal serum level between 3.8 and 5.0 mEq/L. These regulatory tools consist mainly of aldosterone and renal function, although insulin, glucagon, and the sympathetic nervous system play minor roles. As for potassium, the human body contains 50 to 55 mEq/kg; most is intracellular, and only 2% is extracellular; daily dietary intake is 50 to 100 mEq. Generally speaking, the amount absorbed each day equals the amount excreted by the kidney. Losses in the sweat and stool are small. Unfortunately, the renal mechanism for *conserving* potassium is inefficient, and severe gastrointestinal potassium loss may therefore rapidly produce serious hypokalemia. Between 200 and 300 mEq of loss lowers the serum potassium by 1 mEq/L.

Data The laboratory data have returned. The plasma electrolytes are (in mEq/L): Na^+ 131; Cl^- 90; HCO_3^- 33; and K^+ 2.1. Normal values are: Na^+ 135 to 145; Cl^- 98 to 106; HCO_3^- 21 to 28; and K^+ 3.5 to 5.0. The patient has marked hypokalemia; the plasma Na^+ concentration is modestly depressed, and the plasma HCO_3^- level is elevated. The blood pH is 7.50. A complete blood count and urinalysis are both normal.

Logic These data confirm your initial impressions of hypokalemia. The cause is still unknown. Consider the scheme shown in Figure 17.9 as a means to aid in your diagnosis.

You have already excluded those conditions associated with both hypokalemia and hypertension because the patient is normotensive. The slightly alkalotic blood pH and elevated plasma HCO_3^- are consistent with a metabolic alkalosis. As shown in Figure 17.9, a 24-hour urine test for K^+ determination would be helpful. If K^+ excretion exceeds 20 to 30 mEq/24 h with this degree of hypokalemia, renal losses are excessive, and a search should be made for more factors that accelerate renal K^+ loss.★ If excretion is less, then the hypokalemia is due to other mechanisms that are listed in the table.

★Depending on the duration of the hypokalemia, excessive renal loss is suggested by a spot urine sample with a K^+ concentration greater than 20 mEq/L.

Data A 24-hour urine collection is sent to the laboratory for determination of the K^+ concentration, and the result returns 1 day later: 120 mEq/d. The patient's mother, who had arrived from another city to stay with her, confirmed that she had noted no vomiting or diarrhea over the weekend, although she had not eaten well.

Logic This urinary K^+ excretion is excessively high. Returning once again to the schematic outline, six diagnoses are to be seriously considered with this constellation of findings.

Bartter's syndrome is highly unlikely. The manifestations of this recessive inherited disorder begin in childhood and it is characterized by excessive loss of K^+ and Mg^{++} in the urine, episodes of weakness, and retarded growth. It is caused by excessive secretion of renin from the juxtaglomerular apparatus, resulting in hyperaldosteronism.

Although she denies it, repeated self-induced vomiting remains a consideration. A diagnosis of acute hyperventilation is inconsistent with the plasma HCO_3^+ concentration. Acute leukemia seems unlikely on the basis of the physical examination and blood count; its mechanism for lowering the serum K^+ is unknown. She has not taken any antibiotics; furthermore, all antibiotics listed in Table 17.7 are administered parenterally and are therefore unlikely candidates.

Surreptitious drug use appears to be a likely consideration. Diuretic therapy seems very likely; she may still be taking a diuretic, and even if she is not, its effects may continue for 48 hours after cessation.

Data The patient was again questioned regarding possible causes for hypokalemia. When confronted with the findings that suggested excessive urinary K^+ loss, possibly due to diuretics, she admitted that she had begun diuretic use 2 months ago in an effort to lose weight. The mild hyponatremia also resulted from diuretic abuse. She had a job as a waitress in a pharmacy and had access to the drug. She had become lonely since she left home and was hoping to make herself more attractive by losing weight. The patient was begun on KCl therapy and a psychiatric consultation was requested.

Logic Hypokalemia may have a number of adverse consequences. For example, cardiac effects include electrocardiographic changes indicating abnormal repolarization, predisposition to digitalis tox-

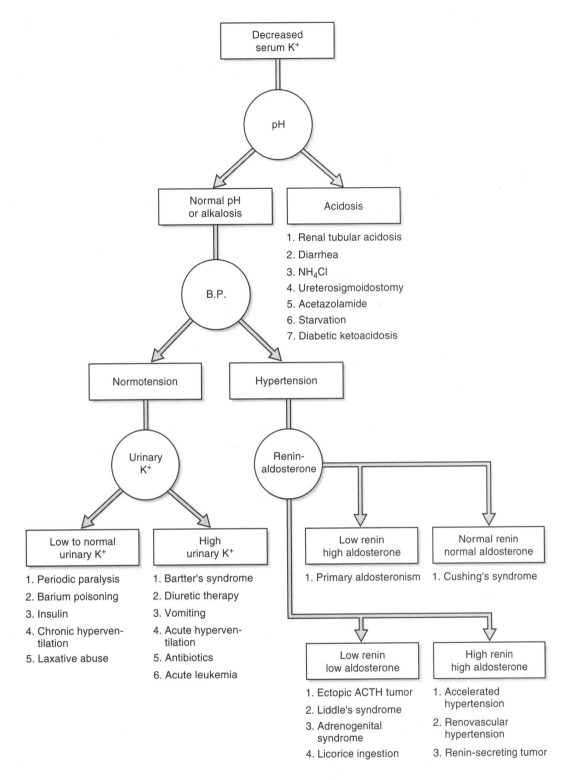

▶ **Figure 17.9.** Scheme for diagnosing the causes of hypopotassemia.

icity, arrhythmias, and, in sudden severe cases, cardiac arrest.

Profound skeletal muscle weakness may be present and sometimes results in paralysis. Renal functional impairment is frequently seen as a *result* of hypokalemia; a decrease in concentrating ability is the most common finding. The potassium level at which disturbances occur is variable, but levels of 2.5 mEq/L or below are dangerous and require attention.

Questions

1. The two major causes of hypokalemia in the patient who has persistent vomiting are:
   (a) loss of potassium in the vomitus.
   (b) movement of potassium into cells.
   (c) loss of potassium in the urine.
   (d) inadequate dietary intake of potassium because of the persistent vomiting.
2. Which of the following are important consequences of hypokalemia?
   (a) Hypoglycemia
   (b) Intestinal hypomotility
   (c) Glucose intolerance
   (d) Muscle weakness
3. Prevention of hypokalemia is particularly essential for patients:
   (a) receiving drugs that accelerate potassium loss.
   (b) receiving digitalis compounds.
   (c) receiving anti-aldosterone medication.
   (d) receiving triamterene for diuresis.
4. Hyperkalemia is even more dangerous than hypokalemia. It can result from:
   (a) the terminal phase of chronic renal failure.
   (b) use of oral potassium in the presence of renal failure.
   (c) Addison's disease.
   (d) immediate use of intravenous potassium in the patient with diabetic coma.

Answers

1. **(b) and (c) are correct.** Although the patient with persistent vomiting loses potassium in gastric juices, the shift of potassium into cells and the urinary loss of potassium, both caused by the associated metabolic alkalosis, are the major causes of hypokalemia in this circumstance.
2. **(b), (c), and (d) are correct.** Intestinal hypomotility and muscle weakness are both well-known effects of

hypokalemia on the smooth and skeletal muscle, respectively. Despite much investigation, the cause is still unclear. Glucose intolerance in the hypokalemic patient results from an impairment of insulin release. Hypoglycemia does not occur.
3. **(a) and (b) are correct.** Diuretics commonly cause hypokalemia in patients with congestive heart failure and cirrhosis of the liver, but not so commonly in ordinary hypertensives. Thus, supplementary potassium is sometimes used in the former. Patients taking digitalis should be watched closely because hypokalemia enhances the potential for digitalis intoxication. Anti-aldosterone medications induce potassium retention, as does triamterene (and also amiloride).
4. **All are correct.** Terminal anuria will cause potassium to rise. Ingestion of oral potassium in a patient who has renal failure may be dangerous; the regulation of potassium excretion does not take place quickly enough. Addison's disease is a hypocorticoid state in which sodium is lost, and potassium is retained. In diabetic coma, even though the total body potassium is depleted, the serum potassium may be low, normal, or high. If given immediately, potassium supplementation may be lethal. Wait until treatment is well under way and potassium is reentering the cells. Then give it orally.

COMMENT A broad knowledge of pathophysiology and an understanding of cause and effect relationships were needed to solve this one. The key clue (hypokalemia) was recognized from the beginning, and the author pursued a self-constructed flowchart as he gathered bits of evidence and arrived at only one possible conclusion. Note that only a few decision points (pH, blood pressure, potassium excretion) were needed to direct him to the terminal branch, where the final twig (diuretic abuse) was found. The author probably had a hunch about what was wrong. This was a healthy but unhappy obese patient who had easy access to oral drugs. *(P.C.)*

PROBLEM-BASED LEARNING Self-education referable to disorders of potassium homeostasis obliges you to cross many modular boundaries. Potassium disturbances occur in gastrointestinal, renal, endocrine, cardiac, and pulmonary diseases—and indeed in any disease requiring treatment with drugs that can effect potassium kinetics. You should learn about:

- Potassium metabolism: its intake, output, distribution, and regulatory mechanisms
- The broad classification of disorders causing disturbances in potassium homeostasis (Table 17.7)
- The clinical features of each disease in that table
- The special roles of diuretics, diabetic ketoacidosis, and diarrheal states
- The effect of steroids and high-steroid states
- How alkalosis and acidosis affect potassium distribution
- Cushing's syndrome, Conn's syndrome, Bartter's syndrome, and Liddle's syndrome
- Symptoms and signs of hypokalemia
- ECG manifestations of both hypo- and hyperkalemia
- Disastrous effects of extremely low or high serum potassium levels
- Causes of hyperkalemia
- When to anticipate and how to manage hypokalemia and hyperkalemia

Suggested Readings

Bradberry SM, Vale JA. Disturbances of potassium homeostasis in poisoning. J Toxicol Clin Toxicol 1995;33(4):295–310.

Howes LG. Which drugs affect potassium? Drug Saf 1995;12(4):240–244.

Kamel KS, Quaggin S, Scheich A, et al. Disorders of potassium homeostasis: An approach based on pathophysiology. Am J Kidney Dis 1994;24(4):597–613.

Steigerwalt SP. Unraveling the causes of hypertension and hypokalemia. Hosp Pract (Off Ed) 1995;30(7): 67–71, 74–75, 79.

 CASE 62

WEAKNESS AND DISORIENTATION

Paul Cutler

Data A 68-year-old man was brought to the outpatient clinic by his wife because he had become disoriented. Although he had always been in excellent health, for the last month or so he had experienced persistent diffuse muscle weakness, lassitude, and "was not himself." Further careful questioning by the intern failed to reveal any significant additional pieces of information. He had had no previous hospitalizations and had recently retired from his position as an accountant. He denied the excessive use of tobacco, had only an occasional drink of alcohol, and took no drugs except for a daily multivitamin tablet. The family history was noncontributory.

On physical examination, the patient appeared his stated age, was well nourished, and was in no obvious distress. Vital signs were: BP, 120/82 with no postural change; pulse, 82; temperature, 37°C; respirations, 16. The skin was free of any lesions and normal in appearance. Examination of the head, eyes, ears, nose, and throat revealed normal findings. The chest was clear to auscultation and percussion. The cardiac, abdominal, and genital examination findings were normal. No evidence of clubbing, cyanosis, dehydration, or edema was demonstrable. There was no apparent muscle atrophy or tenderness. The neurologic examination was unremarkable except for the suggestion of generalized weakness. There was no evidence of focalized areas of weakness.

Logic The intern was puzzled by the chief complaint and the apparent absence of any clues that might suggest a fruitful area to investigate. Because of the history, he thought in terms of a small nonfocalizing cerebral thrombosis, subdural hematoma, brain tumor, generalized cancer, diabetes, uremia, or chronic brain syndrome, but there was nothing in the examination to suggest or confirm any of these. He requested laboratory tests to aid in the evaluation.

Data One hour later the following laboratory results were received: hemoglobin, 13 g/dL; hematocrit, 41%; white blood cell count, 9500/mm^3; differential normal; blood glucose, 90 mg/dL; electrolytes in mEq/L—Na$^+$ 115, Cl$^-$ 79, HCO$_3^-$ 22, K$^+$ 3.2; blood urea nitrogen, 8 mg/dL. Chest radiograph, ECG, and erythrocyte sedimentation rate were normal.

Logic These studies give strong evidence against the various possibilities that first occurred to the intern. Uremia and diabetes may be disregarded in view of the normal data thus far derived. Metastatic cancer appears unlikely because he looks well, and his examination findings are normal.

But the laboratory data are particularly notable for the marked hyponatremia and hypochloremia, mean normal values being Na^+ 140 and Cl^- 100 mEq/L. Is the degree of hyponatremia consistent with muscle weakness, fatigue, and disorientation?

The symptoms and signs of hyponatremia are dependent upon the cause, the magnitude, and the rapidity of onset of the condition. Symptoms include apathy, lethargy, weakness, nausea, vomiting, anorexia, agitation, and disorientation. Physical signs include depressed deep tendon reflexes, disorientation and other evidence of abnormal sensorium, hypothermia, pathologic reflexes, seizures, and coma. The neurologic manifestations usually do not appear until the plasma Na^+ is below 125 mEq/ L. Levels below 115 mEq/L are critical and can result in irreversible brain damage; the reduced plasma osmolality creates an osmotic gradient that favors movement of water into brain cells, which results in cerebral edema.

The diagnostic approach to the patient with hyponatremia should be undertaken with an understanding of the physiology of the renal concentrating and diluting mechanisms and of those factors that affect their function. In addition, the clinical conditions in which one observes hyponatremia should be appreciated. Table 17.8 lists clinical circumstances that may be associated with hyponatremia and a general comment regarding etiology.

It is important to note that the average human body contains 2000 mEq of sodium; that the normal serum sodium concentration varies from 138 to 144 mEq/L; that sodium and its associated anions contribute more than 90% of serum osmolality; that normal serum osmolality is 285 to 295 mOsm/kg H_2O; and that hyponatremia is one of the most commonly encountered electrolyte problems.

More important, the serum sodium concentration and serum osmolality are governed by a delicate interplay between thirst, diaphoresis, osmoreceptors that control the hypothalamic-posterior pituitary antidiuretic hormone axis, and the renal medullary countercurrent system that regulates sodium and water excretion and reabsorption. The management of sodium and water by the kidney depends mainly upon the concentration of antidiuretic hormone, sodium intake, extrarenal sodium loss, corticosteroids, and the kidney's functional integrity.

What laboratory tests might be of benefit?

TABLE 17.8. Classification of Hyponatremic States

Free water intake in excess of normal excretory ability: primary polydipsia
Free water intake in excess of depressed excretory ability
Decreased delivery to diluting segments
Decreased glomerular filtration rate
Volume depletion
Congestive heart failure
Hepatic cirrhosis with ascites
Nephrotic syndrome
Glucocorticoid deficiency
Myxedema?
Decreased solute absorption by diluting segments
Diuretics
Bartter's syndrome
Increased water permeability of diluting segments—vasopressin absent
Glucocorticoid deficiency
Increased water permeability of diluting segments—vasopressin present
Ectopic ADH production
Increased cerebral ADH production due to nonosmotic stimuli
Increased cerebral ADH production due to certain drugs

ADH = antidiuretic hormone.

Pseudohyponatremia may be present when a fall in plasma sodium concentration is not accompanied by a decrease in plasma osmolality. When this occurs, some molecule that does not diffuse freely across the cell membranes is present in the plasma in high concentrations. Glucose is most often responsible, although occasionally lipids and proteins also contribute. Thus, a measurement of the plasma osmolality may be of considerable value. In addition, insight into the state of the renal concentrating and diluting mechanisms can be gained by measurement of the urinary osmolality. Finally, as part of the initial evaluation, serum creatinine and urinary sodium concentrations are helpful, as will be discussed next.

Data The following laboratory results were obtained: plasma osmolality, 240 mOsm/kg H_2O;

urinary osmolality, 425 mOsm/kg; blood urea nitrogen (same as previously recorded); creatinine, 1.0 mg/dL; and urinary sodium concentration, 45 mEq/L.

Logic These values tell us that (1) the patient does not have pseudohyponatremia, (2) the urinary osmolality is inappropriately concentrated for the level of plasma osmolality, and (3) the urine sodium concentration does not suggest an active salt-retaining state.

Data You again return to the patient. How might you most profitably undertake an evaluation that will lead to the correct diagnosis? With the use of the scheme shown in Figure 17.10,

you can evaluate the patient who has true hyponatremia.

Logic As you proceed from the observation of the presence of hyponatremia, the chart shown in Figure 17.10 then separates the disorders into various categories, depending upon the relative state of the extracellular fluid (ECF) volume. The categorization of a particular patient depends upon information derived from the history and physical examination and certain critical laboratory tests that were previously mentioned.

The patient did not have renal insufficiency nor was he in a sodium-retaining state. Furthermore, he was not edematous, nor was any sug-

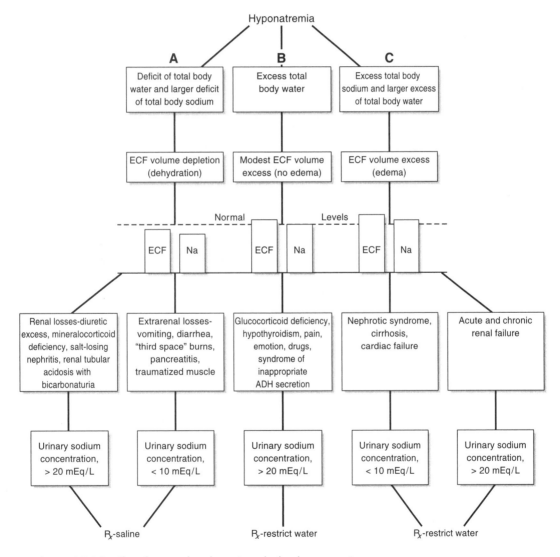

▶ **Figure 17.10.** Clinical approach to the patient who has hyponatremia.

gestion of ECF volume depletion noted, for example, postural hypotension, dehydration, or tachycardia. Thus, he would seem to fall into the middle category, that is, those patients who may have modest ECF volume excess but who are not edematous.

Several of the diagnosis considerations in this group can be reasonably excluded by the data currently available. No suggestion of hypothyroidism or altered emotional state was manifested by the patient's history or physical examination. There was no pain in the history and, as mentioned, except for multivitamins, he denied the use of drugs. Chlorpropamide, clofibrate, vincristine, thiazides, and tricyclic antidepressants may cause clinical pictures that fit this category. Although glucocorticoid deficiency (Addison's disease) cannot be definitely excluded, it seems unlikely without some of the usual stigmata, such as cutaneous and mucosal hyperpigmentation, arterial hypotension, and gastrointestinal complaints. Absolute exclusion of this possibility, however, would depend upon the appropriate measurement of steroid production.

Seemingly this patient would fit into the group of patients with a disorder known as the syndrome of inappropriate antidiuretic hormone production (SIADH). This syndrome, which can be diagnosed only in the presence of an otherwise intact diluting mechanism, is characterized by:

1. Hyponatremia and plasma hypo-osmolality
2. Urine that is less than appropriately dilute
3. Urine sodium excretion that parallels sodium intake
4. Absence of other causes of hyponatremia. (renal, adrenal, thyroid)

In normal people, changes in plasma osmolality are detected by osmoreceptors in the hypothalamus, which in turn controls thirst and the release of antidiuretic hormone (ADH) from the posterior pituitary gland. The normal function of ADH is to promote reabsorption of water from the distal tubule. SIADH is said to exist when, for a variety of mostly unexplained reasons, there is an excessive production of ADH by the posterior pituitary or from an ectopic source.

Table 17.9 lists the causes of this syndrome. Diagnostic considerations should include those studies required to investigate the various possi-

TABLE 17.9. Causes of the Syndrome of Inappropriate Antidiuretic Hormone Production

Malignancies
  Bronchogenic carcinoma
  Adenocarcinoma of pancreas and duodenum
  Carcinoma of ureter
  Lymphoma
  Thymoma
Pulmonary diseases
  Tuberculosis
  Pneumonia
  Aspergillosis with cavitation
  Lung abscess
  Chronic chest infection
Diseases of the central nervous system
  Acute psychoses
  Infections, e.g., encephalitis, meningitis, brain abscess
  Trauma
  Subarachnoid or subdural hemorrhage
  Guillain-Barré syndrome
  Brain tumor
  Systemic lupus erythematosus
  Acute intermittent porphyria
  Stroke

bilities. The relationship between SIADH and most of the causes listed is not entirely clear.

Data The patient was treated with fluid restriction, and his serum sodium level rose to normal levels. In the meantime, a search was made for a cause. A small retrocardiac pulmonary mass, overlooked on the previous chest radiograph, was found. There were no evidences of metastases. The mass was resected, and histologic study disclosed an oat cell (small cell) carcinoma of the lung. This cell type is known to secrete antidiuretic hormone-like substances, so the SIADH should disappear.

However, the prognosis for small cell carcinoma is not good. Most oncologists consider this a medical problem requiring chemotherapy. The disease is already widespread at the time of detection, and surgical resection is generally not curative. But only time will tell. . . .

Questions

1. A patient with severe congestive heart failure who is actively retaining sodium and who is hyponatremic (Na^+ = 128 mEq/L) would be expected to have:
   (a) urine appropriately hypo-osmotic.
   (b) urine hyperosmotic relative to plasma osmolality.
   (c) no reasonable conclusions drawn from the data.
   (d) a normal total body sodium.
2. Hyponatremia will develop in the patient who has SIADH:
   (a) because the amount of antidiuretic hormone present will result in renal sodium wasting.
   (b) but it is unusual unless sodium is restricted in the diet.
   (c) due to a marked increase in total body water and sodium, the amount of water retained being greater than the amount of sodium.
   (d) provided the patient has access to adequate amounts of water.
3. The plasma osmolality in a patient with a plasma sodium concentration of 143 mEq/L and a glucose of 1800 mg/dL is approximately:
   (a) 285 mEq/L.
   (b) 385 mEq/L.
   (c) 520 mEq/L.
   (d) 257 mEq/L.
4. A 38-year-old diabetic was taking an oral hypoglycemic agent for control of his hyperglycemia. Routine plasma electrolytes revealed a sodium level of 120 mEq/L. The blood sugar was normal, and the plasma was not grossly lipemic. Which of the following is most likely?
   (a) The patient has been ingesting too much water.
   (b) The patient very likely has diabetic nephropathy with an inability to appropriately dilute his urine.
   (c) The patient may be ingesting a hypoglycemic agent, chlorpropamide, which can cause water retention.
   (d) Diabetics are known to be profound salt wasters, and sodium depletion may contribute to the hyponatremia.

Answers

1. **(b) is correct.** For a number of reasons, patients who have both congestive heart failure and avid sodium retention cannot appropriately dilute their urine. Thus, the urine will be hypertonic to plasma. The presence of edema essentially always indicates an increase in total body sodium, regardless of the serum sodium level.
2. **(d) is correct.** Hyponatremia will occur only if the amount of water ingested exceeds insensible losses and the obligatory amount required to excrete the urinary solute load. If combined water loss equals the amount of water ingested, hyponatremia will not occur. Sodium excretion, retention, and ingestion are not related to the action of antidiuretic hormone or the SIADH.
3. **(b) is the correct answer** with the information provided. The osmolality can be estimated as two times the sodium concentration plus the contribution of the glucose. The latter can be determined by dividing the number of milligrams of glucose per liter by the molecular weight of glucose, which is 180. Thus, 18,000 ÷ 180 = 100 mOsm/kg H_2O. It is obvious that the glucose in milligrams per deciliter divided by 18 will provide the same answer. This patient is hyperosmolar.
4. **(c) is the most logical choice,** although others, particularly choices (a) and (b), deserve a second look. Chlorpropamide, like a number of other drugs, may impair the renal excretion of water. Choice (d) is not typical of diabetic patients.

COMMENT This presentation could have been caused by many different pathologic states, but a battery of laboratory tests led to the key clue—hyponatremia. A very few additional clinical findings and decision points limited the possible diagnoses to a small handful. SIADH became the obvious underlying pathophysiologic mechanism. A further search disclosed the cause of this syndrome—often not an easy task because of the strange assortment of unrelated diseases in which this syndrome is inexplicably found. *(P.C.)*

Suggested Readings

Spigset O, Hedenmalm K. Hyponatremia and the syndrome of inappropriate antidiuretic hormone secretion (SIADH) induced by psychotropic drugs. Drug Saf 1995;12(3)209–225.
Williams AV. Hyponatremia: Manifestations and treatment. JSC Med Assoc 1992;88(6):285–290.

CHAPTER

18

Gynecologic Problems

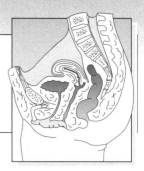

The gynecologist is faced not only with problems peculiar to his or her field but with all the problems of women. This is because he or she has developed the kind of interpersonal relationship that encourages patients to consult him or her for all matters—medical, family, social, and sexual.

After all, the gynecologist was the one who performed the first pelvic examination, discussed contraception, and delivered the children, so it is only natural that he or she should become the primary care physician for many women concerning any matter relating to their emotional or physical health. Such is the confidence and confidentiality that has ideally developed! Consequently, his or her knowledge base must rise far above the pelvis.

Because the field of gynecology revolves mainly around the reproductive organs, sex, pregnancy, and relationships with children and husband, it is logical that psychosomatic factors often play a large role in modifying or even being the reason for the patient's complaints.

Commonly seen problems are those relating to vaginal discharge, acute and chronic pelvic pain, menstrual abnormalities, vaginal bleeding, pregnancy, sexual intercourse, contraception, and menopause. In the case of bleeding, it may be because menses are late, absent, or long. As for pregnancy, the patient consults her physician because she is pregnant, because she fears she is pregnant, or because she is unable to become so. Various symptoms that may or may not be related to menopause can be the cause for the visit. Sexual problems may consist of painful intercourse, frigidity or the opposite state, inability to have an orgasm, or incompatibility.

Perhaps one of the most common reasons for visiting a gynecologist is the periodic checkup for cancer. This usually includes a pelvic and rectal examination, Papanicolaou (Pap) smear, examination of the breasts, and sometimes a com-

plete physical examination, including radiographs and laboratory tests. Indeed, if the gynecologist is the only physician the patient sees, all these procedures are in order.

Although vaginal discharge is one of the most frequent problems encountered, it requires only simple problem-solving skills. The answer should be obtainable by a pelvic examination, Pap smear, gonococcus smear and culture, and potassium hydroxide and wet drop preparations. More sophisticated techniques are needed to identify chlamydia and the human immunodeficiency virus.

As for problem solving in general, the pelvic examination usually provides the answer. However, because there is so often an overlap with endocrine problems, whereby pelvic organ disease can cause systemic endocrine effects, and endocrine disease can cause gynecologic symptoms, that the examination must often be more generalized.

Three more points! First, history taking is not routine and easy: tact, diplomacy, warmth, privacy, and confidentiality are crucial. Second, it is necessary to know what is "normal." This is particularly true for such items as vaginal discharge, the amount of pain with the menses, the amount of blood loss with each menstrual flow, the frequency of intercourse, and the duration of menopause. Last, the physician must always be alert for the presence of the most serious pelvic disease: cancer (cervix, endometrium, or ovary)—especially in women beyond the age of 30. (P.C.)

A MISSED MENSTRUAL PERIOD

Paul Cutler

Data A 42-year-old woman is concerned because her menstrual period is 3 weeks late. She had two full-term pregnancies with normal deliveries at ages 20 and 23. Until 3 years ago, she had successfully used oral contraceptives. At that time she was advised to use an alternative method because of beginning mild hypertension (148/90). She chose a diaphragm and jelly contraceptive that she had used early in her marriage, and now wears her diaphragm regularly with each coital encounter.

The patient's menses began at age 13, were always regular, and lasted 3 to 4 days without dysmenorrhea. The onset of amenorrhea was abrupt, was not preceded by a gradual decrease in amount or frequency of menstrual bleeding, and had never happened before.

Further history discloses recent insomnia, "more nervousness than usual," nighttime perspiration and occasional flushed feelings during the day. These symptoms have been pronounced since she missed her period, but she is unsure when they actually began. She takes no drugs or medications.

Logic When you first hear the chief complaint, a number of common possibilities immediately surface from your knowledge base. But before considering them you remember that absolute menstrual regularity is a rarity. Also, you know from experience that an occasional irregular or missed period usually has no significance, although it may cause profound anxiety.

Patients who are accustomed to absolute regularity may visit you if their menstruation is only 2 weeks late. Others who often miss one or more menstrual periods are not so readily concerned.

For starters, you consider pregnancy, premature menopause, persistent corpus luteum, and psychogenic amenorrhea. Secondary amenorrhea is defined as the cessation of menses after they have already started. One swallow does not make a summer, nor does one missed period fulfill the definition of secondary amenorrhea. Wait a few months and see.

In spite of the regular use of and prior success with mechanical contraception, pregnancy must still be a consideration. It is too early for symptoms or even for confirmation by pelvic examination (unless the pregnancy is tubal). However, pregnancy tests that measure β-human chorionic gonadotropin would now have positive results if the patient were pregnant.

Psychogenic factors are extremely common.

In some unknown way, they affect the hypothalamus, which regulates the release of gonadotropic hormones. Menstrual flow can begin prematurely or not at all. Acute psychologic stress, major or seemingly trivial, can temporarily alter menstrual regularity. Going away to college, getting married, vigorous dieting, an emotional upset, or mental distress of any sort can be implicated, although sometimes no obvious stress factor can be elicited. An acute transient organic illness may also cause a temporary menstrual derangement. Anorexia nervosa may halt the menses too. In our patient, the symptoms could be psychophysiologic, but so far there is no positive evidence for a psychogenic problem, and further questioning about the patient's psychosocial situation is indicated.

Although this patient takes no drugs, it is important to be aware of the fact that amenorrhea may be caused by major tranquilizers, psychotropics, heroin, possibly marijuana, cancer chemotherapy, and the cessation of oral contraceptives.

Premature menopause is less likely. The symptoms fit, but they came on rather suddenly and could be manifestations of anxiety. Also, in menopause the menses usually alter gradually in flow and frequency. They do not suddenly stop. And last, although premature menopause is not unheard of, it is unusual. The average age in our western civilization is 51 years. If hard pressed for a diagnosis, you might obtain a follicle-stimulating hormone level (FSH), because its level is elevated with the onset of menopause. But time and patience will tell the story. A persistent corpus luteum (Halban's syndrome) is another possibility. The pelvic examination could detect an adnexal mass, although a mass could also be a tubal pregnancy. In this instance, ultrasonography may add precision by determining whether the ovarian mass is cystic or solid.

Data Physical examination shows a normal-sized uterus and ovaries, no evidence of vaginal atrophy, no adnexal masses, and no cervical discoloration. The breasts are normal and do not show increased vascularity, engorgement, or Montgomery glands around the nipples. A careful search fails to find galactorrhea. In fact, the entire examination findings are normal. The blood pressure is now 118/60, so her prior pill-induced hypertension is resolved.

Logic There is no objective evidence of pregnancy or menopause, although it may be too early to see such evidence even if those conditions existed. A persistent corpus luteum cyst might be palpable.

The patient did not complain of a milky discharge from the nipples. But had this information been elicited on examination, consideration of the amenorrhea-galactorrhea syndrome would be indicated. This would require a search for a prolactinoma.

Data Careful delicate questioning reveals that she has recently been involved in an extramarital affair for the first time in her 24-year marriage. She states that she has used her diaphragm and contraceptive jelly regularly, but is upset about this continuing relationship and does not know how it will resolve vis-à-vis her marriage. While you were gathering your data base, your assistant performed a pregnancy test, the result of which is negative.

Logic You now have positive data to support a psychogenic reason for the missed period. Pregnancy is ruled out with reasonable certainty. The lack of physical evidence is against pregnancy, and a negative pregnancy test result at this time would be especially reliable if the urine is concentrated. Menopause, still a distant possibility, can be ruled out with time or an FSH level determination.

Data After a frank but tactful discussion with the patient, she is still not satisfied she is not pregnant. So you collect a sample of blood for FSH determination. You also give the patient an injection of 150 mg of progesterone in oil, although you could have given her 5 days of orally active progesterone. Several days later, she develops a bleeding episode similar to normal menstruation.

Logic This simple test induces progestin withdrawal and precludes pregnancy. But it is important to know that the "progesterone challenge test" may be used only after the possibility of pregnancy has been excluded. The test may cause congenital defects if a fetus is present; therefore, the Food and Drug Administration prohibits its use as a test for pregnancy.

In this case the test was used to convince a patient who needed reassurance; the physician was already sure. But in other instances the test can serve as an algorithmic divider in difficult diagnostic situations. Amenorrheic patients who respond with vaginal bleeding have adequate ovarian estrogen function; those who don't respond have poor ovarian estrogen production. Then proceed toward the diagnostic possibilities from this pathophysiologic separator.

Data The FSH test has returned and shows normal levels. Your assistant repeats the pregnancy test, and its result is again negative.

Logic Because the FSH level is high in early menopause, this possibility is excluded. Both you and your patient are now satisfied that the diagnosis is psychogenic amenorrhea. You have solved her problem. She hasn't. . . .

Questions

1. Suppose the same patient sees you for the first time after having missed six consecutive menstrual periods. She has no other symptoms, and her abdomen has not enlarged. Each of the following is possible except which one?
   (a) Pseudocyesis (false pregnancy)
   (b) Stein-Leventhal syndrome
   (c) Hypopituitarism
   (d) Potent psychogenic factors

2. Pseudocyesis may be a form of psychogenic amenorrhea. It occurs in women who firmly believe themselves to be pregnant, and develop most of the signs and symptoms. Which one of the following statements is incorrect?
   (a) The abdomen enlarges, the breast become full, and morning nausea is present.
   (b) Amenorrhea is the rule for 9 months (sometimes longer).
   (c) This condition is seen in women who desperately do or do not want to become pregnant.
   (d) The uterus enlarges, as in true pregnancy.

3. The patient in the case presentation developed hypertension from birth control pills. This was reversible. Other possible complications of birth control pills include all of the following except:
   (a) increased tendency to develop thromboembolic complications.
   (b) enlarged breasts with galactorrhea.
   (c) increased incidence of carcinoma of the breast.
   (d) increased incidence of carcinoma of the uterus.

4. Consider a reverse situation. You see a 64-year-old woman who had her menopause 10 years ago. She is taking estrogen pills for backache and postmenopausal osteoporosis because her physician thinks this may help. Suddenly she has what seems to be a menstrual period. Your course of action should be:
   (a) stop estrogen pills and see what happens.
   (b) do nothing and see what happens.

(c) hunt carefully for cancer of the uterus.

(d) change to an estrogen-testosterone combination.

5. An anxious mother brings you her 15-year-old daughter who has not yet begun to menstruate. The young woman looks normal and feels well. Her breasts are well developed, and she has pubic hair. Which of the following statements is/are false?

(a) Pregnancy is excluded.

(b) The hymen may be imperforate, or she may not have a uterus or vagina.

(c) There may be a chromosomal disorder.

(d) She may simply be a "late starter."

Answers

1. **(a) is correct** because it is not possible. Pseudocyesis is characterized by all the outward signs and symptoms of pregnancy, including enlargement of the abdomen. The Stein-Leventhal syndrome is caused by polycystic bilateral ovarian enlargement resulting in primary hypogonadism. In 80% of patients the ovaries are palpably enlarged on pelvic examination; hirsutism may be present. Hypopituitarism can be caused by postpartum infarction of the pituitary (Sheehan's syndrome), a chromophobe adenoma, craniopharyngioma, or infiltrative disease destroying the pituitary. No menses following childbirth is the hallmark of Sheehan's syndrome. In any event, the gonadotropic hormones are the first to be affected. There is no clinical evidence for a pituitary disorder in this patient. Many cases of secondary amenorrhea are caused by a persistent corpus luteum (Halban's syndrome), which is not included on the list in this case. Case (d) is correct for long periods of amenorrhea as well as for a single missed period. Such a profound psychologic disturbance may be found in schizophrenia. It is interesting to note that the onset of simple severe obesity or severe starvation (as in concentration camps) may be associated with cessation of menses. More recently amenorrhea has been frequently noted in women who jog or train vigorously for distance running or serious ballet careers. This is thought to be due to a shift in the lean-to-fat body mass ratio.

2. **(d) is the only incorrect statement.** Choice (a) occurs for postural, psychologic, and unknown reasons. Ninety percent of patients with pseudocyesis stop having menstrual periods. **Choice (c)** is an obvious truth as potent psychologic factors are invoked. The uterus does not enlarge, nor does the pregnancy test result become positive.

3. **(c) is the incorrect statement,** although this is still debatable. Most recent studies show a slight increase in risk for breast cancer as a result of long-term use of oral contraceptives. There is clearly an increased risk of endometrial cancer and thromboembolic phenomena. The latter include stroke, leg vein thromboses, and pulmonary emboli. Enlarged breasts do occur, and galactorrhea may be discomforting.

4. **(c) is correct.** Regardless of hormone therapy, cancer must be your prime consideration at this age. Perform a Pap smear, cervical biopsy, and diagnostic curettage if considered necessary to rule out cancer of the cervix or endometrium. Although estrogen may indeed cause bleeding, it usually does so after the medication is stopped. A "wait and see" attitude would be dangerous. Changing to another preparation, even though it contains testosterone, would also be ill-advised at this point, because you must look for cancer anyway.

5. **(a) and (d) are false.** Pregnancy cannot be excluded, even if the patient has never menstruated. Although the average age at menarche is 12½ years, the normal range is 9 to 16 years, so this might simply have been a delayed onset were it not for the breasts and pubic hair. The presence of secondary sex characteristics may require the consideration of abnormal sex chromosome mosaics and warrants a buccal smear. As for answer (b) the physician may be subsequently embarrassed to learn that the hymen is closed as the uterus continue to enlarge, or that no uterus exists; a rectal examination may be indicated. In the *absence* of secondary sex characteristics, a search for a hypothalamic-pituitary disorder is indicated or (d) may exist.

COMMENT A physician would easily solve the problem of a missed period by a brief stepwise approach: first, a short menstrual, sexual, and psychosocial history; next, an examination of the pelvis and breasts; third, a pregnancy test. Based on these three easily gathered bits of information, a reasonably certain conclusion could be reached. If necessary, an FSH level determination and a short period of observation would establish the diagnosis. Other problem-solving methods used in this case presentation were: (1) frequent use of cause-and-effect relationships; (2) diagnosis by exclusion; (3) attention to specificity and sensitivity of clues—for example, early pregnancy test, FSH level, palpability of ovaries in Stein-Leventhal syndrome; (4) regard for absence of clues that would be pertinent if other diagnoses existed; and (5) statistical likelihoods. Consider pregnancy as the cause of secondary amenorrhea until proved otherwise. *(P.C.)*

PROBLEM-BASED LEARNING On the surface, this is simply a case of a missed menstrual period—common enough. But the reader should learn all about:

- Complex physiology of the menstrual cycle
- Causes of primary amenorrhea
- Causes of secondary amenorrhea
- Early signs of pregnancy
- Menopause
- Pregnancy tests
- Effects of birth control pills
- Mystery of pseudocyesis
- Psychogenic aspects of menstrual disturbances
- Effects of certain drugs
- Endocrinopathies that cause amenorrhea (pituitary tumors; thyroid, ovarian, and adrenal dysfunctions)
- Newer concepts of prolactinomas, Stein-Leventhal syndrome (polycystic ovaries), and hyperthecosis

There's a lot of gynecology in this case!

Suggested Readings

Aloi JA. Evaluation of amenorrhea. Comr Ther 1995; 21(10)575–578.

Dewailly D, Duhamel A, Robert Y, et al. Interrelationship between ultrasonography and biology in the diagnosis of polycystic ovarian syndrome. Ann NY Acad Sci 1993;687:206–216.

Nattiv A, Agostini R, Drinkwater B, et al. The female athlete triad. The inter-relatedness of disordered eating, amenorrhea, and osteoporosis. Clin Sports Med 1994;13(2):405–418.

 CASE 64

ACUTE PELVIC PAIN

Paul Cutler

Data A 19-year-old female visits the emergency department with the sudden onset of constant moderately severe lower abdominal and pelvic pain that she has had for the past 8 hours. She has a vaginal discharge but says it is no different than usual.

Logic The patient's age, sex, and complaint lead us to many possibilities. Pain is the main clue. The considerations include acute appendicitis, regional enteritis, urinary tract infection, ureteral stone, ovarian cyst (twisted, ruptured, or sudden enlargement), ectopic pregnancy, threatened abortion, and acute pelvic inflammatory disease (PID). We do not know the significance of the discharge because it is usually there. More information is needed.

Data Two years ago a pregnancy was terminated by suction abortion. Menses have since been normal and regular. She has continued to be sexually active with different partners and irregularly uses foam contraception. One week ago she had a more scant menstrual period than usual, and she has had some spotting of blood with the present onset of pain. Requestioning confirms the fact that the pain is constant and not crampy. There has been no nausea, anorexia, vomiting, epigastric pain, dysuria, urgency, frequency, visible hematuria, burning on urination, or other previous surgery.

Logic The type and location of pain, slight menstrual disturbance, and unprotected sexual activity lean us toward a gynecologic disorder. Ectopic pregnancy, ovarian cyst, and PID head the list, but other possibilities have by no means been ruled out. The constancy of the pain is against ureteral colic and threatened abortion. Absence of urinary tract symptoms tends to exclude urinary infection and is against ureteral calculus. The lack of preceding nausea, anorexia, and epigastric pain are points against appendicitis. Ileitis can have many different presentations, although this would be an unusual one, and there is no previous evidence for the disease.

Can she be pregnant, yet have menstrual periods? Rarely so, but possible. Can she have an ectopic pregnancy? She did not miss any period, but the last one was abnormal for her, and she is spotting. So it is definitely possible. Venereal disease always hovers in the background of such a setting. Foam kills sperm, not the gonococcus.

Data Her temperature is 38.7°C, pulse 80, respirations 22, and blood pressure 116/74 in the reclining, sitting, and standing positions. The head and neck, breasts, lungs, and heart are normal. There is no pallor. The abdomen is not distended. Direct and referred tenderness, rebound tenderness, and muscle guarding are present in both lower quadrants. Bowel sounds are normally active. The costovertebral angles are not tender. Pelvic examination reveals normal external genitalia, a well-epithelialized cervix with no lesions, and a mucopurulent discharge coming from the cervical os. This material is sampled for Gram's stain and cultured on Thayer-Martin media. Marked bilateral tenderness and tenderness with cervical motion is noted on bimanual and rectovaginal examination. The uterus is normal in size, shape, and position, and there are no palpable adnexal masses. Culdocentesis yields 5 mL of seropurulent material, which is also prepared for Gram's stain, smear, and culture.

Logic The diagnostic possibilities are narrowing. Localization of the findings to the lower abdomen and pelvis further supports pelvic pathology as the major consideration. Acute appendicitis becomes even more remote in view of the bilaterality of signs. Even a pelvic appendix would give unilateral signs, unless it had ruptured, and an abscess or peritonitis were present.

Several findings would preclude ectopic or tubal pregnancy: moderately high fever, bilaterality, no evidence of hypovolemia, mucopurulent endocervical discharge, and seropurulent culdocentesis material rather than unclotted blood. Also, no adnexal mass is palpated. Against hypovolemia are the absence of pallor and no orthostatic blood pressure changes. Normal pregnancy and threatened abortion are not likely in the presence of a normal-colored cervix and normal-sized uterus.

On the other hand, the data support an inflammatory condition as the most likely diagnosis. The cluster favoring inflammation consists of pain, tenderness, guarding, fever, and purulent discharge. Acute PID should be foremost in our minds.

Data Laboratory studies immediately available show: hematocrit, 42%; hemoglobin, 12.5 g/dL; and white blood cell (WBC) count, 12,300/mm³ with 86% neutrophils. Urinalysis results are normal except for a few WBCs per high-powered field. A Gram's stain of both the cervical discharge and the culdocentesis material shows numerous WBCs, some of which contain gram-negative intracellular diplococci. Radiographs of the chest and abdomen yield normal results. The 18-test blood chemistry profile, ordered routinely on admission, has completely normal results, as expected. (It was really not necessary.) A rapid urine pregnancy test result is negative. (It is always necessary.)

Logic The diagnosis of acute gonorrheal PID is clearly established by the clinical picture and confirmed by the positive results from Gram's stain and presence of leukocytosis. The normal red blood cell count and hematocrit further rule out ruptured ectopic pregnancy with hemoperitoneum. The urinalysis weighs against stone and infection, and you are not surprised to see a few WBCs in the presence of an internal genital infection. One 125-mg dose of azithromycin was given intramuscularly, and the patient was told to take doxycycline for 7 days. She improved markedly in 48 hours. At that time the culture results returned positive for *Neisseria gonorrhoeae*.

Subsequent review of the situation impresses you with the fact that venereal disease must always receive prime consideration in a sexually active unprotected individual having relations with many partners. You still cannot fully explain the scant menstrual period and spotting unless they were related to already existing pelvic inflammation. Although the gonococcus was the proven felon in this case, *Chlamydia trachomatis* may cause the same picture.

Data On questioning the patient again, you learn that her chronic vaginal discharge did change in quantity and nature at approximately the time she became ill. It was more profuse and had become more creamy and foul-smelling. She had douched before coming to see you.

Questions

1. The most specific clue in making this patient's diagnosis was:
   (a) leukocytosis.
   (b) vaginal discharge.
   (c) the sexual history.
   (d) presence of the gonococcus.

2. Suppose that pelvic examination had disclosed a tender 8-cm round mass in the right adnexal area, and no laboratory work had yet been done. Pain and tenderness were limited to the right side, and there was no fever. The most likely diagnosis would have been:
   (a) tubal pregnancy.
   (b) acute appendicitis.

(c) ovarian cyst.

(d) tubo-ovarian abscess.

3. Change the clinical picture a bit. The patient is 28, married, and professes to have only one sexual partner—her husband. He is a traveling salesman and is frequently away from home. The same acute clinical episode happens to the patient while her husband is briefly away. The rest of the history and examination are the same. In addition, you can palpate both ovaries; they are tender, although not enlarged. Your leading impression before laboratory work is:

(a) ruptured ectopic pregnancy.

(b) acute PID.

(c) twisted ovarian cyst.

(d) bilateral oophoritis.

4. Another 28-year-old patient sees you for a dull nagging pain in the right lower quadrant that she has had for several days. She missed her last period and is spotting. On the way to the hospital she fainted several times. The blood pressure is 118/80, dropping to 90/60 when she stands up. Even before doing your examination, you have a pretty good idea that she has:

(a) gastrointestinal bleeding.

(b) pregnancy plus anxiety.

(c) tubal pregnancy.

(d) acute appendicitis.

Answers

1. **(d) is correct.** All the other clues could be and very frequently are present without the patient necessarily having acute PID. Indeed, the gonococcus can be found in asymptomatic patients, but the presence of the venereal organism in the cervix and peritoneal aspirate is positive evidence for the diagnosis in this clinical setting.

2. **(c) is correct.** An ovarian cyst may be twisted on its pedicle and give the acute picture. Tubal pregnancy would not be so large. Acute appendicitis would cause fever and a tender area, but not a large mass in the pelvis. A tubo-ovarian abscess would not be round, and there would probably be some findings on the left side too.

3. **(b) is correct.** Acute PID is still the diagnosis of choice and gonorrhea is a prime suspect. She may be truthful about having a single sex partner, but her husband may be the promiscuous one. Oophoritis is only a part of generalized PID. Diagnoses (a) and (c) are ruled out by the clinical picture just as in the case presentation.

4. **(c) is correct.** The tube is ruptured, and she has already lost considerable blood into the abdomen. The orthostatic blood pressure changes and history of syncope indicate reduced blood volume. A missed period, spotting, and nagging pain all point to a tubal pregnancy rather than gastrointestinal bleeding as the cause for her blood loss. Orthostatic changes are not seen in normal pregnancy or acute appendicitis.

Comment Acute pelvic pain is a common emergency situation that requires a prompt decision regarding medical treatment versus hospitalization and surgery. The array of diagnostic possibilities in a sexually active female is not large. Selected bits of information in the history and examination may often pinpoint the cause. Aside from the blood count, cervical smear, and pregnancy test, the laboratory has little to offer. A pelvic examination may be painful, difficult, and only sometimes fruitful.

But an ultrasound examination of the pelvis, often available in the emergency room, may offer an excellent and highly reliable means for help in the important decision needed here. It may reveal ectopic pregnancy, ovarian cyst, tubo-ovarian abscess, abortion in progress, and so forth, with such a high degree of accuracy that the need for laparoscopy is often eliminated. *(P.C.)*

Suggested Readings

Ault KA, Faro S. Pelvic inflammatory disease. Current diagnostic criteria and treatment guidelines. Postgrad Med 1993;93(2):85–86, 89–91.

Quan M. Diagnosis of acute pelvic pain. J Fam Pract 1992;35(4):422–432.

Quan M. Pelvic inflammatory disease: Diagnosis and management. J Am Board Fam Pract 1994;7(2): 110–123.

CASE 65

ABNORMAL VAGINAL BLEEDING

Paul Cutler

Data · A 47-year-old woman visits her doctor because of abnormal vaginal bleeding. She has not seen a physician since the birth of her last child 5 years ago.

Logic There are numerous causes of abnormal

bleeding. The data base you collect should include her past menstrual history, her method of contraception, and a precise description of the abnormal bleeding. Table 18.1 defines some terms used to describe abnormal bleeding.

Data History reveals she is gravida 7, para 6, ab 1. Her first child was placed for adoption when she was 16 years old. Her current husband (fourth) had a vasectomy after her last delivery, so she is using no other contraception. Menarche was at age 13 and menstrual cycles have occurred every 25 to 30 days until 4 months ago when she missed two menstrual periods. Two months ago she bled heavily for 8 days followed by intermenstrual bleeding of varying degrees. She bled heavily again last week but stopped 2 days ago. She experienced cramps with the bleeding and passed large clots that "left her weak" after passage. She says the blood was bright red.

Logic You can now define the problem more precisely as hypermenorrhea and intermenstrual bleeding (menometrorrhagia) in a 47-year-old woman following 2 months of amenorrhea. You have excluded few diagnostic possibilities except contraceptive complications. The presence of clots in the menstrual flow indicates brisk bleeding. Passage of clots is often associated with cramping and is of no

particular significance in her history. The color of menstrual blood is frequently reported by patients but has little diagnostic importance.

Now that you have some estimate of the blood loss and the relationship to normal menstruation, additional historical information should be obtained. Is the bleeding associated with body function such as coitus, urination, or defecation? Is there abdominal or back pain? How does the abnormal bleeding bother her? Additionally, a review of systems, family history, and medication history should be recorded.

Data The patient states that her bleeding is not related to bodily functions, and she has no pain except with the passage of clots. When she initially missed two menstrual periods she thought she might be pregnant or "going through the change of life" so she took some of her neighbor's "hormone pills" for a few weeks to see if she could induce menstrual bleeding. The first heavy bleeding episode ensued so she quit taking the hormones. Abnormal bleeding continued. She is afraid she has cancer because her mother died of cervical carcinoma that was detected because of abnormal bleeding. She is quite anxious and asks you for some "nerve pills." The remainder of her history is unremarkable.

TABLE 18.1. Terms Used to Describe Abnormal Bleeding

TERM	DEFINITION
Menstrual cycle	Normally 21–35 days
Polymenorrhea	Menstrual cycles more frequent than 21 days
Oligomenorrhea	Menstrual cycles less frequent than 35 days
Duration of menstrual bleeding	Normally 2–7 days
Shortened menses	Less than 2 days
Prolonged menses	More than 7 days
Menstrual blood loss	Normally 30–150 mL
Hypomenorrhea	Less than normal blood loss
Menorrhagia or hypermenorrhea	Greater than normal blood loss
Metrorrhagia or intermenstrual bleeding	Bleeding between menses
Spotting	Light bleeding
Postcoital bleeding	Bleeding after intercourse
Postmenopausal bleeding	Bleeding 1 year after menopause
Perimenopausal bleeding	Bleeding within 1 year of presumed menopause

Logic There are grounds for her fear of cervical carcinoma, because she had an early age of first coitus, has had multiple sexual partners, and is 47 years old—the peak age of incidence for cervical carcinoma. Her bleeding history is not characteristic for cervical carcinoma, because she has had no postcoital bleeding. If she does have invasive cervical carcinoma, there should be a gross lesion visible on pelvic examination. You should now proceed to physical examination in order to try to identify the cause of her abnormal bleeding.

Data Pertinent data are as follows: weight 140 lb, pulse 96, BP 130/70. She does not appear pale but seems quite anxious. She has no evidence of jaundice, petechiae, or easy bruisability. Her thyroid is not palpable, there are no heart murmurs, and no abdominal organs can be felt. The breasts are normal.

Pelvic examination reveals normal external genitalia. Her vagina is supple, pink, and rugated. No blood is seen. She has a small cystocele and urethrocele. The cervix appears parous and has a small ectropion with numerous nabothian cysts. There is no bleeding when cervical cytology is obtained. The uterus is axial and does not seem enlarged or irregular in contour. It is mobile, firm, and nontender. The adnexa are nontender,

and the ovaries are barely palpable. Rectal examination findings are normal, and the stool is brown and tests guaiac negative.

Logic Most abnormal vaginal bleeding is uterine in origin. Vaginal sources of abnormal bleeding are easily seen during examination, and none were detected in this woman. Occasionally, patients are unsure whether blood is coming from the vagina, urethra, or rectum, so examination should be performed while they are bleeding. Such is not the case with this patient.

After the clinical data base has been collected, patients with abnormal bleeding may be grouped into one of four categories for further evaluation and treatment (Table 18.2).

Hyperpolymenorrhea of adolescence can be excluded. Abnormal uterine bleeding usually does not complicate systemic illness until the illness is overt. She has no signs of systemic illness, but determination of the complete blood count, thyroxine (T_4), and TSH might be performed for completeness. She has no indication of pregnancy and no other diagnosable causes of abnormal bleeding. Cervical carcinoma, uterine leiomyoma, and ovarian tumor can be reasonably excluded by the normal examination findings.

Her bleeding abnormality suggests a period

TABLE 18.2. Categories of Patients with Abnormal Uterine Bleeding

Group I. Adolescents with hyperpolymenorrhea: usually due to an anovulation

Group II. Women with detectable disease

    Systemic illnesses—thyroid disease, liver disease, immunologic thrombocytopenic purpura, leukemia, von Willebrand's disease, and so forth

    Pregnancy complications—abortion, ectopic pregnancy, hydatidiform mole

    Gross cervical lesions—polyps, carcinoma, some ectropions

    Uterine leiomyomas

    Other pelvic pathology—functioning ovarian tumors, endometriosis, chronic salpingitis

Group III. No detectable disease: history confusing, short duration, or uncertain, but not suspicious for cancer

    Minor variations from normal

    Related to contraception

Group IV. No detectable disease: history of persistent abnormality or suspicious for cancer

    Patient over age 40

    Abnormality recurrent or present for more than 3 months

    Postcoital bleeding

of anovulation with continued estrogenic stimulation of the endometrium, worsened by the hormone pills (probably estrogen). Although abnormal bleeding is commonly encountered near the menopause, it should never be considered normal and should be completely investigated for possible endometrial adenocarcinoma. Certainly, hormone therapy should never be given without a tissue diagnosis of the disease process.

This patient would be classified as having no demonstrable disease, but her history is suspicious for cancer. Minimum evaluation at present should consist of a complete blood count, urinalysis, cervical cytology, and an endometrial biopsy. The biopsy could be diagnostic of endometrial carcinoma. A diagnostic dilation and curettage (D&C) should also be scheduled in several weeks, after the assumed time of ovulation.

Data Laboratory data are as follows: hemoglobin, 12.4 g/dL; hematocrit, 37%; WBC count, 7,800/mm^3 with a normal differential; and platelets, 240,000/mm^3. Urinalysis results are unremarkable. T_4 and TSH results are normal. The endometrial biopsy report shows focal adenomatous hyperplasia, and cervical cytology results are normal. When the woman returns for these reports, she asks why she needs a D&C and whether or not you will give her hormones.

Logic A D&C is necessary to exclude the possibility of endometrial adenocarcinoma that could coexist with adenomatous hyperplasia. Estrogenic hormones would certainly not be used with this patient.

Data At the time of D&C the patient is anesthetized and pelvic examination is unchanged from 3 weeks previously. The uterus is sounded to 8 cm, and the curettage is performed without complications. Pathologic report is still focal adenomatous hyperplasia.

Logic Your impression of anovulatory bleeding near the menopause has been confirmed. There are now several methods of management for this patient. Many women have no further abnormal bleeding after a D&C so a time of observation could be recommended. Progestins could also be utilized to induce regular bleeding episodes and minimize the chance for recurrent hyperplasia. She is not a candidate for estrogens.

Questions

1. Suppose you decided not to treat the patient with progestins. She returns 8 months later and says she had no bleeding for 6 months after the D&C, but for the last 2 months she has again had heavy and irregular bleeding. Proper management now would be:
   (a) hysterectomy.
   (b) estrogenic hormones.
   (c) progestins.
   (d) D&C.

2. You see a 26-year-old nulliparous woman who has episodes of amenorrhea followed by hyperpolymenorrhea. She is slightly hirsute, and her ovaries are easily palpable. D&C is done in the expected luteal phase, and the pathologic report reveals that endometrial hyperplasia is present. Correct management is:
   (a) observe for future abnormal bleeding.
   (b) induce ovulation with clomiphene.
   (c) give cyclic progestins to induce regular menses.
   (d) give combination estrogen-progestin oral contraceptives.

3. A 56-year-old woman who has been taking estrogen since her menopause comes to see you because of "spotting" for 2 weeks. Her vagina appears well estrogenized, and findings from the remainder of the pelvic examination are normal. Proper management includes:
   (a) stopping estrogen replacement.
   (b) continuing estrogen replacement and adding progesterone.
   (c) cervical cytology.
   (d) D&C.

4. A 24-year-old mother of three comes to see you because her menses have increased in length and flow, and she has had cramps and some intermenstrual spotting since she was fitted for an intrauterine device (IUD) 2 months ago. Pelvic examination findings are normal. Proper management is:
   (a) remove the IUD.
   (b) remove the IUD and do a D&C.
   (c) remove the IUD and give oral contraceptives.
   (d) reassure her that her symptoms are not uncommon and will probably abate.

5. An 18-year-old woman comes to the emergency room with a history of 3 months of amenorrhea followed by 3 weeks of daily vaginal bleeding. A mass arises from the pelvis to the umbilicus. A fetal heart cannot be heard. Her BP is 160/100. The most likely diagnosis is:

(a) uterine leiomyoma.

(b) ovarian tumor.

(c) hydatidiform mole.

(d) threatened abortion.

Answers

1. **(d) is correct.** The woman has perimenopausal meno-metrorrhagia that is probably still the result of anovulation, but some women with adenomatous hyperplasia progress to endometrial adenocarcinoma. A diagnosis should be made before treatment. Hysterectomy is not indicated. Estrogens are contraindicated. Cyclic progestin therapy is warranted if her pathologic diagnosis is still endometrial hyperplasia.

2. **(b), (c), or (d) is correct.** This patient is anovulatory and most likely has polycystic ovary disease. She is at high risk for developing endometrial cancer because her endometrium is being exposed to estrogen and not to progesterone. Her chance for endometrial cancer can be reduced by providing progesterone, and this can be accomplished by inducing ovulation if she seeks pregnancy or by providing progestins alone or in oral contraceptives.

3. **(a), (c), or (d) are correct.** Choices (a) and (c) should of course be done, but a D&C is mandatory. Prolonged estrogen administration may be associated with an increased risk of endometrial adenocarcinoma, and this is best diagnosed by a D&C. Abnormal bleeding is the early warning of endometrial cancer, and this possibility must always be considered whenever postmenopausal bleeding occurs. Choice (b) is unacceptable and perilous.

4. **(d) is correct.** Many women have hypermenorrhea and occasionally intermenstrual spotting during the first few months after they have an IUD inserted. If symptoms persist or are distressing, the device can be removed. A D&C is unnecessary because her cancer risk is quite low.

5. **(c) is correct.** Hydatidiform moles are frequently associated with a uterus larger than expected for the duration of amenorrhea. In addition, most patients with moles have abnormal bleeding, and many develop preeclampsia, as suggested by her blood pressure. A leiomyoma of this size would be quite uncommon in a female of her age. Most abortions occur in the first 12 weeks of pregnancy. An ovarian tumor is always a possibility, but the story presented is more characteristic of a mole. Sonography could give the correct diagnosis in a matter of minutes. Pregnancy complications must always be considered in the patient who has abnormal uterine bleeding.

COMMENT After a detailed analysis of the types of abnormal vaginal bleeding, the author pursues a branched pattern of problem solving based on a systematic list of causes for bleeding. Only a few decision points are needed: the age of the patient, the use of contraceptives, the presence or absence of apparent systemic disease, the pelvic examination, cytologic studies, endometrial biopsy, and D&C. The questions and answers take the reader through different pathways of logic as varied settings for abnormal bleeding are presented. High-yield questions in patients with vaginal bleeding focus on the taking of hormones and the possibility of pregnancy.

The patient's age often alters diagnostic likelihoods. Abnormal vaginal bleeding in teenagers results mainly from hormonal imbalances (dysfunctional uterine bleeding), although complications of pregnancy and ovarian tumors must be considered. From ages 20 to 40, bleeding problems relate mainly to birth control devices and pills, but pregnancy, polycystic ovaries, and hormonal imbalances are important here, too. From age 40 on, and perhaps even earlier, carcinoma of the cervix and endometrium is your principal concern. The few years around the menopause are where the interplay between anovulatory bleeding, endometrial hyperplasia, and endometrial carcinoma exists; alteration of the normal menstrual pattern, taking estrogens for symptom relief, and the high incidence of cancer are three factors that may cause confusion, anxiety, and mistakes at this age.

Remember that idiopathic thrombocytopenic purpura and other coagulopathies often first manifest themselves in young to middle-aged women with profuse menstrual bleeding. A platelet count determination may be indicated. Other diagnostic studies that may be of value in selected instances are hormone assays, Pap smears, D&C, ultrasonography, and laparoscopy.

It must be recognized that abortions, polyps, carcinomas, and other pathologic processes account for roughly one quarter of all cases of abnormal vaginal bleeding. The rest are the result of the hormonal imbalances that stem from the complex hypothalamus–pituitary–ovary relationships responsible for the menstrual cycle, and whoever wishes to understand such problems must know the physiology of all the loops and feedbacks involved. *(P.C.)*

Suggested Readings

Chambers JT, Chambers SK. Endometrial sampling: When? Where? Why? With what? Clin Obstet Gynecol 1992;35(1):28–39.

Feldman S, Cook EF, Harlow BL, et al. Predicting endometrial cancer among older women who present with abnormal vaginal bleeding. Gynecol Oncol 1995;56(3):376–381.

Samsioe G. The endometrium: Effects of estrogen and estrogen-progestogen replacement therapy. Int J Fertil Menopausal Stud 1994;39(suppl)2:84–92.

Thorneycroft IH. Practical aspects of hormone replacement therapy. Prog Cardiovasc Dis 1995; 38(3):243–254.

CASE 66

BREAST LUMP

Paul Cutler

Data During a vicious exchange of volleys at the net, a vigorous 48-year-old athletic lady is struck in the left breast by a tennis ball. Like all women who are informed regularly about breast cancer in the various women's magazines, she is concerned that a breast injury might result in cancer even though this may only be a popular misconception, and there is no scientific evidence thereof. Her concern is heightened by the fact that her older sister had surgery 2 years ago for a malignant breast lump. So she examines herself each day, and on the 25th day she thinks she feels a small lump in the general area of the original injury. She consults her physician.

Logic The patient is correct to be concerned. Breast cancer strikes one woman in nine, and is three times more likely to occur if it existed in a first-degree relative (sister, mother, daughter). First, it is necessary to confirm the lump, and if present, try to decide whether it is malignant or benign. Early diagnosis is the key to cure, and failure to diagnose breast cancer in a timely fashion is one of the most common causes of malpractice litigation.

Data On examination, the breasts are symmetric, and there is no nipple retraction or nipple discharge. There is a 1- × 1.5-cm nontender, movable, rubbery mass in the outer upper quadrant of the left breast, 3 cm from the nipple. There is no axillary or supraclavicular adenopathy.

Logic Breast examination should ideally be done shortly after the menses because the breast will then be less dense and less tender. It is important to examine the breast with the patient in four different positions. Inspection should be done with the patient sitting upright, first with the arms relaxed, then held over the head, then hands on hips and exerting pressure. These maneuvers allow for detection of abnormal contour such as dimpling or retraction. The skin overlying the breast tissue may have changes of prognostic significance. For example, inflammation of overlying tissue carries a worse prognosis.

Palpation of the breast is best done with the patient supine and her arms extended over her head. It is important to remember that the breast extends from the inferior border of the clavicle to the inframammary fold and from the sternum to the mid-axillary line. It is palpated with the flat portion of the three middle fingers while applying three degrees of pressure to all areas of the breast, thereby assessing superficial, intermediate, and deep tissue. The patient must show the examiner the area of question. If the examiner cannot identify the abnormality indicated by the patient, the breast should be re-examined in midcycle. The axillae are palpated with the patient sitting and arms relaxed at both sides.

Physical findings that suggest malignancy are a hard, fixed mass with irregular or indistinct borders; retraction or dimpling of overlying skin or of the nipple; the presence of a bloody nipple discharge; or axillary adenopathy.

Benign lesions such as a cyst, fibroadenoma, intraductal papilloma, lipoma, or fat necrosis may be cystic, sometimes soft, mobile, well-circumscribed, or multiple. Tenderness may be suggested of abscess.

More questions need to be answered.

Data The patient's age at menarche was 13 years. She has been pregnant twice, at ages 28 and 34. She used oral contraceptives between her two pregnancies, but got a tubal ligation after her second child. She completed her menses 2 days ago. She is a nonsmoker and drinks three to four drinks a week.

There has been no discharge from the breast, either serous, milky, or bloody, no pain, her appetite is good, and she feels generally quite well.

Since the age of 40, she has had a mammogram every 2 years. The last one was done almost

2 years ago. All showed reportedly normal findings. As directed by her physician, she does a careful self-examination every month just after her menses, and she never detected any abnormality before.

Logic In addition to the presence of breast cancer in a first-degree relative, other factors that increase the propensity toward breast cancer are nulliparity, late age for the first pregnancy, prolonged exposure to estrogens by early menarche and/or late menopause, current oral contraceptive use, high-fat diets, and postmenopausal estrogen replacement therapy. The latter two have not been conclusively proved.

As many as 5% of patients with breast cancer have been shown to have inherited a specific genetic abnormality involving chromosome 17. Bear in mind, however, that 70 to 80% of breast cancers occur in patients who do not have identifiable risk factors.

Nipple discharge, although not commonly present, can be serous, milky, or bloody. If milky and bilateral, the cause may reside with an endocrine disorder such as prolactinoma. Unilateral discharge, especially if bloody, suggests the presence of an intraductal carcinoma. A nipple discharge that tests negative for hemoglobin is almost always benign, but only a small percentage of breast cancers have a hemoglobin-positive discharge. It must be remembered that many nipple discharges, whether serous or sanguinous, are caused by benign disorders such as an intraductal papilloma.

In addition to the character of the mass itself and the presence of a bloody nipple discharge, other physical evidences that point to cancer are dimpling of skin caused by cancer infiltrating the dermis, fixation of the tumor to the pectoralis muscle or chest wall, retraction of the nipple because of ductal involvement, skin that resembles the texture of an orange peel (*peau d' orange*), the result of plugging of dermal lymphatics, satellite skin nodules, matted axillary nodes, and the presence of any supraclavicular node.

As for lymph nodes, 50% of patients with breast cancer have histologic evidence of lymph node involvement at the time of diagnosis. On physical examination, however, 25 to 35% of those with detectable axillary adenopathy turn out to have histologically negative findings, and an equal number of patients without detectable adenopathy turn out to have histologically positive findings.

The guidelines for mammography are an important issue. Breast cancers are detected either by routine mammography or by the finding of a mass—either by the patient or the doctor. Each year, the percentages found by mammography are on the increase, and their discoveries therefore tend to be earlier. Current thinking is to not screen with mammography until the age of 40, to screen between ages 40 and 49 (debatable), and to screen every 1 to 2 years after age 50. These guidelines do not apply for every patient, and a monthly self-examination is highly recommended by all, even though its benefits in terms of long-term survival have not been proved.

In summary, the propositus has a breast mass, has only one risk factor—cancer in a sibling—and the rest of the history and physical examination points neither in a malignant nor a benign direction.

Further studies are indicated. The options include: (1) ultrasound, (2) mammography, (3) fine needle aspiration (FNA), and (4) open biopsy. The order in which these may be done may vary from patient to patient and from physician to physician.

Data A mammogram reveals a dense, irregularly-shaped, 1-cm solid lesion where it was clinically felt (Fig. 18.1). It shows no calcification in the left breast, but there is an area of coarse calcification in the right breast suggestive of a fibroadenoma. Compared with the study done 2 years ago, the calcification in the right breast has not changed, but the nodule in the left breast is new—that is, almost new. Careful inspection shows a very faint but smaller density in the same spot.

Logic Even though the mammogram is a highly sensitive screening procedure for breast lumps, approximately 10% of them may be missed, especially in patients with dense breast parenchyma (false negatives). On the other hand, when a breast lump has been identified by patient and doctor, the diagnostic mammogram will confirm the lump but may not offer foolproof evidence of whether the lump is benign or malignant.

The screening mammogram consists of two standard views and is meant to detect breast cancer at an early stage in the asymptomatic patient. If mammography is done to evaluate a sign or symptom, it is no longer a screening test—it is a

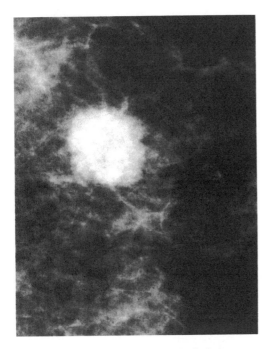

▶ **Figure 18.1.** Mammogram (magnified) shows dense round mass with indistinct microlobulated borders.

diagnostic test and consists of numerous views depending on the reason for the study. It is useful in evaluating the mass for actual size, shape, density, margins, and the presence of calcifications and architectural distortion. It examines the breast for multifocal cancer and the contralateral breast for concurrent pathology. Characteristically the calcification seen in breast cancer consists of clusters of five or more microcalcifications, each less than 1 mm in size, and all in an area less than 1-cm wide.

Mammographic readings may suggest that: 1. the mass is definitely benign; therefore follow the patient; 2. the mass is malignant; excision is indicated; if intraoperative frozen section confirms malignancy, then initiate appropriate treatment; 3. the results are equivocal; proceed with fine needle aspiration (FNA).

This patient seems to fit into the third category. FNA may help determine if the mass is cystic or solid and hopefully may determine the cytology.

Data Before making a final decision, the patient asks whether the nodule, if cancer, may already have spread to other parts of the body. Her physician says "probably not" and explains that because the nodule is small, the disease is yet early, and there is no physical evidence of spread.

Logic This nodule may have been present 2 or even more years ago, although it was seen only in retrospect. Generally, such cancers have a slow doubling time and may not begin to metastasize until they contain 10^6 to 10^9 cells. When breast cancers spread, they go to regional lymph nodes, lung, pleura, liver, bones, and meninges. As such, pleural effusions, bone pains, and jaundice may occur.

Data The patient further asks what may determine her future course after surgery is performed.

Logic The doctor answers that the prognostic factors in this patient, as in any patient who has breast cancer, will depend on: (1) tumor size and spread; (2) menopausal status; (3) atypia of the tumor cells; (4) percentage of tumor cells undergoing mitoses; and (5) the presence or absence of estrogen and progesterone receptors.

Data Together, the doctor and patient review the entire case; the various optional management pathways and their possible outcomes are discussed. The patient opts for a direct and immediate approach. The mass is surgically removed, and at frozen section it is determined that the patient has an intraductal carcinoma in situ, a lesion that accounts for 10% of all breast cancers.

Logic Decisions made on the operating table revolve around whether to do a lumpectomy or modified mastectomy, whether to remove axillary nodes, and whether to offer adjuvant types of therapy.

It appears that the errant tennis ball may have serendipitously called attention to an area of the breast where disease was already in progress. The next scheduled screening mammogram would have detected the early cancer anyway.

Questions

1. The following patients should be followed up on a routine basis, except:
   (a) a 22-year-old woman with a solid mass in whom the biopsy yielded fibroadenoma.
   (b) a 67-year-old woman who had a breast cyst aspirated 1 year ago and has not had recurrence of the mass.

(c) a 40-year-old woman with a mass—the biopsy had a small focus of atypical hyperplasia.

(d) a 52-year-old woman whose aunt died of breast cancer at the age of 65.

2. A 28-year-old pregnant woman notices a nodule in her breast. She has no risk factors or stigmata for cancer. Mammography confirms the lesion. Which of the following statements is incorrect?

(a) Ultrasound should be done, because it may detect abnormal calcifications.

(b) Ultrasound may serve as a guide for FNA, which should be done.

(c) FNA yields nonbloody fluid; the mass does not recur: it was a benign cyst; do routine follow-up.

(d) FNA yields equivocal cytology, and the mass persists; perform surgery.

3. In which of the following clinical descriptions is breast cancer most likely?

(a) A 22-year-old woman with a tender lump

(b) A 68-year-old man with a nontender lump

(c) A 48-year-old woman with tender, lumpy breasts

(d) A 36-year-old man with gynecomastia

(e) A 68-year-old woman with a nontender lump

Answers

1. **(c) is correct.** This patient with evidence of atypical hyperplasia has the greatest likelihood of developing breast carcinoma. It would be prudent to initiate close follow-up and yearly, rather than biennial, mammography. In the 22-year-old patient with benign breast disease, some studies have shown increased likelihood of developing breast cancer over a lifetime. However, the recommendations for follow-up are no different in this patient. In an elderly patient with a benign cyst, no alteration in follow-up is necessary after the first-year follow-up physical examination. In the case of the last patient, the recommended follow-up of annual mammography and physician examination would not be changed even if a first-degree relative (aunt is not a first-degree relative) had breast cancer.

2. **(a) is correct,** because it is the only incorrect statement. Ultrasound does not detect microcalcification. All other statements are correct. Ultrasound may serve as a good stereotactic guide for FNA. The nature of the aspirate and the fate of the nodule determine management in either direction.

3. **(b), possibly (e).** Choice (a) is probably a benign cyst or abscess. Choice (c) represents "chronic cystic mastitis" in which cancer is no more common than in other women. Men who have gynecomastia are not predisposed to cancer. This is a statistical call, but the likelihood is probably greater in the individual man with a lump. Many nodules in older women turn out to be benign fibroadenomas. One percent of all breast cancers occur in men.

Suggested Readings

Bassett LW, Hendrick RE, et al. Quality determinants of mammography. Clinical practice guideline No. 13. AHCPR Publication No. 95–0632. Rockville, MD: Agency for Health Care Policy and Research. Public Health Service, US Department of Health and Human Services. October 1994.

Ernster VL, Barclay J, Kerlikowske K, et al. Incidence of and treatment for ductal carcinoma in situ of the breast. JAMA 1996;275 (12):913.

Fajardo LL, et al. Mammography in clinical practice. IM 1995;36–44.

Harris JR, et al. Breast cancer (Parts I, II, and III). N Engl J Med 1994;327:319–328, 473–480.

CHAPTER 19

19

Musculoskeletal Problems

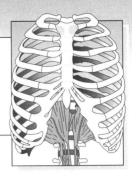

Here, a symbiotic relationship often exists between the rheumatologist and the orthopedic surgeon. However, in most cases there is no overlap, and the problem lies clearly in one field or the other.

The orthopedic surgeon is usually faced with problems related to trauma, deformities, bone tumors, or pain syndromes. Backache, neck pain, and shoulder pain are common situations with which he or she must deal. A branch of the history and physical examination is usually sufficient. Diagnosis depends mainly on what is seen by retinal multicolor or radiographic chiaroscuro. A few additional physical maneuvers may be necessary. But sometimes the problems are much more complicated (e.g., backache), and extensive studies are needed. Visceral diseases may first manifest themselves with what appears to be an orthopedic complaint. Aneurysms cause backache, and lung cancer can cause a painful shoulder. Or the seeming orthopedic problem may really be part of a systemic medical disease (e.g., metastases, Paget's disease, atherosclerosis).

Front-line diagnostic advances in orthopedic surgery include *magnetic resonance imaging (MRI)* and the *computed tomographic (CT) scan* for disc delineation; high-resolution radiographic techniques for the study of bone disease by *densitometry; radioisotope scans* for bone inflammations and metastases; *arthroscopy* for looking directly inside joints; and *arthrography* for radiocontrast study of the joint contents. Total joint replacement must be mentioned, because it represents a miraculous advance in the management of joint diseases. Diagnostic certainty must exist before such interventions are undertaken.

With the advent of "Olympianism" for all ages and both genders, almost everybody plays tennis and golf, cycles, skis, jogs, or performs aerobics or isometrics. This creates a swarm of diagnostic problems—proudly called "athletic in-juries"—in both athletes and amateur exercisers. One wonders whether such activity is more costly than beneficial.

Arthritis can affect one or many joints, can be acute, subacute, or chronic, or can be part of a systemic disease like systemic lupus erythematosus (SLE), sarcoidosis, gout, or rheumatoid variants. For every patient who has SLE seen by the primary care physician, there will probably be 15 patients with rheumatoid arthritis (RA), 15 patients with gout, 100 patients with degenerative osteoarthritis, and far more patients with aches and pains of unknown cause. Such is the approximate relative frequency of joint diseases.

But certainly the realm of the rheumatologist extends far beyond the synovial cavity. Joint diseases are most often part of multisystem disorders with far-reaching immunologic significance and consequences. Hundreds of scientists labor to unravel the mysteries of antigen-antibody complexes with only modest success.

As we approach the end of the 1990s, the quest for specific diagnostic markers and clusters continues. Rheumatoid arthritis, rheumatoid variants, and SLE still overlap and are often difficult to define and diagnose. None has a known cause or cure, and their manifestations are body-wide. The unknown still clouds the pathophysiology of one of the world's oldest recorded diseases—gout—and the reasons for its acute episodes are still not fully understood.

Immunologic disorders of connective tissue overlap and often coexist with similar diseases of the liver and kidney. The burgeoning field of immunology keeps broadening as it engulfs many other organs within its domain—brain, heart, lung, liver, kidney, gastrointestinal tract, endocrine glands, blood, lymph nodes, and so forth.

The existence of fibrositis or fibromyositis, alleged by some to be the most common cause of diffuse aches and pains, is still in dispute and con-

419

sidered to be a myth by many. Drugs continue to be incriminated in the causation of more and more diseases, especially the collagen–vascular disorders.

On the success side of the ledger is the exquisitely precise detail offered by magnetic resonance imaging in diseases of bone, joints, and the spinal column; the better and broader use of joint fluid for diagnosis; and the more widespread recognition of newer entities like Lyme disease and apatite arthritis—yet another crystal-induced arthropathy. *(P.C.)*

 CASE 67

PAINFUL SWOLLEN JOINT

Paul Cutler

A third-year medical student (MS III) presents the following case to her attending physician (MD) on ward rounds. The method of presentation closely parallels the sequence of problem solving used.

MS III Last night we admitted an unmarried 34-year-old traveling salesman who had just returned from a convention in Las Vegas with a very painful hot swollen right knee. The joint was extremely tender and inflexible, and he could not bear any weight on it; the skin over and around the joint looked purplish red and inflamed. This condition came on rather suddenly.

MD Were you sure that the inflammation was in the joint itself rather than in the periarticular tissue?

MS III Yes. We considered various extra-articular inflammations such as cellulitis, bursitis, tendinitis, and an inflamed Baker's cyst. But the clinical picture was typical for arthritis. The patient appeared to have an effusion. Furthermore, he had pain on both active- and passive-assisted motion, so we were sure that the trouble was within the joint.

MD Sounds like typical acute gout! Why did you admit him to the hospital?

MS III There were some other features that worried us. He felt chilly, had a temperature of 38°C, and told us that he had had a chronic recurrent urethral discharge for several years for which he had many times received penicillin. His occupation, unmarried status, and trip to Las Vegas may have influenced us too much.

MD In almost all cases, a single hot joint is caused by either infection or a crystal-induced disease. So what were your provisional hypotheses?

MS III I thought mainly in terms of gout and acute suppurative arthritis, probably gonococcal.

MD What data did you then get to substantiate or disprove your hypotheses?

MS III As for gout, he never had any similar joint problem; his father and older brother do have gout, but they get it in their big toes. Also, he never passed any kidney stones and does not have any tophi in his ears. The blood studies have not returned yet, so I do not know the serum uric acid level. Yesterday, before the acute joint episode started, he had a tremendous dinner: a 1–lb steak and a whole bottle of wine.

MD Well, so far you have given me several important clues for gout: the meal preceding the attack, the family history, and the appearance of the joint. But you have presented some negative clues, too. What speaks for or against a suppurative joint?

MS III First I milked his urethra and found no discharge. His throat was not sore, and his anorectal examination findings were normal. He has no other infectious foci; I looked carefully for skin pustules. He had no high fever or frank chills. He denied having had sexual intercourse in the previous 2 weeks. The leukocyte count was 13,000/mm^3 with 84% polymorphonuclear leukocytes (PMNs), and the urinalysis showed 5 to 10 white blood cells (WBCs) per high-powered field, but otherwise its findings were normal.

MD Of course, the absence of observable discharge at the moment does not rule out urethritis or prostatitis. But the point you make about the absence of high fever and chills is a good one. He certainly has an excess of WBCs in the urine, and the blood leukocytosis could go with either condition. The clues you gave were mainly negative and weigh against infection. But if the gonococcus is suspected, a look is not enough. Cultures of the urethra, anus, blood, throat, skin vesicles if present, and the cervix in women will have positive findings from at least one site in 95% of patients. The synovial fluid culture is only 50% sensitive.

And speaking of bacteria, the gonococcus is not the only villain. Septic joints are usually associated with fever and chills and often infection elsewhere. *Staphylococcus aureus* and *Staphylococcus pyogenes* are probably the most common organisms causing suppurative arthritis in such instances. In children, *Haemophilus influenzae* is usually at fault; the staphylococcus organism favors intravenous drug users, and gram-negative bacilli predominate in immunosuppressed persons.

Tell me, did you consider other possibilities like pseudogout and Reiter's syndrome?

MS III Yes, we did, but not for long. Pseudogout occurs in older persons and does not come on with such explosiveness. Reiter's syndrome usually involves two or more joints and is associated either with active nongonococcal urethritis or with diarrhea, as well as with conjunctivitis and mucocutaneous lesions. Except for possible urethritis, these features are not present here.

MD So the location of joint involvement and the number of joints involved influenced your reasoning?

MS III Yes, to some extent. Gout usually involves only one joint. The gonococcus and other bacteria that invade the bloodstream often cause multiple mild transitory joint involvement, but then settle down in one, two, or sometimes several joints.

Gout can affect any joint, but the first metatarsophalangeal joint is most common (75%); the ankles and knees may also be affected early. Bacteria are not too particular, although the knees and hips are common sites. Pseudogout favors the knee. An important fact I learned is that gout can involve the soft tissues near a joint and can simulate cellulitis. So many a patient with gout mistakenly receives an antibiotic.

MD I noted that the patient seems quite comfortable today; his temperature is normal, and his knee does not look so bad. What happened?

MS III We aspirated some fluid from the knee shortly after he was admitted last night. It was cloudy yellow and had a decreased viscosity and poor mucin clot. There were 20,000 WBCs/mm^3, most of which were PMNs. We are waiting for the fluid glucose determination. A culture was begun at the bedside, and a Gram's stain showed many PMNs, but no bacteria. Under polarized light microscopy, negatively birefringent needle-shaped crystals, 2 to 10 μm in length, were found free in the synovial fluid and inside leukocytes.

MD That proves the diagnosis of gout, does it not? The presence of typical monosodium urate crystals tells you that the patient has a crystal-induced arthritis. The calcium pyrophosphate

dihydrate crystals of pseudogout are rodlike or rhomboid in shape and are weakly positive birefringent.

There is a third uncommon crystal-induced arthritis. Calcium hydroxyapatite crystals can be found in some cases of arthritis. These crystals are too small to be seen with the ordinary light microscope; they can be identified by electron microscopy or radiographic diffraction studies (Table 19.1).

Why did you proceed with synovial aspiration even before the serum uric acid level result was returned?

MS III The uric acid level would not have been conclusive. First of all, the patient might have hyperuricemia, yet have an unrelated suppurative joint. Next, he might have gout, yet the uric acid level could be within normal limits. In addition, the definitive diagnosis of infectious arthritis can be made by identifying the organism in the synovial fluid. So we decided to go ahead.

MD An excellent thought! Approximately 5% of patients with gout have serum values under the upper limit of normal (7.0 mg/dL $\pm$ 0.2 mg) as demonstrated by population studies. Furthermore, 20% of patients with pseudogout have hyperuricemia, and large numbers of patients with hyperuricemia never develop gout. Remember too that the presence of urate crystals in the joint fluid does not necessarily exclude the added presence of another articular disease.

MS III Here come the results of the blood chemistry tests ordered last night. All findings are normal, except the serum uric acid level, which is 12.2 mg/dL. The blood glucose level is 100 mg/dL, whereas the synovial fluid glucose level is 70 mg/dL. We have already started treatment with colchicine, and the patient is improved this morning.

MD I am glad to see that you ordered an old but effective remedy even though your diagnostic techniques are very modern. Hippocrates described gout 2500 years ago, Galen noted tophi,

TABLE 19.1. Crystal Arthropathies

Monosodium urate—gout
Calcium pyrophosphate—pseudogout
Calcium hydroxyapatite

and 3500 years ago the Ebers Papyrus mentioned a drug that was probably colchicine; it was brought to this country by Benjamin Franklin, who suffered with gout. Can you tell me about the pathophysiology of gout?

MS III Yes. I had time to do some reading during the night. It is caused by monosodium urate crystals and is associated with *hyperuricemia*. This results from an overproduction of uric acid in some patients with primary or familial gout; many of these individuals have a disturbance in urate excretion by the kidney as well. But defective elimination by the kidney is solely responsible for *most* cases of gout.

Myeloproliferative states including leukemia, lymphoma, multiple myeloma, pernicious anemia, and polycythemia vera—especially under treatment—release large amounts of nucleoprotein that is degraded to uric acid. This may also cause gout. I suppose I should mention drugs that may cause hyperuricemia and precipitate an acute gouty attack, especially in gout-prone individuals. These include diuretics, ethambutol, nicotinic acid, pyrazinamide, and alcohol.

The exact cause for acute arthritis in most hyperuricemic patients is not clear, although it often seems to be precipitated by surgery, trauma, emotional upset, dietary excess, or alcohol. Often there is no clear-cut trigger event.

MD You have not mentioned a radiograph of the joint. Was it not done?

MS III Yes, but it did not help much. It showed some soft-tissue swelling, but no bone changes. The fact that there was no calcium in the cartilage (chondrocalcinosis) weighs against pseudogout, although I was not inclined toward that diagnosis anyway.

MD I note that the glucose level determinations have returned. This joint fluid is clearly a group II fluid. Do you know the classification?

MS III I believe that there are three groups: I, II, and III—depending on the cell count, ratio of synovial fluid to serum glucose, viscosity, and the presence of bacteria by Gram's stain or culture. Group I fluids are noninflammatory, have less than 5000 WBCs per cubic millimeter, glucose ratio > 0.90, high viscosity, and no bacteria. Group II fluids are aseptic inflammatory, have 5000 to 50,000 cells per cubic millimeter, glucose ratio $> .50$, low viscosity, and no bacteria. Group III fluids are septic inflammatory, have 20,000 to 200,000 cells per cubic millimeter, glucose ratio < 0.50, low viscosity, and test positive for bacteria on Gram's stain or culture. In groups II and III fluids, the cells are mostly PMNs, except for tuberculosis, where lymphocytes predominate. A fasting blood glucose level is used for comparison.

Group I fluids are found in normal joints and in hypertrophic osteoarthritis; group II fluids are seen in gout, pseudogout, Reiter's syndrome, acute rheumatic fever, rheumatoid arthritis, and systemic lupus erythematosus; group III fluids occur in septic and tuberculous joints.

MD Very good! I got more than I expected.

A point about the study of joint fluids! Do not hesitate to aspirate if in doubt. If carefully done, it is simple, without risk, and yields quality information. You may be surprised. Chronic gout mimics rheumatoid arthritis. Patients who have known gout or degenerative joint disease may develop a suppurative joint. Gout and pseudogout may coexist. At least once in the lifetime of an arthritic patient, a joint must be aspirated. And even in a previously diagnosed case, arthrocentesis may again be indicated if symptoms persist despite good treatment.

A word more about the nature of synovial fluid. Normal joints contain at most a few milliliters; the fluid is clear, colorless, and highly viscous—due to its high hyaluronic acid content. Inflamed joints (from bacteria or crystals) have effusions that are xanthochromic and cloudy, and are less viscous because of decreased amounts of hyaluronic acid and mucopolysaccharides. The mucin clot test assesses the ability of synovial fluid to wrap itself into a firm ball on exposure to 5% acetic acid. Effusions from inflamed joints have abnormal mucin clot formation because of the decrease in mucopolysaccharides; the clot is friable and fragments easily.

Suppose you saw a 65-year-old woman with a painful stiff knee for 3 years. What would you consider, and what would you do?

MS III I would think more in terms of hypertrophic osteoarthritis or degenerative joint disease because it is so common, especially in this age group. Tuberculosis would be a far less likely possibility. The radiograph and joint fluid for each condition would be characteristic.

MD Do gender and age enter very much into the logic of determining the type of arthritis?

MS III Very much so! More than 90% of gout and ankylosing spondylitis is seen in men. Pseudogout is also more common in men. Sjögren's syndrome, rheumatoid arthritis, and systemic lupus erythematosus are far more common in women.

MD I agree with your evaluation of pseudogout. But it merits more discussion. It is usually asymptomatic and is simply a radiographic finding. Calcification of cartilage is seen in radiographs of the knees, symphysis pubis, wrists, elbows, hip, spinal discs, and so forth. Clinically the disease may be manifested by an acute or subacute monarticular or polyarticular arthritis. It can thus mimic any of the common joint diseases—gout, rheumatoid arthritis, or degenerative joint disease. Aspiration reveals positively birefringent calcium pyrophosphate dihydrate crystals seen by polarized microscopy. This disease process is closely related to aging. But when found, it is sometimes associated with hyperparathyroidism or hemochromatosis.

One last item. You have mentioned those clues that were pertinently positive or negative to your provisional hypotheses. What about the rest of the examination?

MS III After the prime diagnosis was established and treatment was begun, the rest of the history and physical examination were completed. Except for obesity and hypertension, no other problems were uncovered.

MD An excellent job! Remember that a patient may have hyperuricemia for years without ever developing symptoms, that he may have uric acid stones instead of or before arthritis, and that he may progress into the stage of chronic tophaceous gout. This severe form of chronic destructive and deforming arthritis is unusual with today's forms of good treatment. We also see less tophi today for the same reason. These urate aggregates were formerly common and were seen in the helix, antihelix, extensor surface of the forearms, and around any involved joints. Sometimes they eroded the skin and exuded a milky or chalky material. When seen they are diagnostic.

Gout is such a fascinating disease! A few more points are worth mentioning. Careful questioning uncovers a family history in 70% of patients. The natural history of the disease is notable. The first attack of gouty arthritis comes after many years of hyperuricemia; in 90% of patients it affects one joint first, but it may affect several. Ultimately almost all patients experience podagra—involvement of the first metatarsophalangeal joint. Do not confuse this with an inflamed bunion!

Recurrent attacks occur in 1 to 10 years. Between episodes all is well except for the ongoing ravages of hyperuricemia. Eventually the attacks get longer, more severe, and polyarticular, and the disease becomes chronic and persistent. Good treatment should circumvent the latter situation.

The related problems are many. *Nephropathy* occurs in 90% of patients. Its mechanism is controversial, but it is associated with urate deposits in the interstitial tissue and tubules. This may be manifested simply by albuminuria or by serious obstructive and inflammatory nephropathy leading to renal failure. *Nephrolithiasis* is frequent. The stones consist of uric acid, but sometimes calcium stones are seen; perhaps the uric acid crystals act as a nidus for calcium deposition. Obesity, hypertriglyceridemia, diabetes mellitus, and hypertension are commonly associated with gout.

Perhaps less overlooked today than before, Lyme disease may present unusually with a single inflamed joint. There should be a history of tick-bite or tick exposure, and a very noticeable rash within the past year. Immunologic tests are almost 100% sensitive, but there are false-positive results, too.

This patient can be discharged from the hospital and referred to ambulatory care. Be sure to note that he needs care for obesity and hypertension—as well as for gout!

COMMENT In the first minute of patient contact, this capable student generated several initial hypotheses. Then she immediately sought specific clues to reject or confirm her hypotheses just as the experienced clinician does. As if guided by radar, she "hit the bull's eye" with confirmatory irrefutable tests. And last, after diagnosis and treatment were well established, she filled in the rest of the data base. Note that statistical likelihoods, overlap, coincidence, test specificity and sensitivity, gender, age, and the number and location of involved joints all entered into her very mature logical approach.

The problem of monarticular arthritis is generally best solved by an algorithmic or flowchart application of logic. Only basic skills and two or three tests are needed. On the basis of the clinical picture you can be reasonably sure of the diagnosis. But arthrocentesis and detailed fluid examination are almost invariably indicated and should produce a definite diagnosis. If not, a therapeutic trial with colchicine or antibiotics may be indicated if the joint is "hot." Otherwise, a "wait-and-see" strategy followed by a synovial biopsy in 4 to 6 weeks is indicated for the "cold" chronic undiagnosed joint. This may uncover a granulomatous disease or pigmented villonodular synovitis. *(P.C.)*

PROBLEM-BASED LEARNING The student who presented and discussed this case had obviously learned very much about the patient, his disorder, and related disorders before the presentation. Her performance was excellent. To do likewise, you must learn about:

- Gout and its pathophysiology, symptoms and signs, differential diagnosis, precise diagnosis, and complications
- Gouty nephropathy in particular
- Asymptomatic hyperuricemia and what to do about it
- Acute suppurative arthritis, its features, and its microbiology
- Gonorrhea, where to look for it, and how it affects joints
- Pseudogout and apatite-induced arthropathy
- Causes of secondary gout (diseases and drugs)
- Synovial fluid aspiration, the three general types of fluids and their features, and the type of fluid that characterizes various diseases
- Polarized light microscopy for crystal identification
- Reiter's syndrome
- Radiographic features of various joint diseases

Suggested Readings

Baker DB, Schumacher HR Jr. Acute monoarthritis. Current Concepts 1993;329:1013.

Goldenberg DL. Bacterial arthritis. Curr Opin Rheumatol 1995;7(4):310–314.

Joseph J, McGrath H. Gout or "pseudogout": How to differentiate crystal-induced arthropathies. Geriatrics 1995;50(4):33–39.

Rasaratnam I, Christophidis N. Gout: "A disease of plenty." Aust Fam Physician 1995;24(5):849–851, 855–856, 859–860.

Smith JW, Piercy EA. Infectious arthritis. Clin Infect Dis 1995;20(2):225–230.

CASE 68

SHOULDER PAIN

James D. Heckman and Michael A. Wirth

Data A 53-year-old left-handed carpenter comes to your office complaining of left shoulder pain that he has had for 3 months. The shoulder is especially symptomatic when he uses the arm at or above shoulder level. At first, the pain was intermittent, but now it is persistent and so severe that he is unable to work.

Logic Carpenters and certain other heavy laborers are prone to early degenerative changes in the joints of the dominant extremity. The patient's job and hobbies often give clues to the cause of musculoskeletal pain. Pain often results when the extremity is used in the overhead position when there are lesions in the rotator cuff. The rotator cuff is the name given to the group of muscles, ligaments, and cartilage that holds the shoulder together.

Most episodes of shoulder pain are the result of local inflammatory changes in the shoulder joint complex. These changes may be due to any of a wide variety of problems, including subdeltoid bursitis, bicipital tendonitis, rotator cuff injury, calcific tendonitis, osteoarthritis, rheumatoid arthritis, fracture, subluxation, dislocation, tumor, impingement syndrome, gout, and septic arthritis. On occasion, pain can be referred to the shoulder from a distant lesion (cervical radiculopathy, coronary artery disease, carpal tunnel syndrome, lung cancer, subdiaphragmatic abscess). Our first goal is to localize the pain.

Data The pain is constant and aching in nature. It is fairly well localized to the anterior portion of the shoulder and deltoid muscle, and it occasionally runs down the arm to the elbow. The pain is aggravated by any shoulder motion but particularly by abduction and forward flexion. The range of motion in the involved shoulder is only slightly diminished compared with the other side. Sensation and circulation in the arm are normal. Partial pain relief is obtained by resting the arm in a sling and taking aspirin. Hot packs applied to the shoulder give temporary relief. In addition to activity-related pain, the patient complains of discomfort that frequently awakens him from sleep.

Logic The additional data indicate that the pain is the result of local inflammation in and around the shoulder joint complex. "Bursitis" is a term used to describe this local inflammation. There are several different causes of shoulder bursitis. Inflammation in the rotator cuff is usually secondary to compression between the humeral head and the undersurface of the acromion (the outermost tip of the scapula at the top of the shoulder). With prolonged impingement and inflammation, the rotator cuff ruptures, producing weakness of abduction and atrophy of the cuff muscles. This pain and weakness constitute the "rotator cuff syndrome." After rupture of the cuff, there is a permanent communication between the shoulder joint and the subdeltoid bursa.

A number of problems commonly involved in "bursitis" of the shoulder cause pain that is increased by motion of the joint and relieved by limitation of motion and application of heat. Frozen shoulder, or adhesive capsulitis, results in a painful restriction of motion; the patients are frequently women older than 40 years of age, and range of motion is typically limited on one side. The biceps tendon runs through the shoulder joint, just deep to the rotator cuff. Repetitive activity of the biceps (as in carpentry) may produce inflammation in the tendon, which results in pain in the same area. However, primary bicipital tendonitis is uncommon, and inflammation of the biceps tendon is secondary to other disorders in 95% of patients.

Although night discomfort is generally considered an ominous finding because of its association with malignancy, this is a common complaint in patients with shoulder bursitis, especially when they sleep on the involved side.

Data The patient denies any recent injury to the shoulder or neck. He does remember one episode of acute shoulder pain 5 years ago after pitching baseball. This lasted approximately 2 weeks and then completely resolved. He has no pain in any other joints. There is no numbness, paresthesia, or weakness in the left upper extremity.

Logic It is very important to know if there has been any trauma to the shoulder. Fracture, subluxation, and dislocation are frequent causes of local joint pain. No history of injury virtually eliminates trauma as a possible cause in this patient. Conversely, if the patient had remembered an episode of forceful abduction and external rotation of the shoulder in the past, recurrent subluxation or dislocation of the shoulder would be a definite possibility. The incident of transient pain 5 years ago, after moderate shoulder activity, supports the pattern of a local recurrent inflammatory process in that area.

The fact that the patient has not had pain, heat, or swelling in other joints now or in the past allows us to think less in terms of polyarticular disease (rheumatoid arthritis, gout, pseudogout, degenerative arthritis). Although some of these diseases can initially exhibit monarticular symptoms, it is unusual for them to do so in the shoulder.

The absence of neck pain and no history of neck injury are very important. Remember that diseases of the cervical spine, especially osteoarthritis with radiculitis, often present with pain in the shoulder, particularly over the area of the trapezius muscle. But there is usually some associated numbness or weakness of the involved limb, which is not the case here.

Carpal tunnel syndrome may sometimes start as a pain radiating to the shoulder from the wrist. Numbness and weakness in the median nerve distribution will usually be prominent complaints as well. This syndrome is caused by compression of the median nerve in the rigid and narrow carpal tunnel at the wrist. It is occasionally seen after wrist fracture and can sometimes be associated with hypothyroidism or rheumatoid arthritis. Again, these factors do not apply.

Data The patient has been self-employed for 32 years and has four children, two of whom are still in college. Because he has been in "great" health, he has not seen a physician in years. He has smoked two packs of cigarettes per day for 35 years, but has no other bad habits. He specifically denies any chest pain, fatigue, shortness of breath, anorexia, or weight loss; however, he does have a morning cough that produces a small amount of clear phlegm. This has not changed during the last year, and there has been no hemoptysis.

Logic With musculoskeletal problems, it is especially important to assess the patient's motivation regarding his job. Very often a significant amount of secondary gain can be derived from physical impairment. Because our patient is self-employed and has burdensome family financial obligations, it is doubtful that he is seeking disability compensation.

Cardiopulmonary disease is a common cause of shoulder pain, especially in this age group. But if the patient had angina, he would have episodic chest pain radiating to the left shoulder that comes on exertion and may be accompanied by fatigue and/or dyspnea. This is not the case here. However, his smoking history should raise a red flag. Shoulder pain is a common presentation of lung carcinoma arising in the medial part of the apex (Pancoast's tumor). The mild chronic cough is probably from smoking but must be checked. He has no hemoptysis, weight loss, anorexia, or fatigue to suggest cancer. It is important to note that shoulder pain of visceral origin (lung cancer, heart disease, diaphragmatic disease) is not worsened by shoulder movement. Thus far, we have a healthy middle-aged man with disabling pain in his dominant shoulder that probably has a local cause.

Data Physical examination is performed. The patient appears healthy, has good color, and is muscular and slightly overweight. Complete examination findings are normal except for those in the shoulder area. The cervical spine shows no deformity or difficulty with full flexion, extension, rotation, and left- and right-sided bending. He has no pain or symptoms on axial compression of the cervical spine, and there is no tenderness to palpation.

Logic The absence of abnormalities in the heart and lungs reinforces the absence of major symptoms there. Inspection, palpation, and the performance of range of motion of the cervical spine require less than 1 minute. After these normal examination findings have been established, we can be virtually certain that the origin of the pain is not in the cervical spine.

Data On inspection of the shoulder, there is wasting of the muscles over the scapula. The shoulder is otherwise normal in appearance without swelling, erythema, or deformity. Comparison with the normal shoulder demonstrates no other discrepancy in appearance.

Logic The limbs are paired organs, and one limb should always be compared with its opposite member, which is usually a normal mirror image. All of the examinations (inspection, palpation, range of motion, strength, and even radiographs) should be performed on both limbs using the opposite normal limb as a control. Wasting of the muscles of the rotator cuff (supraspinatus, in-

fraspinatus, teres minor, and subscapularis) indicates probable tear of part or all of the cuff and reinforces our impression that the problem lies within the shoulder joint. Paralysis of the suprascapular nerve or a C5-C6 nerve root lesion could produce this positive finding, but this is rare without trauma and without positive cervical spine findings.

Data On palpation, there is slight tenderness over the distal clavicle and acromioclavicular joint. Localized tenderness is noted over the anterolateral acromion, greater tuberosity of the humerus, and biceps tendon, but there is no exquisite tenderness or discomfort on the posterior or lateral aspects of the shoulder.

Logic Localized tenderness is the single most helpful diagnostic finding in evaluation of musculoskeletal problems. Careful gentle palpation of the bony landmarks in the area of pain will usually demonstrate localized tenderness. By knowing what musculotendinous or ligamentous structures pass over or around these landmarks, or insert into them, the physician can pinpoint the involved structure.

In this patient, the area of tenderness is the inferior edge of the anterior and lateral acromion. This is the location of the subacromial bursa, and tenderness there points to inflammation in the bursa and probably a lesion of the underlying rotator cuff. Exquisite point tenderness in the region of the greater tuberosity usually indicates calcific tendonitis. Most patients who have calcific tendonitis will respond to nonoperative management, but may require needling and steroid injections. In cases of suspected calcific tendonitis, the diagnosis is easily made with anteroposterior internal and external rotation radiographs of the shoulder.

Data Range of motion of the shoulder shows extension to 30 degrees, external rotation to 30 degrees, and internal rotation to 60 degrees. On passive forward flexion, there is severe pain in the shoulder, especially from 60 to 120 degrees. Actively, the patient can flex to only 120 degrees because of severe pain. Abduction is limited to 100 degrees actively and passively. Strength is graded as 4/5 during external rotation with the arm at the side and during forward flexion.

Logic Normal active and passive range of motion would be a good indication of the absence of disease within and around the joint, but this patient has significant limitation of range of motion. He demonstrates the classic findings of the impingement syndrome: pain on forward flexion due to impingement of the humeral head on the undersurface of the acromion. This coincides with our findings on inspection of a probable rotator cuff tear in which the rotator cuff has become caught between the humeral head and acromion and has gradually worn away, allowing the humeral head to press against (impinge on) the acromion on forward flexion.

Data   The remainder of the limb is examined and no deformity is seen or palpated. There is a full range of motion of the other joints. Circulation, sensation, and motor function are normal.

Logic   Completion of the upper extremity examination shows no other disease process.

Data   Radiographs in the anteroposterior and lateral projections of the shoulders show no evidence of fracture or dislocation. A special view (30-degree caudal tilt) taken at an angle that shows a profile of the acromion demonstrates a spur on its anteroinferior rim. On the left side, there is mild degenerative arthritis of the joint of the acromion and the clavicle and narrowing of the space between the acromion and the humeral head (Fig. 19.1). There are no lesions present within the bones. The glenohumeral joint appears normal. Chest radiographic findings are normal.

Logic   The radiographs of the shoulder support the physical findings (remember the importance of always obtaining radiographs in two planes at right angles to one another). The patient has early degenerative arthritis of the acromioclavicular joint, which explains the moderate tenderness in that area. Routine anteroposterior radiographs do not usually demonstrate an anterior acromial spur. However, a radiograph of the shoulder taken at an angle will adequately demonstrate this finding in the majority of patients (Fig. 19.1). Narrowing of the acromiohumeral space results from a chronic tear of the rotator cuff—the spacer effect is lost—and from spurring of the acromion. The absence of other bony lesions reassures us that there is no bone tumor. Such a tumor most likely would have been a metastatic lesion, and in the middle-aged and older individual, this possibility must always be remembered. Similarly, the chest radiographs rule out a Pancoast tumor. Although rare, the grave consequences of

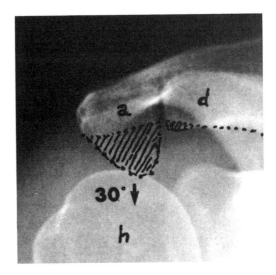

► **Figure 19.1.** The radiograph beam is aimed at the shoulder from 30 degrees above the horizontal plane, thus allowing better visualization of the acromioclavicular joint where the major pathology lies. The radiograph demonstrates the acromial spur: a = acromion; d = distal clavicle; h = humeral head; cross-hatched area shows the spur. The broken line defines the normal clavicle and acromion.

such tumors require that we search diligently for them.

The diagnosis of impingement syndrome with chronic cuff tear and subacromial bursitis is now virtually certain. A final simultaneously diagnostic and therapeutic step can be made.

Data   Arthrocentesis of the shoulder joint is performed. Ten milliliters of clear yellow joint fluid with fair viscosity is aspirated. The shoulder joint is injected with 10 mL of 1% lidocaine and 40 mg triamcinolone. Following injection, the patient has complete relief of pain and a full passive range of motion of the shoulder. Laboratory evaluation of the joint fluid shows: aerobic and anaerobic cultures—no growth; WBC count, 5000/mm^3 with 50% polymorphonuclear leukocytes and 50% lymphocytes; glucose, 108 mg/dL; rheumatoid factor (RF) absent; antinuclear antibody (ANA) absent; and examination for crystals—no monosodium urate and no calcium pyrophosphate.

Logic   Arthrocentesis provides us with the best material for examination in a patient with joint pain. The cultures demonstrate the absence of septic arthritis. This is supported by the low

WBC count and the normal glucose level. The absence of crystals rules out gout and pseudogout, and absent rheumatoid factor and antinuclear antibody make the possibility of collagen disease very remote.

The ability to relieve joint pain by instillation of a local anesthetic confirms our suspicion that the source of the pain is inflammation in the shoulder joint. By careful questioning and precise examination, we have been able to localize the source of the patient's pain. Trauma, systemic disease, and tumor have been eliminated. Inflammation of the subdeltoid bursa due to rupture of the rotator cuff leading to chronic impingement of the humeral head on the acromion is the most likely diagnosis.

Questions

1. The usual cause of acute shoulder pain in a 20-year-old man who sustains an abduction and external rotation stress to the joint is:
   (a) impingement syndrome.
   (b) subluxation or dislocation of the shoulder.
   (c) shoulder separation.
   (d) shoulder-hand syndrome.
2. The tumor most apt to cause shoulder pain in a 60-year-old woman is:
   (a) osteogenic sarcoma.
   (b) synovial sarcoma.
   (c) metastatic carcinoma.
   (d) enchondroma.
3. A 39-year-old woman is initially seen with a 6-day history of right shoulder pain after a car wreck. On examination, she demonstrates weakness of grip strength and decreased sensation in the little and ring fingers of the right hand. It is likely that we will find additional abnormalities on further examination of the:
   (a) chest.
   (b) cervical spine.
   (c) shoulder.
   (d) wrist.
4. A 68-year-old woman has shoulder pain after falling on her outstretched hand. The probable diagnosis is:
   (a) acute rotator cuff tear.
   (b) rupture of the biceps tendon.
   (c) fracture of the surgical neck of the humerus.
   (d) dislocation of the shoulder.

Answers

1. **(b) is correct.** Anterior dislocation and subluxation of the shoulder occur very commonly in this age group, and the mechanism of injury is almost always abduction and external rotation stress. Impingement syndrome occurs in older individuals after years of repeated stress, particularly of forward flexion. Shoulder separation means acromioclavicular separation, and although common in this age group, it usually occurs from a direct blow to the point of the shoulder. The shoulder-hand syndrome is a chronic problem not usually related to acute injury; it frequently follows myocardial infarction.
2. **(c) is correct.** The most likely tumor in the older woman is a metastatic lesion to the proximal humerus. The metastasis usually comes from the breast, lung, kidney, or gastrointestinal tract. An enchondroma is a benign, usually asymptomatic, tumor. Osteogenic sarcoma is the most common primary sarcoma of bone, and approximately 10 to 15% occur in the proximal humerus. However, this malignant lesion is uncommon in adults unless the patient has underlying Paget's disease. Synovial sarcoma is also rare, especially in the shoulder joint.
3. **(b) is correct.** The cervical spine is very frequently injured in car wrecks, and a nerve root injury in the neck often causes shoulder pain and a neurologic deficit in the limb. Shoulder injury with damage to the brachial plexus might cause these findings, but injury of the brachial plexus is uncommon.
4. **(c) is correct.** The prevalence of osteoporosis among elderly women makes fracture the most likely result of trauma to the shoulder. Seventy-seven percent of proximal humerus fractures occur in women, and the incidence increases exponentially with age greater than 50 years. The muscles and supporting ligaments are much less likely to be injured in a fall.

COMMENT On the basis of a key clue, various possibilities were considered. Bayes' theorem established periarticular inflammation as the most likely possibility: all other possibilities were ruled out, and the most likely one was proved. False-positive indicators (cough, cigarette smoking) were present. The type of pain, relationship to shoulder motion, and occupation were important clues. Cause and effect was frequently invoked. An anatomic approach was used in the physical examination. The diagnosis was reasonably certain, but an invasive diagnostic procedure (arthrocentesis) was done to clinch the diagnosis and employ a therapeutic trial at the same time. A decision tree could easily have been used here. A few selected questions and examination techniques, radiographs, and joint aspiration, and the problem would have been very rapidly solved. Age, sex, and history of injury weighted our thinking in the questions and answers. *(P.C.)*

Suggested Readings

Rockwood CA, Lyons FR. Shoulder impingement syndrome: Diagnosis, radiographic evaluation, and treatment with a modified Neer acromioplasty. J Bone Joint Surg 1993;75A(3):409–424.

Rockwood CA, Matsen FA. The Shoulder. Philadelphia: WB Saunders; 1990. [This is an all-inclusive text on the shoulder.]

 C A S E 69

PAINFUL STIFF JOINTS

Paul Cutler

Data Difficulty in performing the duties of her occupation brings a 37-year-old secretary to your office. For the past 3 years she has had intermittent episodes of pain, stiffness, warmth, and swelling of the hands and wrists. Each bout lasted for several months and then subsided. Now she has similar symptoms in her knees and elbows too. The present illness began 2 weeks ago, and she not only finds it impossible to type but can hardly get out of bed and do her morning chores.

Logic Symmetric polyarthritis brings to mind many diseases: rheumatoid arthritis (RA), systemic lupus erythematosus (SLE), acute rheumatic fever, Reiter's syndrome, other connective tissue diseases like scleroderma and dermatomyositis, and sarcoidosis.

Rheumatic fever can be eliminated almost immediately because of the length of the illness and the frequency of recurrences; it is an acute febrile illness lasting only 6 to 8 weeks. The presentation of sarcoidosis embodies different complaints (lymphadenopathy, dyspnea), and most of the other diseases mentioned are not nearly so prevalent as RA and SLE.

RA is the most common, has its peak incidence in women of this age, behaves precisely this way, and thus becomes your first provisional hypothesis. It is a joint disease whose cause is unknown, and it is manifested mainly by inflammation of synovial linings of the proximal interphalangeal and metacarpophalangeal joints, erosion of their articular cartilages, and eventual deformity and fixation.

Next in order of likelihood is SLE. It too has a predilection for the same population subset and usually begins in the same manner, but it is only one twentieth as common as RA. It becomes your second hypothesis.

With the information already on hand, you lean toward RA. But in thinking of RA you realize that this disease, whose main features are in the synovial cavities, has widespread extra-articular manifestations. It may be associated with inflammations of various layers of the eyeball; diffuse vasculitis; generalized amyloidosis; cardiac manifestations (pericarditis, coronary arteritis, valvulitis); pulmonary indicators (effusion, nodules, fibrosis); hematologic omens (normocytic anemia of chronic disease, hypochromic anemia from aspirin-induced blood loss); splenomegaly (Felty's syndrome); renal abnormalities signaled by proteinuria (vasculitis, amyloidosis, proliferative glomerulonephritis, treatment with gold, penicillamine, and nonsteroidal antiinflammatory drugs, and papillary necrosis from analgesics); and carpal tunnel syndrome resulting from compression of the median nerve by realigned carpal bones.

Data The patient has seen various physicians in the past, each of whom treated her for "arthritis," although no type was ever specified. She had received pills, tablets, injections, and physiotherapy with partial benefit. Between the last few episodes, she did not become symptom-free as before, but continued having some residual pain and stiffness, especially on awakening.

Logic Degenerative joint disease, or hypertrophic osteoarthritis, is by far the most common form of arthritis. It too may affect multiple joints, but it occurs in older age groups, is not usually associated with inflammation or constitutional symptoms, and tends not to be so episodic.

Crystal-induced arthritis was not considered from the start. Gout is unusual in young premenopausal women, it tends not to affect the small joints of the hands at first, nor is it so symmetrically polyarticular. Pseudogout involves mostly large joints and is seen in older individuals.

The patient has had a variety of treatments, some of which may have helped, but it is difficult to judge this by her history. Note that she is no longer symptom-free between bouts of arthritis. Further inquiry must aim toward proving or disproving one of the two principal hypotheses. The difficulty in doing this lies in the fact that both diseases (RA and SLE) have similar presentations, and both have systemic manifestations and laboratory abnormalities in which there is considerable overlap.

The American Rheumatism Association (ARA) has adopted criteria for the diagnosis of and distinction between RA and SLE. These criteria also help differentiate RA and SLE from other arthritic diseases that may resemble them. Table 19.2 lists the criteria for RA, and Table 19.3 lists the criteria for SLE. Note the number of criteria considered to be diagnostic when they are present in concert.

Sad to say, the criteria for RA may not be reliable in all cases, especially the early, the atypical, or the complicated ones. There can be overlap with other diseases bearing a family resemblance. Therefore, the sensitivity and specificity of this supposedly diagnostic set are not spectacular.

Textbook cases of SLE are simple to diagnose. For example, visualize a young woman with fever, polyarthritis, serositis, malar rash, marked albuminuria, and a high-titer antinuclear antibody test. Often, however, the case is not so typical, and it has features that overlap with other autoimmune disorders. Only *some* earmarks may be present. The 1982 ARA criteria tried to simplify the diagnosis and required the presence of

TABLE 19.3. Criteria for Systemic Lupus Erythematosus (Revised 1982, American Rheumatism Association)[a]

1. Malar rash
2. Discoid rash
3. Photosensitivity
4. Oral or nasal ulcers
5. Arthritis (two points)
6. Serositis (pleuritis, pericarditis)
7. Renal disorder—proteinuria or abnormal casts
8. Seizures or psychosis
9. Hematologic disorder—hemolytic anemia, or leukopenia, or lymphopenia, or thrombocytopenia
10. Immunologic disorder—positive LE cell preparation, or high anti–DNA titer, or false-positive serologic test result for syphilis
11. ANA titer abnormal

[a]If four or more criteria are present simultaneously or serially, the diagnosis is established.

any four salient points. But this attempt to establish paradigms does not work. It, too, overlooks early atypical cases, and some patients whose symptoms seem to fit do not have the disease. So these criteria also are not only insensitive, but they are not even specific.

Data During the past year, she has noted malaise, weakness, and easy fatigability. For the past 2 weeks she has not felt well and thinks she has had some fever. She has never noted any color changes in the fingertips on immersing them in cold water. There has been no diarrhea; blood in the stool; abdominal cramps; rashes of any kind, including any on the face; cough; sharp chest pain; shortness of breath; convulsions; mental changes; eye problems; dryness of the mouth and eyes; loss of hair; or cutaneous sensitivity to sunlight. Other than aspirin for her arthritis, she now takes no medication.

Logic The constitutional symptoms of fever, weakness, and malaise are common to both diseases. Raynaud's phenomenon is not present; it is seen in 20% of SLE patients and uncommonly in RA. Arthritis that is occasionally associated with inflammatory bowel diseases (ulcerative colitis, regional ileitis) can be ruled out by the lack of gastrointestinal symptoms. Absence of a facial

TABLE 19.2. Criteria for Diagnosis of Rheumatoid Arthritis (Revised 1988, American Rheumatism Association)[a]

Morning stiffness (1 hour)
Arthritis in 3 joints or more
Arthritis in hand joints
Symmetric arthritis
Rheumatoid nodules
Serum rheumatoid factor
Typical radiographic findings

[a]Diagnosis exists if four criteria are present.

rash and no evidence of cerebral disease weigh against SLE because each of these symptoms occurs in one quarter to one half of patients. Neither is there a history of patchy alopecia or sunlight sensitivity, which are peculiar to SLE. No symptomatic evidence is present for lung or pleuropericardial disease; these are more common in SLE but can be found in both diseases. There is nothing in the history to suggest uveitis, keratoconjunctivitis, or sicca syndrome—each sometimes seen in RA.

Moreover, the patient takes no medication other than aspirin; hydralazine, procainamide, certain anti-epileptics, and, rarely, other drugs can cause pictures identical to SLE.

So far there are no distinguishing clues, but the absence of those frequently found in SLE (rash, cerebral symptoms, and pleuropericardial disease) makes this diagnosis even less likely.

Physical examination in any patient with joint disease often discloses an abundance of findings. These vary with the type of arthritis and have different diagnostic significance. Look for alopecia, photosensitivity, sicca syndrome, Sjögren's syndrome, eye inflammations, temporal arteritis, heliotrope of the eyelids, oral or nasal ulcers, psoriasis, Raynaud's phenomenon, vasculitic lesions, decreased neck and spinal flexion, nodules over the elbow, erythema nodosum, the special rashes of SLE and Lyme disease, carpal tunnel syndrome, anemia, splenomegaly, and of course abnormalities of the joints themselves. Do not forget the CREST syndrome seen in scleroderma, a disease that often produces a polyarthritis. This acronymic syndrome consists of calcinosis, Raynaud's phenomenon, esophageal abnormalities, sclerodactyly, and telangiectasia.

Data The patient seems a bit pale, and her temperature is 38.2°C. There is swelling, tenderness, slight redness, and warmth of most proximal interphalangeal joints, the metacarpophalangeal joints, the wrists, knees, and elbows. She can hardly walk, cannot shake hands, and has great difficulty getting in and out of a chair.

Her eyes appear normal, and there is no rash across the cheeks nor nodules on the extensor surfaces of the elbows and hands. The blood pressure, heart, and lungs are normal; in particular, there is no evidence of pleural effusion, and no friction rubs or murmurs are heard. The rest of the examination is normal, too.

Logic Pallor, fever, and symmetric subacute polyarthritis are present. These are nondiscriminatory. Although it may be too early to see the characteristic hand deformities of RA, if these deformities are present, RA becomes likely; SLE is less often the cause of subluxations and ulnar deviation of the fingers (Fig. 19.2). The absence of findings in the head and chest corroborates the lack of symptoms there and does nothing to alter likelihoods. Subcutaneous nodules commonly seen in RA (20%) are not present. The absence of a heart murmur is of no special help; systolic murmurs are common in SLE and rare in RA.

Although found in 10% of patients with both diseases, splenomegaly is not noted here. Neither is lymphadenopathy. An important discerning clue will be the presence or absence of renal disease because it is uncommon in RA (amyloidosis) and common (50%) in SLE. The laboratory may help. So far, SLE has not been proved because only one criterion—arthritis without deformity—is noted to be present.

An abundance of tests helps in the differential diagnosis. Each must be interpreted with caution because sensitivity and specificity are variable. A *blood count* usually discloses anemia; if there is leukopenia too, suspect Felty's syndrome and search again for an enlarged spleen. The *erythrocyte sedimentation rate* is very rapid in polymyalgia rheumatica (temporal arteritis), moderately rapid

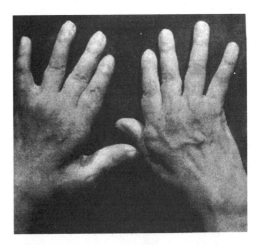

▶ **Figure 19.2.** Hand of patient with advanced rheumatoid arthritis. Note swelling of metacarpal-phalangeal joints, proximal interphalangeal joints, wrist, and ulnar deviation of some fingers.

in any active inflammatory arthritis, and normal in degenerative joint disease. A 1:160 *ANA titer* is more than 90% sensitive for SLE, but the test result may sometimes be positive in RA, too. The *anti-DNA antibody* test correlates well with SLE and is fairly specific. However, the *rheumatoid factor* (latex test), although having positive results in 75% of RA patients, is not very specific; its results are positive in 5% of normal individuals, in 20% of the elderly, and often in other types of arthropathy. Be wary of a diagnosis in an older patient with diffuse aches and pains who happens to have a positive latex test result. The *LE cell preparation* is 80% sensitive for SLE, but its results are also positive in 10 to 20% of patients who have RA. *Serum complement* is decreased in active SLE but normal in RA (Table 19.4).

The radiograph is not so valuable as you might think. In early cases it shows nothing. In late cases where the radiograph is helpful, the diagnosis has long since been made by other clinical features.

Data The following studies are done: complete blood count shows mild "anemia of chronic disease," normal WBC count and differential, and adequate platelets; urinalysis results are normal; erythrocyte sedimentation rate is rapid (40 mm/h); serologic test result for syphilis is negative; and the 18-test blood chemistry profile findings are normal.

Logic Anemia is common to both diseases, but hemolytic anemia and cytopenia are frequent in SLE. The normal urinalysis findings speak for RA; had there been much protein and cellular casts present, SLE might have moved into the first position. Also, 15% of patients with SLE have a

TABLE 19.4. Incidence of Positive Antibody Tests in RA and SLE

TEST	RA (%)	SLE (%)
ANA	10–25	99
Anti–DNA	5	>50
LE cells	10–20	60–80
Hypocomplementemia	0–10	75
RF	>75	20
False-positive VDRL	0	20

ANA = antinuclear antibody; RF = rheumatoid factor; VDRL = Venereal Disease Research Laboratory.

false-positive serologic test for syphilis. The rapid erythrocyte sedimentation rate is almost always present in both conditions. Kidney function is normal. Autoimmune processes exist in both diseases, but there are many more demonstrable antibodies in SLE. Further tests are needed.

Data The ANA test result is positive; anti-DNA test result is negative; LE cells are not present; serum complement is normal; and the RF test result as measured by latex agglutination is positive. Levels of creatine phosphokinase and serum aminotransferases are normal. (Note that the test for LE cells is no longer commonly done, because it has been replaced by more specific antibody tests.)

Logic There is much overlap in most of these tests regarding both diseases. In fact, some tests have results that are occasionally positive in other diseases or in nondisease. The problem is evident, as shown in Table 19.4. However, even without using formulas and Bayesian equations, it can be seen that the patient's test results lean more heavily toward RA. Had the ANA test result been negative, there would have been no question about the diagnosis of RA, because this test is very highly sensitive for SLE. Also, had serum complement been low, RA would have been rendered most unlikely. Normal muscle enzymes rule out the already unlikely and rare disease, dermatomyositis.

No discussion of joint diseases can exclude one of the newest members of the family—Lyme disease. This spirochetal disease is transmitted by the tick, *Ixodes dammini* and was first noted in the area of Lyme, Connecticut. It affects mainly the young and is characterized by erythema chronicum migrans and recurrent arthritis. Notably, 25% of those individuals with arthritis do not have skin lesions, and arthritis is seen in only 50% of patients.

Data To complete the work-up: a chest radiographic finding is normal, and radiographs of the involved joints show only periarticular swelling and bone demineralization, and the electrocardiogram (ECG) results are normal.

Logic The chest radiograph lays to rest any possibility of lung or pleural disease. A normal ECG finding does not aid in diagnosis, although sometimes a conduction abnormality caused by a critically located rheumatoid nodule is seen in RA. The joint radiographs at this stage are the same for both diseases, and synovial fluid aspiration would have shown a group II fluid in both instances. With all the evidence on the scales, RA weighs in the heavier.

Data The patient is told she has rheumatoid arthritis and is placed on a carefully prescribed regimen of high-dose aspirin, rest, and physiotherapy. The use of gold or methotrexate will be considered.

COMMENT Because RA and SLE have different complications, prognoses, and treatments, it is advisable to be sure which of these two closely related diseases is present. The overlap of criteria and the less than ideal sensitivity and specificity of tests and procedures used to diagnose these two diseases make their distinction all the more difficult. However, on the basis of criteria set up by the ARA, this differentiation may often be possible.

Although provisional hypotheses were formed early, it was difficult to prove one or the other decisively, even with all the clues at hand. Statistical probability gives RA the overwhelming Bayesian likelihood, although the clinical picture is inconclusive; the laboratory tests lean more toward RA. The patient's future course may mandate a change in diagnosis and perhaps in treatment too. No wonder her previous physicians would only label this disease as "arthritis." This writer is not so sure either . . . . *(P.C.)*

Suggested Readings

Gruppen LD, Palchik NS, Wolf FM, et al. Medical student use of history and physical information in diagnostic reasoning. Arthritis Care Res 1993;6(2):64–70.

Maini RN, Elliott MJ, Charles PJ, et al. Immunological intervention reveals reciprocal roles for tumor necrosis factor-alpha and interleukin-10 in rheumatoid arthritis and systemic lupus erythematosus. Springer Semin Immunopathol 1994;16(2–3):327–336.

Reveille JD. The molecular genetics of systemic lupus erythematosus and Sjogren's syndrome. Curr Opin Rheumatol 1992;4(5):644–656.

C A S E 70

BACKACHE

Paul Cutler

Data A 52-year-old man comes walking slowly into your office, stooped over and holding his hand to his back. He puts his hands on the arms of a chair, slowly lowers himself into it and exclaims, "Doctor, I have had this terrible back pain that shoots down my hip and into my leg for the past 2 weeks!"

Logic Back pain is one of the most common symptoms seen in practice. Epidemiologic studies show that 80% of persons in North America will experience some extent of back pain during their active lifetime. In industrial workers the yearly incidence of back pain is 50 in 1000 workers.

When faced with the previously described scenario, you immediately recall the many different causes of back pain: (1) viscerogenic, (2) vascular, (3) neurogenic, (4) psychogenic, and (5) spondylogenic. The last category is by far the largest. It includes all those cases of backache that are directly related to the spinal column and its many components: bones, muscles, tendons, ligaments, fascia, discs, and nerves. The anatomy and biomechanical features of the back must be understood.

To solve this problem, three important issues must be quickly settled: the exact location of the pain, the presence or absence of radiation down a leg, and the relation of back and leg activity to the pain. Pain down the leg is called "sciatica" because it tends to follow the course of the sciatic nerve. It usually starts in the low back or buttock, and then radiates down the posterior thigh into the calf and plantar aspect of the foot. Sometimes it can radiate from the posterior thigh into the anterior compartment and dorsum of the foot.

Viscerogenic back pain is caused by penetrating ulcers or pancreatic or renal disease, is localized near the area of the disease, does not radiate down the leg, is not worsened by back motion, and is almost always accompanied by other manifestations of the disease. Kidney pain is in the flank or costovertebral angle, off to a side, whereas pancreatic or ulcer pain is high in the midback. Prostate or uterine disease can cause low back pain but, again, no radiation or worsening by movement—unless the disease is metastatic carcinoma to the spine.

Vascular causes include abdominal aortic aneurysms that give rise to boring pain where they exist, and peripheral vascular disease that causes pain in the lower extremity. The latter disease can be confusing in that the leg pain can include hip and buttock pain too, but it is easily distinguishable because pain is brought on by walking, relieved by stopping, and is not related to bending or lifting.

Spinal canal tumors can present with sciatic pain, but often the pain is at night, and activity is required for relief. True sciatic neuritis can be caused by diabetes mellitus. Pure psychogenic pain is uncommon, but organic pain patterns can be confused by psychogenic overtones.

Data As the patient enters your office, you skim over your notes of his previous visits. He is a self-employed businessman running a shoe store, and he has been having financial problems. His wife has threatened to leave him. Ulcer symptoms have been intermittently present for 10 years, although radiographs done twice were inconclusive. He has been overweight for years.

Recently he consulted a urologist for hesitancy and increasing frequency of urination. Cystourethroscopy was done, but he does not know the results; he was unable to keep his reappointment because of back pain. His mother had diabetes that she got in her 60s. Also, he had three previous visits because of back pain in the past few years. Each episode occurred after heavy gardening, radiated to the right gluteal area, and resolved with rest.

Logic You have been barraged with a series of clues that may be relevant to his back pain. Psychosomatic components may be present. Malingering is unlikely because, being self-employed, he has nothing to gain financially from his illness. However, back pain could be a means of getting sympathy or an excuse for business failure.

Although he may have an ulcer, it would not cause pains such as he has. The urologic problem worries you. Prostatic cancer with metastasis is possible. And cystoscopy can cause vertebral osteomyelitis via Batson's venous plexus. The family history of diabetes is a concern; diabetic neuropathy can present as sciatic neuritis, although back pain would be absent.

Many backaches seen in the primary care physician's office are transient and caused by a back strain or "sprain." This may relate to an injury of a ligament, tendon, or muscle caused by a specific activity like lifting, bending, or twisting. But remember that this minor episode may be the first manifestation of discogenic disease. The potential for such minor injuries can be increased by conditions that put extra strain on the spine. These include obesity, severe

spinal deformity (scoliosis, kyphosis, lordosis), poor body posture, and, occasionally, significant leg length differences. Some say that the latter conditions alone can cause backache, but this is debatable. At any rate, these predisposing conditions can be readily detected on examination.

Osteoarthritis of the spine can and does cause backache. But osteoarthritis is such a common radiographic finding in persons without backaches that its presence is difficult to assess. Bony overgrowth can entrap nerve roots in the intervertebral foramina and produce pain radiating down the leg. It is difficult to be sure the radiograph findings correlate with the clinical picture.

Even though it is uncommon, be alert for tuberculosis of the spine. And persistent back pain can be a sign of a more common disease—metastatic cancer. Radiograph, isotope scan, and MRI may be needed. The entity of "muscular rheumatism" (fibrosis or fibromyositis) has not been proved to exist, although the term is frequently used to describe short-lived pain around the back; it remains a subject for dispute.

This patient has backache with sciatica. Disc degeneration is the most common cause of this type of pain. His previous episodes of back pain could all be classified as mechanical or spondylogenic in that they were relieved with rest and aggravated with activity. They could be described as "lumbosacral strains" in that they resolved quickly with rest, but they may also suggest an ongoing process of degenerative disc disease. Shrinkage and degeneration of the disc itself allow abnormal disc motion and microtears in the annulus; eventual disc protrusion into the spinal canal takes place.

Data The present episode started 2 weeks ago when he was lifting a tire from his trunk. A short while later he felt midline low back pain, which then radiated to his right buttock and down the posterior thigh into the anterior portion of his calf to the dorsum of his foot. He went to bed and has been quite comfortable lying down. The pain returns when he stands to resume his activities. If he coughs or strains, the same pain shoots down his right leg.

Examination of the vital signs, head, neck, chest, and abdomen is normal. He points to the lower lumbar spine as the site of his pain. There is slight curvature of the back and markedly decreased range of motion. By flexing the back, he can only reach his knees with his fingertips. This action aggravates the pain. He can toe walk, but on heel walking he finds it impossible to lift up his right foot. Straight leg raising is limited to 20 degrees as compared with 80 degrees on the left. Lasègue's sign is present on the right. There is tenderness along the course of the right sciatic nerve in the buttock and popliteal space. He has markedly decreased power in the dorsiflexors of the ankle and the extensor hallucis longus, with hypesthesia to pinprick over the lower anterolateral calf and dorsum of the right foot. Patellar and Achilles reflexes are normal. Good pulses are felt in both legs and feet.

Logic There is a foot-drop on the right with signs of sciatic nerve irritation and L5 nerve root compression as shown by the neurologic abnormalities, nerve tenderness, limitation of straight leg raising, and positive Lasègue's sign. Sensory abnormalities also conform to the L5 dermatome. The reflexes remain normal because the knee-jerk is an L2-L3-L4 reflex arc, and the ankle-jerk is an S1-S2 reflex arc.

Psychogenic causes are clearly ruled out. No vascular disease is detected in the abdomen or extremities. A herniated disc between L4 and L5, with L5 nerve root compression, is almost certain. A spinal canal tumor can cause the same symptoms and the initial trauma history could be coincidental. The prostate and possibility of diabetes are yet to be evaluated.

Data Radiographs of the lumbar spine show a narrowing of the L5-S1 disc space with osteophyte formation. No osteolytic or osteoblastic lesions are seen. Fasting and 2-hour postprandial glucose levels are normal. Erythrocyte sedimentation rate, acid and alkaline phosphatase, calcium, phosphorus, protein electrophoresis, blood count, and urinalysis findings are normal.

Logic The osteoarthritis seen on radiograph does not correspond to the site of the known neurologic lesion. Disease between L5 and S1 would affect the first sacral nerve root and give a different picture. The normal findings from the complete blood count, erythrocyte sedimentation rate, and radiographs tend to rule out vertebral osteomyelitis, although it is a little early to be sure of the radiographs. Normal levels of proteins essentially preclude multiple myeloma, and normal phosphatase levels weigh against any bone-destroying lesion. The normal acid phosphatase level does not rule out prostatic cancer.

Data A rectal examination should have been done earlier. It shows a diffusely enlarged, smooth prostate gland. No nodules are felt. A telephone call to the urologist confirms the impression of benign prostatic hypertrophy based on his examination and a normal prostate-specific antigen test result.

Logic You are now more secure because most carcinomas of the prostate are detectable on digital examination. The urologist helps allay your concern too. There is still the possibility of a spinal canal tumor.

Data The patient is told that he probably has a herniated lumbar disc. He is advised to rest in bed at home and is given an analgesic and muscle relaxant. An electromyogram and MRI scan are performed on an outpatient basis.

The MRI shows normal disc space at the L3-L4 and L5-S1 levels. At the L4-L5 disc level there is a diffuse bulge of the disc with focal herniation on the right side. This pushes against the dural sac on the right and obliterates the epidural fat planes (Fig. 19.3).

Electromyography shows spontaneous fibril-

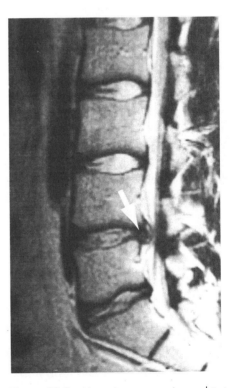

▶ **Figure 19.3.** Magnetic resonance image detects herniated L4-L5 disc.

lations in the muscles supplied by the L5 nerve root as well as positive sharp waves at rest. There is also a decrease in the number and amplitude of action potentials on voluntary activity.

Logic MRI, which is considered to be superior to CT for spine and spinal cord imaging, confirms the clinical impression of disc herniation. It precisely locates and delineates the extent of the lesion. A radionuclide bone scan of the lumbar area for prostatic metastases is deemed unnecessary. The electromyogram merely confirms what you already know; under the circumstances some physicians might consider it equally unnecessary.

Data He does not improve with 2 weeks of bed rest at home, so he is hospitalized. A myelogram is performed. It shows an indentation of the dye column with probable impingement on the L4–L5 level. On running the dye proximally and distally, no other lesions are seen.

Logic The myelogram confirms the single lesion and excludes other concomitant lesions. Some clinicians might consider myelography to be superfluous and would rely wholly on MRI. Most patients improve on a conservative regime. He is given an H_2-receptor antagonist for the heartburn that began to recur a week ago. Now you advise 2 more weeks of conservative management with enforced and supervised bed rest and wait and hope for signs of improvement. Surgical options will be explored if symptoms continue.

Questions

1. Suppose that the man in the case just discussed is initially seen with a history of severe back pain and bilateral leg pain. He is unable to void and has not had a bowel movement for 1 week. Examination reveals a patulous anal sphincter with an absent bulbocavernosus reflex. Your most likely diagnosis would be:
   (a) abdominal aneurysm.
   (b) central disc herniation.
   (c) benign prostatic hypertrophy with urinary obstruction.
   (d) spinal cord tumor.

2. A 28-year-old construction worker complains of low back pain that does not radiate. It has been slowly increasing in severity during the past year. Examination shows no neurologic abnormality, slight decrease in range of movement of the back, and decreased chest expansion. Based on these findings, you would consider the diagnosis of:
   (a) degenerative osteoarthritis.
   (b) lumbar strain.
   (c) ankylosing spondylitis.
   (d) Scheuermann's disease.

3. A 12-year-old girl is initially seen with back pain of 1 week's duration. No neurologic defect can be demonstrated, but she has marked loss of lumbar lordosis with tight hamstring muscles. Straight leg raising can be done to only 20 degrees bilaterally. In your differential diagnosis at this time you would consider:
   (a) disc herniation.
   (b) spondylolisthesis.
   (c) vertebral osteomyelitis.
   (d) idiopathic scoliosis.

Answers

1. **(b) is correct.** A central disc herniation can produce compression of the sacral nerves with bowel and bladder dysfunction in addition to the pain described. You are dealing with a surgical emergency. The sacral nerves are mainly unmyelinated parasympathetic fibers that are very susceptible to pressure. Permanent dysfunction can result. Choice (d) should also be considered because the presentation of a spinal cord tumor can be exactly as described. However, one would expect more night pain and not so much mechanical pain. Choices (a) and (c) can be ruled out because of the leg pain as well as the neurologic abnormalities.

2. **(c) is correct.** Measurement of chest expansion is an important part of the back examination. With decreased chest expansion in a young man, the possibility of ankylosing spondylitis should always be considered. This disease process starts in the sacroiliac joints, has a presentation of back pain, and spreads to the costovertebral joints, producing stiffness and decreased chest expansion. An erythrocyte sedimentation rate and radiographs of the sacroiliac joints would help confirm the diagnosis. The HLA-B27 test may also be of help. Choice (a) does not occur at the age of 28, and choice (b) is an acute event that tends to settle down over a short period of time and not linger for a year. Also, the decreased chest expansion would not be expected with a lumbar strain. Choice (d) is a gradually progressive thoracic kyphosis found in adolescents. It may produce thoracic pain, but the pain generally abates by the end of spinal growth, and this patient's age would rule it out.

3. **(a), (b), and (c) are all correct.** Idiopathic scoliosis or lateral curvature of the spine usually starts to appear approximately at the age of 10 and progresses during spinal growth. This condition, however, is rarely associated with pain. Children with (a), (b), and (c) tend to have a presentation of this sort, irrespective of the cause of the pain. Disc herniation can occur and has been reported in patients as young as 10 years old. The presence of a neurologic deficit would be more suggestive, but in its absence disc herniation still cannot be ruled out. Spondylolisthesis, where there is slippage of one vertebral body under the one below, usually has a presentation exactly as described previously. This can be identified by doing oblique radiographs of the lumbar spine to show a defect in the pars interarticularis as well as a standing lateral radiograph to show the degree of slippage. Vertebral osteomyelitis can also have a presentation in this manner; fever, leukocytosis, and rapid erythrocyte sedimentation rate would also be present. A radionuclide bone scan may help in the first 2 weeks; conventional radiographic findings become positive later.

Suggested Readings

Albeck MJ, Hilden J, Kjaer L, et al. A controlled comparison of myelography, computed tomography, and magnetic resonance imaging in clinically suspected lumbar disc herniation. Spine 1995;20(4):443–448.

Jonsson B, Stromqvist B. Motor affliction of the L5 nerve root in lumbar nerve root compression syndromes. Spine 1995;20(18):2012–2015.

Weber H. The natural history of disc herniation and the influence of intervention. Spine 1994;19(19): 2234–2238.

Wetzel FT. Surgery for herniated vertebral disks. JAMA 1996;275(7):513–514.

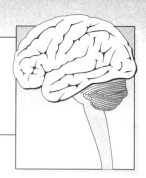

When a toastmaster says "our guest for tonight needs no introduction," he or she usually proceeds to give the guest speaker's full biography. It would seem on the surface that neurologic problem solving needs no introduction either, for nowhere in medicine are the signs and symptoms so clearly and understandably related to the underlying neuroanatomic alterations. Certain findings may limit the disease to an entire level of the spinal cord; in other instances you can be sure the disease is in the right frontal lobe.

But locating the disease site is not tantamount to naming the disease process. Different diseases can affect the sites just mentioned. The transverse myelitis syndrome can be caused by trauma, tumor, viral infection, or vascular occlusion, whereas cerebral thrombosis, brain tumor, or brain abscess can affect the right frontal lobe. And "there is the rub!"

The relative importance of presenting neurologic problems and the amount of emphasis on teaching them, as in most other organ systems, depends on their frequency, seriousness, and treatability. It is better to find a rare serious disease that is amenable to treatment than to exhaust your diagnostic acumen in labeling a rare, relatively benign disease for which no treatment exists.

But, as in other systems, a few common problems account for most of what the primary physician sees. Statistics show that the most frequently presenting issues are headaches; dizziness; pain syndromes (e.g., backache); alterations in consciousness or mentation; strokes; seizures; neuropathies; multiple sclerosis; and Parkinson's disease. Situations needing urgent care include coma, meningitis, status epilepticus, and head trauma. The most readily treatable problems include seizures, transient ischemic attacks (TIAs), migraine, subdural hematoma, Parkinson's disease, and meningitis.

Neurologic problems may be solved at a glance (Parkinson's disease, stroke); by pattern recognition (TIAs, meningitis, multiple sclerosis); by a stepwise approach with early hypothesis generation and testing (coma, polyneuropathy, brain tumor); or they may require a detailed data base (obscure atypical headaches).

Often a diagnostic procedure such as computed tomography (CT), magnetic resonance imaging (MRI), cerebral arteriography, radionuclide brain scan, ultrasound, or lumbar puncture furnishes the ultimate clue.

The introduction of high-technology tests has virtually eliminated standard radiologic procedures, and has altered the diagnostic process in neurologic diseases perhaps more than in any other disease category. For example, CT and MRI, although expensive, are cost-saving procedures that save days of observation, and have essentially phased out radionuclide scans, ultrasound, pneumoencephalograms, and other procedures of the recent past. Although CT scans define anatomic detail, MRI scans do so also, and in some instances in a superior fashion. The positron emission tomographic (PET) scan yields physiologic and biochemical data, and at this time this scan is still primarily research-oriented.

The decision as to which imaging procedure is best for each suspected lesion awaits the establishment of clear-cut guidelines and protocols. For reasons of cost, availability, and utility, a CT scan (with or without contrast enhancement) remains the procedure of choice in most instances. It should not be used for the routine work-up of simple headaches, minor head trauma, syncope, dizziness, or every garden-variety typical cerebral thrombosis. But it *is* especially valuable for *severe head trauma* and *suspected neoplasm*. It can distinguish hemorrhage from edema, subarachnoid aneurysmal leak from intracerebral bleed, and, in most instances, cerebral hemorrhage from cerebral thrombosis. In so doing, lumbar puncture may not be needed, and decisions on anticoagulation therapy can be made. Furthermore, the CT scan detects subdural hematoma, intracranial aneurysm, tumor, abscess, and arteriovenous malformations. It is usually requested when an adult experiences an unexplained seizure, be it generalized, partial, or focal. MRI may be equally useful for intracranial lesion identification, but it seems to surpass the powers of CT in lesions of the spinal column and spinal cord. *(P.C.)*

HEADACHE

Herschel L. Douglas

Data You see a 22-year-old woman in your office who complains of headache for 6 months. Actually, she had had occasional dull headaches for several years; these began in the occiput and progressed into a bandlike constriction of the head, were stress related, and occurred in the early evening.

For the last 6 months, however, the nature of the headaches changed. They consist of severe left temporal throbbing pain that starts in the morning, and are preceded by a few minutes of feeling "strange in the head." After several hours, the pain loses its throbbing character and becomes more generalized, although still severe. She requires rest in a quiet, dark room, is usually nauseated, and often vomits. These headaches occur at irregular and unpredictable intervals of 2 to 14 days.

Logic Headache is one of the most frequent symptoms seen in office practice. It is humanity's most common pain and occurs, in one form or another, in more than 90% of persons. You should be familiar with its usual causes and their clinical manifestations. The diagnosis is often easily established on the basis of history alone, although physical examination and, rarely, diagnostic procedures, must be done before initiating treatment.

First, let us eliminate the headaches that almost everybody gets occasionally: the "ice cream headache" from rapid swallowing of cold food, the headache from too much noise, the one from an emotionally upsetting situation, the "hang-over" or "morning after" headache—in short, headaches with obvious causes.

Post-traumatic headaches can mimic any type of chronic recurrent headache. They may continue for months to years after the initial trauma, and their intensity and duration cannot be correlated with the degree or severity of the initial trauma. Indeed, headaches may follow seemingly trivial injury and their mechanisms are usually unexplainable.

Solving the headache problem may involve a consideration of many factors: age and gender; duration of the problem; statistical incidence of the various types of headache; duration of each individual headache; presence of tenderness, aura, or psychosocial factors; time of day and day of the week on which the headache occurs; and the presence or absence of visual symptoms, gastrointestinal symptoms, photophobia, or pulsatile pain.

Patients with mild recurrent headaches for many years do not commonly consult the physician; they take analgesics for relief. Those with a sudden-onset severe, single headache usually *do* see the physician; they may have an acute problem such as meningitis, any febrile illness, subdural hematoma, acute suppurative sinusitis, brain abscess, subarachnoid hemorrhage, acute glaucoma, and so forth Their problems are readily recognized by the associated symptoms and physical signs.

Too often there is a tendency to blame headaches on mild coincidental hypertension, "eye strain," "bad teeth," or "sinuses" when such is not the case. Also, momentary head pains lasting 1 or 2 seconds are ubiquitous, meaningless, and without known cause.

However, you must be concerned about the 60-year-old patient who has had severe headaches for days to weeks (possible polymyalgia rheumatica or temporal arteritis); the patient whose headaches are of recent vintage, are getting worse and are associated with morning vomiting (expanding intracranial lesion); and the patient who has recent focal neurologic abnormalities together with headache (e.g., double vision).

In the world of chronic recurrent headaches the great majority (almost 80%) are muscle contraction-tension headaches. Approximately 20% are vascular in origin—migraine or cluster; these persons *do* visit the doctor because their headaches are often excruciating and disabling. The remaining small percentage result from brain tumors, sinusitis, and ocular disorders. The eyes cause headaches when there is glaucoma, hypermetropia, astigmatism, or difficulty with convergence. Sinus headaches are not so common as television commercials lead you to believe. Therefore, chronic recurrent headaches present a spectrum of diagnoses and causes that include:

1. Muscle contraction-tension headaches
2. Vascular headaches: (1) migraine with aura, (2) migraine without aura, and (3) cluster headaches (Horton's headache, histamine cephalalgia)
3. Combination of 1 and 2
4. Psychogenic headaches
5. Diseases of the sinuses, eyes, or teeth
6. Hypertension
7. Temporal arteritis
8. Cervical osteoarthritis

Again, note that well over 90% of chronic recurrent headaches are caused by items 1 and 2. In fact, elements of 1 and 2 often compound each other. It is not surprising to see the headache patient wander from one specialist to another, because each specialist places the headache outside his or her domain. Headaches related to special senses are uncommon but should be easy to recognize.

Data Closer questioning elicits the story that the patient's second type of headache began shortly after her marriage. At that time a CU-7 intrauterine device was inserted and this was contrary to her religious convictions. Her headaches are worse before menses, and her mother had similar "sick headaches" from the time she was a young woman until after the menopause. The recent courtship and marriage have been happy and without emotional disturbance, significant worries, or stress. There are no complaints of nervousness, anxiety, insomnia, crying spells, loss of libido, loss of self-esteem, or feeling blue. She does not smoke or drink alcohol, drinks no coffee, and takes no medicines regularly.

Logic The very common tension headache is related to sustained contraction of the occipitofrontalis muscle and causes the type of pain that this patient had for several years before the headaches changed in character. Often it is described as head-tightness, a bandlike or viselike feeling, a drawing sensation, or soreness. It may be over the entire head, the front, back, or either side, but it is non-pulsatile, not associated with nausea, and likely to be relieved by analgesics, heat, and massage. Nervous headache, psychogenic headache, and tension headache are probably synonyms. They occur against the backdrop of an aggressive, frustrated, anxious, or depressed person who is confronted by an emotional tension state.

Psychogenic headaches (item 4) may overlap with muscular tension headaches. Even if 1 and 4 are separate varieties, they have similar symptoms and are related to concurrent stigmata of anxiety, tension, depression, or conversion.

Although you cannot be certain that her original headaches could be listed under item 1 or 4, or both, you do know that the headaches the patient has had for the past 6 months are vascular in origin. The description is characteristic of migraine without aura, which accounts for 90% of vascular headaches. The onset is usually near important milestones in life's responsibilities—for example, puberty, college, marriage, menopause. It is most often unilateral, with no (or vague) premonitory sensations, is pulsatile and throbbing, and progresses to a steady ache with nausea. The pain can be excruciating and disabling and the family history is 60 to 80% positive.

All of these elements are positive in your patient and you now have a well-substantiated working diagnosis. Other forms of vascular headache have not yet been eliminated, nor have certain organic diseases been ruled out. Invasive, expensive, time-consuming tests are not needed. First complete the history with a systems review, and do a physical and neurologic examination.

Data The systems review discloses the absence of: unrelenting progression of headache, gait disturbance, vertigo, memory loss, visual changes, diplopia, paresthesia, and motor weakness—before, during, after, or between headaches. Results of physical and neurologic examinations are entirely normal, including the blood pressure and fundi. No bruits are heard over the eyeballs or cranium. Complete blood count, urinalysis, and sedimentation rate are normal.

Logic Armed with this additional information, you are now in a position to rule out various previously mentioned causes of headache:

- *Intracranial tumor.* Here the headache is generally progressive and unrelenting, but not necessarily continuous. After 6 months you would expect additional symptoms, some neurologic abnormalities, or even abnormal fundi.
- *Chronic subdural hematoma.* This may be preceded by a history of head trauma, although the trauma may be minor or forgotten, and no history may be obtainable. Alcoholism or drug obtundation is often associated with injuries of the head. The pain is deep-seated and steady. By this time, other symptoms and signs like dizziness, altered sensorium, and hemiparesis might be expected.
- *Brain abscess, meningitis, and encephalitis.* These are acute illnesses with a single constant headache, fever, meningeal irritation—a "sick" patient—and progression of symptoms and signs.
- *Subarachnoid hemorrhage.* Sudden onset of severe headache followed by unconsciousness is a completely different story from that of the patient in this case. Aneurysms or other vascular malformations may cause such an acute critical illness.
- *Temporal arteritis* (polymyalgia rheumatica). This rarely occurs under age 50; is associated with a tender, palpable temporal artery; episodes of homolateral blindness and signs and symptoms of diffuse arteritis—for example, fever, malaise, anemia, muscle aching and tenderness; and a very rapid erythrocyte sedimentation rate.
- *Hypertension.* Your patient is normotensive and has no history of hypertension. But remember that even though headaches are more common in hypertensive persons, there is little or no correlation between blood pressure levels and the presence or severity of the headache.
- *Cervical osteoarthritis.* This disorder not uncommonly causes occipital headaches that radiate to one side or the other and are usually related to motion of the head and neck. They are more common in middle-aged and elderly individuals.

From the easily obtainable data base you conclude that the patient has vascular headaches—migraine without aura. The next step would be a prophylactic diagnostic and therapeutic trial with an ergot preparation. Because the pathophysiology of migraine invokes intracranial arterial dilation plus humoral mechanisms, a combination vasoconstrictor/serotonin inhibitor is used for prevention. If this drug causes a diminution of severity and frequency of headaches, your conclusion will be further confirmed. But with any long term follow-up, be alert for changes in pattern of symptoms or new symptoms that could herald additional problems or hint that the original diagnosis may have been wrong. Remember that ergot preparations may have serious side effects, and the patient will need careful supervision. A decision is made to reserve preventive medication for future use if acute treatment is not effective.

Data You discuss the entire situation with the patient, tell her your conclusions, and begin to explore some of the psychodynamics, when she suddenly asks: "Are you sure there is nothing wrong with my eyes or sinuses? My sister gets sinus headaches, and my 58-year-old mother gets headaches when she reads."

Logic The patient seems reluctant to accept a psychophysiologic diagnosis. Perhaps she is properly skeptical. Many diseases of the special senses can cause headaches. But these are much less common than patients or many physicians believe.

Glaucoma or an error in refraction can cause ocular headaches. In the first instance, the fundi may show cupping of the disc, and tonometry should be done. In the latter instance, headaches are brought on by strain of the muscles of accommodation during reading.

Sinus headaches are usually located near the involved sinus, although the pain may radiate to another part of the cranium. They occur mostly in the morning and are altered by head position, and evidence of sinus disease is present on examination, for example, swollen turbinates, mucopurulent nasal discharge, tenderness over the sinus, and radiographic evidence of a fluid-filled sinus, sometimes with an air-fluid level.

Headaches from a tooth abscess or disease of the temporomandibular joint are easily detected by simple examination techniques.

You recall that specific foods may act as trigger mechanisms for migraine headaches and make a mental note to ask the patient about such a possibility.

Data On questioning her, you learn she has already been informed of this concept; she has kept a careful food diary and has been unable to correlate the headaches with any particular food.

To reassure both the patient and yourself, you recheck the fundi, test ocular tension with a tonometer, and check for visual acuity. Then you carefully inspect the inside of the nose, elicit no tenderness over the sinuses, and transilluminate them in a dark room. The patient opens her mouth, and you inspect and tap the teeth, look at the gums, and feel and listen over the temporomandibular joints. All of these maneuvers give normal results. So you again explain the diagnosis to the patient.

She seems more reassured, but states: "My neighbor gets migraine headaches, and they are not like mine."

Logic Your interpersonal skills are being further tested. Many patients with migraine are rigid, ambitious, perfectionistic, and have self-conflicts, frustrations, and anxieties. They need extra attention, care, and patience.

You explain that there are three types of vascular headache. The one she has is *migraine without aura*.

In *migraine with aura* (the type she has not), constriction of a cerebral vessel causes transient contralateral neurologic manifestations for approximately a half-hour before subsequent vasodilatation results in homolateral headache. The initial vasoconstriction may be associated with scintillating scotomata, flashing lights, shining spots, zigzag lines, geometric apparitions, nasal congestion, lacrimation, and transient oculomotor ophthalmoplegia, hemianesthesia, hemiplegia, or hemianopsia. Approximately 15 to 30 minutes later, the vessel dilates and causes throbbing headache in the hemicranium (mi-graine) on the side of the vascular disturbance, usually opposite from the neurologic signs or symptoms. Systemic complaints such as nausea, vomiting, and diarrhea are common ("sick headaches"). Serotonin, catecholamines, 5-hydroxy indoleacetic acid, prostaglandins, kallikreins, and bradykinins may be implicated in the vascular episodes, but their roles are not clear.

It is the frequently associated neurologic symptoms and signs that often stampede the physician into hunting for a nonexisting intracranial lesion or epilepsy. This is especially true when the postspasm headache is mild or hardly noticed. In rare instances the patient who has migraine with aura develops a stroke or is found to have an arteriovenous malformation.

In migraine with aura the headache is more often unilateral and briefer than in migraine without aura. Many times there is a childhood history of motion sickness and frequent nausea. In both types of migraine, the family history is usually positive and the incidence is greater in women.

Data The patient is still not satisfied. She says her neighbor is a 45-year-old man, and his headaches are not like either of the migraines you described.

Logic You hypothesize that the man may have cluster headaches (Horton's headache, histamine cephalalgia)—the third type of vascular headache. These almost always occur in middle-aged men. The patient is suddenly awakened at night by severe supraorbital pain, eye pain, tearing, and nasal congestion. The pain is excruciating, but last only a short time—perhaps up to 2 hours—goes away, and returns the next night. It may recur for a few to many consecutive nights, and then not reappear for months to years. That is why it is called "cluster" headache.

Data When this situation is explained to the patient, she realizes that her neighbor indeed has cluster headaches and not migraine. She is now convinced, and you begin preventive therapy.

Logic Fortunately for both of you, she did not ask you to rule out a brain tumor. You had already done so in your own mind, but had she inquired, you might have been tempted to practice "defensive medicine" and request a skull radiograph, electroencephalogram (EEG), CT, or even MRI—against your better judgment.

You think about elusive "migraine equivalents" and are glad they do not exist in your patient. These consist of a variety of intermittent recurrent syndromes that are allegedly also manifestations of migraine. Included are episodic nausea, vomiting, diarrhea, and abdominal pain; periodic thoracic, pelvic, or extremity pain; bouts of fever; paroxysmal vertigo; and recurrent psychic equivalents, such as episodes of confusion.

Try explaining these to a patient—or to yourself.

Comment This problem was reasonably easy to solve. The author tracked one key clue, considered all the possibilities, and then, on the basis of a careful history, arrived at a tentative solution. This probability was further confirmed by age, gender, and statistical likelihood. Recognition of the total migraine pattern helped too. Other possibilities were ruled out by historical and physical features that were pertinently negative or absent. No paraclinical tests were needed.

The same conclusion—migraine without aura—could have been reached by constructing a diagnostic tree or flowchart, asking some appropriate questions, and performing a few maneuvers. Example of such decision points are: (1) Are the headaches constant or intermittent? (2) Is there nausea, photophobia, lacrimation, or throbbing? (3) Are there other neurologic symptoms? (4) Do the headaches occur on awakening, on reading, in the evening, or during sleep? (5) Describe the fundi and blood pressure. The answer to each question decides which branch to follow toward the answer. *(P.C.)*

PROBLEM-BASED LEARNING To understand all about headaches, you must have a broad knowledge of the conditions that may cause them. Even though the great majority are benign, you cannot afford to overlook the unusual instance where the problem is serious and potentially either fatal or curable.

Therefore you must learn all about:

- Relative prevalence of different types of headaches
- Muscle contraction-tension headaches
- Psychogenic factors related thereto
- Vascular headaches, including classic migraine and cluster headaches
- Headaches related to cerebrovascular accidents (hemorrhage, thrombosis, embolus, subarachnoid hemorrhage) and the clinical pictures of these illnesses
- How afflictions of the ears, eyes, nose, sinuses, teeth, and cervical spine cause headaches, and their associated clues
- Temporal arteritis (polymyalgia rheumatica)
- Post-traumatic headaches, including subdural hematoma, its clinical characteristics and diagnosis, plus other less definite varieties of headache resulting from head trauma
- Manifestations of brain tumors and other expanding intracranial lesions
- Evidence for meningeal irritation or infection

- Ophthalmoscopic signs of glaucoma and increased intracranial pressure
- Testing the visual fields and extraocular motions, performing tonometry, and indeed doing a complete neurologic examination
- Technologic procedures used to diagnose intracranial disease
- Pharmacologic effects of analgesics, ergotamine preparations, in particular methysergide, and newer anti-migraine drugs

Although such a broad base of knowledge is not needed for the management of most patients with headaches, better physicians (and students) know all that has just been stated. Their patients with tension headaches will not be given ergot preparations or β-adrenergic blockers, migraine patients will not have CT scans performed, and the rare brain tumor will not be overlooked. *(P.C.)*

Suggested Readings

Blau JN. Headache history: Its importance and idiosyncrasies. Headache Quarterly 1990;(2):129.

Rapoport AM, Sheftell FD. Headache disorders, a management guide for practitioners. Philadelphia: WB Saunders; 1996.

Rasmussen BK, Jensen R, Olesen J. A population-based analysis of the diagnostic criteria of the International Headache Society. Cephalgia 1991;11:129.

CASE 72

DIZZINESS

Paul Cutler

Data Leaning on her daughter, a 64-year-old woman totters into your office and tells you that she has been troubled with recurrent episodes of "severe dizziness." When these occur, the room suddenly seems to spin around, and she must hold onto things to steady herself. She feels as if she is about to be "thrown to the floor," and on occasion the ground seems to rise up or suddenly quiver. The sensations are terribly unpleasant and frightening and are sometimes accompanied by nausea and vomiting; she must lie down for several hours or more until they pass. Such an episode is just subsiding, and she wants you to see her during one. Another physician told her she had "hardening of the arteries," but she is not satisfied with this diagnosis.

Logic There are three principal questions to be resolved: Is this truly vertigo? Where is the lesion? What is causing it?

Vertigo is defined as a hallucination of movement of the surroundings or the person him/herself. It must be distinguished from lightheadedness, confusion, absence seizures and partial complex seizures, feelings of unreality, presyncope or syncope, and incoordination and loss of position sense, because each of these symptoms conjures up a different list of diagnostic possibilities. For example, loss of position sense can be caused by posterior column disease or peripheral neuropathy wherein movements are incoordinated, and the patient feels unsteady, but vertigo is not present. Lightheaded feelings or presyncope may occur in the cardiac patient who has transient decreases in cardiac output. And nonspecific gait disturbances that can be confused with vertigo are common in the elderly. By description, the propositus does have true vertigo.

It is more difficult to locate this lesion because vertigo can be caused by diseases of the middle ear, inner ear, eighth cranial nerve, vestibular nuclei, cerebellum, forebrain, eyes, or arteries. Each anatomic site can be afflicted with a variety of illnesses (Table 20.1).

Each of these lesions has its own special characteristics. To locate the site and determine the cause, it is often helpful to know whether the vertigo occurred once or many times, whether it is continuous or intermittent, and whether it is accompanied by headaches, nausea and vomiting, hearing loss and tinnitus, nystagmus, or other neurologic defects.

Before proceeding, a brief sketch of some diagnostic possibilities is in order:

Benign positional vertigo is extremely common, perhaps the most common cause of vertigo; it lasts up to a minute or so and is associated with changes in position such as rolling over in bed or getting up. It is theorized that it results from free-floating calcium carbonate crystals in a semicircular canal.

Motion sickness, air sickness, and height vertigo are considered physiologic, and momentary 1-second episodes of dizziness on bending over or straightening up occur in many persons and are meaningless.

TABLE 20.1. Causes of Vertigo Classified by Anatomic Site and Lesion

SITE	LESION
Middle Ear	Suppurative otitis
	Cholesteatoma
Labyrinth	Acute vestibular neuronitis
	Benign positional vertigo
	Ménière's disease
	Acute labyrinthitis
Eighth cranial nerve	Acoustic neuroma
	Drugs (quinine, quinidine, salicylates, aminoglycosides)
	Disabling positional vertigo
Vestibular nuclei	Tumor, stroke, ischemia, multiple sclerosis
Cerebellum	Tumors or vascular lesions with associated vestibular nuclei involvement
Forebrain	Certain tumors, migraine, epilepsy (especially in the temporal lobe), psychogenic causes
Eyes	Ocular nerve palsy, adjusting to bifocals
Arteries	Vertebrobasilar transient ischemic attacks

Vestibular neuronitis is suggested by several episodes of vertigo, each lasting approximately 1 week, recurring over a period of a year, unaccompanied by other symptoms, and allegedly caused by a virus. This entity is a common cause of vertigo.

Sudden complete unilateral deafness plus vertigo suggests an *acute labyrinthitis* of bacterial, viral, or vaso-occlusive origin. This condition is uncommon.

Disabling positional vertigo is a newly described entity. It occurs when the patient is up and about, and, as the name implies, it is quite incapacitating. No causes can be found. In such instances, the problem is thought to arise from compression of the eighth cranial nerve by arteries or veins, and microsurgical decompression is allegedly curative. But wait a few more years before final judgement is passed on this newly described disease and its cure.

In elderly patients, think especially about vascular disease, tumors, transient decreases in cardiac output, anemia, and medications. Seemingly trivial items such as the slow adaptation to new shoes, new eyeglasses, or a new cane may cause disturbances in equilibrium that the patient equates with dizziness. Sedatives and hypnotics such as phenobarbital and diazepam may cause sensations that may also be interpreted as dizziness.

Vertebrobasilar ischemia should be suspected when episodes of dizziness occur in conjunction with diplopia, dysarthria, dysphagia, "drop attacks," or transient focal motor or sensory loss.

Data The symptoms have been present for a month. They seem to develop suddenly, last from minutes to hours, and then subside. On at least one occasion, the patient's speech was transiently slurred. She has had no aural discharge, headaches, seizures, blackouts, visual changes, impairment of hearing, tinnitus, weakness, or paresthesias. In fact she emphasizes that she felt absolutely well before 1 month ago, and she takes no medications.

Logic One positive and several negative clues may be helpful. Slurred speech suggests the possibility of a transient lesion in the brain stem involving the motor nerves as well as the vestibular nuclei. Meniere's disease is characterized by recurrent bouts of vertigo in a patient who already has impaired hearing and tinnitus; the absence of the latter two are strong points that weigh against this diagnosis. An acoustic neuroma (cerebellopontine angle tumor) is unlikely without associated hearing loss. The absence of headaches, seizures, and aural discharge weighs against migraine, epilepsy, and ear infection. Multiple sclerosis is unlikely without evidence of demyelinization in other areas of the brain, too, but sometimes dizziness may be the first and solitary manifestation.

Data The past history indicates intermittent hypertension that is not currently being treated. At age 14 she had a minor concussion following a fall from her father's ice wagon, and she had a hysterectomy 20 years ago. The family history is not remarkable and on eliciting a systems review, she reports a history of transient episodes of bilateral leg weakness in the past 6 months. She attributed this to her age. These short spells nearly resulted in falls, but the patient always regained strength immediately.

Logic The hypertension may be meaningful in

that it hastens cerebrovascular disease. Too much time has elapsed for the childhood concussion to relate to the vertigo. But the spells she describes are alarming and could result from transient ischemia in the posterior circulation.

Data Before beginning the history you checked her for nystagmus; it was present then but seems to be subsiding now. In fact, she is feeling much better. The entire physical and neurologic examination findings are normal, except for the blood pressure, which is 180/100 in both arms. There is no cerumen in the auditory canals, the eardrums are normal, hearing is normal, and there are normal responses to Weber's test and the Rinne test. Romberg's test finding is negative with both open and shut eyes; rapid alternating movements, tandem gait, finger-to-nose, and heel-to-shin tests have normal findings.

No bruits are heard in the carotid, supraclavicular, or occipital regions, and the carotid pulses are equal and full. The heart is not enlarged and exhibits no murmurs or abnormal rhythm. There is no dysarthria, dysphonia, or cranial nerve palsies. Peripheral sensation, reflexes, and motor function are normal.

Logic Nystagmus is seen with many forms of vertigo and is only slightly discriminatory. It may result from lesions of the inner ear, vestibular nerve, brain stem, or cerebellum. There are many kinds of nystagmus—jerky, pendular, end-position, oblique, rotatory, vertical, horizontal, and positional; each has different significance in locating the lesion and identifying the cause. An analysis of this subject is too detailed for this book. But it is good to remember that not all nystagmus is pathologic; end-position horizontal nonsustained nystagmus is usually a normal finding.

The absence of bruits weighs against significant extracranial cerebrovascular disease. No neurologic deficit was noted in the nerves of the brain stem. Normal cerebellar function and position and vibration sense weigh against disease in the cerebellum and posterior columns; anyway, these conditions cause disequilibrium rather than vertigo. Equal blood pressure in both arms and the absence of a supraclavicular bruit weigh against the subclavian steal syndrome, a form of transient ischemia in the vertebrobasilar system.

The diagnosis is uncertain, and serious possibilities exist, but the patient now appears quite well. A medical and neurologic work-up is indicated. Hospital policy denies her admission to the hospital, so she is to be studied on an ambulatory basis.

Data Complete blood count, urinalysis, VDRL test, 18-test chemistry profile, chest radiograph, and electrocardiogram (ECG) are normal. A 24-hour Holter monitor is applied, and no arrhythmias are found. The EEG shows minor background slowing that is not believed to be significant; no paroxysmal features are seen. Computed tomographic brain scan is normal; no tumors are apparent. A lumbar puncture reveals normal cerebrospinal fluid, including a normal protein electrophoresis result.

Logic The Holter monitor results argue against paroxysmal cardiac arrhythmias that might cause transient cerebral ischemia. Normal spinal fluid protein findings weigh against multiple sclerosis. A normal CT scan is very strong evidence against an intracranial neoplasm. The CT scan makes both the skull radiograph and the isotope scan obsolete in cases of this sort because it is far more reliable. You might also question the need for a lumbar puncture.

Because several features point to transient ischemic attacks resulting from arteriosclerosis and marked insufficiency in the posterior cerebral circulation, arteriography is scheduled for the next day.

As for the choice of imaging procedures, aortic arch arteriography is rarely needed if MRI is available. Although CT detects tumor or infarct, MRI does it earlier and better. MRI angiography (MRA) can determine vertebral artery patency and occasionally can image the posterior inferior cerebellar arteries. Transcranial Doppler flow study can establish vertebral artery patency, but its sensitivity for stenotic lesions is limited. The patient is scheduled to have the posterior cranial circulation assessed by MRA.

Data Two hours before the scheduled test, the patient complains of dizziness and difficulty with speaking and swallowing. Examination reveals a marked change. There is now right and left gaze nystagmus and slight upward nystagmus as well. She has uncontrollable hiccups. The right pupil is constricted. Pinprick is poorly appreciated in the right lower face, whereas it is not perceived in the left arm and leg. Yet the strength and reflexes are normal, and the plantar response is bilaterally flexor. Gait is slightly ataxic, and the patient sways from side to side on Romberg's testing without falling in either direction. She is admitted to the hospital.

Logic These findings are typical of sudden involvement of the lateral portion of the right side of the medulla and signify vascular occlusion of the right posterior inferior cerebellar artery (Wallenberg's syndrome). The descending fibers of the fifth cranial nerve nucleus, the vestibular nuclei, cerebellar tracts, and motor nerves originating in the medulla have been affected on the side of the lesion. Also, involvement of descending sympathetic fibers is causing a homolateral Horner's syndrome. There is damage to the spinal lemniscus that has already crossed over, thus giving sensory impairment on the contralateral half of the body.

A brain stem stroke has occurred. You may now surmise that the episodes of vertigo, attacks of weakness ("drop attacks"), and incidents of slurred speech were the results of transient ischemia in the posterior circulation.

Data An MRA shows complete occlusion of the right vertebral artery and its posterior inferior cerebellar branch (Fig. 20.1).

Logic Periods of transient ischemia preceded the eventual infarction of the lateral medulla. The degree of neurologic deficit and the prognosis depend in some measure on the amount of collateral circulation shunted to the affected area by the anterior cerebral circulation via the circle of Willis and the contralateral vertebral artery.

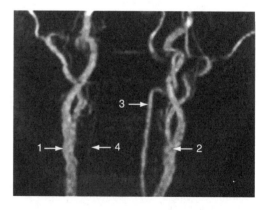

▶ **Figure 20.1.** Magnetic resonance angiography shows occlusion of the right vertebral artery. **1.** Right carotid artery. **2.** Left carotid artery. **3.** Left vertebral artery. **4.** Ghost of right vertebral artery.

You may wonder why no bruit was heard in the supraclavicular area before the complete occlusion, but you decide that either you did not listen in the correct place, that it may have been absent because of 100% occlusion, or that this was just one of those false negatives you have heard so much about.

It is imperative to point out that vascular disease is not the most common cause of vertigo, even in the elderly. Primary vestibular dysfunction (neuronitis) is far more common. Although relatively benign, its symptoms are very severe, the cause is unknown, and no other neurologic deficits are present. Meniere's disease is common, too. And in the 20s, 30s, and 40s, think also in terms of multiple sclerosis, but in that event look for evidence of associated neurologic lesions.

Comment   Vertigo is a common key clue. As with many neurologic diseases or symptoms, the first task is to locate the lesion by associated clues. The second is to determine the pathology by more clues and further studies. The specificity and sensitivity of diagnostic studies and the importance of age as a factor in the logical process are many times woven into the discussion.

While a complete data base was obtained, the author clearly had two principal provisional hypotheses: a medullary lesion and vestibular neuronitis. He leaned toward the former because of the possible existence of other symptoms of medullary origin (slurred speech). But with the large number of other possibilities, he chose to gather a complete data base rather than pursue individual hypotheses separately. It was wise to do so, because he discovered a very important clue in the systems review: imminent "drop attacks."

You may justifiably question the wisdom of the diagnostic procedural sequence in this case. Episodic vertigo, an episode of slurred speech, and several imminent "drop attacks" suggest a vascular lesion in the posterior cerebral circulation that is threatening to occlude completely. Under these circumstances, a Holter monitor, skull radiograph, EEG, and CT scan are considered superfluous by most clinicians. An arteriogram performed at the preocclusive stage may also be considered askance. It is risky, and its results may not appreciably alter management. If a threatening vascular lesion *is* found by MRA, or if the clinical picture suggests its existence, anticoagulants or anti-platelet-aggregation agents may

be used; however, their efficacy is under scrutiny, especially in women.

In almost all cases of vertigo, biochemical tests, EEG, radionuclide scans, CT scans, and traditional angiography are either of no help or only rarely of value. The CT scan has its prime value if a cerebellopontine angle tumor is suspected, but you must remember that only 10% of patients with acoustic neuromas have vertigo; their hallmarks are usually deafness and tinnitus. MRA would appear to be exquisitely sensitive for the presence of severe extracranial vascular disease.

In most cases the primary care physician can identify the cause of vertigo. Anxiety, vestibular neuronitis, benign postural vertigo, drug toxicity, Meniere's disease, and so forth are easily diagnosed. But in doubtful or possibly serious cases, electronystagmography (including caloric stimulation) and audiometric tests are indicated. It may be wise to refer the dizzy patient to an otoneurologist if the diagnosis is in doubt, if there is need for further tests, or if there is suspicion of a tumor or impending stroke. *(P.C.)*

Suggested Readings

Linstrom CJ. Office management of the dizzy patient. Otolaryngol Clin N Am 1992;25(4):745–780.

Luker J, Scully C. The lateral medullary syndrome. Oral Surg Oral Med Oral Pathol 1990;69(3):322–324.

Ruckenstein MJ. A practical approach to dizziness. Questions to bring vertigo and other causes into focus. Postgrad Med 1995;97(3):70–72, 75–81.

Warner EA, Wallach PM, Adelman HM. Dizziness in primary care patients. J Gen Intern Med 1992;7(4): 454–463.

CONVULSIONS

Paul Cutler

Data   Just after finishing lunch, a 50-year-old unmarried woman suddenly became unconscious, fell to the floor, and was noted to be making severe jerking movements of her entire body. She was taken to the hospital by the emergency rescue squad.

Logic   Unless the patient has known idiopathic epilepsy, hospitalization may be advised after sudden and unexpected loss of consciousness in an adult, especially when it is accompanied by seizure activity. Only rarely does a doctor observe the patient's seizure, and reliance must be placed on a description by others. The patient, however, may give evidence of a bitten tongue, a broken tooth, and incontinence. These are good indicators of what transpired. Such an episode may indicate the presence of a serious disease and can have a variety of causes:

- Withdrawal from drugs (alcohol, sedatives, narcotics)
- Effect of medication and toxins (excessive heroin, cocaine, stimulants, lead, arsenic)
- Transient insufficiency of cerebral blood flow (TIAs, cardiac arrhythmias)
- Appearance of an anatomic lesion in the intracranial cavity (tumor, abscess, hematoma, infarct, metastasis)
- Biochemical derangement secondary to systemic disease (hypoglycemia, hypocalcemia, hyponatremia, uremia)
- Idiopathic epilepsy
- Infection (meningitis, encephalitis)
- Previous head trauma

Therefore, the first questions asked of the patient (or those close to the patient) are directed at these eight categories to see which is at fault so that proper early treatment and more definitive evaluation can proceed.

Bear in mind that in young adults (ages 16 to 35) the most common causes of seizures are trauma, tumor, alcoholism, and cocaine. The common cause of seizures in older adults are cardiovascular diseases, metabolic derangements, alcoholism, and brain tumor.

Data The patient had been behaving normally before lunch and had been having a routine day up to that point. She had the reputation of being a very stable and healthy person. Her appetite was good. She was not known to be using any drugs—prescribed, over-the-counter, or illicit. Furthermore, she never smoked, drank only decaffeinated coffee, had alcoholic beverages sparingly on festive occasions, and had never in her life been observed to be intoxicated. There was no known incident of head trauma.

The shaking spell lasted 3 minutes, she was unresponsive for 15 minutes, and at the hospital 30 minutes later was conversing normally and felt well. There had never been a similar episode.

Logic The technology of our times has produced a proliferation of substances that can affect brain function, and technology produces these substances in such abundance that they are readily available. The stresses of our times have created a perceived need for such drugs. Alcohol may be taken daily to allay anxiety and produce euphoria. The dose may escalate to one or two fifths of liquor daily over the years. A sudden discontinuation can cause a seizure. Alcoholism may also cause seizures by virtue of previous head trauma (which is common) and by acute intoxication, as well as by 24 hours of abstinence ("rum fits").

Sedative drugs such as barbiturates, benzodiazepines, chloral hydrate, glutethimide, methaqualone, and opium derivatives act similarly when suddenly discontinued. Stimulants such as cocaine, ephedrine, methamphetamine, and the like can also cause convulsions when taken in excess. The patient's history negates any drug-related seizures.

A temporary reduction in blood flow can cause syncope, convulsions, or other neurologic manifestations. This possibility would be rendered more plausible if there were a history of palpitations immediately preceding the attack or if there were a background for cerebral arteriosclerosis as evidenced by hypertension, arterial bruits, or additional brain symptoms.

Other cardiovascular causes for cerebral ischemia include acute myocardial infarction, episodic complete heart block from various causes, extracranial vascular stenosis with TIAs, atrial fibrillation, and mitral stenosis. Each of these conditions can cause temporary decreases in cerebral blood flow or cerebral emboli. A physical examination usually detects these problems.

The possibility of an intracranial anatomic lesion still exists and we need further data. A stroke is unlikely because everything returned to normal in short order. But the possibility of a space-taking lesion is still present. After 50 years of age, *cerebrovascular diseases and tumors,* either primary or metastatic, assume greater prevalence in the list of causes for seizures.

Medication and toxic substances like lead or arsenic usually cause behavioral changes much before the seizure, and their effects are present for a considerable time afterward. This patient's excellent condition both before and after the attack precludes these causes. Lead intoxication can cause an unexpected seizure in an adult, but it also causes wrist-drop, emotional changes, and anemia. Arsenic gives a characteristic picture too. The effects of toxic substances are usually widespread and produce a clinical template that should suggest the possibility to the clinician. But if the cause for a seizure is not discovered promptly, laboratory tests for common toxic substances in the blood and urine are necessary. In fact, these tests should be requested as soon as the patient is seen.

Idiopathic epilepsy begins in childhood, and its onset at age 50 would be most unlikely. If present, the EEG finding would be positive in more than half of patients, and a family history is common. The EEG finding in the set of all patients who have idiopathic epilepsy is positive in 70% of patients during the interictal phase; it is almost always abnormal during a seizure. It is noteworthy that some patients who do not have epilepsy have falsely positive abnormal EEGs.

Seizures can come on within 2 years after head trauma with prolonged unconsciousness, but there is no such history here. Other causes must be sought.

Data In the emergency room a fresh bite mark was noted on her tongue, but there was no evidence of urinary or fecal incontinence. She had skipped breakfast that morning because she was too busy, but she had skipped meals on many previous occasions and never felt any ill effects. There were no preceding palpitations or cardiac awareness, but she did report a "funny feeling" in the epigastrium that "came up" (here she gestured with her hand to show an epigastric sensation rising up to the level of her throat), at which time she "blacked out." At the same time, "my foot began to shake" (. . .the right foot only!). She was amnesic for the next 30 minutes and does not recall the ride to the hospital.

Logic Rapidly developing hypoglycemia can cause a seizure. This can occur from insulin administration, an insulin-secreting tumor, or an alcoholic binge. None is likely here. Insulinomas cause convulsions that are preceded by milder manifestations of hypoglycemia; these attacks come after a missed meal or during the night, not immediately after a meal. Reactive or functional hypoglycemia causes mild sympathomimetic but

not cerebral manifestations. The patient describes what sounds like a preseizure aura, and shaking of the right foot sounds like a key clue.

Focal or partial seizures usually imply focal pathology in the brain such as tumor, scar, or vascular malformation. Generalized seizures are usually idiopathic, toxic, or metabolic. But because partial seizures can eventually march into generalized convulsions, it is important to inquire for evidence of a focal onset.

Data She recalled that her right foot was shaking at the onset of the seizure. As this question was pursued, she further related that she seems to have had a weak feeling in the right foot for 5 months, although it functioned quite well. Then it began to tremble occasionally and in the past 2 months she had actually developed clonic motions of the foot and ankle (as she described them); during the same period she could not walk on the right foot as well as she felt she should. This was attributed to "neuralgia." Review of systems brought out the fact that she had been experiencing mild brief headaches recently; these were episodic, a little worse in the morning, but, as with the foot, she tended to ignore them.

Logic An important aspect of gathering data about a seizure is the sequence of events leading up to it. In this instance, you can be suspicious about the part of the brain controlling the right foot. The seizures seem to originate in a focal area of the brain—the parasagittal area of the left frontal lobe's precentral gyrus. Transient ischemia is an unlikely cause of such a localization. Metastases would give a more progressive picture. Abscess is unlikely in the absence of a demonstrable source, and it too would not be so chronic and stable. Meningitis and encephalitis are acute infectious diseases in which the patient is sick—not so here. A brain tumor looms high on the list of possibilities. It is estimated that 16 to 20% of adults who have their first seizure after the age of 35 will demonstrate a mass lesion.

Data The general physical examination findings were normal. In particular, there were no "running" ears, extracranial arterial bruits, evidences of meningeal irritation, or primary tumor sites (thyroid, breast, and so forth). The neurologic examination findings were entirely normal except for the right leg; there, the reflexes were hyperactive, and there was weakness of dorsiflexion of the toes and foot, faint ankle clonus, and a

Babinski's sign. There were no sensory disturbances. The head jolt test was moderately positive on both sides and she localized the sensation to the front of her head.

Logic The findings tended to confirm what was already suspected from the history: an intracranial lesion over the foot area of the left motor cortex. Further study is indicated.

Data The skull radiographs were almost normal; there were no fractures or evidence of increased intracranial pressure. Although there was no enlargement of venous channels or the middle meningeal artery channel, this is not always a reliable negative finding in patients with meningiomas, a common type of brain tumor. However, there was a faint hyperostosis in the parasagittal area where we now suspect an intracranial lesion to be.

Chest radiograph and ECG were normal. The fasting blood glucose, 5-hour glucose tolerance test, complete blood count, urinalysis, blood urea nitrogen, serum calcium and sodium, and antinuclear antibody test results were normal or negative. The urine and blood test results were negative for toxic substances.

Logic Simple skull radiographs are usually no longer ordered in these circumstances. CT or MRI (with and without contrast) are the modalities of choice.

Hypoglycemia, hypocalcemia, hyponatremia, and uremia might already have been disregarded because each should have had an accompanying indicative clinical picture. Vasculitis and collagen disorders are unlikely too without added clues. The cerebrospinal fluid was not studied because a lumbar puncture is dangerous if a mass lesion is suspected.

Some of the studies already done and some that you are about to do are for confirmation purposes only, because you are now reasonably certain of the diagnosis. The faint hyperostosis seen on the skull films bolsters your conviction. Two studies are still under consideration.

Data Magnetic resonance demonstrated a 5- to 6-cm mass on the screen. It was solitary, and there were no satellite lesions. By virtue of the shape, location, and history, the mass was thought to be a meningioma (Fig. 20.2). An arteriogram was deemed not necessary.

Logic No doubt the meningeal tumor pressing on the motor cortex is the cause of the seizure. In retrospect, she had been having brief partial

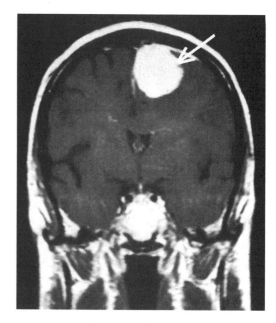

▶ **Figure 20.2.** Contrast-enhanced magnetic resonance image showing parasagittal meningioma in the left frontal lobe.

seizures of the right foot for at least 2 months but was stoic and did not seek medical advice.

Data Surgery and histologic study confirmed the diagnosis. The tumor was successfully removed. The patient has some residual weakness in the right foot, but still walks well and is free of seizures while using anticonvulsant medication.

Questions

Test your judgment by matching each of the following 10 clinical pictures with a lettered diagnosis that *explains convulsions.* Then name the *single diagnostic measure* needed to prove each situation.

Diagnosis
   (a) meningitis
   (b) insulinoma
   (c) metabolic acidosis
   (d) epilepsy
   (e) hyponatremia
   (f) cerebral ischemia
   (g) brain tumor
   (h) stroke
   (i) subdural hematoma
   (j) drug withdrawal

1. Twenty-four-year-old heavyweight boxer complains of severe headaches for 3 days and gradually lapses into stupor
2. Fifty-eight-year-old woman with chronic insomnia, emotional problems, and frequent visits to different physicians.
3. Twenty-two-year-old army recruit with sore throat, headache, and macular rash
4. Sixty-eight-year-old man with diabetes and hypertension.
5. Obese patient with good appetite and weak sweaty spells
6. Fifty-two-year-old woman who had a mastectomy 1 year ago
7. Fifty-six-year-old man with recent acute myocardial infarction, whose pulse intermittently drops to 20 per minute
8. Sixteen-year-old female with gingival hyperplasia and the same kind of spells her mother had
9. Fifty-six-year-old man who smokes heavily and has a chronic cough, muscle cramps, anorexia, nausea, and agitation
10. Forty-two-year-old woman with polyarthritis, a facial rash, nausea, anorexia, and drowsiness.

Answers

1. **(i).** Head injury and subdural hematoma are likely; CT scan is indicated.
2. **(j).** It is likely that she takes sedative drugs from different sources but ran out of medication and has drug withdrawal; a history should suffice.
3. **(a).** Meningococcal meningitis is seen in army recruit camps. The patient probably also has evidence of meningeal irritation. A lumbar puncture is indicated.
4. **(h).** The man's age and background make him a candidate for cerebral thrombosis, which may have its onset with a convulsion. A neurologic examination may provide help.
5. **(b).** The picture suggests hypoglycemia from a beta-cell tumor. A fasting blood glucose level and simultaneous insulin immunoassay should tell the tale.
6. **(g).** A brain metastasis is likely; a CT scan will detect it.
7. **(f).** Adams-Stokes attacks occur under these circumstances. An ECG offers proof, and a pacemaker is needed.
8. **(d).** Idiopathic epilepsy is likely in view of the family history. The phenytoin she probably takes causes gingival hyperplasia. In 70% of patients the EEG finding is corroborative.
9. **(e).** Hyponatremia resulting from inappropriate antidiuretic hormone secretion is suggested by the symptoms; an oat cell lung carcinoma is likely. Order a chest radiograph.
10. **(c).** The picture suggests systemic lupus erythematosus resulting in uremia. A positive antinuclear antibody test result is expected; so is an elevated creatinine level.

Note: In a few instances, the answer is justifiably debatable because your logic may properly provide a different diagnosis. Such disagreements were deliberately introduced to encourage you to think.

COMMENT A single key clue—a convulsive seizure—had to be fleshed out by the author as he elicited information from the complete history that the patient thought was not important or significant. These were the symptoms referable to the right foot.

But first he formed a list of possibilities and quickly eliminated the absurd, the impossible, and the improbable. Left with the cluster of a seizure and involvement of the upper motor neuron supply to the right foot, the diagnosis became fairly evident. The one hypothesis that was most likely, most serious, and for which most can be done was chosen and then proved by carefully selected studies.

Nowadays, a 50-year-old healthy woman with a single seizure has a CT or MR brain scan done promptly. If the scan shows presence of tumor, the problem is solved. If the scan result is negative, you must proceed through the traditional diagnostic sequence described in this case. Even though the scan is expensive, it often supplies the answer quickly, avoids other studies, and is therefore cost- and time-efficient. *(P.C.)*

Suggested Readings

Devinsky O, Thacker K. Nonepileptic seizures. Neurol Clin 1995;13(2):299–319.

Devinsky O. Seizure disorders. Clin Symp 1994;46(1): 2–34.

Drury I, Beydoun A. Seizure disorders of aging: Differential diagnosis and patient management. Geriatrics 1993;48(5):52–54.

Morrell MJ. Differential diagnosis of seizures. Neurol Clin 1993;11(4):737–754.

PARALYSIS

Paul Cutler

Data Over a period of 48 hours, a 68-year-old right-handed woman gradually developed paralysis of the left side of her face and her left arm and leg. The arm, face, and leg became weak and then paralyzed in that order.

She was brought to the hospital where she was found to have left-sided hyperreflexia, Babinski's sign, and inability to move her left arm, leg, and the lower two thirds of her face. There was no loss of consciousness or disturbance in sensation, and the other cranial nerves were intact. Speech was preserved.

Logic On the surface this appears to be a "garden variety" stroke involving the right lenticulostriate artery, which supplies the corticobulbar and corticospinal tracts in the internal capsule. Because only the lower part of the face, arm, and leg (and sometimes the tongue) have unicortical innervation, the classic picture is as presented.

One feature of the stroke is disturbing. It evolved slowly. Although the initial clinical impression still favors a vascular accident, the slow evolution persuades you to consider other possibilities such as brain tumor, abscess, metastasis, or hematoma. Furthermore, a stroke can be caused by embolus, thrombosis, or hemorrhage for which treatment may vary.

It is not always a simple matter to distinguish between these three types of stroke because of overlapping clinical features. But it is most important to do so, for although anticoagulants or thrombolytic agents may benefit patients with emboli or thrombosis, they may be fatal for those with hemorrhage. Therefore it may be necessary, perhaps early on, to rely on imaging procedures. Although CT easily detects hemorrhage, it may not visualize an infarct until 48 hours or more after its occurrence. On the other hand, MRI, although more expensive and less universally available, confirms the presence of an infarct resulting from thrombosis or embolus within one hour of its onset. An added benefit of early imaging lies in its ability to identify or exclude a space-taking lesion.

The clinical manifestations of a *cerebral embolus*

have a sudden onset. They may be minor and transient if the embolus is small and lodges in a distal tiny vessel, or they may be major and lasting if the embolus is large and occludes a larger, more proximal vessel. Though not always substantiated, a site for the origin of the embolus must exist—usually in the heart or carotid arteries.

Cerebral artery thrombosis occurs more slowly, usually over a period of several hours, often noted on awakening, and almost always against a backdrop of diabetes and hypertension. The postulated mechanism is capillary rupture into a preexisting atheroma with subsequent thrombus formation, vascular occlusion, and cerebral infarction.

Cerebral hemorrhage is sudden. Often the patient develops severe headache and vomiting and lapses quickly into coma. Hypertension is present. The putamen, basal ganglia, and internal capsule are usually involved by the process and the neurologic picture is commensurate. Most cases are fatal.

The clinical findings in each case depend on which artery is involved, the consequent area of brain damaged, and the status of the collateral circulation. Stroke syndromes can be identified by studying the blood supply to the brain. For example, occlusion of the left middle cerebral artery results in right-sided hemiplegia, hemianesthesia, homonymous hemianopsia, and aphasia—if the patient is right-handed. The vertebrobasilar system supplies the occipital and temporal lobes, pons, medulla, cranial nerve nuclei, cerebellum, and long tracts coming from or going to the spinal cord. Occlusion in this system is usually devastating and is marked by varying combinations of vertigo, cranial palsies, hemianopsia, hemiplegia, and hemianesthesia.

Data Additional history revealed a draining left middle ear infection for 20 years, treated hypertension for 15 years, diabetes mellitus controlled by diet for 10 years, recent trouble with an irregular heartbeat, and a mastectomy 2 years ago. She smokes 30 cigarettes daily and has a chronic cough that is often productive of purulent sputum. The rest of the systems review, family history, and patient profile added nothing significant.

Logic The additional history raises many possibilities. Chronic suppurative otitis media is a good source for a brain abscess. So are the bronchitis and bronchiectasis that she may very well have. Hypertension and diabetes accelerate cerebrovascular disease and may predispose to thrombosis, and hypertension can certainly cause a cerebral hemorrhage. The irregular heartbeat makes you consider a cerebral embolus from a clot in the heart. Both the chronic cough and the mastectomy raise the specter of a metastatic brain lesion from the lung or breast. This case may not be so simple as it first appeared.

Although strokes usually appear suddenly, as their name implies, it is important to remember that a stroke may sometimes evolve slowly as this one seems to have done. On the other hand, a space-taking lesion, although present and asymptomatic for a while, may suddenly produce symptoms by occluding an adjacent vessel or by bleeding within itself.

Special terms are often applied to the varying clinical courses of strokes. A *stroke* represents the acute onset of a neurologic deficit that is vascular in origin and clears very slowly if at all. A *transient ischemic attack* represents an acute neurologic deficit that clears completely within 24 hours. A *stroke in evolution* develops in a stuttering, slow mode over a period of hours rather than minutes or seconds. A *completed stroke* is one in which the neurologic pattern of damage has been fully expressed and has become stable.

Data Physical examination shows a conscious, alert apprehensive patient. The vital signs are: temperature, 37°C; respirations, 18 per minute; pulse, 106 and irregular; and blood pressure, 190/110 in both arms. There is a purulent discharge from the right ear. No bruits are heard in the neck and no attempt is made to feel the carotid arteries. The fundi show grade 2 hypertensive and arteriosclerotic changes. A right radical mastectomy scar is noted, but there are no nodes or masses palpable anywhere in the axillae, scar, other breast, or supraclavicular areas. There are coarse inspiratory rales and fine expiratory wheezes at both lung bases. The apex beat is strong and displaced downward and to the left. There are no murmurs or gallops, but the apical rate is irregularly irregular, and there is a pulse deficit of 12 beats per minute. The fingers show beginning clubbing, but the rest of the examination findings are normal.

Logic Additional diseases are present. The patient has otitis media with chronic ear drainage; probable bronchiectasis based on the history, rales, wheezes, and clubbing; and hypertensive cardiovascular disease with atrial fibrillation. There is no evidence of recurrent cancer. Each of these problems could relate to her stroke. Although there is no history of trauma, subdural hematoma is a possibility to be reckoned with.

Hematomas generally cause headache and disturbed sensorium before or coincident with paralysis. Fever and leukocytosis accompany brain abscess 50% of the time.

In order to assess the situation immediately, a CT brain scan is ordered. This procedure will visualize a tumor, abscess, or subdural hematoma, if present. In the event that the patient has had a stroke, the scan will demonstrate an intracerebral hemorrhage if that is the cause, but it may be too soon for a cerebral infarction, whether caused by embolus or thrombosis, to be apparent.

Data A CT scan if performed with dye enhancement. It is normal. Or almost normal! Although there is no indication of a mass lesion and the pineal gland is in the midline, the radiologist reports a small lucent area in the left cerebrum. This is not compatible with the clinical picture, but a repeat study in the near future is suggested.

The chest radiograph shows cardiac enlargement and a few questionably enlarged nodes in the left hilum, but it is otherwise normal. A complete blood count, urinalysis, and 18-test blood chemistry profile are all normal except for a blood glucose of 190 mg/dL. The ECG shows left ventricular hypertrophy and atrial fibrillation.

Logic Although the neurologic picture unfolded slowly, there is no mass lesion present. The blood glucose is in keeping with the history of diabetes mellitus and the ECG abnormalities result from long-standing hypertension. Atrial fibrillation concerns you, for it raises the possibility of cerebral embolization that may recur. Clots tend to form in the auricular appendages of atria that are not contracting; frequently they dislodge and embolize. You feel that the clinical picture suggests thrombosis more than embolus, so for this reason and because of the hypertension, you decide against the use of anticoagulants.

The questionably enlarged hilar nodes and the seemingly inconsequential finding noted on the CT scan are put on the back burner for a few days. These studies will be repeated later. You elect not to do a lumbar puncture because the only reason for doing so is if hemorrhage or meningitis is suspected—not the case here. Furthermore, there is no need for an isotope scan, electroencephalogram, or cerebral arteriography. The picture seems clear-cut except for some questionable abnormalities noted on radiography.

In recent years, emboli have been recognized to be much more common than was once thought. The latest figures show that the approximate incidence of thrombosis to embolus to hemorrhage is 2:2:1.

It is notable that in patients with cerebral thrombosis, 60% have hypertension, 25% have diabetes mellitus, and 50% have clinically evident vascular disease elsewhere (heart or legs). Atheroma formation and sclerosis with ulceration and partial obstruction occur at the bifurcation of the common carotid artery, the origin of the internal carotid artery, the carotid siphon, and the origins of the anterior and middle cerebral arteries, as well as in the cerebral and basilar arteries—especially in the atheroma-prone individuals.

Patients with cerebral thrombosis often have minor prodromes. If severe narrowing already exists, an infarct may be precipitated by thrombosis at the atheroma site, an embolus, or a low flow state, especially if there is associated poor collateralization around the circle of Willis. A low flow state may be caused by a decreased cardiac output, a more proximal arterial narrowing, a drop in blood pressure, sleep, or certain body or neck positions.

In fact, sclerosis, thrombosis, emboli, low flow, and inadequate collateral circulation frequently seem to perform in concert to produce strokes or TIAs. It is often difficult to decide which is the prime cause of the cerebral infarct.

Emboli strike like a bolt out of the blue. They originate in more proximal atherosclerotic lesions, primarily the internal carotid artery, or in the heart. If an embolus is suspected because of sudden onset and the absence of atherogenesis accelerators, search the heart for atrial fibrillation, mitral stenosis, mitral prolapse, recent myocardial infarction, and infective endocarditis. The site of lodgment of the embolus varies with the size of the embolus and determines the neurologic picture. A large embolus may land in the internal carotid artery; a smaller one may strike the middle cerebral artery; and an embolus as small as 2 mm may end in a tiny artery and result only in a TIA.

TIAs are common. They probably result from microemboli composed of fibrin and platelets; these are formed on the ragged intima of stenotic carotid arteries. The transient neurologic picture they cause depends on where they land. TIAs recurring in the same area of the brain are probably the precursors of a cerebral thrombosis at an atheroma site. If the TIAs occur in different parts of the brain they are almost certainly caused by multiple emboli originating outside the brain. This makes sense!

Be aware that TIAs herald strokes. But the incidence of subsequent stroke is not so high as you might think. A single TIA may not recur, or it may recur infrequently or frequently. The stroke rate is 4 to 8% per year, perhaps higher.

If emboli are suspected, yet the carotid arteries are normal, ultrasound may detect silent mitral stenosis, mitral valve prolapse, or clots adherent to the valves or endocardium. You can see that an individualized diagnostic protocol and a unique decision tree must be constructed for each patient.

Data The patient is digitalized to slow the ventricular rate. Antihypertensive medication is altered. Supportive treatment is given and the diabetes is controlled. By Day 3, the patient is able to move her big toe and seems to have improved slightly.

Logic Her slight improvement is gratifying. But there are still one or two doubts in your mind that were planted by the radiographic reports.

Data A repeat CT scan again shows no evidence of a mass lesion or hemorrhage, but it does show an area of decreased density approximating the location of the internal capsule in the right cerebral hemisphere (Fig. 20.3). This area has the appearance of an infarct. The distinction between thrombosis and embolus cannot be made. Furthermore, the small questionable lucent area noted on the left side is no longer evident.

The chest radiograph is also repeated, and this time the patient is more cooperative. Hilar nodes are not enlarged.

After detailed instructions to the family, the patient is sent home to recover.

Logic Note how the CT scan made it possible to be certain, exclude other possibilities, omit other studies, decrease hospital stay, and cut overall costs. The two questionable radiographic abnormalities were somewhat counterproductive in

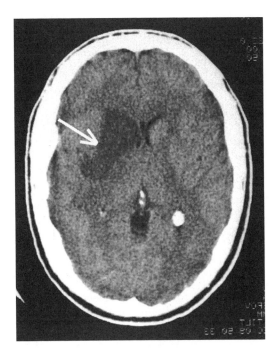

▶ **Figure 20.3.** Computed tomography shows area of decreased density in area of right internal capsule.

this regard; they were misleading bits of false positive information.

You are completely satisfied with the diagnosis of cerebral thrombosis—well, almost completely. The presence of atrial fibrillation is worrisome. If a cervical bruit was also present, there would be even more concern for embolization.

The entire romance of bruits, carotid stenosis, emboli, and their treatment with anticoagulants or surgery has not yet been fully written. It is a fascinating story about which much has recently been published. A bruit in the area of the carotid bifurcation, especially if accompanied by a palpable thrill, indicates significant (50 to 90%) diametric narrowing. If asymptomatic, perhaps nothing need be done; but if the bruit is found in association with a TIA, most physicians would recommend surgery, whereas some would opt for anticoagulant therapy.

If you suspect a patient has had a TIA, search for a source first in the neck vessels. Bruits may be heard not only in the area of carotid bifurcation but also in the root of the neck where the common carotid and vertebral arteries begin. Also listen for a bruit in the vertebral arteries just medial to the mastoid processes.

Doppler ultrasound studies are useful in de-

termining the degree of stenosis, but aortic arch arteriography is still the gold standard test that defines the carotid artery defect, pictures the circle of Willis, and assesses the cerebral circulation. It may be supplanted by MRA.

Data At home, over the next 10 days, gradual improvement is noted. Ambulation and physiotherapy have been started. You impress your patient with the need to give up cigarettes, adhere to her diet, and continue with antihypertensive medication. Although you do not suspect an embolus, you are not absolutely certain, so the patient is advised to take ticlopidine too.

The pros and cons of long-term therapy with warfarin sodium are discussed with the patient and her family; its use is vetoed. There were too many unanswered questions. Did the atrial fibrillation cause the stroke? Will warfarin sodium prevent future strokes? What are the risks?

Problem List
1. Cerebral thrombosis
2. Essential hypertension
3. Diabetes mellitus
4. Chronic suppurative otitis media
5. Chronic bronchitis
6. Hypertensive cardiovascular disease
7. Atrial fibrillation
8. Status post-mastectomy
9. Cigarette abuse

Questions

1. Suppose the patient in this case study was noted to be still sick on Day 5. The neurologic picture is the same, her sensorium is clouded, the temperature is 38.7°C, and respirations are 28 per minute. You should:
   (a) start antibiotics.
   (b) request cerebral arteriography.
   (c) examine the chest and repeat the chest radiograph.
   (d) request blood and urine cultures.

2. On Thursday, 5 days after the big football game, the star halfback develops a gradually worsening, persistent headache in the left hemicranium. Neurologic examination reveals no abnormalities. The best thing to do is:
   (a) watch him carefully.
   (b) lumbar puncture.
   (c) arteriography.
   (d) CT.

3. A 62-year-old man is admitted to the hospital with the sudden onset of paralysis of the right arm and leg. Hyperactive reflexes confirm a corticospinal tract lesion. But he also has paralysis of the entire left side of his face (cannot wrinkle his forehead or blow out his left cheek, and the left corner of his mouth droops). There are no other abnormalities noted. The diagnosis is:
   (a) cortical infarction on both sides.
   (b) pontine infarction on the left side.
   (c) internal capsule infarction on the left side.
   (d) internal capsule infarction on the left side plus an old facial palsy on the right side.

4. A 28-year-old patient complains of sudden paralysis of both legs. There are no other symptoms. Neurologic examination findings are normal. Reflexes are equal, there are no pathologic reflexes, and sensation is intact, but the legs are limp. The patient has:
   (a) infectious polyneuritis.
   (b) thrombosis of an artery supplying the spinal cord.
   (c) multiple sclerosis.
   (d) hysteria.

Answers

1. **(c) and (d) are correct.** Pneumonia or urinary tract infection is likely in sick bedridden patients such as this one. Depending on the probable site of infection, the immediate initiation of appropriate antibiotics might also be considered a correct action. Arteriography would be worthless.

2. **(d) is correct.** It has the highest specificity and sensitivity for a suspected subdural hematoma. To watch the patient might be dangerous, because brain damage can result. A lumbar puncture is neither specific nor sensitive for this diagnosis, and it may be harmful. Arteriography is an excellent test, but it is invasive, bears risk, and is costly. Although expensive, computed tomography will tell you what you need to know at little risk, and it will be less costly in the long run.

3. **(b) and (d) are correct.** Bicortical infarcts are statistically unlikely; moreover, both sides of the face would be involved. Choice (c) would affect the right lower two thirds of the face. An infarct in the pons could catch the uncrossed corticospinal tract and the emerging fibers of the seventh cranial nerve (crossed paralysis). Also, be aware that the facial palsy may be old, and the thrombosis may be new. Note how (b) locates the lesion by noting where the longitudinal disease site crosses the vertical disease site—a fine example of anatomic diagnosis.

4. **(d) is correct.** Choice (a) tends not to appear so abruptly, often has accompanying sensory symptoms, and has diminished-to-absent reflexes. The blood sup-

ply to the spinal cord is not such as to selectively affect only the upper motor neurons to the legs; even if it were, the reflexes would be hyperactive, and Babinski's sign would be present. Multiple sclerosis can concurrently involve any areas of the nervous system, but if the nerve supply to both legs were involved in the spinal cord, hyperreflexia would exist. Inquiry into the psychodynamics is indicated. It is important to remember that true paralysis or weakness can result from lesions in the long motor pathway, lower motor neuron, nerve root, peripheral nerve, myoneural junction, or muscle.

COMMENT The patient's acute illness began with what at first appeared to be a common type of stroke, and despite various distracting possibilities, turned out to be so. The running ear, breast cancer, cough and expectoration, and the heavy smoking history were unrelated to the principal diagnosis. Much significance was attached to the gradual onset of symptoms.

In order to solve this problem and to offer proper management, it was first necessary to decide if the cause of the illness was vascular or the result of a space-taking lesion. Brain imaging, as in other neurologic disorders, was of paramount importance. Next, if the illness was vascular in origin, was it embolus, thrombosis, or hemorrhage?

Sir Thomas Bayes is your consultant, and he tells you that cerebral thrombosis is the most likely cause of a slowly developing hemiplegia in a bruitless elderly person who has diabetes and hypertension—atrial fibrillation notwithstanding. You may disagree with this conclusion. (P.C.)

Suggested Readings

Brown RD Jr, Evans BA, Wiebers DO, et al. Transient ischemic attack and minor ischemic stroke: An algorithm for evaluation and treatment. Mayo 2Clin Proc 1994;69(11):1027–1039.

Furlan AJ. Transient ischemic attacks: Recognition and management. Heart Dis Stroke 1992;1(1):33–38.

Poole RM, Chimowitz MI. Ischemic stroke and TIA: Clinical clues to common causes. Geriatrics 1994; 49(6):37–42.

Smucker WD, Disabato JA, Krishen AE. Systematic approach to diagnosis and initial management of stroke. Am Fam Physician 1995;52(1):225–234.

Geriatric Problems

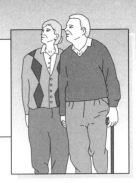

Perhaps the most moving description of old age to be found anywhere is in the *Book of Ecclesiastes* 12:1–8. Problems of the elderly, such as blindness, depression, tremors, unsteadiness, deafness, light sleep, fear of stumbling, and lack of opportunity are beautifully depicted in allegoric verse:

"Before the sun, and the light, and
the moon,
And the stars, are darkened,
And the clouds return after
the rain;
In the days when the keepers of the
house shall tremble,
And the strong men shall bow themselves,
And the grinders cease because they
are few . . ."

Read—where it is written.

But today, the portrayal of old folks is not so bleak. Whereas one was old at 50 a century ago, with the advent of the means of preserving one's ability to see, hear, chew, and locomote, even persons age 70 are no longer "old." There can be no doubt that today's lifestyle of continuing education and work, exercise, and hobbies for those in their 60s and 70s contributes very much to the ongoing vigor of many older persons.

Prominent symptoms. Although older persons may have the usual symptoms resulting from virtually every disease, some are especially common. *Dizziness* requires an accurate description of what is happening, for it may refer to feeling weak, lightheaded, or "funny," as well as to true vertigo. *Constipation* can be a vexing problem. Usually it results from an improper diet or poor habits, but it may augur a colonic neoplasm. *Insomnia* is a common complaint, often the result of daytime naps or pressing concerns. *Loss of appetite* is worrisome; be wary of cancer and de-

pression. The patient may complain of *falling*—once or frequently; this can be a Chinese puzzle. Was it simply because a rug slipped, or was it the result of a transient ischemic attack? *Syncope* is also frequent; cardiovascular causes are both common and serious.

Note how many symptoms are "cannot symptoms," such as cannot sleep, cannot eat, cannot chew, cannot swallow, cannot move bowels, cannot urinate, cannot see, cannot hear, cannot walk, and cannot breathe.

Especially common diseases. Because heart disease, cancer, and stroke are the three leading causes of death, you can expect them to be the most common diseases of the elderly. They are, and this simple truth must always weight your logic. No matter what the clinical presentation, one of these three illnesses must be seriously considered, because it often hides behind what may seem at first to be another disease.

Commonly seen neuropsychiatric disorders include anxiety, depression, acute confusional states, dementia, alcoholism, melancholia, and loneliness. For the special senses you see cataracts, glaucoma, presbyopia, deafness, and vertigo. Continuing into the gastrointestinal tract, the elderly person suffers from inability to chew because of lost teeth; cancer from the mouth to the anus, but mainly in the stomach, pancreas, colon, and rectum; cholelithiasis; diverticulitis; and last but not least, hemorrhoids.

Cardiovascular diseases include mainly ischemic heart disease, congestive heart failure, arrhythmias, and peripheral vascular disease. In the lungs, chronic obstructive pulmonary disease and cancer lead the list. As for hematology, anemias of all sorts, especially those of chronic disease and chronic blood loss, are rampant. And in the endocrine system, diabetes is very common, perhaps occurring in 1 in 10 patients. Indeed, diabetes and hypertension, singly or combined, will be the underlying problems in a high percentage of older patients seen in the office or hospital. It is interesting to note that hyperthyroidism in the elderly is often undiagnosed because its presentation is in many ways atypical, and hypothyroidism is often overlooked because its manifestations overlap with and are mistaken for those features that indicate that the patient is "getting older."

It is important to recall that older patients are highly prone to *adverse drug reactions* and that these may be the cause for or may modify the presenting symptoms, thus confusing the physician. In fact, adverse drug reactions and drug-drug interactions are among the most common problems in this age group. These patients may have multiple diseases, take various medications, and take them at ill-conceived intervals—a perfect background for confusion and mistakes, even if the patient were young.

To Solve or Not. Inevitably, the issue of whether or not to pursue a diagnosis, and how vigorously to pursue it, arises for the elderly patient. There is no simple "yes" or "no" answer. An 80-year-old may have right upper quadrant pain, easily withstand a cholecystectomy, and live on for another 10 fruitful and enjoyable years.

On the other hand, an 80-year-old with metastatic cancer should not have a coronary arteriogram for the investigation of chest pain. Nor should an 80-year-old with proven advanced triple vessel coronary artery disease have an extensive survey for suspected cancer. No matter what the results of such studies, you would do nothing anyway.

Do not push too hard with diagnostic studies in the very old because their tolerance for such study is limited. The illness you are pursuing has probably already made the patient frail. If he or she has occult gastrointestinal bleeding that has already stopped, and colonoscopic and gastrointestinal radiographic findings are normal, it might be both more discreet and valorous to give iron for the anemia rather than do visceral angiography or computed tomography with contrast. Often the diagnostic procedure causes more distress than the illness, and you should not gamble with the vitality of the patient by subjecting him or her to more tests than he or she can tolerate with reasonable safety.

Such attitudes may come more naturally to those who have practiced medicine for many years and have seen much of life and death. But such ideas may be heretical to many of today's interns or residents who, with a plethora of diagnostic tools, have not yet learned that they are not omnipotent and that nature may often take its course despite their actions.

CASE 75

INCONTINENCE

Karen Kelly

Data A television commercial dealing with inadequate bladder control brings your 75-year-old female patient to your office for help and advice. She saw you a month ago for her routine annual checkup, but did not mention incontinence and you did not ask about it. She says she frequently wets her undies and wears protective pads at all times. Now she wants to know if anything else can be done.

Logic Typical of many patients with incontinence—the involuntary loss of urine—she had never before brought this up as a problem, perhaps because of shyness, embarrassment, or because she thought it was natural with old age. Up to 30% of community-dwelling elderly, and more in nursing homes, are incontinent of urine. Incontinence affects 5% of men and 25% of women older than age 65 and costs 10 billion health dollars each year. Yet only a minority of persons who have this condition consult physicians or receive evaluations.

Although incontinence is common, it should never be regarded as part of aging; it is often treatable or curable. It may signal an important *acute* medical condition such as an infection (Table 21.1). *Chronic* incontinence generally has other causes and often leads to embarrassment and isolation, and perhaps in the more debilitated patient to rashes, bedsores, catheterizations, infections, falls, and fractures. Institutionalization may result when a demented or otherwise disabled person, previously cared for at home, becomes incontinent.

Data The problem is not acute, but it has gradually gotten worse over the past few years. She notices that when she feels the urge to urinate, she often cannot hold it and will wet herself. She denies dysuria (painful voiding), unusual frequency, an increase or decrease in urine volume, swollen legs, or vaginal symptoms such as itching, burning, and discharge. Occasionally she is incontinent at night.

TABLE 21.1 Causes of Acute Incontinence

Urinary tract infection

Certain medications

Acute delirium

Stool impaction

Marked hyperglycemia

Other than a β-adrenergic blocker for moderate hypertension, she takes no medication, has no serious medical problems, has had no surgery, had three vaginal deliveries, and is 25 years postmenopausal.

Logic Normal bladder function is under control of the parasympathetic nervous system via the pelvic nerves at the S2, S3, and S4 levels of the spinal cord. A full-sensation from stretch receptors in the bladder trigone is transmitted to the spinal cord and then to the cerebral cortex for conscious awareness. When the person is ready to urinate, the cortex releases its inhibitory effect on the urination reflex, the sphincter relaxes, and the detrusor contracts.

In this regard it is notable that incontinence is often seen in patients with strokes, Alzheimer's disease, and brain tumors because cortical inhibition to urination via the reticulospinal tracts is lost or impaired, resulting in detrusor instability.

There are various types of incontinence: (1) total, (2) stress, (3) urge, and (4) overflow; combinations can occur.

Total incontinence occurs without the patient's knowledge and consists of almost continuous or repeated wetting. This situation may be seen in neurogenic bladders and in patients in whom the urinary sphincter is bypassed, such as in vesicovaginal fistulas.

Stress incontinence occurs when the woman coughs, sneezes, strains, laughs, or lifts a heavy object. It results from pelvic relaxation and weak sphincter control, usually associated with a cystocele, rectocele, or urethrocele in a multigravida. Estrogen deficiency in the postmenopausal state may be a contributing factor in that it leads to weakened sphincter tone and a change in position of the bladder neck. Small quantities of urine are passed, and incontinence occurs only rarely at night.

Urge incontinence consists of a sudden urge to urinate and the inability to hold it long enough to get to the toilet. It is a common type and can be caused by bladder and urethral infections and neurologic diseases, but may also be idiopathic.

Overflow incontinence exists when the bladder overdistends and small amounts of urine are repeatedly and involuntarily passed. This type most often occurs in men with large obstructive prostate glands. But sphincter control may be compromised in men and women who have hypotonic or neurogenic bladders as in diabetic autonomic neuropathy, uremia, hypothyroidism, chronic alcoholism and collagen vascular diseases. All causes produce a dilated and usually palpable bladder.

The patient's general state of good health and the absence of frequency and dysuria, as well as of vaginal symptoms, are points against the presence of urinary tract or vaginal infection.

In some cases of incontinence, the problem may reside in the facts that the bed is too far from the bathroom, or that arthritis may prevent a quick trip to the toilet or the rapid loosening of clothing.

A voiding diary may help clarify the history by listing all episodes of urination, whether or not there was incontinence, and the quantity and circumstances of each voiding.

Data The blood pressure is 158/90. Otherwise, findings from the complete physical examination are normal, including the other vital signs, head and neck, heart and lungs, abdomen, and extremities. The findings from neurologic examination, including cranial nerves, reflexes, and sensation, are normal. The pelvic examination showed thinning and dryness of the vaginal mucosa, and there was slight protrusion of the bladder into the anterior vaginal wall on straining, but no clear-cut cystocele, urethrocele, or rectocele. Rectal examination findings were normal. In trying to induce stress incontinence, the patient is asked to stand with her legs apart and cough. Leakage on this maneuver suggests stress incontinence. There is none.

You ask her to void and then catheterize her to measure postvoid residual (PVR). She voids 250 mL. The PVR is 25 mL (normal is less than 50 mL). Sequential multiple analyzer (SMA)-6 and urinalysis findings are normal.

Logic These findings rule out urinary tract infection, neurologic diseases such as stroke and Parkinson's disease, stress incontinence from relaxation of the pelvic floor, overflow incontinence, diabetes, and renal dysfunction.

Most cases of incontinence are acute and transient and either resolve themselves or are easily treated. Of the rest, most can be either helped or cured by a variety of available measures.

Acute and treatable causes include: (1) urinary tract infection; (2) medication such as furosemide, anticholinergics, psychotropics, sedatives and hypnotics, α-adrenergic agents, and alcohol; (3) state of acute delirium; (4) stool impaction; and (5) sudden marked hyperglycemia.

Infection causes bladder irritation. Medications act by either causing retention with overflow, decreasing sphincter control, or by causing excessive urine to be formed. In delirious states, the patient is not consciously aware of the signal to urinate. The mechanism by which stool impaction causes incontinence is unknown. Sudden massive elevation of blood glucose causes an overwhelming amount of urine to be formed and passed.

This patient has chronic urge incontinence based on detrusor overactivity; the muscle of the bladder wall contracts excessively at low bladder volumes. No primary cause is identified, so it is most likely idiopathic. The medication she takes for the blood pressure is not on the list of those possibly causing incontinence.

Data You start her on a program of voiding every 1 and 1/2 hours. She is asked to keep track of her voiding and to record any accidents. If continence is obtained, the interval is gradually extended by one half hour at a time. If favorable results are not obtained, consideration can be given to the use of estrogens and Kegel exercises to tighten the pelvic floor and urethral sphincter.

Questions

1. Acute incontinence associated with polyuria may be caused by which of the following?
   (a) Hyperglycemia
   (b) Hypercalcemia
   (c) Hypernatremia
   (d) Hyperthyroidism
   (e) Diuretic administration
2. A variety of medications can lead to or aggravate incontinence. Match the following drugs with their respective mechanisms:

(a) diuretics	1. overflow
(b) anticholinergics	2. delirium
(c) α-adrenergic blockers	3. polyuria
(d) β-adrenergic blockers	4. outlet incompetence
(e) narcotics	5. don't cause incontinence

3. A demented patient is noted to be newly incontinent. Which of the following might be helpful in evaluation?
   (a) Urinalysis
   (b) Glucose
   (c) Postvoid residual
   (d) Rectal examination
   (e) Temperature

Answers

1. **(a), (b), and (e) are correct.** All conditions cause polyuria, which can overwhelm the ability of even normal elderly persons to maintain continence. Hypernatremia is typically caused by dehydration, which lowers urine volume. Excess thyroid hormone has no effect.
2. (a) 3. (b) 1. (c) 4. (d) 5. (e) 2.
3. **All of the aforementioned.** Acute incontinence is a nonspecific sign of acute medical or functional problems. It should never be ignored, and proper work-up consists of looking for likely underlying problems, including such things as urinary tract infections, hyperglycemia, fecal impaction, acute obstruction, and infections of any cause that may lead to delirium and incontinence. A review of new medications is also important.

Suggested Readings

Fantl JA, Wyman JF, McClish DK, et al. Efficacy of bladder training in older women with urinary incontinence. JAMA 1991;265:609–613.

National Institute of Health Consensus Development Conference. Urinary incontinence in adults. J Am Geriatr Soc 1990;38:265–272.

Resnick NM. Initial evaluation of the incontinent patient. J Am Geriatr Soc 1990;38:311–316.

CASE 76

NOCTURIA AND FREQUENCY

Paul Cutler

Data He comes to the doctor only to have his blood pressure checked, but when this 58-year-old man was about to leave the office, his wife reports that for several months he has been getting up three to four times a night to urinate. She is worried about it. You ask the patient to elaborate. He notes that in addition to his night-time peregrinations, he has to strain to void and sometimes he presses his lower abdomen to complete voiding. He denies polydipsia, dysuria, and hematuria, and jokes that like the rest of the body, his urine stream is slowing down, too.

Logic In a male patient of this age, the foremost consideration should be benign prostatic hypertrophy (or hyperplasia). Its symptoms include increased urinary frequency (normal is 3–5 times per day and 0–1 time per night), nocturia, decreased caliber and force of stream, and later on, hesitancy, intermittent stream, sense of incomplete emptying, and dribbling. Urgency and incontinence occur along the way. This symptom complex is called "prostatism."

Prostatic enlargement is an age-related phenomenon. By age 55, one of four men develop difficulty in voiding. The prevalence of symptoms doubles by age 75. On autopsy, 90% of men 80 years old and over have prostatic hyperplasia.

The strategic anatomic location of the prostate gland in the area of the bladder neck and posterior urethra and its subsequent hypertrophy create an obstruction to the voiding process. As obstruction worsens, intravesical pressure must increase in order to void and the bladder wall hypertrophies.

In any individual the need to urinate arises when the bladder is almost full and the stretch receptors in the bladder wall are activated. As the bladder hypertrophies, it loses compliance and receptors may be activated sooner. Later, as obstruction worsens, the bladder becomes unable to empty on voiding, and although the bladder capacity may be 300 or more milliliters, only 100 mL is voided, and there is a residual volume of 200 mL.

The term "polyuria" refers to the excretion of more than 3000 mL of urine per 24 hours, and it may occur in the following pathophysiologic situations:

- Inadequate vasopressin—as in diabetes insipidus and some pituitary tumors
- Failure of renal tubules to respond to vasopressin—as in some kidney diseases—for example, pyelonephritis, analgesic abuse, obstructive uropathy, sarcoid, sickle cell disease—as well as a result of drugs like lithium and demeclocycline

- Solute diuresis—as in severe uncontrolled diabetes mellitus
- Natriuresis as a result of "salt-losing nephritis" and the administration of diuretics
- Primary polydipsia or compulsive water drinking.

It is notable that polyuric states are almost always associated with nocturia and an increased frequency of urination, unless the bladder capacity is unusually large. An additional cause for nocturia exists in patients having edema from any one of a variety of diseases (congestive heart failure, cirrhosis, nephrotic syndrome, venous insufficiency of the lower extremities) and in whom fluid shifts from the dependent areas to the general circulation and out through the kidneys when supine.

In this patient, as in all patients who have urinary tract symptoms, there must also be concern for urinary tract infection (urethritis, cystitis, pyelonephritis) as well as for carcinoma of the prostate, neurogenic bladder, urethral stricture, and side effects from medications.

When considering the pathophysiology of polyuric states, it is wise to remember that the increased thirst (polydipsia) in uncontrolled diabetes mellitus or diabetes insipidus is a consequence of the severe diuresis, whereas, in compulsive water-drinking, the diuresis is a consequence of the large fluid intake.

Although all polyuric states can result in nocturia and daytime frequency, it should be noted that benign prostatic hyperplasia (BPH) does *not* cause polyuria. Rather it results in nocturia and frequency because smaller than normal amounts are voided each time.

Data The patient has been on a β-adrenergic blocker for his hypertension and takes no over-the-counter medications. There is no history of stroke, diabetes, arthritis, urethritis, or pelvic trauma. The urinary bladder was not palpable, and the prostate was moderately enlarged, rubbery, not nodular, nontender, and without areas of induration. The findings from neurologic examination were normal; in particular, anal tone and perineal sensation were normal.

Logic A neurologic cause for his symptoms is very unlikely because the neurologic examination findings are normal, and he does not have an insensitive distended bladder in association with overflow incontinence. Urethral stricture is also unlikely at his age and in the absence of a vene-real disease history. He takes no medications such as diuretics, antihistamines, anticholiner-gics, tricyclic antidepressants, or narcotics that may cause obstructive-like symptoms.

The size of the prostate gland does not clearly correlate with the degree of obstruction and its related symptoms. What seems to be normal size may mask cases of obstruction where the hyper-plasia is mainly in the periurethral area, whereas the prostate may be huge yet without prominent symptoms.

In benign hyperplasia, the prostate, if en-larged, is generally uniformly so; it is firm or rub-bery. Cancer, on the other hand, occurs most of-ten in the lateral lobes and appears as a stony-hard nodule, or if more advanced, a diffusely hard and nodular gland. It is important to note that hyper-plasia does not predispose to cancer.

The precise cause of BPH is not known. The gland is composed of stromal and epithelial cells; androgenic stimulation (via 5α–dihydrotestos-terone) and age are prerequisites for prostate en-largement. The smooth muscle of the prostatic urethra and bladder neck is innervated by α-adrenergic nerves. These concepts are the basis for the medical therapy that is currently available.

Data The doctor sends the patient to the labo-ratory for some tests and gives him the American Urologic Association (AUA) Symptom Index Questionnaire. Over the next month, he is to monitor the times of voiding and the amount voided each time, as well as the various associ-ated symptoms that may be present, such as ur-gency, hesitancy, intermittency, double stream, weak stream, or burning.

Logic The Agency for Health Care Policy and Research has developed a set of guidelines for the management of BPH, which recommends that, in a typical patient, the diagnosis of BPH re-quires:

- Patient's history (include AUA symptom score)
- Focused physical examination (rectal exami-nation)
- Urinalysis
- Serum creatinine level determination

Data Urinalysis revealed no squamous epithelial cells; specific gravity, 1.010; pH, 6.5; no glucose; no protein; 1 white blood cell (WBC) per high-powered field; 0 red blood cells; no casts; and no bacteria. A fasting glucose level was 75 mg/dL; creatinine level was 1.2 mg/dL; and prostate-specific antigen level (PSA) was 3.0μg/L.

Logic These tests exclude urinary tract infection, impaired renal function from obstructive uropa-thy (hydronephroses), and diabetes mellitus (DM), at least diabetes as a cause of the symptoms that the patient has.

Frequently, common diseases occur together, and when BPH and poorly controlled DM co-exist, it may be difficult to decide which of the two (or perhaps both) is causing the nocturia and frequency. For concurrent diabetes to cause or worsen symptoms, the blood glucose must be high and the urine must contain considerable glucose. But if diabetes is well controlled, it does not contribute to the symptoms of BPH.

There is significant controversy over the util-ity of the PSA in screening for cancer of the prostate, and the limit of normal varies with the age of the patient. The PSA is glycoprotein-specific to the prostate gland, and there may be overlapping values in cancer, BPH, and prostati-tis. Up to 3.0 μg/L is regarded as normal; 3 to 10 μg/L is considered equivocal; and more than 10 μg/L suggests cancer. Clearly, the results may be falsely positive for cancer that is not present and falsely negative for cancer that is present.

Studies have demonstrated that occult carci-noma is present in 10 to 20% of patients with prostatism, that the PSA helps to detect one third of cancers that a digital rectal examination (DRE) would miss, and that PSA alone as a screening tool would also miss some carcinomas detectable only with DRE. Some investigators believe that using the annual rate of change of the PSA or the PSA density (PSA/prostate mass by ultrasound) improves the specificity of the serum PSA.

Data The patient returns in 1 month and scores a 12 (moderate severity) on the AUA symptom index scale.

Logic The AUA has developed a standard symp-tom scoring tool known as the AUA Symptom Index, which is a seven-item questionnaire. The patient keeps score, and a severity assessment is based on the patient's symptom score. The score is classified as mild (0–7), moderate (8–19), and severe (20–35). This score is then used to deter-mine therapy and to monitor the patient's response to treatment. A patient who has a mild score can be observed and reviewed in a year; someone with moderate-to-severe symptoms would require further intervention.

Data The doctor reviews therapeutic options with the patient—medication or surgery. Before deciding, the patient wants to know if cancer has been absolutely eliminated from the possibility. The doctor says that it is highly unlikely because of the findings from the DRE and the low PSA level, but to be sure he advises that transrectal ultrasound (TRU) of the prostate be performed (Fig. 21.1). This procedure was done. The prostate was noted to be diffusely and homogeneously enlarged, but no hypoechoic densities could be seen.

Logic No further tests were indicated. TRU with or without biopsies are generally done if the DRE findings are positive (hard, irregular, or nodular prostate) or if the PSA level is elevated. In this case it was done because reasonable diagnostic certainty was sought by the patient. The acid phosphatase level is elevated when prostate cancer has spread distantly into bones.

Magnetic resonance imaging and computed tomography are sometimes done to define the extent of the tumor and to detect spread to nodes. Other tests are used on a case-by-case basis. These include uroflowmetry to determine maximal urine flow rate, postvoid residual volume by ultrasound, and pressure flow studies if

neurogenic bladder is suspected. Intravenous pyelography is done if there is hematuria or if hydronephroses are possible. Cystoscopy is rarely indicated.

Data The patient opts for medical treatment. Therapy is begun with an α-adrenergic blocker, and he is to return in 6 months for follow-up.

Logic Medical therapy consists of two groups of medications: the 5α-reductase inhibitors (finasteride) and the α-adrenergic blockers (prazosin, doxazosin, terazosin). The 5α-reductase inhibitors act by inhibiting the conversion of testosterone to 5α-dihydrotestosterone, which is a more potent androgen. In doing so, the epithelial cells of the prostate will atrophy. Therapy with finasteride has been shown to increase urine flow rate and to shrink the prostate. However, 3 to 6 months of therapy are needed to note improvement. The side effects are decreased libido, erectile dysfunction, and sometimes ejaculatory dysfunction. There is some concern that because finasteride lowers PSA it may interfere with the utility of PSA as a screening test for prostate carcinoma.

The α-adrenergic blocking agents relax smooth muscle at the bladder neck and the prostatic urethra to facilitate micturition. Their effect is noted as early as within 2 weeks of therapy. Their side effects are postural hypotension and dizziness. In this patient an α-adrenergic blocker is appropriate because he is hypertensive and because he indicates symptoms of significant retention (that is, pressing on his abdomen to complete voiding).

Data The patient returns in 6 months and says his stream is much improved and the nocturia has decreased to once a night. But he still feels the need to press on the lower abdomen to evacuate completely. In addition, he thinks that he may have passed a stone in his urine; once he had sharp pains in the penis while urinating and heard a pinging sound in the toilet bowl. On examination after voiding, the bladder is palpated above the level of the symphysis pubis.

Logic Even though some of his symptoms seem to be improving, the patient is referred to a urologist because of the large residual volume and the history of what sounds like the passage of a small bladder stone.

Data Urodynamic studies are performed, and the patient's peak urine flow rate is 9 mL/sec. He is scheduled for a transurethral resection of the prostate (TURP).

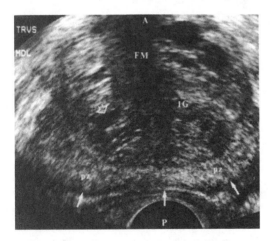

► **Figure 21.1.** Transrectal ultrasound shows characteristic benign prostatic hypertrophy. Open arrow points to small cyst. A, anterior; P, posterior; PZ, normal peripheral zone (closed arrows); IG, inner gland hypertrophy.

Logic The low urine flow rate, when added to the other complicating factors, makes surgery a reasonable choice. More than 300,000 surgical procedures for BPH are performed annually in the United States, making it, except for cataract extraction, the second most common surgical procedure for men older than 65 years of age. Other new therapeutic options, still to be evaluated, include laser ablation, balloon dilatation, stents, and hyperthermia.

Data TURP is successfully done, and the patient returns in 6 months for follow-up. The prostatic tissue was benign. He had occasional episodes of incontinence postoperatively, but this has resolved. So has his nocturia and frequency.

Questions

1. Which of the following situations may arise as a consequence of long-standing prostatic hypertrophy?
   (a) Urgency, frequency, dysuria, fever
   (b) Hematuria, suprapubic pain, dysuria
   (c) Weakness, pallor, azotemia
   (d) Suprapubic discomfort and inability to void
2. Which of the following clinical situations should be considered for TRU and transrectal prostate biopsy?
   (a) DRE notes hard nodule left lobe of prostate, PSA 1
   (b) DRE notes hard nodule right lobe of prostate, PSA 20
   (c) DRE notes normal prostate, PSA 20
   (d) DRE notes stony hard prostate, PSA 1
3. Arrange the following events in correct pathophysiologic sequence.
   (a) Enlarged bladder
   (b) Overflow incontinence
   (c) Hypertrophy, bladder wall
   (d) Acute retention
   (e) Nocturia and frequency
   (f) Obstruction to flow

Answers

1. **All are correct.** Choice (a) represents urinary tract infection; obstruction and residual urine predispose to bacterial colonization. Choice (b) suggests bladder stone formation and passage, also a consequence of obstruction and stagnation. Choice (c) sounds like obstructive uropathy with impaired renal function. Choice (d) indicates complete obstruction and acute urinary retention requiring quick intervention. Alcohol, infec-

tion, and use of tranquilizers may precipitate acute retention.
2. All require further study because cancer is a strong possibility in each instance. Choices (a) and (d) could represent false-negative PSAs. In (c) the high PSA is worrisome even though the DRE is normal.
3. **(f), (e), (c), (a), (b), (d).** Obstruction is the initiating factor. Acute retention is at the end of the line.

Comment This problem was easily solved. The symptoms and findings on rectal examination were enough to decide on diagnosis and treatment. In the universe of 58-year-old men, benign prostatic hypertrophy is by far the most common cause of this small cluster of clues.

In the subsequent development of this case, the pathophysiology of diuresis, urine excretion, polyuric states, benign prostatic hypertrophy, and cancer of the prostate were analyzed, and the special diagnostic roles of the prostate-specific antigen, transrectal ultrasound, and transrectal biopsy were explored.

It is notable that two advisory agencies have issued guidelines for the management of such patients, a trend that will no doubt expand under future managed health care programs. *(P.C.)*

Suggested Readings

Klein EA. An update on prostate cancer. Cleve Clin J Med 1995;62:325–338.

McConnell, et al. Benign prostatic hyperplasia: Diagnosis and treatment. Clinical Practice Guideline No. 8, AH CPR Publication No. 940582, Agency for Health Care Policy and Research, Public Health Service, U.S. Department of Health and Human Services, February, 1994.

Monda JM, Oesterling JE. Medical treatment of benign prostatic hyperplasia: 5 alpha-reductase inhibitors and alpha-adrenergic antagonists. Mayo Clin Proc 1993;68:670–679.

Pressman RM, Figueroa WC, Kendrick-Mohamed J, et al. Nocturia: A rarely recognized symptom of sleep apnea and other occult sleep disorders. Arch Intern Med 1996;156.

Robers RG. Novel idea in BPH guideline: the patient as decision maker. Am Fam Physician 1994;49(5):1044–1051.

CASE 77

DEMENTED OR DEPRESSED

Karen Kelly

Data Unpaid bills scattered about the house and the nauseating odor of rotting food in the refrigerator prompt the patient's son to bring his 78-year-old mother to the doctor. She lives alone, and although he visits weekly and has noticed forgetfulness and what he feels are signs of old age, he quite suddenly realized that she may no longer be able to take care of herself. He comments that he believes she is depressed, has lost interest in her usual activities, and her memory has been bad.

Logic Although depression can be related to apparent memory loss and lack of interest, so can dementia. First it is imperative to get a more detailed history and to evaluate the patient's mood and mental status.

Data She denies any problems, is vague about the unpaid bills, and although she admits her memory is not what it used to be, she says, "I am almost 80, you know." She denies insomnia, loss of appetite, and feeling sad or hopeless about the future. She smiles during the interview, particularly when discussing her grandchildren (Fig. 21.2).

Logic So far, there is no evidence for depression. The things the son mentions, then, are more likely to be signs of dementia.

Dementia is the acquired global impairment of cognitive abilities of sufficient severity to affect normal function. It must be distinguished from the "minor forgetfulness of old age," which is normal. Symptoms are of gradual, almost imperceptible onset. Insight is lost early, so the patient is usually unaware of the changes, and the history is invariably given by a relative. Unusual behavior includes loss of interest in social contacts and conversations, lapses of memory, failure to remember names and appointments, difficulty in learning new information, failure to remember recent events, and giving up hobbies. As the disease progresses, mistakes are made in dress and everyday life. Appearance deteriorates, and personal hygiene is neglected. Eventually, the afflicted person is unable to care for him- or herself, does not recognize friends or relatives, repeats questions, and may wander off and get lost.

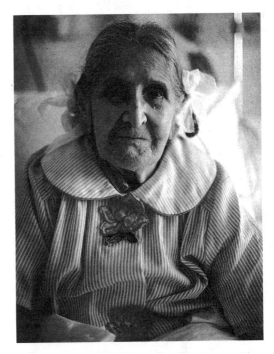

▶ **Figure 21.2.** The patient appears to be comfortable, is neatly and tastefully dressed, and does not seem to be depressed.

Cognition may be evaluated in a more formal way with the Folstein Mini-Mental Status Examination (MMSE). This is a standardized set of questions that can be completed in under 10 minutes. Many but not all demented patients are unaware of the degree of their disability, so the patient's comment that she is fine should not deter further evaluation. Nor should her age be a dissuasion. Dementia may be more common with advancing age, but it is never normal.

Data Her MMSE score is 21. She does not know the date, the day of the week, or the month. She cannot remember any of three objects and cannot copy a figure. She cannot count back from 100 by 7's. However, she can spell the word "world" backward, and her language is preserved. She is a college graduate who taught school until her retirement.

Logic The MMSE assesses cognitive function by measuring orientation, memory, attention, language, and visuospacial skills. It is 87% sensitive and 82% specific for a diagnosis of dementia.

These results, along with the history from her son, are consistent with mild dementia. A college graduate her age should score 26 or above. She has obvious short-term memory loss, as well as visuospacial difficulties. Forgetting to pay bills and to clean out the refrigerator indicate that normal function is impaired. And because she does not appear to be depressed, her altered functional states are no doubt caused by dementia.

Dementia is the major cause of long-term disability in old age and affects more than 20% of persons older than age 80 (some 4 million persons in the United States alone), filling this country's nursing homes and institutions, and consuming huge slices of public and private dollars.

Commonly, concerned relatives bring you an older person who is acting strangely, is incoherent, disoriented, forgetful, and cannot manage his or her clothing and hygiene. This represents full-blown senile dementia. The picture may have existed for days, weeks, or months, and the patient may be coming from home or from a nursing home where the family or staff can no longer cope.

There are many causes of dementia, and the physician's next task is to seek out and pinpoint the likely cause in this patient (Table 21.2). The two principal causes are *Alzheimer's disease* (ALZ) and *multi-infarct dementia* (MID), which account for some 50% and 20% of cases, respectively. Many other diseases account for the rest. Because some in the latter group are either curable or may be arrested or slowed by treatment, it is advisable to look for a specific, remediable cause.

Neurologic space-occupying or destructive lesions may result in dementia. These include tumors such as frontal lobe meningioma, subdural hematoma, and metastatic carcinoma. Unusual chronic central nervous system infections or inflammations such as syphilis, sarcoid, Creutzfeldt-Jakob disease (caused by an abnormal protein), and

TABLE 21.2. Causes of Dementia

Alzheimer's disease
Multi-infarct dementia
CNS infections, inflammations
Space-occupying intracranial lesions
Injury (pugilism)
Metabolic-endocrine
Alcohol and drugs
Depression

human immunodeficiency virus infection in younger patients may also result in dementia, but usually these are associated with additional neurologic and physical evidence.

Many medical diseases, and sometimes their treatments, may cause dementia. Some are remediable. These include the vitamin B_{12} deficiency of pernicious anemia, hypothyroidism, chronic and repeated episodes of hypoglycemia in the overtreated diabetic, hepatic encephalopathy, uremia, and chronic cerebral anoxia from severe heart or lung disease, as well as those conditions associated with serum levels of sodium and calcium that are high enough or low enough to cause cerebral manifestations.

Medications are in a class by themselves because they are such common offenders. Even the correct dose of digoxin, chlorpropamide, indomethacin, steroids, phenothiazines, barbiturates, and anticholinergies may cause mental abnormalities, especially in the presence of polypharmacy and drug-drug interactions. Virtually no drug is exempt from this list, so a good and complete medication history, including over-the-counters, is important.

Repeated cerebral contusions as a result of pugilism may cause a "punch-drunk" state of dementia. Brain injury from an automobile accident may similarly do so.

And last, chronic alcoholism may result in dementia. Here, a history from the patient, often difficult to elicit, as well as added information from family or friends, is important.

These possibilities should all be excluded by additional history and selected subsets of the physical and neurologic examinations.

Data She has no significant medical history and takes no medications whatsoever. She never smokes and drinks only occasionally. The review of systems is mostly negative, but she admits to occasional incontinence and some hearing loss. She had a hysterectomy for fibroids in her 40s.

Physical examination reveals: weight, 140 lb; height, 5 ft 4 in; blood pressure, 140/85 without orthostatic changes; pulse 80 and regular; temperature 98.2°F; no thyromegaly; no pallor; normal heart and lungs; liver not enlarged; normal abdomen; and no edema. Peripheral pulses are full everywhere, and there are no carotid bruits. The results of a careful neurologic examination are normal, except for the mental status.

Logic   There are no illnesses found that may cause dementia. She has no evidence of generalized vascular disease to suggest the added presence of cerebrovascular disease. There are no stigmata of liver disease, and the normal vital signs and good color negate uremia, myxedema, and pernicious anemia.

The absence of neurologic abnormalities weighs heavily against an intracranial space-occupying lesion and certainly against the possibility of MID. She has never had a stroke or a transient ischemic attack. MID usually results from repeated cerebral infarcts, bilateral emboli originating in the heart or in the carotid arteries, or as a result of diffuse vasculitis. It is episodic, and tends to occur in patients with hypertension, diabetes, and cardiovascular disease. Its onset may be relatively sudden. Most often there are residual neurologic findings such as hemiparesis, hemianopsia, pseudobulbar palsy, or positive Babinski's signs.

ALZ therefore becomes the working diagnosis for this patient by virtue of the clinical picture, the commonness of the disease, and the exclusion of other possibilities. Over a period of several years there is a gradual loss of cortical tissue in the temporal, parietal, and frontal lobes, associated with neurofibrillary tangles and senile plaques, especially in the hippocampal area (Fig. 21.3). Biochemically there is decreased activity of neurotransmitters and, as observed by positron emission tomography, a diffuse decrease in the metabolism of oxygen and glucose. The disease may have genetic implications, but this has not been conclusively proved to date.

The actual brain mass is not a determining factor. Atrophy of gyri occurs normally with the aging process as neurons are lost, but this alone does not cause intellectual decline. On the other hand, patients known to have ALZ may have normal brain size.

With most dementia illnesses, the patient may demonstrate a positive palmomental reflex, which was not, however, present in this patient. This primitive reflex consists of homolateral contraction of the mentalis and orbicularis oris muscles on stroking the palm.

Data   Findings from laboratory studies of electrolytes, complete blood count, calcium, vitamin B_{12}, folate, thyroxine (T_4), and thyroid-stimulating hormone (TSH) are normal. CT of the head

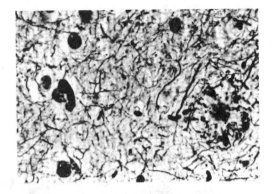

▶ **Figure 21.3.** Tissue sample from a patient with Alzheimer's disease. Prominent senile plaques on left, neurofibrillary tangles on right; disruption of cortical architecture.

is unremarkable and shows no evidence of tumor, hematoma, or infarct; there is mild cortical atrophy.

Logic   Metabolic, endocrine, and gross intracranial lesions are virtually excluded.

Although there has been much talk of reversible dementia, it is unusual to see a patient with a truly reversible dementia. Rather, sometimes there are medical conditions or medications that are aggravating an underlying dementia. Treating the medical problems or discontinuing medications may improve, but not cure, the problem.

Data   You meet with the son and the patient to discuss your findings.

Logic   Making the diagnosis is just the first step. As with any serious diagnosis, the news should be given gently in a setting where adequate time for reaction and questions is allowed.

The patient and family will need counseling regarding her present and future needs. Currently she seems to need more assistance with housework and bill paying. The son may be able to provide this. As time goes on she may need further supervision and help, so it will be important to follow her periodically to reassess her safety and social needs.

You also advise further testing of her hearing. The hearing loss, although not the cause of her problem, may further decrease her functioning and correcting it may improve things somewhat.

Questions

1. You notice that a long-time patient of yours is beginning to repeat herself. You ask about memory, but she denies problems. Physical examination is unrevealing. The best next step is:
   (a) CT of brain.
   (b) talk to family.
   (c) MMSE.
   (d) T_4 and TSH level determinations.
   (e) hearing test.
2. One of your previously well patients is hospitalized with pneumonia. You come in to see her the next day, and she is asleep. When you wake her up, it is clear that she does not recognize you and is confused about where she is. Neurologic examination is unremarkable except for her abnormal mental status. The most likely diagnosis is:
   (a) dementia.
   (b) psychosis secondary to the hospitalization.
   (c) delirium.
   (d) stroke.
3. Many demented patients have behavioral problems that pose challenges for caregivers and can even endanger the patient. Which one of the following behaviors is most likely to cause safety problems?
   (a) Wandering
   (b) Repeating oneself
   (c) Losing household items
   (d) Insomnia
   (e) Incontinence of urine
4. Which of the following is *least* likely to be an early sign of dementia?
   (a) Trouble balancing the checkbook
   (b) Repeating oneself
   (c) Losing household items
   (d) Complaint of memory loss by the patient
   (e) Forgetting the names of medications

Answers

1. **(b).** All of the proposed tests are reasonable once the diagnosis of cognitive loss is made. The first step is to do a systematic assessment of mental state. Talking to family members will be important to confirm problems and assess functioning once the diagnosis is made. A CT scan, hearing tests, and thyroid function tests should also be done as part of the evaluation.
2. **(c).** Delirium is a syndrome of acute global confusion usually precipitated by medical problems or medica-

tions. It is characterized by cognitive loss in the setting of drowsiness or agitation. The onset is usually acute, and a precipitant is identifiable. Delirium is not uncommon in elderly, ill hospitalized patients. It is usually reversible with proper treatment of the medical problem or removal of the medication (usually a sedative, analgesic, or anticholinergic).

You cannot make a diagnosis of dementia because the patient is acutely ill and has signs of delirium (drowsiness). There is no reason to think that she is psychotic because this usually causes hallucinations, but not cognitive loss. A stroke is a possible cause of her delirium, but it usually would have a presentation involving focal neurologic signs.

3. **(a).** Wandering can result in a patient getting lost and injured or taken advantage of. The other behaviors can be annoying to caregivers, but are not generally dangerous.
4. **(d).** Most, although not all, demented patients are unaware of the deficit. In fact, a complaint of memory loss, especially when out of proportion to objective memory loss, is often a sign of anxiety or depression. All the other symptoms *are* typical early signs of a dementia process.

Suggested Readings

Clarfield AM. The reversible dementias: Do they reverse? Ann Intern Med 1988;109:476–486.

Howell T, Watts DT. Behavioral complications of dementia: A clinical approach for the general internist. Gen Intern Med 1990;5:431–437.

Katzman R, Jackson JE. Alzheimer's disease: Basic and clinical advances. J Am Geriatr Soc 1991;39:516–525.

 CASE 78

ERECTILE DYSFUNCTION

Paul Cutler

Data "Do not tell my first wife I was here," says a 68-year-old man who comes to her doctor's office. He goes on to tell the doctor his story: He has not been to a physician for 3 years, since his own physician retired. During that time he has gained some 10 to 15 lb because his new wife is such a good cook. However, she is 25 years his junior, and as the interview progresses, it becomes clear that he is really concerned about difficulty in having and maintaining an erection. He says, "Doctor, I am old, but not that old!"

Logic Many patients hesitate to present the problem of erectile dysfunction to their physicians. It is believed to affect almost 10 million American men, and its prevalence increases with age, affecting at least one of four men older than age 65.

Impotence is strictly a male problem. It is defined as the consistent inability to form and maintain an erect penis—all of the time, or in at least three quarters of attempts.

In cases of sexual dysfunction, it is essential to analyze the sexual history very carefully, because the problem may consist of one or many of the following components: (1) loss of libido; (2) disinterest in the partner; (3) premature ejaculation; (4) lack of orgasm; (5) lack of ejaculation; (6) increase in length of postcoital refractory period; (7) erectile dysfunction; and (8) psychologic causes.

Data Further conversation with the patient determines that he still has a strong sexual urge, but the problem lies entirely with his inability to achieve an erection.

Logic Normal sexual function invokes an extremely complex interplay between the brain, spinal cord, autonomic nervous system, integrative centers at the S2-S4 levels and in the pelvic plexus, and the blood vessels and striated and smooth muscles of the pelvis and genitalia in such a way as to bring about the desired cycle of tumescence, orgasm, ejaculation, and detumescence.

Erection occurs when erotic sensory impulses from the eyes, ears, nose, skin, and imagination are relayed from the brain to centers in the lower spinal cord and pelvic plexus so as to relax smooth muscle in the penis and allow for an increased flow of blood into its lacunar spaces. The amount of blood in the penis represents a balance between blood in and blood out, and alterations in blood flow to and from the penis are the commonest organic causes of impotence. As engorgement takes place, a corporal veno-occlusive mechanism, acting in concert with compression of venules against the firm fibrous bands of the corpora, results in a decrease in the venous outflow and thereby rigidity. Local factors such as nitric oxide, prostaglandins, and endothelins play a role in this process.

Although not a problem in this patient, libido—the drive to have sexual intercourse—is in large part dependent on the presence of androgens, and it may be impaired by sickness, drugs, and unpleasant factors in the sensory environment. Premature ejaculation is seldom organic and usually results from anxiety. Absence of ejaculation can be caused by retrograde ejaculation, androgen deficiency, and drugs such as guanethidine.

Erectile dysfunction may have any of many causes (Table 21.3). Endocrine causes include primary or secondary hypogonadism, prolactinoma, and diabetes mellitus. There is a long list of medications (Table 21.4), some commonly used, that may play a role; included are antihypertensives, especially those that are sympatholytic; cimetidine; finasteride; and monoamine oxidase inhibitors. It is interesting that angiotensin converting enzyme inhibitors, calcium channel blockers, and vasodilators have little or no adverse effect. Thiazide diuretics are thought to produce

TABLE 21.3. Causes of Erectile Dysfunction

Endocrine diseases
Drugs
Penile diseases
Neurologic diseases
Vascular diseases
Psychologic causes

TABLE 21.4. Medications that Cause Impotence

Diuretics (especially thiazides)
β-adrenergic blockers
Tranquilizers
H_2-blockers
Gemifibrozil
Antidepressants
Cytotoxic agents
Antiandrogens (finasteride)
NSAIDs
Anticonvulsants
Metoclopramide

NSAIDs = nonsteroidal anti-inflammatory drugs.

impotence by decreasing testosterone levels and by causing zinc deficiency.

Marked fibrosis of the connective tissue on the dorsal surface of the penis, a not uncommon occurrence, may hinder tumescence and even distort penile shape, thus resulting in impotence (Peyronie's disease).

Neurologic diseases of various kinds may also interfere with normal sexual function at different levels of the nervous system—the temporal lobe, spinal cord, pelvic plexus, and autonomic nerves.

Vascular disease sometimes plays a significant role. The inadequate delivery of blood to the penis may occur in those with severe atherosclerosis of the pelvic arteries. Leriche's syndrome exists when both iliac arteries are occluded at the aortic bifurcation; symptoms include claudication and impotence.

Data More history! The patient has had mild-to-moderate hypertension for at least 10 years, managed with a diuretic at first; more recently a calcium channel blocker was added. Three years ago, he was found to have "a trace of sugar" and was told to restrict carbohydrates and lose weight. He did not.

He is not depressed; in fact he claims to be a pretty happy individual except for this problem. He has marked interest in his "young and attractive" wife as a sexual partner, although he admits to some performance anxiety and fear of failure. There is no current marital discord, he has no worries, is not fatigued, and believes that he is generally in good health, although there are times—especially before attempted intercourse—when he thinks about his first wife and feels some guilt about their breakup.

On a more intimate level, he says that even though he cannot perform successfully in bed, he is still able to masturbate on occasion, and that he often has a moderate erection on awakening.

Logic The diuretics he takes for hypertension may play a role; the calcium channel blocker does not. Diabetes is one of the three most common causes of impotence: diabetes, medications, and vascular diseases (these three account for the majority of cases of organic impotence). It does so in two ways: vascular disease and autonomic and sensory neuropathy.

In addition to a detailed medication list, questions should be asked about angina and claudication (seeking evidence of vascular disease), thy-

roid disease, hyperlipidemia, neurologic diseases, and psychologic assessment.

Atherosclerosis affects the entire body, including the penile arteries. Consequently, its presence makes a patient more likely to be at risk of impotence on a vascular basis.

Although the patient is neither depressed nor anxious, he offers clues suggesting that psychologic factors may be at the root of his problems. Although these were once thought to be the major causes of impotence, organic problems relating to diabetes, medications, and neurologic and vascular disorders seem to currently play more prominent roles.

The ability to successfully masturbate and to have nocturnal emissions and morning erections seem to point away from organic disturbances and in the direction of psychogenic impotence, although these are not completely reliable indicators.

Data The patient says he has smoked one pack of cigarettes each day for the past 25 years and has 3 to 5 glasses of wine per week in the evenings, including weekends. He has never used recreational drugs. He has been married for a total of 28 years, has two healthy children, and has worked as an accountant in the same company for 20 years. His job is secure and is not a source of stress.

Logic Substance abuse (especially opiates) and cigarette smoking are common contributing factors to erectile dysfunction. The excessive use of alcohol—not the case here—can cause autonomic and sensory neuropathy as well as hypogonadism. Cigarette smoking helps to increase vascular disease; one study showed that smoking two cigarettes will inhibit the erection that is achievable by intracorporeal papaverine.

Data The physical examination reveals a comfortable, well-dressed, mildly obese male; height, 69 in; weight, 180 lb; temperature, pulse, and respiration normal; and blood pressure, 158/90 in both arms. The fundi show arteriovenous nicking. There are no bruits in the neck. There is an S_4; S_1 and S_2 are normal, and there are no S_3, murmurs, or rubs; the lungs are clear.

His abdomen is soft, nontender, and without masses, organomegaly, or bruits. Genitourinary examination reveals bilaterally descended testicles of normal size and consistency. Anal sphincter tone is normal, the prostate gland is somewhat enlarged although without nodules or induration, perineal sensation is normal, and the bulbocavernosus reflex is intact. There are no signs of feminization, and there are no fibrotic plaques on the dorsum of the penis. The femoral, popliteal, and dorsalis pedis pulses are symmetric and bounding bilaterally, and the complete neurologic examination findings are normal.

Logic A careful physical examination is critical. The fundi show evidence of long-standing hypertension, and the S_4 likely results from left ventricular hypertrophy. There is no clinical evidence of atherosclerosis, neuropathy, or endocrine disorders.

Data Urinalysis reveals: specific gravity, 1.018; pH, 6.0; 1+ glucose; no protein; and no WBCs. Serum cholesterol level is 200 mg/dL, and triglycerides level is 272 mg/dL. The fasting serum glucose level is 164 mg/dL, and the prolactin and testosterone levels are within normal range.

Logic Hypogonadism and prolactinoma are excluded. Mild diabetes is confirmed. Lipids are unremarkable. The association between diabetes mellitus and impotence was described nearly two centuries ago. As many as half of all male diabetics will develop impotence in the first 10 years after diagnosis. In some patients, impotence occurs even before the diagnosis of diabetes is made. However, erectile dysfunction does not clearly correlate with the duration of the disease.

Data Even though diabetes is present, the patient is considered to have psychogenic impotence because there is no evidence of vascular disease or neuropathy. He is advised to stop smoking and to stop the diuretic because these two items may be playing an additional role.

Several months later, the patient returns; his diabetes is now well-controlled with diet, and he has lost 8 lb. He no longer takes a thiazide diuretic. He quit smoking on learning of its possible role in his erectile dysfunction. He had been to a psychologist in the interim to explore the possibility of psychogenic factors, but did not benefit from counseling. His problem still exists, and he is not convinced that there is no organic problem.

Logic The doctor reconsiders the case. Could this yet be an organic problem? Can he be helped? How important is this entire matter to the patient? To what lengths should he go? If he

succeeds at masturbation and nocturnal tumescence, could it still be organic?

Data "It is important!" Both the patient and his wife are interested in resuming a normal sexual relationship. A further search is indicated.

The penile-brachial pressure index (PBPI) is 0.5. The nocturnal tumescence test (NTT) suggests that the erections are not adequately rigid. A trial of papaverine injection therapy achieved mild erection that quickly detumesced.

Logic The PBPI compares the pressure in the penile artery to the pressure in the brachial artery, and is therefore a measure of arterial blood flow. A neonatal sphygmomanometer and an ultrasonic stethoscope are used. The ratio should be more than 0.6. Test results suggest restriction of arterial flow to the penis.

The NTT is expensive and tedious. It can be performed in a sleep laboratory with a strain gauge or at home with a monitoring device. Normally, tumescence occurs for 100 minutes each night during rapid eye movement (REM) sleep.

The patient seems to have elements of both functional and organic causes for his impotence—not a simple situation to diagnose or to treat, but perhaps a common concurrence.

Further observation, testing and therapeutic trials, as well as counseling from a sexual therapist are all in order. Consideration will be given to intrapenile papaverine injections, vacuum constriction devices, surgical arterial reconstruction, a penile prosthesis, and a trial of yohimbine. Before a course of action is taken, all options and their risks will be discussed with the patient and his wife.

Questions

Decide whether the following statements are true or false:
1. The younger the patient, the more likely that impotence is psychogenic.
2. The older the patient, the more likely that impotence is organic.
3. If libido persists, the cause of impotence is organic.
4. If nocturnal erections occur, the cause of impotence is psychologic.
5. If libido is lost, the cause of impotence is psychologic.

Answers

1. **T.**
2. **T.**
3. **F.** Libido may persist, yet other psychologic factors may be at the root of impotence.
4. **F.** This statement is generally true, but as in the case just presented, other factors may be simultaneously present.
5. **F.** Loss of libido may occur for organic reasons such as chronic or debilitating illnesses and hypogonadal states.

COMMENT This is yet another symptom that patients may be reluctant to mention or discuss with their doctors. Although it would seem that the distinction between psychogenic and organic factors should be easy to make, this is commonly not so, as in this patient. Often, there is a mixture of the two, and the physician must resort to a variety of tests and trials, none perfect and none without risk, in order to satisfy the requirements of the couple. *(P.C.)*

Suggested Readings

Kaiser FE, Korenman SG. Impotence in diabetic men. Am J Med 1988;85(suppl 5A):147–152.

Morley JE, Kaiser FE. Impotence: The internist's approach to diagnosis and treatment. Adv Int Med 1993;38:151–168.

NIH Consensus Conference: Impotence. JAMA 1993; 270(1):83–90.

CASE 79

FALLS

Karen Kelly

Data A concerned son brings his 76-year-old widowed mother to your office. She lives alone and sustained a fracture of the wrist when she fell last week.

Logic He is right to be concerned. Falls are a common problem in the elderly population. An estimated one in three elderly persons living in the community will fall annually. Falls result in significant morbidity and even mortality. Among the complications are fractures, most commonly in the hip, wrist, and pelvis; subdural hematoma; soft tissue injury; and death. Moreover, after falling, the elderly patient becomes fearful, may lose independence, and may reduce his or her activities. Recurrent falls are a common reason for admission to a nursing home or other long-term facility.

It is important not to view falls in the elderly patient as an inevitable and therefore untreatable problem. A systematic approach to the etiology of falls must be undertaken in order to prevent further events and their complications.

Data The patient has had non–insulin-dependent diabetes for nearly 14 years and systolic hypertension for 5 years. Her medications include glipizide 2.5 mg a day and hydrochlorothiazide 25 mg a day. Her grandchildren had been visiting the evening before the fall. When she went to make breakfast, she stepped on a small toy and slipped. She tried to break her fall by putting her hand down on the floor first. Although she had never fallen before last week, she did trip a few times on the stairs at home and also occasionally on the street.

Logic A detailed history is the first step in evaluating the patient who falls. This must include specific questions regarding prior falls or near falls and the situation surrounding the fall.

Under-reporting of falls is common. Patients and their families dismiss them as either accidental or expected as a result of aging. In addition, patients are concerned that this may limit their independence, and that if family members become aware of recurrent falls, they may consider sending the patient to a long-term care facility.

Distinction must be made between falls, syncope, seizures, dizziness, narcolepsy, and coma. The U.S. Preventative Services Task Force defines "falls" as referring strictly to events that lead to the *conscious* subject coming to rest inadvertently on the ground.

To maintain body balance while in motion, there is a complex interaction between muscles, joints, nerves, vision, hearing, reflexes, cerebellum, cardiovascular system, gravity, and Newton's laws. Balance may become impaired with age by disease of any or at times many of those factors, and as the ability to adapt rapidly to an environmental change becomes lessened.

Falls result from a disordered interaction between the patient (intrinsic factors) and the environment (extrinsic factors).

Intrinsic factors having to do with problems arising within the patient include alterations in visual acuity (cataract, new glasses, adjustment to bifocals, need for refraction), as well as impaired hearing, peripheral neuropathy from diabetes and alcohol, and lessened mobility from stroke, Parkinson's disease, or arthritis. The patient may have orthostatic hypotension and fail to adjust the pulse and blood pressure to sudden changes in position. In pernicious anemia, posterior column disease may cause loss of proprioception. Medication that the patient takes for another disorder is a common offender. These include diuretics, antihypertensives, some antibiotics, sedatives, hypnotics, psychoactives, anticonvulsants, and some antiarrhythmics. At times, urinary urgency associated with prostate disease may precipitate a quick run to the bathroom.

Extrinsic factors include poor lighting, slippery or wet floors, stairways, especially those without handrails, storage facilities that are difficult to access, absence of grab-bars and other assistive devices, cracks in the pavement, bed too high or too low, sliding rugs, and improperly fitted footwear.

Falls are rarely the result of a single cause. Usually they result from a combination of a variably impaired patient facing an environmental challenge.

Data At no time did the patient lose consciousness and she denies feeling dizzy at the time of the fall. There has been no polyuria, nocturia, polydipsia, fevers, chills, chest discomfort, palpitations, or shortness of breath. She has been eating and drinking as usual. She thinks she may be developing cataracts because objects look hazier and several of her neighbors recently had eye surgery. Her son assures you there is adequate lighting throughout the apartment; however, he is not certain she uses it. She has not seen an ophthalmologist in more than 2 years. At that time she was told everything was "fine."

Logic *Syncope* is the sudden temporary loss of consciousness associated with the inability to maintain postural tone, followed by spontaneous recovery without cardioversion. If she had fainted, the problem solver would be confronted by an additional array of diagnostic contenders, such as aortic stenosis, cardiac arrhythmia, and transient cerebral ischemia. This is an important consideration because syncope may result in a significant increase in morbidity and cardiovascular mortality and requires additional evaluation.

Dizziness (or vertigo) is a sensation of irregular or whirling motion either of one's self or of external objects. If present, another list of diagnostic possibilities such as the effect of medication, middle ear and inner ear disease, pontine angle tumor, cerebellar disease, and vertebrobasilar insufficiency must be considered.

The absence of other symptoms points against the possibility that the diabetes is poorly controlled, that she has an infection, and that she has significant heart disease.

Even well-controlled diabetes can predispose to peripheral neuropathy as well as visual disturbances not allowing her to sense her surroundings. In other words, she may not be able to feel and/or see the ground, or the steps, or the toy. She is at risk for orthostatic hypotension from the autonomic dysfunction caused by diabetes, or volume depletion from her diuretic.

As for medications in this case, the patient takes only two drugs. The diuretic seems guiltless, unless it has caused an electrolyte imbalance. The antidiabetic tablet does not seem to bear on the problem; furthermore she has taken it for years. Polypharmacy is common in the elderly and drug interactions can result in more falls. Thus, only medications that are absolutely necessary should be prescribed—for all patients. It is also advisable to use only short-acting medication, at the lowest possible dose to achieve the desired effect. A history of alcohol is often forgotten, but may predispose the elderly patient to falls.

Data On physical examination, the patient is a thin, well-dressed woman. She is not in an orthostatic state as judged by blood pressure or pulse. Fundoscopic examination reveals no papilledema, nor any proliferative retinopathy. The red reflex in her left eye is decreased. Visual field testing results are normal. Her ear canals are packed with cerumen. She has no carotid bruits. Cardiac examination reveals normal S_1 and S_2 without any murmurs, rubs, or gallops. Her pulmonary and abdominal examination results are normal. She has a cast on her left wrist. On neurologic examination, she is alert and oriented. She achieves a perfect score on the Mini-Mental Status Examination. She has symmetric 4+ motor strength, but has diminished vibratory sensation and proprioception in both lower extremities. She was able to get up from her chair easily, walk 10 feet, turn around, and sit down. But she did look at the floor while walking.

Logic At this point, it seems that this patient fell as a result of multiple factors, both intrinsic and extrinsic. Intrinsic factors include a proprioceptive defect and visual disturbance. The evaluation of mental status is simple and is necessary to assess cognitive function in order to detect errors in judgement and to plan intervention.

A functional assessment of the patient's balance and gait can be done in a few minutes by the "Get Up and Go Test" as done in this patient. A person with Parkinson's disease, for example, may have difficulty getting up from a chair and take small steps. On the other hand, someone with autonomic dysfunction may get light-headed after standing up. Posterior column cord degeneration and its subsequent decrease in position and vibration sense is common in the elderly and exists in this patient, even in the absence of vitamin B_{12} deficiency. It may result in gait and balance disturbances. The need to look at the floor on walking indicated compensation for not knowing where her legs were.

Motor strength often decreases with age. Physical therapy to increase muscle strength can be integrated into the treatment plan. The elderly patient's vision may be checked in the office by a Snellen's chart. However, she should be sent to an ophthalmologist to be examined for retinopathy, macular degeneration, glaucoma, and cataracts. Correcting visual disturbances is necessary to avoid falls, and disimpacting an ear canal full of cerumen is likely to help increase sensory input.

Data A visiting nurse makes a home visit and finds that the lighting in the apartment consists of 25- to 40-watt bulbs, and the area near the kitchen sink where the patient fell has a mat on it that is dark in color and not secured onto the floor. The stairway leading to the front door is also poorly lit. In the patient's bathroom, there is a cloth mat on a tiled floor. For sentimental reasons, the patient uses her husband's slippers at home. They are too big for her, and the rubber soles are nearly gone.

Logic Although some information regarding environmental factors can be obtained from the patient and the family, an objective assessment by someone who knows what to look for can provide additional useful information. The majority of falls occur in the home; thus it should be investigated. There are checklists available to guide such a survey. Risk factors for falls such as poor lighting, loose rugs, improperly placed furniture, lack of grab bars in the bathroom and on stairwells, and poorly fitting shoes are just a few of the easily modifiable extrinsic factors.

Data Findings from the patient's electrocardiogram, serum chemistry, complete blood count, and vitamin B_{12} level are all within normal limits. Her diabetes has been well controlled for at least the past 2 years. She is seen by an ophthalmologist and undergoes a cataract extraction. An occupational therapist visits the home with her son, appropriate changes are made in the lighting, and the loose rugs are removed. After some convincing, the patient agrees to wear proper, closed slippers.

Logic The management of falls is a multi-disciplinary approach. The laboratory tests are needed to ascertain whether the diuretics are causing electrolyte disturbance. In a patient with peripheral neuropathy, it is valuable to rule out vitamin B_{12} deficiency as its cause. Therapeutic and diagnostic intervention should be directed by the patient's history and physical examination findings: for instance, correction of visual problems and alteration of the environment in order to minimize the risk of future falls. In addition to preventing the morbidity and mortality associated with falls, interventions should be aimed at preserving the patient's independence without compromising safety.

Questions

1. A 65-year-old plumber has fallen three times; each fall was preceded by transient loss of consciousness. Which of the following situations might be causing him to fall?
   (a) Grade 3/6 systolic aortic ejection murmur
   (b) Takes diuretic and a β-adrenergic blocker for hypertension
   (c) Soft systolic bruits heard beneath the mandible
   (d) Untreated hypertension—160/90
   (e) PR interval .10 seconds, QRS interval .12 seconds
2. Which of the following clinical pictures may result in falls in an elderly patient being treated for diabetes?

(a) Blood glucose level 180 mg/dL, urine glucose 2+, no acetone

(b) Hyperactive reflexes, loss of position sense in legs

(c) Positive tilt test, incontinent, bloats on eating

(d) Retinal microaneurysms

(e) Chronic alcoholism

Answers

1. **(a), (b), (c), and (e) are correct.** They might represent aortic stenosis, orthostatic hypotension, transient ischemic attacks, and the Wolff-Parkinson-White syndrome with paroxysmal arrhythmias. Untreated mild hypertension should not cause syncope.

2. **(b), (c), and (e) are correct.** They represent posterolateral sclerosis and dysautonomia, each a complication of diabetes; the diabetic patient, like any other, is not immune to alcoholic intoxication. Mild diabetes alone should not cause syncope, and microaneurysms themselves do not affect vision unless they result in retinal hemorrhages.

COMMENT After first clarifying the circumstances and nature of the fall, it was crucial to know if it was accompanied by loss of consciousness or dizziness, because each of these symptoms has its own list of diagnostic contenders. However, the fall was not accompanied by either of these two symptoms. Next, a search was made for the various defects within the patient's own health status that might predispose to falls, as well as a search through the long list of potential hazards in her environment. The identifiable causes in this patient, as in most patients, turned out to be a combination of intrinsic and extrinsic factors, only some of which were remediable. *(P.C.)*

Suggested Readings

Cutson TM. Falls in the elderly. Am Fam Physician 1994;49(1):141–156.

Ruberstein LZ, et al. The value of assessing falls in an elderly population. Ann Intern Med 1990;113(4): 308–316.

Tinetti ME, Speechley M. Prevention of falls among the elderly. N Engl J Med 1989;320(16):1055–1059.

CHAPTER 22

Multisystem Problems

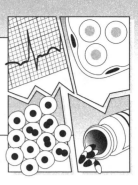

Until now, each chapter has dealt mainly with problems within a single category of medicine. Sometimes, a clinical presentation might have resulted from disease in any of several systems (e.g., pulmonary or cardiac). This chapter will deal further with symptoms whose origin may be in any one of many systems, whose diagnosis may be a single multisystem disease, or whose diagnosis may be multiple.

Recall, for instance, that the patient whose chief complaint is fatigue may suffer from any one or more of a wide variety of ailments, ranging all the way from depression to cancer—with numerous other possibilities in every organ system in between.

The acquired immunodeficiency syndrome (AIDS) is a prime example of how one disease may affect any or every organ system and may therefore be seen by the physician in many different ways. Indeed, AIDS is a diagnostic contender in many of the cases and in almost every chapter of this book.

Other clinical presentations—such as syncope, strange behavior, prolonged fever, and coma—conjure up a long list of possibilities that roam through every body system.

Always bear in mind that, whatever the cause of the chief complaint turns out to be, patients frequently have more than one disease, and it is common to find that hypertension, diabetes, arthritis, or duodenal ulcer are also present—a concurrence of high-incidence diseases.

Problems of this sort almost always require the initial formation of a differential diagnosis for the chief complaint. This is formed by culling the various diseases that should be stacked by system in the shelves of your brain. The mechanics of forming the differential diagnosis were discussed in Chapter 3 and should now be reread.

Multisystem problems are usually solved by collecting a complete patient data base and then selecting relevant clues. The entire gamut of problem-solving techniques may be called upon: clusters can be formed, key clues sought, and clues pointing to a specific organ are helpful. Once you have found a leading clue, you may branch into a subset of data. A single question to the patient with longstanding fever—"Did you drink any goat's milk or eat goat's milk cheese during your recent travels through the Middle East?"—may direct you to the solution. Brucellosis may then be confirmed by specific laboratory tests, and a complete data base can thus be sidestepped or delayed.

Unless a key clue is uncovered in the history or physical examination, extensive tests and procedures are usually needed to exclude most possibilities and prove one. Here is your opportunity to exercise restraint and use thoughtful selectivity in ordering diagnostic procedures. (P.C.)

CASE 80

WEAKNESS, WEIGHT LOSS, ANOREXIA

Paul Cutler

Data You see a 62-year-old man who has had weakness, weight loss, and loss of appetite for 5 months. Prior to that time, he was perfectly well.

Logic This common triad is always ominous, especially in the patient's age group. It usually indicates serious organic disease or a depressive reaction. The symptoms are not specific and point to no particular organ or illness. By culling the various modules of pathophysiology stored in your brain, you compose a list of common problems to consider:

1. Cancer (stomach, lung, colon, pancreas, prostate, kidney)

2. Tuberculosis (pulmonary or generalized)
3. Depression
4. Uremia
5. Hematologic disease (chronic anemia, leukemia, myeloma, lymphoma)

Less common causes, such as the malabsorption syndrome, a connective tissue disorder, or Addison's disease, must also be considered while sifting through the clues that follow.

As you approach the patient for additional information, the signs and symptoms of the various diagnostic possibilities are whirling through your mind. Each positive or negative clue will give more or less credence to a diagnosis, and you hope to harvest a combination of findings that will fit the template for one of the listed possibilities.

Data The patient has been working hard at his printing job and had taken on additional responsibilities as a church elder and Sunday school teacher. He attributed his symptoms to too much pressure but nevertheless continued in these activities because he enjoyed them. However, during the past month his anorexia got worse, and he noticed that his clothes felt loose; a scale revealed a 30-lb weight loss in 5 months. In the week before coming to your office, he began to have severe, constant backache unrelated to activity or motion and unrelieved by heat and aspirin.

Logic It now appears that the backache is what really drove him to your office. He seems to deny the importance of the other symptoms. Severe weight loss, lack of evidence for depression, and the recent unrelenting backache cast an aura of organicity upon the situation. Remember the possibility that the backache may be unrelated to the other symptoms.

Data A review of systems is negative. In particular, the patient has had no polyuria, polydipsia, nocturia, urgency, thin stream, or dysuria. There has been no indigestion, early satiety, abdominal pain, change in bowel habit, or black stools. He has had no fever, chills, night sweats, cough, chest pain, hemoptysis, or dyspnea; no pain, stiffness, or swelling of joints; and no heat intolerance, insomnia, palpitations, or tremor. He is not aware of family, financial, or emotional problems and is not depressed, although he admits to being a bit worried about not feeling well.

Logic This long series of pertinent negative historical data leads you away from diabetes mellitus, prostatic obstruction, carcinoma of the stomach and bowel, tuberculosis, carcinoma of the lung, connective tissue disease, thyroid disease, and depression—in that order.

Diabetes as a cause of weight loss is unlikely anyway, because polyphagia rather than anorexia would be expected. Carcinoma of the prostate could metastasize body-wide, yet not be large enough or located so as to cause urethral obstruction. The absence of frequent greasy stools and the presence of anorexia weigh against malabsorption. Because there are no gastrointestinal (GI) symptoms, cancer along this tract is less likely, although it certainly cannot be ruled out. Cancer of the stomach, pancreas, or colon could each display a presentation with a downhill course from generalized spread before causing localized symptoms. The absence of pulmonary symptoms is strong evidence against pulmonary tuberculosis or cancer; there, a lesion producing such a rapid, relentless course would probably cause local symptoms, too. Depression seems even more remote.

Data Examination discloses a chronically ill patient who is emaciated and shows signs of severe weight loss. He is 70 inches tall, weighs 138 lb, and has normal vital signs. There is no jaundice, cyanosis, or clubbing, but the conjunctivae, mucous membranes, and nail beds are pale. The rest of the complete physical examination findings are normal. There are no palpable lymph nodes and no palpable abdominal masses or organs. A satisfactory rectal examination cannot be done because the rectum is filled with hard feces. No reason for the back pain is found on orthopedic and neurologic examination.

Logic Weight loss is confirmed by the emaciation (loss of subcutaneous fat—that is, sunken cheeks, hollowed temples, and deeply wrinkled, loose skin over the arms and abdomen). The patient is anemic, and you clearly have a serious organic problem to manage. The absence of large nodes and spleen weighs against most forms of leukemia. The absence of jaundice, large liver, and supraclavicular nodes whispers against metastatic cancer. An enema must be given, and the rectal examination redone. Uremia is virtually excluded by normal fundi, normal breath odor, and absence of hypertension. Pernicious anemia merits little further consideration because of the normal appearance of the tongue and the absence of neurologic and GI symptoms and signs; also, this disease is not usually characterized by weight loss. Further help is needed.

Data Studies are done. The complete blood count shows 3 million red blood cells per cubic millimeter; hemoglobin, 9 g/dL; hematocrit, 27%; and white blood cell count, platelets, and blood smear results normal. The urinalysis, chest radiograph, electrocardiogram (ECG), and purified protein derivative skin test findings are normal or negative. Stool examination is negative for excessive fat (Sudan III fat stain), ova, parasites, and occult blood. Test results from blood chemistry (glucose, urea nitrogen, creatinine, electrolytes, protein electrophoresis, calcium, phosphorus) are normal. Radiographs of the lumbosacral spine and pelvis show numerous osteolytic and osteoblastic lesions (Fig. 22.1).

Logic The solution is at hand. In the presence of a normochromic normocytic anemia, you are not surprised to find the stool negative for excessive fat and occult blood. Steatorrhea and chronic GI bleeding usually cause macrocytic and microcytic anemias, respectively. Malabsorption as well as a bleeding mucosal GI lesion are now most unlikely. Normal proteins and urinalysis virtually exclude multiple myeloma; also, myeloma causes osteolytic, not osteoblastic lesions. Leukemia, lymphoma, tuberculosis, and uremia are now very unlikely.

The radiographs indicate bone metastases. Cancer probably explains the backache, the anemia, and the entire picture. The primary source of the cancer must still be located. Because osteoblastic bone lesions are usually caused by prostatic cancer, your suspicion is strong, and you aim directly for this target.

Data Repeated enemas eventually clear the rectum, and a stony-hard nodular prostate is palpated. Acid and alkaline phosphatase levels are both 10 times normal. The prostate specific antigen (PSA) level is elevated—22 μg/L. Bone marrow aspiration shows sheets of small malignant cells.

Logic Had a proper rectal examination been possible at the start, the problem would have been quickly and easily solved. Usually, prostatic symptoms are present and guide you in the correct direction. But in this case, as in many others, there is no encroachment upon the urethra, and therefore no dysuria or frequency.

PSA is a very sensitive test. Cancer is rare with levels less than 3 μg/L. True positives and false positives exist between 3 and 10 μg/L. Values greater than 10 μg/L are highly suggestive of prostate cancer. An elevated alkaline phosphatase level is not specific; but an elevated acid phosphatase level is specific and indicates that the cancer has extended beyond the prostate to bones and elsewhere. The anemia is at least partly caused by bone marrow infiltration and replacement by cancer cells.

Consideration must now be given to patient education, and a decision regarding optimal treatment in this case must be made. Transrectal ultrasound and prostate biopsy will determine local extent of disease and cell type. Both will help in the selection of proper treatment.

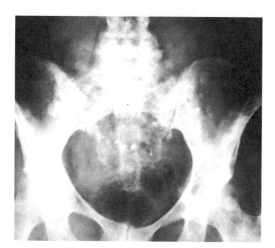

▶ **Figure 22.1.** Pelvic and lumbosacral radiographs showing osteoblastic and osteolytic lesions of metastatic prostatic carcinoma.

Questions

1. You see a patient with a similar initial presentation who shows no evidence of cancer of the prostate, and repeat stool examinations are positive for occult blood. You would then suspect cancer in the GI tract. All except which one of the following might be true?
   (a) Barium enema demonstrates cancer of the cecum.
   (b) The anemia is hypochromic.
   (c) The alkaline phosphatase level is elevated.
   (d) A bleeding duodenal ulcer is the cause of the patient's problem.

2. Had there been no evidence for cancer of the prostate, no anemia, and had the stool been repeatedly negative for occult blood, you might have given serious consideration to cancer of the pancreas. If the latter disease were present, which one of the following statements would be false?
   (a) GI radiographs are usually of no help.
   (b) Jaundice may be present.
   (c) Pancreatic function tests are the diagnostic procedure of choice.
   (d) A left pleural effusion may be present.
3. In a patient who has weakness and weight loss, yet has a good appetite and no other symptoms, consider:
   (a) diabetes mellitus.
   (b) hyperthyroidism.
   (c) malabsorption.
   (d) all of the aforementioned.
4. You see a 60-year-old woman who has weakness, anorexia, and weight loss. She lost her husband 1 year ago, seldom sees her children, and has no hobbies or friends. The complete data base is otherwise normal. Advise her to:
   (a) take mood elevators.
   (b) return in 3 months for re-evaluation.
   (c) see a psychiatrist.
   (d) have superficial psychotherapy and return frequently for re-evaluation.

Answers

1. **(d) is correct.** It is the only unlikely answer. Even though a duodenal ulcer could also be present, it would hardly cause anorexia and weight loss. Cancer of the cecum often has such a presentation. A hypochromic iron deficiency type anemia results from chronic GI blood loss. The alkaline phosphatase level could be elevated from liver or bone metastases originating in any primary GI cancer.
2. **(c) is correct** because it is false. Such studies are neither sensitive nor specific. The choice procedure today is the computed tomographic (CT) scan, although some physicians prefer ultrasound, endoscopic retrograde pancreatography, and an eventual guided biopsy. Ordinary GI radiographs are not helpful unless the lesion is large and located in the head of the pancreas. Under these circumstances, jaundice from common bile duct obstruction is also usually present. A left pleural effusion may be the only hint of cancer in the pancreatic tail just under the left hemidiaphragm.
3. **(b) is correct.** There may be no other symptoms, but plenty of signs. For diabetes to cause this cluster, polyuria and polydipsia would also have to be present. Malabsorption fits the cluster, but if weight loss were present, there would be considerable loss of fat in the stool resulting in frequent greasy stools, which is not present here.
4. **(d) is correct.** Depression is probably the principal issue. If so, patience, understanding, mild medication, and revisits should suffice. Furthermore, revisits are indicated to detect new clues should they appear. Cancer and depression are frequently confused. Do not be lulled into complacency. Have your patient make a serious conscious effort to eat well and gain weight. Choice (a) is satisfactory, but not without psychotherapy. Three months is too long a time between visits, either for depression or should something else be wrong. If the patient does not improve, psychiatric consultation would be indicated, along with a complete medical re-evaluation.

COMMENT Nonspecific presentations of this sort must often be solved by the traditional method of gathering a complete data base and sifting through the clues. Many diseases in numerous organ systems can have presentations such as this one. But even here, shortcuts are possible.

Although weakness, weight loss, and anorexia are each nonspecific, the triad is ominous and conjures up a distinct differential diagnosis. Then added bits of information in the history and physical examination narrow the list by eliminating most possibilities (proof by exclusion) and suggesting very few. Noteworthy is the use of the pertinent negative clue. During the data-gathering process, anemia and backache are added to the cluster and augur the presence of a malignant disease.

In this case, the problem solver could have thrown out a huge fishnet to see what he or she could catch, or could have been more selective in his or her approach. The entire work-up was done on an outpatient basis. Had the rectal examination been immediately achievable, the diagnosis would have been quickly evident. Had alkaline phosphatase and acid phosphatase level determinations as well as prostate-specific antigen assay been included in the initial chemical battery, the final diagnosis might have been more readily apparent; the test result would have prompted a search for bone or liver metastases. In this instance, the value of complete battery screening is clearly seen.

GI radiographs and high-technology tests were not needed. But if the prostate gland and spine radiographs had been normal, a search for GI cancer or lymphoma would have necessitated such radiographs and at least a computed tomographic scan.

The absence of lower urinary obstructive symptoms in the presence of a large hard prostate gland is somewhat of a surprise and represents a false-negative historical clue that was initially misleading. But carcinoma of the prostate gland is common in men older than age 60, and the laws of probability are thereby obeyed. *(P.C.)*

PROBLEM-BASED LEARNING Such case presentations can be solved simply, or may require that the problem solver have a large information base. You should know all about:

- The array of diseases that may have similar presentations
- The common carcinomas of men—lung, prostate, and GI tract—and their clinical features
- Carcinoma of the prostate in particular—its metastatic features and serum markers
- The reliability of testing modes for prostatic cancer—acid phosphatase, PSA, and biopsy
- How to best test for occult pancreatic cancer (e.g., the relative values of ultrasound computed tomographic scan, guided biopsy, endoscopic retrograde cholangiopancreatography, and so forth)
- Why cancer causes general symptoms of weight loss and anorexia

Suggested Readings

Brawer MK. The diagnosis of prostatic carcinoma. Cancer 1993;71(suppl 3):899–905.

Choyke PL. Imaging of prostate cancer. Abdom Imag 1995;20(6):505–515.

Gittes RF. Carcinoma of the prostate. N Engl J Med 1991;324(4):236–244.

Oesterling JE. Using prostate-specific antigen to eliminate unnecessary diagnostic tests: Significant worldwide economic implications. Urology 1995;46(suppl 3A):26–33.

Smith JA Jr, Scaletsky R. Future directions in tumor marker technology for prostate cancer. Urol Clin N Am 1993;20(4):771–777.

CASE 81

THE GREAT IMITATOR

Paul Cutler

Data You receive a telephone call. "Doctor, why is my daughter not getting better? You saw her for a cough and fever over a week ago and said she had a virus. She is still coughing and has a little phlegm, but this morning her temperature was 101."

Logic Quickly you review the facts: Her daughter is 23 and seems to be in generally good health. She had never been really sick before except for the infectious mononucleosis (IM) she had 3 years ago. You recall that at that time she had a fever, sore throat, headache, and diffuse lymphadenopathy. She got better in approximately 2 weeks, and except for fatigue and lethargy that lasted an additional month, and an unexpectedly negative Monospot test, there was nothing unusual about the case.

Two weeks ago, her examination was normal except for a slight fever and a few scattered rales at each lung base.

Data Both mother and daughter come into your office. The young woman looks sick. Vital signs are as follows: temperature, 100.8°F; pulse, 110; respirations, 24; and blood pressure (BP), 110/80. Respirations are a bit labored. More rales are present than before, although otherwise the examination has not changed. The blood count is normal, and the chest radiograph shows faint bilateral interstitial infiltrations in both lungs (Fig. 22.2).

You perform an intradermal tuberculosis test, send a sputum specimen to the laboratory for Gram's stain and all kinds of cultures, prescribe a broad-spectrum antibiotic, and ask the patient to return in 2 days.

The purified protein derivative (PPD) test result is negative. The Gram's stain and cultures of sputum show the usual normal throat flora. However, the Wright-Giemsa stain as well as immunofluorescent and immunoperoxidase stains show the presence of *Pneumocystis carinii* (Fig. 22.3).

The patient is hospitalized and treated for *Pneumocystis carinii* pneumonia (PCP) with trimethoprim-sulfamethoxazole (TMP-SMX). Recovery is slow but sure.

Logic PCP suggests the possibility of the acquired immunodeficiency syndrome, which is

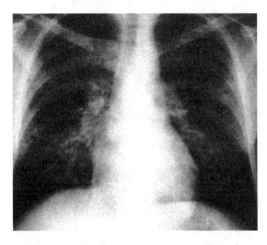

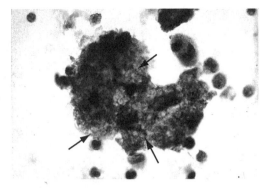

▶ **Figure 22.3.** Sputum shows large number of tiny round cystic organisms whose walls take special stains (*Pneumocystis carinii*).

▶ **Figure 22.2.** *Pneumocystis carinii* pneumonia. Diffuse bilateral interstitial infiltrates in a "ground glass" pattern.

caused by the human immunodeficiency virus (HIV-1). It occurs to you that the IM-like illness may have represented the initial viremia that some 50% of patients who have AIDS experience after the virus is introduced into the body by certain homo- and heterosexual practices, intravenous drug abuse, or exposure to HIV-contaminated blood and blood products.

The initial episode is usually followed by a long latent period that lasts for several to as many as 10 years, during which time the infected individual's immune mechanisms are gradually eroded: this results in a huge variety of infections by both the usual bacterial offenders and also opportunistic organisms that include viruses, usually inoffensive bacteria, fungi, and protozoa.

Data The situation and its possible causes are discussed openly with the patient and her mother. She has a boyfriend, but insists that other than some heavy petting, she has never had sexual intercourse with him or anybody else. There is no history nor physical evidence that she takes intravenous drugs. Although she currently works as a receptionist in a physician's office, she had tried her hand as a laboratory technician some 3 years ago, but quit because she did not like it.

Permission is obtained for an AIDS test. Both the enzyme-linked immunosorbent assay (ELISA) and Western blot test results return with positive findings. There are 300 CD4-positive lymphocytes per cubic milliliter. *The patient has AIDS!*

Logic Although no clearly definable point of vi-

ral entry could be identified in this case, exposure to contaminated blood by an inexperienced laboratory technician must be postulated. However, a claim of virginity must always be suspect, and it is advisable that the boyfriend be tested.

The negative PPD finding is of questionable reliability, because it may be falsely negative when an immunocompromised state exists, such as in this patient. But in cases other than AIDS, immunity to infection may be compromised in a variety of clinical circumstances, such as: (1) breaks in the epithelial barrier by burns, intubation, or catheters; (2) congenital defects, such as IgA deficiency, hypo- or agammaglobulinemia; and (3) acquired defects (such as in systemic lupus erythematosus [SLE] and multiple myeloma), the administration of steroids, cancer chemotherapy, administration of anti-rejection drugs, granulocytopenia, and asplenia, as well as in AIDS.

As for the AIDS virus, HIV-1 is the retrovirus that is primarily responsible for causing most worldwide cases of AIDS. HIV-2 is a genetically similar, although not identical, less virulent virus that causes a like disease seen mainly in Africa. Both viruses are transmitted in the same ways. These viruses are distinct from the human T-cell lymphotropic virus (HTLV-1 and -2) that relates to some unusual forms of lymphoma/leukemia.

There are basically three ways in which AIDS is associated with disease processes. *First,* the virus itself directly infects various body organs such as the brain, bone marrow, and lymph nodes, causing a wide spectrum of diseases. *Second,* the virus attacks the various elements of the body's immune system—T and B lymphocytes, macrophages, and monocytes—resulting mainly in a progressive loss of CD4−T lymphocytes, and immunodeficiency. In turn, a broad array of opportunistic infections (Table 22.1) and some neoplasms such as non-Hodgkin's lymphoma and Kaposi's sarcoma may flourish. And *third,* problems almost invariably arise as a result of complications from treatments used for the infections and neoplasms.

The lymphocyte story is complex. Normal blood contains 1500 to3000 lymphocytes per cubic millimeter, of which 70 to 80% are T cells that trace their ancestry to the thymus, and of which 10 to15% are B cells whose origins are in the bone marrow. Lymphocytes are further classified into subtypes according to cell surface markers. The CD4 molecule on T cells acts as a receptor for the AIDS virus. This results in a gradual depletion of CD4-positive T cells from normal values of 800 to1200/mm^3 down to worrisome levels of 500/mm^3, and then to critical levels of 200/mm^3 or less where opportunism becomes rampant. Dangerous levels may be detected not only by the total CD4 count, but also by a decreased ratio of CD4 to CD8 cells from a normal of 1.5–2.0.

As occurred in this patient, the first clinical manifestation of AIDS may be in the form of an opportunistic infection such as PCP.

After lengthy discussions about transmission, treatment, and prognosis, the patient is discharged from the hospital, told to take one TMP-SMX tablet daily, and to return to the office in 1 month.

Data The patient returns 2 years later. In the interim period, she has been treated in several AIDS clinics, as well as by two or three private physicians. She has gone steadily downhill, first with a recurrence of PCP only 2 weeks after you last saw her, then with episodes of severe gastroenteritis caused by *Mycobacterium avium-intracellulare,* and more recently, a critical episode of meningitis caused by *Cryptococcus.*

At this visit she complains of fever, sweats, anorexia, weight loss, and diarrhea. Examination reveals pallor, extreme cachexia, white, cheesy exudate lining the tonsillar fauces, diffuse lymph node enlargement, and a tender abdomen.

Logic After having suffered through many inevitable opportunistic infections, the patient is now approaching a terminal state with a "wasting syndrome," a common endpoint for those with AIDS. She is suffering with multiple infectious diseases.

Data You begin again with a possibly effective antibiotic, depending on what organisms are most likely; obtain cultures of blood, urine, sputum, and stool; and await the results of cultures before altering treatment.

TABLE 22.1. Opportunistic Infections and their Principal Target Organs in AIDS[a]

OPPORTUNISTIC ORGANISMS	PRINCIPAL AREAS INVOLVED
Protozoa	
Pneumocystis carinii	Lung
Toxoplasma gondii	CNS
Cryptosporidia	GI tract
Microsporidia	GI tract
Isospora belli	GI tract
Giardia lamblia	GI tract
Fungi	
Candida albicans	Mouth
Cryptococcus neoformans	Meninges
Histoplasma capsulatum	Lung
Coccidioides immitis	Lung
Virus	
Herpes	Skin
Cytomegalovirus	Retina, GI tract
Epstein-Barr virus	Lymphoma
JC virus	PML
Bacteria	
Mycobacterium avium intracellulare	Disseminated disease

[a]The usual pathogens in persons without AIDS affect AIDS patients with much greater frequency.
AIDS = acquired immunodeficiency syndrome; CNS = central nervous system; GI = gastrointestinal; PML = progressive multifocal leukoencephalopathy.

Comment In the first part of the 20th century, the maxim put forth by wise clinicians was "he who knows syphilis knows Medicine." But in the last part of this century, it has become evident that "he or she who knows AIDS knows Medicine." Testimony to this statement is offered by the fact that several standard textbooks of medicine devote more than 50 pages to this disease, far more than are given to any other single disease. The various complications, the almost countless types of opportunistic infections, and the large number of target organs make it impossible to cover very much in a case such as is presented here.

AIDS is a viral infection having an inoculation, an initial viremia, and a long latent period, which lead into viral involvement of almost all organ systems, a profound defect in cellular immunity, multiple opportunistic infections, unusual types of malignancies, and eventual fever, wasting, and inevitable death.

How strange that the epidemics at either end of this century should be primarily venereal in origin. *(P.C.)*

Suggested Readings

Bylund DJ, Ziegner UH, Hooper DG. Review of testing for human immunodeficiency virus. Clin Lab Med 1992;12(2):305–333.

Coodley GO. A checklist for evaluation of HIV-infected patients. Postgrad Med 1993;93(4):101–104, 107–108.

Havlir DV, Richman DD. Viral dynamics of HIV: Implications for drug development and therapeutic strategies. Ann Intern Med 1996;124(11):984–994.

Hirsh HL. AIDS and the emergency room physician and staff. Leg Med 1994:201–228.

Stein DS, Korvick JA, Vermud SH. CD4+ lymphocyte cell enumeration for prediction of clinical course of human immunodeficiency virus disease: A review. J Infect Dis 1992;165(2):352–363.

 CASE 82

FAINTING SPELLS

Paul Cutler

Data Repeated episodes of fainting bring a 62-year-old priest to the doctor. During the most recent one, he fell and broke his nose. He was admitted to the hospital to be observed and tested in a carefully controlled environment.

Logic Fainting or syncope is a transient loss of consciousness that usually lasts no more than a minute or two. It must be differentiated from seizures, coma, and milder sensations such as giddiness, lightheadedness, and "graying out," or presyncope. Seizures are episodes of loss of consciousness associated with convulsions. Coma is a prolonged period of unconsciousness. The other states mentioned may be milder, incomplete forms of syncope, or unrelated to any disorder associated with loss of consciousness.

Data The patient has had approximately 12 such episodes in the past 2 months. They come on quite suddenly without any premonitory symptoms; he faints and then "comes to" in approximately a minute or so. Others have observed several of the spells and tell him he lies motionless and quickly wakes up with no aftereffects. The episodes come at no particular time of day and do not seem to be related to any special event like eating, not eating, exercising, walking, urinating, coughing, suddenly standing up, shaving, or turning his head to the side. So far as he can recall, each episode occurred while he was sitting or standing, although he thinks one happened in bed.

A month ago he visited a physician who examined him and told him he could find nothing wrong. When advised to have further study, the patient said he was too occupied with his work but would consider it if the fainting recurred.

Logic You are anxious to see if he has carotid sinus syncope but prefer to have him in a controlled environment before pressing on his carotid sinus. Because he is a priest and wears a high, stiff collar, your first hypothesis is based more on a hunch than on logic and statistics. The history obtained so far has given you much to think about, and even more that you should not think about.

The causes of syncope range from benign emotional factors to malignant arrhythmias resulting in sudden death. A single fainting spell is commonly caused by a vasovagal reflex associated with fright, fear, or other passionate peaks. The relationship is obvious, and these patients rarely reach the doctor. However, studies of large groups of patients who have syncope reveal that one third to one half remain undiagnosed. In roughly half of those for whom a cause is found, the origin is cardiovascular, and these have a more serious prognosis than the diagnosable noncardiac cases or the undiagnosed cases.

The reasons for fainting are myriad, but they revolve mostly around five basic mechanisms: cerebral ischemia, decreased cardiac output, peripheral vasodilatation, reflexes, and altered composition of blood going to the brain, each alone or in combination. In these categories you must consider:

1. Transient ischemic attacks (vascular disease)
2. Heart disease: aortic stenosis, atrial myxoma or thrombus, paroxysmal tachycardia, sinoatrial disease (sick sinus syndrome), atrioventricular (AV) block with Stokes-Adams attacks, angina pectoris, left ventricular failure; pulmonary embolus
3. Carotid sinus syncope
4. Orthostatic hypotension
5. Gastrointestinal hemorrhage
6. Hysteria
7. Decreased PO_2, PCO_2, or glucose in blood
8. Syncope induced by cough, urination, or fluid removal from chest, celom, or bladder
9. Epilepsy (without seizures)
10. The common faint

On the basis of the information thus far, many of the listed possibilities can be ruled out. Carotid sinus syncope and orthostatic hypotension occur only in the erect position. In the former instance, the patient stimulates a sensitive sinus by shaving, turning his head, wearing a stiff collar, or by unknown means; this lowers the blood pressure and often slows the pulse so that insufficient blood reaches the brain.

Orthostatic hypotension occurs in old, debilitated, or bedridden patients whose blood pressures drop when they stand up, resulting in cerebral ischemia. It is also seen in patients who have diseases of the autonomic nervous system that preclude rapid adjustments by arterial constriction; included are some patients who have diabetes, amyloidosis, and generalized dysautonomia. These patients (especially the last group) often have other evidences of autonomic disturbance affecting sphincter control, pupils, potency, and so forth. In addition, marked orthostatic blood pressure changes causing syncope can occur when drugs are given to treat hypertension or when there is acute or chronic volume depletion.

Older persons may already have modest decreases in cerebral blood flow because of hypertension, diabetes, and atherosclerosis. In addition, they often have inactive baroreceptors and sluggish sympathetic reflexes that impair mechanisms

for homeostasis. These factors make them more susceptible to faint with postural change, carotid sinus sensitivity, inadvertent Valsalva's maneuvers, and moderate drops in blood pressure seen in myocardial infarction, gastrointestinal hemorrhage, and paroxysmal tachyarrhythmias.

Healthy young soldiers may faint after prolonged motionless standing at attention during military displays—a dramatic yet benign form of syncope.

Gastrointestinal hemorrhages would not recur so frequently. Hypoglycemic syncope could occur from serious illness like insulinoma and severe liver disease; the episodes would come early in the morning or after a missed meal—not as in this case. Functional hypoglycemia that occurs 2 to 3 hours after a meal seldom, if ever, causes neurologic symptoms.

There is no demonstrable relationship to any of the activities previously mentioned, so reflex syncope from cough, urination, and removed fluid can be discarded. Aortic stenosis is unlikely because exercise does not bring on an episode.

Myxomas and ball-valve thrombi in the left atrium can cause intermittent occlusion of the mitral valve and transient syncope; it must be considered.

Data Other than for mild diabetes that is well controlled by diet, he has been in good health. He has no chest pain, dyspnea, or orthopnea, but he occasionally feels a palpitation in his chest. His memory is good, and he says that he is still an effective, capable priest; this is confirmed by his peers. He is obviously not emotional or disturbed and wants to return to work as soon as possible. The systems review is negative.

Logic He has no symptoms of heart disease. The composite picture being formed of his personality would lead you to exclude hysteria as a viable cause of his problem. Also, the fact that he injured himself refutes that possibility.

As with attacks of any type, it is always good to examine a patient during an attack if possible. Checking the pulse, blood pressure, and ECG at these times is often helpful. Hysterical individuals have normal pulse and blood pressure. Those with cardiac causes usually do not.

Further points to consider are whether there are preceding symptoms. An aura suggests epilepsy. The common faint is induced by pain, an unpleasant sight, or an emotional disturbance and is preceded by sweating, pallor, tachycardia, and presyncopal "grayness." Transient ischemic attacks may be preceded by or accompanied by other neurologic symptoms like visual disturbances, sensory changes, aphasia, motor weakness, or vertigo, depending on the brain area involved. Numbness, tingling, and "difficulty in breathing" precede the giddiness and syncope of hyperventilation (alkalosis with low PCO_2). None of these factors is present here.

The occurrence of a single or many episodes is a key point. One faint can be caused by a gastrointestinal hemorrhage, a myocardial infarction, or a pulmonary embolus, but multiple episodes are not likely to have such causes. The rapidity of onset tells you much. Arrhythmias and cardiac arrest cause sudden syncope. Reflexes that induce vasodilatation and hypotension act slowly.

Overlap sometimes exists in that Stokes-Adams attacks and hypoglycemia may cause seizures too and may thus be confused with epilepsy. The length of time that the syncope lasts may be distinctive. For example, most cases of syncope recover in 1 or 2 minutes. But syncope caused by aortic stenosis, hypoglycemia, or hysteria lasts longer.

Data Finally, you examine the patient and go directly to the carotid sinuses and arteries. There are no bruits or thrills over the carotid, vertebral, or subclavian arteries, and pressure applied on each carotid sinus separately for 5 seconds causes a drop in blood pressure from 130/80 to 110/70, and a fall in pulse rate from 54 to 50. The patient is sitting up during the test, and he experiences no abnormal sensations.

Logic The absence of bruits weighs against significant extracranial vascular disease, but this clue must be carefully weighed. Many older patients have bruits that are not clinically important. On the other hand, if stenosis exceeds 90%, there is not enough blood flow to cause a bruit. So this sign is neither highly sensitive nor specific.

Note that syncope resulting from extracranial cerebrovascular disease may result from disease of the vertebral as well as from the carotid arteries. So look for bruits in the subclavian triangle and suboccipital areas in addition to the site of the carotid bifurcations. Do not forget the special type of vertebrobasilar insufficiency caused by the subclavian steal syndrome.

As for carotid sinus pressure, many older persons have sensitive sinuses and will exhibit circulatory changes, but usually no syncope. This is especially true if there is associated heart disease. Even if you can induce syncope, it does not necessarily mean that this mechanism is the cause of the patient's syncope. The true cause may still be occult. However, if the carotid sinus is not sensitive and no symptoms are induced, then this mechanism is not the cause of the syncope. It can be seen that this test needs careful, deliberate interpretation, because it has false positives, but is not apt to have false negatives.

Hypothesis 1 is rejected. Now you proceed with the rest of the examination, having selected transient ischemic attacks or sudden decrease in cardiac output as your likely alternative possibilities.

Data Physical examination reveals the following vital signs: blood pressure, 130/80; pulse, 54; respirations, 14; and temperature, 37°C. The fundi, head and neck, heart, lungs, abdomen, rectum, genitalia, peripheral pulses, and neurologic examination are completely normal. In particular, there are no heart murmurs, thrills, or arrhythmias.

Logic The mild bradycardia is the only abnormality noted. Aortic stenosis, already rendered unlikely by the absence of exertion-induced episodes, can be eliminated because there is no murmur, thrill, or abnormal apical and carotid impulse characteristic of this condition. He has no ventricular failure or angina by symptoms or signs. There is no reason why he should have a low PO_2 (or PCO_2), because conditions causing such profound blood gas disturbances would be obvious to the naked eye. More studies are needed.

Data After lying flat for 15 minutes, he suddenly stands up. The BP hovers within 10 mm of his reclining BP for a full minute, so you discontinue this test. An electroencephalogram is normal and shows no epileptogenic focus. The chest and skull radiographs are normal. Fasting blood glucose level, blood pH, PO_2, PCO_2, and urea nitrogen level are normal. The 5-hour glucose tolerance test shows expectedly elevated levels at 1, 2, and 3 hours and no hypoglycemic phase. ECG shows a sinus bradycardia but is otherwise normal in all respects. Complete blood count and urinalysis are normal. An echocardiogram

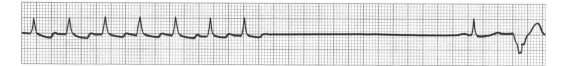

▶ **Figure 22.4.** Paroxysmal atrial tachycardia followed by prolonged asystole—"sick sinus syndrome."

shows no mitral valve disease or evidence of a left atrial tumor or clot.

Logic Orthostatic hypotension, epilepsy, hypoglycemia, and atrial myxoma are ruled out. Mild diabetes is confirmed. Blood gases are normal as predicted. The ECG offers no help except for the mild bradycardia, which may be insignificant. A 20-mm or more drop in systolic pressure with accompanying symptoms would have represented a positive test for orthostatic hypotension.

Data A continuous ECG monitor solves the problem. Three brief episodes of paroxysmal atrial tachycardia are noted; each is followed by a sinus pause of 5 to 6 seconds. One episode occurred while the patient slept; one occurred while he was sitting, and he experienced no unusual sensations; but the third took place while he was walking around, and he almost blacked out. There was no evidence of altered AV conduction (Fig. 22.4).

Logic When testing for the causes of syncope, especially in the elderly, be wary of false-negative and false-positive results. Because arrhythmias are so common in this group, the detection of arrhythmias by the Holter monitor does not mean the arrhythmia is necessarily the cause of recurrent syncope. Furthermore, this procedure is not highly sensitive because nothing may happen during the 24 hours. But if syncope occurs *in conjunction with* a recorded arrhythmia, this is convincing evidence.

The patient no doubt has a *sick sinus syndrome* with paroxysms of tachycardia depressing his sinoatrial (SA) node so that it does not fire when called upon to do so. Had the asystole lasted a bit longer he would no doubt have fainted. Bradycardia and sinoatrial block are also often present.

Causes for this syndrome are not completely categorized. It may relate to myocardial disease in and around the SA node, disease of the artery to the SA node, coronary, hypertensive, or rheumatic heart disease, or unknown causes.

Data A transvenous pacemaker was passed. Very poor SA node recovery time was noted after atrial pacing. Also, a prolonged HV (His-ventricle) conduction time was detected on the bundle of His study. Therefore, it was decided to implant a permanent state-of-the-art dual chamber demand pacemaker. Antiarrhythmic drugs were considered because their use is safe with a pacemaker in place, but the decision was made to wait and see.

Since then, the patient has been free of syncope for 6 months, feels perfectly well, and is back at work. The precise cause of the disease in his SA node and ventricular conduction system remains obscure.

Questions

1. In the past 25 years, this patient's illness has been increasingly recognized and therefore apparently more common. Which of the following statements is incorrect?
   (a) Syncope results from paroxysmal tachycardia.
   (b) Syncope results form asystole following the tachycardia.
   (c) The sick SA node may result in bradycardia and/or SA block.
   (d) Carotid sinus sensitivity and AV conduction delays are common accompaniments.
2. "Low blood pressure" is falsely blamed for many symptoms. True orthostatic hypotension is associated with a profound drop in blood pressure when the patient changes from a reclining to a standing position and may or may not be accompanied by syncope. It can occur in:
   (a) hypertensive patients under treatment.
   (b) patients with blood volume depletion.
   (c) patients who have Addison's disease or pheochromocytoma.
   (d) patients with spinal cord diseases.
3. The Stokes-Adams attack is a long-known cause of syncope or convulsions. Which one of the following statements about it is false?

(a) Complete heart block with episodes of asystole, ventricular tachycardia, or ventricular fibrillation is the usual mechanism.

(b) Coronary artery disease is the principal cause.

(c) Idiopathic disease of the conduction system is the principle cause.

(d) The ECG may not show complete heart block between attacks.

Answers

1. **(a) is incorrect.** Although tachycardia can cause syncope, in these cases it is usually the post-tachycardia asystole that results in transitory unconsciousness. Choices (c) and (d) are true statements, although the causes are not perfectly clear. Generally it is difficult to speed such a patient's pulse with exercise or drugs. Drugs given to suppress the arrhythmias may make the SA disease worse, hence the need for permanent demand pacing.

2. **All are correct.** Drug therapy for hypertension may prevent the adequate vasoconstrictor action that adjusts for position change, allowing hypotension to develop. The tilt test is used to detect volume depletion in hemorrhage or severe dehydration in like manner. In choice (c), both are known to be true by induction. In severe spinal cord disease, the autonomic control of vessels and sphincters may be lost.

3. **(b) is false.** Coronary disease is not the main cause. Degeneration of the conduction system (Lenègre's disease) is. Choice (a) represents the usual mechanisms for attacks but, interestingly, (d) is also true, and the ECG may show lesser degrees of conduction system disease between attacks. Occasionally the interval ECG is normal.

COMMENT A crucial item of medical logic must be mastered here. Abnormalities that are found or induced may not necessarily be the cause of the patient's syncope. Modest orthostatic drops in blood pressure, arrhythmias noted by Holter monitor, and carotid sinus sensitivity may be *clinically relevant only if they induce syncope*. These aberrations are so common, especially in the elderly, that their mere presence does not necessarily imply a cause-and-effect relationship. Other conditions may account for the fainting spells. The same logic holds true if you find a cardiac conduction disturbance or a cervical bruit. These too

are so common that their presence may mislead you; other causes of syncope may be operative.

Most cases of diagnosed syncope can be solved by the history and physical examination alone. When necessary, you can also do a blood count, serum glucose and electrolytes, arterial blood gases, and ECG. In unusual instances, you may need to do Holter monitoring, a ventilation-perfusion scan, an electroencephalogram, or programmed electrical stimulation of the heart. Brain scans are almost always fruitless.

This was a difficult presentation to solve. The author used at least 12 of the strategies and methods described in Chapters 3 to 6 in order to reach a conclusion. Try your hand at identifying these techniques, and then compare your answers with the list printed at the end of Case 83. Afterward, you should reread this case and see if you can detect where and how each of the listed strategies was used. *(P.C.)*

Suggested Readings

Farrehi PM, Santinga JT, Eagle KA. Syncope: Diagnosis of cardiac and noncardiac causes. Geriatrics 1995;50(11):24–30.

Hart GT. Evaluation of syncope. Am Fam Physician 1994;51(8):1941–1948, 1951–1952.

Kapoor WN. Work-up and management of patients with syncope. Med Clin N Am 1995;79(5):1153–1170.

C A S E   83

STRANGE BEHAVIOR

Paul Cutler

Data A woman of approximately 40 is brought to the emergency department by an employee of the YWCA because "she has been acting strange all day." Alcoholic intoxication is suspected because of the odor of her breath and the presence of several empty bourbon bottles in her room at the "Y." She is furtively alert and constantly changes her sitting position, does not seem to comprehend your questions, and appears to be listening intently for some sound.

Logic You suspect an alcohol-related problem, but she does not seem to be merely drunk. Because alcohol has been recently ingested, you tend to minimize problems of the withdrawal syndrome and focus rather on alcohol's acute and chronic toxic effects.

Chief among the possibilities from the available data are pathologic intoxication and acute alcoholic hallucinosis. The former is usually manifested by violent behavior following the consumption of even small amounts of alcohol, but is part of a spectrum that includes the possibility that this woman simply acts strangely whenever she drinks.

Acute alcoholic hallucinosis typically comes several hours after a severe drinking bout but may develop during its course. It is thought that alcohol in this case allows the appearance of latent schizophrenic symptoms. Indeed, schizophrenia and alcoholism may coexist, and the delineation and separation of the two must be determined by a longitudinal history. None of these conditions is likely to pose an immediate threat to life, although psychiatric hospitalization is often necessary for alcoholic hallucinosis.

Data You decide that further analysis of her problems is less urgent than that of the man with chest pain whom the nurse insists you see immediately. You ask the nurse to prepare the woman for an examination to be performed when you are able.

Logic But while you listen to the heart of the patient with chest pain, your mind drifts back to the woman just seen. Could she be developing an alcohol withdrawal syndrome, even though she still has the odor of alcohol on her breath? Something does not seem to fit, so having read about a similar patient seen last week, you rethink the possibilities.

Patients who are seen with the seemingly sudden onset of strange behavior, delirium, or acute confusional states call to mind a wide assortment of disorders. These abnormal states are manifested by disturbances in perception, memory, thinking, concentration, orientation, insight, and mood, often coupled with bizarre movements and tremors.

A few, some, or many of these manifestations can be seen in any of the following clinical situations: (1) drug interaction or drug intoxication; (2) drug withdrawal, especially from sedatives; (3) alcohol intoxication; (4) alcohol withdrawal syndromes; (5) postsurgical states and acute severe medical illnesses, especially when complicated by fever or occurring in the elderly; (6) diseases specifically affecting the nervous system, such as encephalitis, meningitis, subdural hematoma, cerebral thrombosis, and brain tumor; postictal states; hypoglycemia; and trauma.

Medications well known to cause confusion in some patients include bromides, opiates, barbiturates, amphetamines, atropine, hyoscine, steroids, and antidepressants such as amitriptyline.

You recall that confusional states seeming to start suddenly may merely be *noticed* all at once. In retrospect, a family member may tell you that "Dad has not really been right" for several days, weeks, or months, but it suddenly became much worse. If the problem is therefore more long-standing, think of: hepatic encephalopathy or uremia; hyper- or hypo- states of osmolarity calcemia, natremia, or thyroid function; pernicious anemia; and chronic brain syndromes of the multi-infarct or Alzheimer's types.

Data The nurse records the vital signs: oral temperature, 38.5°C; blood pressure, 144/85; radial pulse, 105. She further notes that the patient is very restless and seems "startled" when her body is touched. The patient complains of headaches, which prompts the nurse to test for a stiff neck; this is absent.

When informed of the temperature elevation and lack of nuchal rigidity, you request a complete blood count with white cell differential, clean-catch urinalysis, chest radiograph, serum glucose, serum calcium and sodium, and urea nitrogen. Had you not been so scholarly and selective, you would have simply ordered an 18-test blood chemistry profile. The results will be available in approximately 45 minutes, at which time you expect to be seeing the patient again. You decline the nurse's suggestion of acetaminophen for the patient.

Logic Knowing that the patient is febrile raises additional diagnostic possibilities. In the presence of altered mental status, infection of the central nervous system must be a consideration. An important factor is that the patient did not appear acutely ill; adults who have bacterial meningitis are almost always in a toxic state: they look sick. This feature accounted for the relatively slow pace of assessment.

The white blood cell count is a good screen for bacterial infection in this age group, and a differential count showing a leftward shift could provide further diagnostic support. The urinalysis and chest radiograph are screening tests for common sites of infection and are ordinarily indicated in the evaluation of infection without obvious source. The measurement of glucose, calcium, sodium, and urea nitrogen is routine in the evaluation of acutely altered function of the central nervous system.

The symptom of headache is consistent with subdural hematoma, another problem associated with alcoholism, because such patients often get hurt after a fall or brawl.

Data The samples are obtained. You have just assessed the cardiac patient when you receive a "stat" page to the radiograph department. You rush over and find that your "alcoholic" patient has had a grand mal seizure; the onset was not observed. Her blood pressure and pulse are about the same. She is awake and shows little or no postictal depression. There is a minor laceration on her tongue, but no evidence of sphincteric incompetence. You note that she has no sign of recent or remote cranial trauma, and the tympanic membranes and fundi are normal; the pupils are 3 mm in diameter, equal, and react directly and consensually to light. There is no nuchal rigidity, and both Kernig's and Brudzinski's signs are absent. Movement of all extremities is forceful, and the tendon reflexes are very brisk, although clonus is absent. You cannot assess the plantar reflexes because of withdrawal. If anything, she seems more in contact with her surroundings, and she says that she still has a terrible headache, which she knows "will only get better with some Fiorinal."

Limited general physical examination reveals: several spider angiomas on the upper trunk; normal thyroid, lungs, and heart; a smooth, soft, nontender liver felt 3 cm below the costal margin in the midclavicular line; no abdominal tenderness or masses; and stool negative for occult blood. Admission is planned, and the patient is prepared for lumbar puncture.

Logic Note the form of the physical assessment. Because an acute neurologic event has just occurred, the immediate focus is on whether there is some intracranial process that needs instant action to save the patient's life. There is no evidence for this, so the search then must focus on abnormalities of major organ systems that could have caused the seizure. When you have an acutely ill patient in the radiograph examining room, only the most basic physical assessment should be done.

The tentative hypothesis that the patient was simply suffering from the acute toxic effect of alcohol is now disproved with the occurrence of a seizure. The headache, fever, and seizure suggest intracranial infection or bleeding, but the patient's relatively good appearance and lack of meningeal signs are difficult to reconcile with these serious possibilities.

Examination of the cerebrospinal fluid is nevertheless indicated because missing the diagnosis of bacterial meningitis would be a fatal error. The absence of ophthalmoscopic evidence for increased intracranial pressure permits removal of cerebrospinal fluid with relative safety. A lack of lateralizing signs serves to reduce the probability of a subdural hematoma, but is by no means definitive because the injury may have left few or no external traces and motor changes are usually late manifestations. The presence of symmetric hyperreflexia could be a valuable sign implying bilateral upper motor neuron lesions; however, the uncertainty about the plantar reflexes weakens this proposition.

In view of the chronic headaches followed by strange behavior, a computed tomographic scan might have been more discreet before doing a valorous lumbar puncture. But the time of night, the temporary unavailability of technical skill, the need for transport to the radiology department, and the anticipated lack of patient cooperation induce you to proceed with the lumbar puncture. This decision may have been made more on the basis of rationalization and prejudice than on wisdom and sound medical judgment.

In addition to structural lesions of the nervous system, hepatic or uremic encephalopathy may also cause hyperreflexia with extensor plantar reflexes. As yet, no data are available to rule out renal failure. Is there hepatic insufficiency? The liver is described as being 3 cm below the costal margin, but this is not necessarily abnormal, because the determinant of hepatomegaly is the total span. The qualitative features of the palpable liver were normal, arguing against acute hepatic enlargement, cirrhosis, or infiltrative disease. The lack of a palpable spleen is consistent with a lack of portal hypertension but is not decisive, because spleens are often difficult to palpate. Spider angiomas are a sign of major hepatic disease, but small numbers of them may be seen in normal individuals, more often in women.

Fever, tachycardia, altered mental status, and even seizures may be features of thyrotoxicosis, but the normal-sized thyroid and absence of other clinical features weigh against this condition. The normal auscultatory examination of the heart and lungs serves to minimize the possibility of infection of those sites, and of the heart as the source of a cerebral embolus.

Data Lumbar puncture produces crystal-clear, colorless fluid at normal pressure, containing no microscopic abnormalities; it is sent for glucose and protein determination, and culture. The previously obtained laboratory data are available: hematocrit, 40%; hemoglobin, 13.3 g/dL; white blood cells (WBCs), 7800/mm³ (differential not performed); the urine is negative for glucose and protein, ketones are 2+, and there are three to four WBCs per high-powered field, no casts, and many vaginal epithelial cells. The urea nitrogen is 14 mg/dL; the glucose is 88 mg/dL; the calcium is 9.7 mg/dL; and the serum sodium is 135 mEq/L. The senior resident arrives in the emergency room and, after studying the available data and briefly examining the patient, proposes what in 48 hours proves to be the correct diagnosis.

Logic The grossly normal cerebrospinal fluid rules out bacterial meningitis and minimizes the possibility of many other intracranial processes under consideration. The normal blood urea nitrogen, glucose, and calcium rule out encephalopathy due to uremia, hypo- or hyperglycemia, and parathyroid disorders. The normal WBC count minimizes the possibility of serious infection, and the lack of anemia reduces the likelihood of several categories of major systemic disease. The urine specimen was contaminated by vaginal secretions, but the lack of many WBCs weighs against the diagnosis of pyelonephritis. The ketonuria probably reflects the effects of fasting.

Data In seeking further information about the patient's prior medical history from both the patient and her roommate, the resident learned that she had no local physician and was living at the YWCA because she had just come to this city. She stated she drank liquor to help her headaches because her usual medication had to be prescribed by a doctor. Usually she drank "only one shot at most three times a week."

For approximately 6 months she had been taking self-increased doses of Fiorinal (contents aspirin 325 mg, caffeine 30 mg, butalbital 50 mg), and most recently was using 16 to 20 tablets or capsules per day (the manufacturer cautions no more than six daily). She had been accustomed to getting prescriptions from each of five physicians, but had run out of the drug 2 days ago.

Logic Butalbital is a barbiturate. Doses in this range could produce physical dependence and an abstinence (or withdrawal) syndrome on sudden cessation. Hyperreflexia and seizures are common features of this syndrome. Bizarre mental states including frank psychosis may occur. Mild elevation of temperature is frequent.

Data The neurologic findings were further amplified by demonstrating a flexor plantar response upon stroking the foot, appropriately after "spanking" the sole to reduce light tactile sensitivity, and by the finding of a glabellar reflex. The BP dropped to 90/78 when she stood up.

Logic The glabella is just above the point where the eyebrows come closest together. A glabellar reflex, the non-extinguishing contraction of one or both orbicularis oculi muscles after tapping the glabella, is seen in virtually only sedative-hypnotic withdrawal and in some cases of parkinsonism. Orthostatic hypotension is another common feature of the barbiturate withdrawal syndrome. And a flexor plantar response is to be expected in the absence of long tract disease.

Data This woman's abstinence syndrome was treated by standard methods of gradual withdrawal. She was seen by an empathic house officer who was not content with the low probability estimate for an intracranial space-occupying lesion and aimed for certainty. So extensive studies, including a computed tomographic scan and electroencephalogram, were done and failed to yield a structural cause of her headaches. But strong evidence of psychoneurotic depression was elicited by additional interview. Tests of hepatic function were normal and there were no positive bacterial cultures. The patient participated briefly in a group psychotherapeutic process after discharge but was lost to follow-up.

Logic We readily accept the danger of drugs, but not of alcohol—which is just another drug. Alcoholic patients are prone to develop numerous complicating diseases. Some have already been mentioned. Aside from pathologic intoxication and various withdrawal syndromes, they may get nutritional diseases such as pellagra, beriberi, polyneuropathy, and Wernicke-Korsakoff syndrome. There is a high incidence of liver disease and alcoholic gastritis. During an episode of intoxication, the patient may develop a Mallory-Weiss syndrome from vomiting or a subdural hematoma from trauma, may suffocate from aspiration or a "café coronary," or may kill or be killed in an automobile accident. Severe hypoglycemia can result from a spree of drinking without eating. Alcohol may cause thrombocytopenia, acute pancreatitis, and acute muscle necrosis.

And as if all this were not enough, there are various brain diseases of uncertain pathogenesis associated with alcoholism: cerebellar degeneration, cerebral atrophy, and pontine myelinosis. And remember the marital discord, disturbed family relations, and altered work performance!

The alcoholic is damned if he does and damned if he does not. Withdrawal syndromes include severe tremulousness, hallucinosis, "rum fits" or withdrawal seizures, and, most serious, delirium tremens. The latter disorder usually occurs 2 to 4 days after enforced cessation of alcohol consumption. Characteristically, a patient is admitted to the hospital with pneumonia or sent to jail to dry out, seems to be doing well, and goes rapidly into a state of delirium combined with tremors—a picture well known to almost everybody. Such incidents are thought by some to be humorous and inspire many jokes. In fact, they are serious, may be fatal, and require urgent care.

Problem List
1. Chronic tension headaches
2. Barbiturate dependence
3. Barbiturate withdrawal syndrome
4. Alcoholism: to be evaluated

COMMENT Physicians often behave as though they do not like to care for alcoholics, perhaps in part because of the failure of the conventional medical approach. Probably because of this bias and the fact that the patient did not look very sick, there was little initial effort at assessment. This is an example of how the diagnostic process may be clouded by a too obvious clue: the smell of alcohol. Many tales are told about drunkards who die in jail or are dismissed from the emergency room only to die at home. These persons all smell of alcohol, but the real problem is overlooked. Always remember that devotees of Bacchus have a predilection for some diseases but are subject to all.

Assessment became more active with the report of fever, but the dramatic seizure really catalyzed vigorous and appropriate data gathering. It was not until these failed to yield solutions that a few questions and tests of a specific hypothesis gave the answer—drug withdrawal. Even so, additional studies were needed to pinpoint the reason for taking so much medication.

This case demonstrated the processing of abundant clues—true positives, pertinent true negatives, a misleading false positive, and several key clues. Cluster formation, differential diagnosis, hypothesis generation, and pruning the differential all took part in the evolution of a diagnosis. The problem solvers made decisions on the sequence of testing, and alternative strategies were weighed.

In today's fast-moving emergency departments, this patient might have been managed with a brief history and a scant selective physical examination followed by a toxicology screen, an 18-test blood chemistry profile, a blood alcohol level, a CT scan, and a lumbar puncture—all in a matter of a few hours. Economy, order, and thoroughness are thereby replaced by speed and accuracy. Even so, despite the use of high-technology procedures and tests, additional history and examination data were needed. The procedures told you what the patient *did not* have. The history and physical examination told you what she *did* have. *(P.C.)*

Answers to Comment on Case 82

1. Positive clues
2. Pertinent negative clues
3. Key clue
4. False clue
5. Decisive clue
6. Sensitivity and specificity of clues
7. Early hypothesis generation
8. Proof by exclusion
9. Pinpointing the diseased organ
10. Traditional method
11. Hunch
12. Varied cause-and-effect relationships

Suggested Readings

Geurian K, Burns I. Detailed description of a successful outpatient taper of phenobarbital therapy. Arch Fam Med 1994;3(5):458–460.

Landry MJ, Smith DE, McDuff DR, et al. Benzodiazepine dependence and withdrawal: Identification and medical management. J Am Board Fam Pract 1992;5(2):167–175.

Sellers EM, Schneiderman JF, Romach MK, et al. Comparative drug effects and abuse liability of lorazepam, buspirone, and secobarbital in non-dependent subjects. J Clin Psychopharmacol 1992;12(2): 79–85.

CASE 84

FATIGUE

Kenneth R. Epstein

Data Progressively worsening fatigue brings a 55-year-old man to your office. He was well until 7 months ago when, some time following what he thought was a viral infection, he noted that he could no longer keep up with his busy work schedule as an accountant. He was tired all the time. Due to this fatigue, he had been forced to take an increasing number of days off from work. On weekends he could no longer complete 18 holes of golf, an activity he had previously done easily every Saturday morning.

Logic Patients often describe their fatigue in terms such as "no pep," "no energy," "out of steam," "tuckered out," or simply "tired all the time." It is important that both doctor and patient be on the same wavelength when it comes to the use of varying words to describe a symptom. Words like fatigue, lassitude, malaise, and weakness are often used interchangeably, and although their definitions seem to be similar and overlapping, there are shaded differences of meaning.

Fatigue is defined as a tired feeling and a sense of weariness that may or may not be related to or worsened by task performance. Motor strength is apt to be normal if tested. *Lassitude* is a feeling that consists of listlessness and languor, a desire to sit and dream, perhaps even laziness or mental inertia. *Malaise* is a feeling of not being well, of being sick and out of sorts. *Weakness* consists of lack of motor strength and a decreased ability to perform certain physical tasks. This may be generalized as in the case of anemia or heart failure, or it may be limited to special muscle groups such as an arm or a leg. Distal extremity weakness may signal a neuropathy; proximal muscle weakness may herald a myopathy.

Data Additional questions reveal that the patient feels tired all the time and is just as tired when he gets up in the morning as when he goes to bed. He denies being weak and says he still has ample strength when called upon to perform a vigorous physical task.

Logic The distinction between fatigue and weakness has not been clearly made, and it is possible that the two coexist in this case, as well as to varying degrees in some others. At a quick glance it appears that the patient has fatigue and not motor weakness. The onset of symptoms after a viral infection may be either significant or coincidental.

Fatigue is a very common complaint in the doctor's office. Chronic fatigue is said to occur in up to 20% of patients attending general medical clinics. This symptom has no predilection based on age, race, education, or occupation, and although such complaints are more common in women than in men, patients of both genders will be seen with fatigue. *Acute fatigue* usually lasts less than a month and may follow an infection such as infectious mononucleosis, a period of prolonged exertional activity, or poor sleep. *Chronic fatigue* lasts more than a month, and has a long differential diagnosis that may include many medical or psychiatric illnesses (Table 22.2).

TABLE 22.2. Causes of Fatigue

Medical disease
chronic infection
malignancy
anemia
heart failure
hypothyroidism
certain drugs
Psychiatric diseases
depression
anxiety
somatoform disorders
Chronic fatigue syndrome

Medical illnesses that are associated with chronic fatigue include chronic infections, malignancies, congestive heart failure, connective tissue diseases, endocrinopathies, and anemias. Fatigue caused by organic disease is usually less severe on awakening, worsens during the day, and tends to be continuous and progressive over time.

Psychiatric illnesses include the affective disorders such as depression, anxiety, and somatoform disorders. Fatigue of psychiatric origin is present equally on awakening and at other times of the day, does not seem to worsen as the day progresses, is not relieved by rest, and tends to be intermittent or remittent over time. It may improve on the weekends or on a vacation if factors in the daily environment are the cause for anxiety or depression.

Over-the-counter and prescribed drugs may be causes for chronic fatigue. Common offenders include antihistamines, sedatives, hypnotics, psychotropics, and some antihypertensives such as β-adrenergic blockers and methyldopa.

A good psychiatric and medical history plus a thorough examination should allow the physician to arrive at a diagnosis for 85 to 90% of patients. One symptom or one sign may direct your line of inquiry. In a significant number of patients, the physician cannot diagnose a clear-cut medical or psychiatric illness, and the chronic fatigue remains unexplained. Some of these patients will meet the Center for Disease Control's (CDC) diagnostic criteria for the chronic fatigue syndrome (CFS) (Table 22.3).

Data The patient states that he has always been

TABLE 22.3. CDC Case Definition of the Chronic Fatigue Syndrome (CFS)

A CASE OF CFS MUST FULFILL MAJOR CRITERIA 1 AND 2, AND EIGHT OF THE SYMPTOM CRITERIA, OR SIX OF THE SYMPTOM CRITERIA PLUS TWO OF THE PHYSICAL CRITERIA

Major Criteria

1. New onset of persistent or relapsing, debilitating fatigue in a person with no previous history of similar symptoms, that does not resolve with bed rest, and decreases daily activity by > 50% for > 6 months.

2. Other clinical conditions that may produce chronic fatigue must be ruled out, based on history, physical examination, and selected laboratory tests.

Minor Criteria

Symptom Criteria

1. Mild fever (<38.6°C) or chills

2. Sore throat

3. Painful cervical or axillary lymph nodes

4. Unexplained generalized muscle weakness

5. Muscle discomfort or myalgia

6. >24 hours of generalized fatigue after levels of exercise that were easily tolerated previously

7. Generalized headaches

8. Migratory arthralgias without arthritis

9. Neuropsychologic complaints (photophobia, transient visual scotomata, forgetfulness, irritability, confusion, difficulty thinking, inability to concentrate, depression)

10. Hypersomnia or insomnia

11. Onset of symptom complex over a few hours to days

Physical Criteria

1. Low-grade fever (<38.6°C orally or 38.8°C rectally)

2. Nonexudative pharyngitis

3. Palpable or tender cervical or axillary lymphadenopathy, 2 cm

CDC = Centers for Disease Control.

an active person, juggling his time between his accounting practice and his family, and still finding time to play golf on most weekends. He admits that over the past year he has found it more difficult to find the proper balance, and worries that he has not spent enough time with his children. However, with the addition of several new, large accounts to his business, he has had even less time to spend with his children than he had had in prior years. Four months ago, he missed his daughter's performance in the school play due to a business trip, and still feels quite badly about this.

Logic He admits to increased stress over the past year and seems unhappy with certain aspects of his life. It is possible that his fatigue is a manifestation of depression, and it is important to look for symptoms of a major depressive disorder.

Depression should not be considered a diagnosis by exclusion. The patient usually has multiple symptoms that may be elicited by a well-done history. These include a depressed mood, feelings of guilt, hopelessness, dissatisfaction, crying spells, palpitations, anorexia, early morning awakening, headache, feeling sad, blue, or lonely, decrease in libido, loss of interest in work and social activities, "life not worth living," and even a wish for self-destruction by suicide. The following may be precipitating factors: major life change such as marriage, divorce, parenthood, death of spouse, loss of job, or other forms of severe emotional stress. The diagnosis is made by history, but must then be verified by normal findings from the physical examination.

Data Approximately 6 months ago he began to have trouble sleeping: he had difficulty falling asleep and then awakened several times during the night. He also noted increased irritability, and states that he was previously easy-going, but noticed that he would yell at his wife and business partner over trivial issues.

Five months ago, he noted that his ankles and knees were stiff and painful in the mornings. His thighs and lower back also were frequently painful, although he did not notice any swelling, tenderness, or warmth over any joint. He developed bifrontal headaches on an almost daily basis, and states that all these symptoms developed rapidly. He can actually pinpoint the week that his fatigue and the other symptoms began because 1 week before these symptoms, he had a flulike illness with fever, sore throat, swollen glands, nausea, and loss of appetite. He recalls that most of the flu symptoms resolved, but he continued to have a mild sore throat and cervical lymphadenopathy.

On review of systems, he disclaims any other respiratory, cardiac, gastrointestinal, or genitourinary complaints. He says that his weight has been stable, and his appetite remains good. He denies feeling sad, but is frustrated at how poorly he feels physically. Occasionally he gets increased myalgias at night, and feels like he has a fever, but his temperature is usually 99.0 to 99.5°F.

His medical history reveals arthroscopic knee surgery 10 years ago and an appendectomy at age 16. He does not smoke, and has one or two beers on summer weekends.

Logic Sleep disturbances and increased irritability lead you to keep depression in mind. However, he does not have appetite changes, weight change, or feelings of sadness. The predominance of joint and muscle symptoms make you consider the connective tissue diseases in the differential diagnosis.

There is nothing in the history to suggest cancer or a chronic infection, such as fever, chills, weight loss, loss of appetite, or associated localizing symptoms that might point to the site of a disease process.

A complete physical examination may be helpful at this point. A single abnormality may help to pinpoint any disease process that may exist.

Data The patient is an alert, tired-appearing man who does not look sick and is in no acute distress. The vital signs, special senses, head, and neck are normal, except for slight posterior pharyngeal erythema and minimal shotty anterior cervical and inguinal adenopathy. The lungs, heart, abdomen, and genitalia are normal. A slightly enlarged, homogeneous prostate gland is noted on rectal examination. There are no masses felt, and the stool is negative for occult blood. The neurologic examination findings are normal.

Logic The lymph nodes and prostate are within normal range. There is no clear-cut evidence of an infection or neoplastic cause for his symptoms. Perhaps the laboratory can offer a clue.

Laboratory tests can be divided into two categories. The first are those needed for routine screening, given the patient's age and gender. Appropriate tests in a 55-year-old man include complete blood count; serum chemistries to include glucose, creatinine, and cholesterol; urinalysis; and prostate-specific antigen. He should be advised to have flexible sigmoidoscopy and undergo fecal occult blood testing.

The second category are those tests indicated by the chief complaint of fatigue. There are very few "routine" tests indicated in the evaluation of patients with chronic fatigue. Many clinicians would order tests for erythrocyte sedimentation rate (ESR), thyroid-stimulating hormone (TSH) and thyroxine (T_4), and liver function to try to exclude hypothyroidism and chronic hepatitis. The ESR is usually elevated if infection or widespread cancer is present, and a normal ESR often serves as a reasonably dependable screening test in such cases.

Additional testing should be based on clinical suspicion. A "fishing expedition" looking for the cause of a patient's fatigue is not useful. Because of the various aches and pains, it would be reasonable to order antinuclear antibodies and rheumatoid factor. However, the laboratory seldom is helpful in cases where the cause is not already apparent by the history and examination.

Data These tests are ordered, and their results are all normal. The patient is upset by the normality of his examination and laboratory tests. He says that he really does feel poorly, and is afraid that the physician will say that his symptoms are "all in his head."

Logic In many cases, no organic cause of a patient's fatigue is found. In the absence of clinical suspicion, further laboratory or radiologic testing is not indicated and could be potentially detrimental to the patient. This patient may have somatic manifestations of depression. However, his symptom complex, particularly with a relatively rapid onset after a viral illness, suggests CFS.

The patient does not meet all the CDC criteria for the diagnosis of CFS (see Table 22.3). Although the fatigue is long-standing and does not resolve with rest, daily activities have not been reduced by 50%. Medical conditions have been virtually excluded but, because of multiple psychologic symptoms, a psychiatric diagnosis is still possible. Also notable is the fact that at least eight of the symptoms listed in the criteria are present in this patient.

The CDC criteria were developed for epidemiologic and research purposes and not for clinical use, and the majority of individuals thought to have CFS do not meet the criteria. The cause of this syndrome is quite controversial, and there are many who feel that the symptom complex is entirely psychiatric in origin. On the other hand, the frequent onset with a viral infection, followed by fatigue, depression, or other psychiatric illness suggests the presence of an immunologic dysfunction.

Data The patient is told that he may have CFS, and the disorder is explained. He is reassured that the condition is not life-threatening, that most patients get better over time, and that he will be followed up closely for any changes in his condition. The physician does not underestimate the patient's discomforts and appreciates that the symptoms are real.

Recommendations for treatment are made. Medications are designed to offer symptomatic relief: a nonsteroidal anti-inflammatory drug for the aches and pains; a tricyclic antidepressant to help the insomnia and depression; or a selective serotonin reuptake inhibitor such as fluoxetine for hypersomnia and psychomotor retardation if these symptoms are prominent. Last, the patient is cautioned to avoid unproven methods of treatment.

Suggested Readings

Buckwald D, Umali P, Umali J, et al. Chronic fatigue and the chronic fatigue syndrome. Ann Intern Med 1995;123(2):81–88.

Komaroff AL. Clinical presentation of chronic fatigue syndrome. Ciba Foundation Symp 1993;173:43–54.

Wilson A, Hickie I, Lloyd A, et al. Chronic fatigue syndrome, science and speculation. Am J Med 1994;96:544.

CASE 85

SUDDEN COMA

Paul Cutler

It is 8:15 AM, July 3, and the attending physician is making rounds with two fledgling interns.

MD I believe the patient we just saw with myocardial infarction is doing well. Whom shall we see next?

Intern 1 We just got a call from the emergency department. A comatose patient is arriving by ambulance. He will be on our service, so we have to see him right away. Would you care to join us?

MD Of course. Let us all go down and see what is wrong.

ER Nurse Glad you got here so quickly, doctors! This man does not look too good.

Intern 1 Does he have any family or friends with him?—And where is the ambulance driver?

Nurse They are just leaving, but I will get them.

MD Good thinking. You can often find the answer from a relative or friend or the ambulance driver in a minute when it might take you all day to find out what is wrong by yourself. Suppose you Jim (intern 2), get as much historical information as you can while Maria (intern 1) assesses the patient's vital signs and cardiorespiratory status. Maintenance of ventilation and circulation comes first.

Intern 1 The patient is really comatose. I think he is approximately 50 years old. He does not respond to my voice or noxious painful stimuli. His pupils are equal, small and respond to light. The pulse is 110 but strong, the BP is 116/80, and the respirations are 18/min with good depth. I do not see any cyanosis. The rectal temperature is 37.5°C.

MD That is good. His circulation and respiration seem adequate, so he is not in shock and does not have cardiac or respiratory failure. What is more, the absence of fever weighs against meningitis. Now you can slow down a bit, but first do a Dextrostix test on a drop of capillary blood to rule out hypoglycemia. Draw some venous blood for determinations of glucose, creatinine, and toxicology screen, and save a tube of blood in the refrigerator for possible future use. Before withdrawing the needle, inject 50 mL of 50% glucose to rule out hypoglycemia if the Dextrostix test result is inconclusive. Also, inject 0.4 mg of naloxone hydrochloride intravenously; you should see a salutary effect in 2 minutes if the patient has taken an overdose of morphine, heroin, or opioids. Get some arterial blood for determination of pH, pO_2, and pCO_2. Then get a urine sample; analyze it yourself, send a sample to the laboratory for further toxicology screening, and leave the catheter in place. Don't forget the blood chemistries, a complete blood count, chest radiograph, and ECG.

As you can see, we are asking the laboratory to help eliminate acidosis, diabetes mellitus complications, hypoglycemia, hyponatremia, drug intoxication, and uremia. Some physicians advise against giving glucose routinely, but as far as I am concerned it cannot hurt, can help, and can give you the solution if the patient wakes up quickly.

The pupillary reactions tell us he has not had a massive cerebral or pontine hemorrhage; in that event one pupil would be unilaterally dilated and fixed or both would be constricted. Bilateral fixed dilatation would be alarming and might suggest extensive brain damage and impending death.

Suppose you proceed with your examination and ask the ER nurse to help you.

Intern 2 We just got them in time—they were about to leave! The patient has no family and lives alone, but I got lots of information from his friend who lives in the next-door apartment. They are used to having breakfast together. He knocked on the door at 7 AM, found it open, and discovered the patient unconscious on the floor beside his bed. Last night while they were watching television together, he seemed perfectly well. They split two six-packs and said good night. The patient is 58 years old, a known diabetic for 15 years, takes pills for his diabetes, and his friend hinted that the patient sometimes "drinks a lot" to forget his divorced wife and children whom he never sees. He has never been known to have "fits" or "convulsions." The ambulance drivers had nothing to add; all they did was pick him up and bring him in. By the way, I asked the friend to check the apartment for any medicine bottles and let me know what he finds.

MD That tells us a lot. The most common causes of coma are stroke, drug overdosage, diabetic complications, and trauma. If you review the various disease systems, you can appreciably lengthen this short list to include meningitis, encephalitis, myxedema coma, hysteria, the postictal state of epilepsy, brain tumor, brain abscess, uremia, hepatic coma, CO_2 narcosis, and shock from sepsis or massive myocardial infarction.

A "stroke" can be caused by thrombosis, hemorrhage, embolus, or subarachnoid hemorrhage. Trauma can result in a skull fracture, concussion, or subdural hematoma. Diabetes may be complicated by ketoacidotic coma, hyperosmolar coma, or hypoglycemia. Drug overdosage, in my experience, is usually caused by barbiturates, glutethimide, benzodiazepines, or heroin, although many other narcotics, sedatives, hypnotics, or mood changers can be the offending agents. Lately we have seen many patients who are unconscious from taking combinations of several drugs—anything they can get their hands on—including alcohol. We are not sure how "alcoholic" he is, but I would be willing to bet that he drinks a lot, so we must be alert for alcoholic intoxication, hypoglycemia, and cranial trauma—the by-products of drinking. All those possibilities can be eliminated quickly with a multibranched but not necessarily thorough data base (Table 22.4).

The fact that the patient had no preceding acute illness or gradual downhill course tells us the coma came on suddenly. This tends to rule out diabetic ketoacidosis, uremia, myxedema coma, brain tumor or abscess, hepatic coma, CO_2 narcosis (respiratory failure), and infectious disease. The absence of previous seizures weighs against epilepsy. All these illnesses would have had symptoms and specific clinical pictures preceding the onset of coma.

Where the patient is found may guide you. If he is picked up in an alley near a bar, foul play or acute alcoholic intoxication are suspect. Think of a stroke if he was known to be well earlier in the day and was later found unconscious at home. On the other hand, if he has not been feeling well and has not been seen for several days, gradual-onset diseases like diabetic coma, uremia, and meningitis are to be considered. So knowing when the patient was last seen to be well helps our logic too.

Do not get locked into a wrong hypothesis. Two common diseases often coexist and may even relate to each other. An alcoholic patient may develop uremia. A comatose diabetic patient may have taken an overdose of drugs, suffered a stroke, or been mugged. Many a patient with alcohol on his breath has been jailed or sent home to die because the main illness was obscured.

Maria, tell us what you found.

Intern 1 First we searched his pockets and found no medicine bottles or pills. His wallet contains a card saying he is diabetic and printed material suggestive of membership in Alcoholics Anonymous. So I did not know what his beer drinking really means. A catheterized urine sample showed nothing other than a trace of glucose. The Dextrostix test showed ample glucose, so I did not give him any. I did give him the naloxone hy-

TABLE 22.4. Common Causes of Coma

Stroke
  Thrombosis
  Hemorrhage
  Embolus
Trauma
  Skull fracture
  Cerebral contusion
  Intracranial bleed
Overdose
  Opioids (heroin)
  Benzodiazepines
  Barbiturates
Metabolic
  Diabetes mellitus
    hypoglycemia
    ketoacidosis
    hyperosmolality
  Hyponatremia
  Uremia
  Hepatic failure
Alcohol
  A class by itself

drochloride; it had no effect. He is well hydrated and has a laceration on the back of his head that is not bleeding. He is not incontinent and has not bitten his tongue. There are no signs of meningeal irritation and no needle marks on his forearms. The fundi, heart, lungs, abdomen, extremities, genitalia, and rectum are normal, and the stool is negative for occult blood. In particular, there is no evidence of chronic liver disease or complications of diabetes. The neurologic examination is normal, but he has doll's-eye movements.

MD He certainly does not have cirrhosis of the liver even though he does drink, but that is not surprising because only 20% of alcoholics get cirrhosis. You have pretty well ruled out meningitis and subarachnoid hemorrhage, so you can see there is no need to do a lumbar puncture routinely on every unconscious patient. One look at the patient tells you he does not have myxedema.

He has neither Kussmaul's nor Cheyne-Stokes respirations, which weighs against any type of acidosis or a large cerebral hemorrhage. Besides, he has no neurologic evidence of a stroke. And diabetic ketoacidosis is unlikely in the absence of dehydration and Kussmaul breathing. What do you think of the laceration on his scalp?

Intern 1 Either he fell out of bed, or it represents inflicted trauma. I favor the fall because the trauma is not great. And, oh, yes I forgot; his breath had no odor of alcohol or acetone, nor did it resemble the breath of uremic or hepatic coma.

MD Can you tell the difference?

Intern 1 Yes. While in medical school, I smelled the breath of a patient with hepatic coma; I will never forget it. The others are easy to identify.

MD How can you tell that the unconscious patient did not have a stroke?

Intern 1 He does not have a hemiplegic posture, the reflexes and muscle tone are equal bilaterally, and there is no Babinski's sign. Neither cheek blows out when he exhales, and the face is symmetric.

MD Very good! What does the presence of doll's-eye movements mean?

Intern 1 I am not sure. Would you explain it?

MD The eyes of a normal person whose head is slowly rocked side to side will move slightly in the opposite direction and then drift back slowly. In the patient who is stuporous or comatose from toxicity, metabolic disease, or cerebral disease, these movements are generally retained but exaggerated so that the eyes rotate more and return more slowly. If there is no movement at all, or only one eye moves, the lesion can be located in the pons, and the cause for unconsciousness is therefore more serious.

I am a little concerned about the scalp laceration. It could have resulted from falling out of bed. On the other hand, somebody who has a stroke may fall and injure his head at the same time. The reverse is true too. The same incident that caused the laceration might have brought about a subdural hematoma. Foul play is always a consideration. Maybe we ought to do a lumbar puncture in this case in order to be sure.

Intern 2 Do you think we should get a computed tomographic (CT) scan of the cranium and brain first?

MD Not a bad idea! It *is* costly and I think we should be able to arrive at a diagnosis without it.

But if cerebral thrombosis, cerebral hemorrhage, cerebral embolus, and subdural hematoma are viable possibilities, the CT scan may supersede other procedures and be of great help. These diagnostic possibilities seem unlikely to me, but in view of the laceration we had better *do the scan before the lumbar puncture.* There is no telling what you might find. I have seen an occasional patient with a brain tumor that suddenly bled, a patient with cerebral metastases who was comatose, and a few with unsuspected subdural hematomas. In these cases a lumbar puncture might be dangerous and unnecessary.

Suppose Jim and I see some other patients. We will return in an hour, Maria; the chemistries should be back by then too. Looks like you do not have any diabetic complications or stroke. Trauma and drugs are both possible.

(*It is 10:20 AM.*)

MD Maria, we have just seen three patients: one with chronic obstructive lung disease, one with cirrhosis and bleeding, and a third for evaluation of a possible ectopic pregnancy. What have you found?

Intern 1 The CT scan was normal so I did a lumbar puncture that revealed clear, colorless fluid under normal pressure; I sent the fluid to the laboratory for studies. There is no change in the physical examination. The ECG was normal. Tests have come back from the laboratory. The complete blood count, urinalysis, blood pH, PCO_2, PO_2, creatinine and other chemistries are normal, the blood glucose is 164 mg/dL, and the toxicology screening results are not back yet. The chest radiographic finding was normal.

MD I suppose we can put diabetic complications and all causes for acidosis to rest. Subdural hematoma is essentially excluded now that the spinal fluid is not xanthochromic and the CT scan is normal.

It is a bit late to mention it now, but while we were seeing the last three patients, it suddenly dawned on me that a lumbar puncture really was not necessary in this patient. The only reasons for doing it—possible meningitis and subarachnoid bleeding—would have already been ruled out by the clinical picture and the CT scan.

We now know what the diagnosis is not, but we do not know what it is! Where do we go from here?

Intern 2 Sir, I just got a telephone call from our

patient's neighbor. He found two pill bottles in our patient's bathroom: one says, "tolazamide: take 1 tablet before breakfast and dinner" and the other says, "secobarbital: take 1 capsule at bedtime for sleep." The first bottle has pills in it; the second is empty. I got the prescribing doctor's name and we are trying to get him on the phone now.

Intern 1 The laboratory just called. The patient has a high barbiturate level in his blood. That clinches it. We will start him on intravenous fluids, watch his blood gases carefully, and make sure he does not get into respiratory difficulty.

Intern 2 The doctor was in his office. He says the patient saw him 3 days ago because he could not sleep, so he prescribed ten sleeping capsules. That means that the most he could have taken last night was seven or eight capsules, a sublethal dose. His physician then told me that the patient was depressed over his living pattern, missed his wife, and just heard she had remarried.

MD Well, I guess I will go back to my office. It is clear I am not needed here. The patient should be well by tomorrow. Do not forget to have a psychiatrist see him.

Comment If this were June 3 instead of July 3, the seasoned intern would have preferred handling this case by himself. By June he would know the common causes for coma in the population with which he works. He would also know that the performance of life-maintaining maneuvers precedes diagnosis, and he would be familiar with the more unusual causes of coma, too.

With no verbal information from the patient, the problem solvers had to flesh out the clinical picture from other important sources such as the neighbor, ambulance driver, and treating physician.

Diabetes, alcoholism, and a scalp laceration were misleading false-positive clues. Many pertinent negative clues were also present. The decisive clue related to the various circumstances surrounding barbiturate intoxication.

Although there are very many causes of coma, attention was given mainly to the common ones; the less likely and easily recognizable ones were discarded almost by inspection alone. The laboratory took care of the rest.

Because drug overdose, stroke, and trauma are such common causes of coma, many emer-

gency room protocols require intravenous naloxone hydrochloride, a toxicology drug screen, and a CT scan for every unconscious patient—unless the cause for the clinical picture is obvious.

Many decision paths or flowcharts have been made for the solution of coma, but they are of necessity very complicated, rigid, and incomplete. Especially in the comatose patient, a flexible, self-constructed flowchart should be utilized by the physician who must meet each somewhat varying problem of unconsciousness with a different "think as you go" approach. (P.C.)

Suggested Readings

Lindberg MC, Cunningham A, Lindberg NH. Acute phenobarbital intoxication. South Med J 1992;85(8): 803–807.

Samuels MA. A practical approach to coma diagnosis in the unresponsive patient. Cleve Clin J Med 1992;59(3):257–261.

Samuels MA. The evaluation of comatose patients. Hosp Prac (Off Ed) 1993;28(3):165–182.

CASE **86**

PROLONGED FEVER

Paul Cutler

Intern We need some help on a difficult problem. The patient is a 48-year-old construction worker who has had documented fever for 2 to 3 weeks. Many temperature readings are between 38.3 and 39°C. He has had no previous illnesses or operations and complains only of fever, malaise, and fatigue. We have checked him for a week and do not have a diagnosis yet.

MD You have just defined the Petersdorf and Beeson criteria for a fever of undetermined origin (FUO). Its features are: (1) illness of more than 3 weeks, (2) fever higher than 38.3°C on several occasions, and (3) diagnosis uncertain after 1 week of hospital study. I think these criteria are good but not explicit enough. Fever should be the principal symptom and, although there may be nonspecific associated symptoms like malaise, fatigue, weight loss, or even chills, there should be no symptoms present that point to an organ or system—for example, arthralgia, abdominal pain, and so forth.

Remember, too, that former criteria for FUO

definition are now obsolete because most of today's patients who have FUOs, except for immunocompromised patients, can be adequately studied in an ambulatory care facility. New technology permits far more studies in several days than were conceivable 20 years ago. By the third outpatient visit, in addition to various cultures, radiographs, and blood and urine tests, the patient may already have had ultrasound, CT, MRI, and gallium scan of the abdomen, to be followed perhaps by needle aspiration, biopsy, or catheter drainage—all without becoming an inpatient. Often, less than a week is required to turn an FUO into an FKO (fever of known origin). The time needed for the study will vary with the aggressiveness of the physician, the complexity of the case, and the compliance of the patient.

How did the illness begin?

Intern He was first seen in the emergency department and was thought to have nothing more than a viral infection. We are seeing a lot of that. So we sent him home on aspirin. When he returned 5 days later, still with fever, he was referred to the ambulatory care clinic for further care. There, he is my patient.

During the past week, his fever has been well documented. The temperature rises to 38.5 to 39°C every day and there are no new symptoms. The physical examination has remained normal; we check him carefully every day. Normal or negative studies include a complete blood count, urinalysis, six blood cultures, two urine cultures, chest and abdominal radiographs, ECG, and complete blood chemistries, except for the alkaline phosphatase level, which is twice the upper normal value. The erythrocyte sedimentation rate is elevated: 26 mm/h, and the intermediate strength PPD test result is positive.

MD I assume you have already asked all the appropriate questions and sought the physical findings that go with febrile disease?

Intern Yes. There is no dyspnea, cough, expectoration, disorientation, stiff neck, sore throat, joint pains, frequent or painful urination, nausea, vomiting, diarrhea, or abdominal pain. The patient has had no unpasteurized cow's or goat's milk products and no recent dental work or urethral instrumentation. Although he has had no recent contact with tuberculosis, his sister died of that disease 25 years ago. He has no evidence of

meningeal irritation, no heart murmur, rash, jaundice, arthritis, enlarged liver, spleen, or nodes.

MD You just rattled off a lot of negative information. Can you tell me why you mentioned these items and what their absence or negativity means?

Intern I have listed what I feel are pertinent negatives. That is, they tend to exclude certain possibilities. The absence of dyspnea, cough, and expectoration weighs against advanced fibrocaseous pulmonary tuberculosis being a cause of fever. Meningitis is unlikely in the absence of disorientation, stiff neck, sore throat, and signs of meningeal irritation. No joint pains, arthritis, or rash weigh against an autoimmune collagen disorder. Infective endocarditis is less likely if there has been no dental work or urethral instrumentation. The other negative findings weigh against brucellosis, enteric fevers, and leukemias or lymphomas.

MD That is good reasoning! Well, the patient does not look sick nor does he look like he has lost weight. He should be weighed daily. He has no other serious disease and is not immunosuppressed, so we are not in any great hurry to make a diagnosis. No need rushing in with invasive procedures just yet. Time may be better than tests. Few syndromes give rise to more abuse and ineffective use of diagnostic procedures than do prolonged fevers.

We have got to consider the anxiety of the patient and the yield, risk, and cost of each procedure against the morbidity, risk, and cost of the illness. It might be wiser from the economic and patient morale standpoints to proceed rapidly. But remember that many FUOs will diagnose themselves by the appearance of a new symptom or sign as we observe the patient. Still other patients get well without a diagnosis ever having been made.

The rapid erythrocyte sedimentation rate and elevated alkaline phosphatase level are nonspecific markers for disease, but the latter suggests liver or bone involvement. An absence of leukocytosis and chills weighs against an occult abscess; the absence of a heart murmur and negative blood culture results weigh against endocarditis. The positive PPD skin test result is a bit confusing. His sister had tuberculosis 25 years ago, so he may have become positive then. I do not know what to make of it. If the results were negative, it would have been more helpful, because anergy is uncommon, even in miliary tuberculosis. Has he received any antibiotics, or is he taking medication?

Intern Before he came under our care he was given penicillin and tetracycline by a physician, but he is taking no medication whatsoever now.

MD Previous antibiotics may make it difficult to get a positive blood culture even if endocarditis exists; and it is interesting to note how often medications of any kind can cause fever. Antibiotics, barbiturates, iodides, phenytoin, propylthiouracil, allopurinol, methyldopa, procainamide, and quinidine are common offenders.

Well-defined FUOs are caused mainly by "the big three": infection in 40% of cases, malignancy in 20%, and collagen-vascular disease in 15% (Table 22.5). Infections include tuberculosis, infective endocarditis, and localized but hidden infection such as perinephric, subphrenic, prostatic, tubo-ovarian, and hepatic abscesses. Less common infections are cytomegalovirus disease, histoplasmosis, coccidioidomycosis, typhoid, paratyphoid, and undulant fevers, chronic meningococcemia, and gonococcemia.

As for malignancies and tumors, the most common types that cause fever are lymphomas, Hodgkin's disease, and leukemias, although renal cell carcinoma, hepatoma, atrial myxoma, and metastatic cancer in the liver may also present with fever as the sole manifestation for some time.

The likelihoods depend on the subset with whom you work too. In my own experience, malignancy is the most common cause of FUO, infection a close second, and collagen disorders a distant third.

I once saw an elderly male patient with widely spaced episodes of chills and fever recurring over a period of 6 months. Each time he got better with a "shot of penicillin" and asked me to give him the same thing. His regular physician was away. But by this time he already had constipation and red rectal bleeding too. Barium enema and subsequent surgery disclosed a carcinoma of the sigmoid colon in an area of diverticulitis with multiple microabscesses that were seeding his bloodstream. Who would think that cancer could cause chills and fever?

Intern That is a strange one! How about the third category?

MD Collagen-vascular diseases are far more common in women, and include SLE, polymyal-

TABLE 22.5. Causes of FUO

CAUSE	OCCURRENCE %
Infection	40
Malignancy	20
Collagen-vascular disease	15
Miscellaneous	15
No cause found	10

FUO = fever of undetermined origin.

gia rheumatica, periarteritis nodosa, rheumatoid arthritis, and hypersensitivity angiitis; fever may sometimes be the sole symptom in these diseases long before other manifestations appear, but this is not usual. You should obtain some immunologic marker test results.

And don't forget a large miscellaneous group that makes up the remaining 20%! Each is most uncommon by itself, but must be considered if one of the preceding triad is not found. In this list are factitious fever, habitual hyperthermia, drug fever, active cirrhosis or hepatitis, inflammatory bowel disease, malaria, periodic fever (familial Mediterranean fever—FMF), nonspecific granulomatous disease, Whipple's disease, atrial myxoma, and the undiagnosed cases. All of these conditions can present with FUO, although sooner or later additional signs appear.

Go after the common causes first, then consider the rare. Do not do anything highly invasive. I will be back in a few days.

(Four days later)

Intern Glad you returned! The patient has been studied from top to bottom and we still do not have the answer.

MD Tell me about it.

Intern Blood, urine, and stool cultures are all still negative and some have been incubating for as long as 10 days. Radioisotopic liver-spleen and liver-lung scans, abdominal sonogram, and computed tomography show no evidence of subphrenic, hepatic, or perinephric abscess. The scan and physical examination now suggest that the liver may be a little enlarged—14 cm on vertical percussion. A whole-body scan with gallium 67 detects no evidence of intra-abdominal malignancy or infection. Prostatic examination findings are again normal. Serologic study results for fungi and cytomegalovirus are negative, and agglutination test results for enteric pathogens are negative. A Giemsa stain of a thick blood smear for malaria parasites is negative too.

The intravenous pyelogram and barium enema are normal. Rheumatoid factor, antinuclear antibody, and anti-DNA antibody test results are negative, and there is no eosinophilia. An echocardiogram shows no evidence of atrial myxoma, and there is no mitral murmur.

Although there have been no new symptoms or findings, the nurse reports a 4-lb weight loss in 2 weeks. I think we have to get to the bottom of this soon. We have pretty much ruled out the various possibilities you discussed. What about factitious fever, cyclic fever, and habitual fever?

MD They are unusual. I am sure you that have already eliminated factitious fever by being continuously present while the temperature is being taken. But devious patients can fool you by warming the mouth in advance. To get around this, you can take the temperature of a simultaneously voided urine sample or take the temperature by instantaneous probe. Also, factitious fever does not follow a diurnal pattern, and it drops suddenly without diaphoresis.

Cyclic fever or familial Mediterranean fever (FMF) occurs in persons who come from the Mediterranean basin, is usually accompanied by signs of serositis, and is cyclic and familial, as the name implies.

Habitual hyperthermia is a normal situation found mostly in young women in their twenties or thirties who have easily detectable psychoneurotic traits. They may have temperatures as high as 38°C daily, and although this is not pathologic, such patients often undergo extensive fruitless studies for FUO.

Drug-induced fevers are becoming more commonly recognized, but this patient is not taking medications and antibiotics were stopped a while ago, so that possibility may be excluded.

I would agree with you that more aggressive studies are indicated. Suppose we get biopsies of the liver, bone marrow, and gastrocnemius muscle. The liver is a good place to biopsy if diffuse visceral disease is expected, and the bone marrow gives essentially the same information. A muscle biopsy is for detecting vascular disease. Hold off on possible laparotomy or a therapeutic trial. Exploratory surgery is rarely necessary now that there are so many new diagnostic techniques.

(Three days later)

Intern We have the answer! The muscle and bone marrow biopsies were normal. But the liver biopsy showed multiple caseating granulomas typical of miliary tuberculosis (Fig. 22.5). The pathologist even found tubercle bacilli in them. I was surprised at the normal chest radiograph, but, on reading, I found this to be common early in the disease.

MD That is correct. You can begin treatment now, and you should see some good results in 2 to 3 weeks. There is some difference of opinion on the value of liver biopsy in FUOs, but I do not think there can be any dispute here.

This case reemphasizes the need to "think common." There are several dozen causes of FUO, but tuberculosis, endocarditis, occult bacterial infection, lymphoma, cancer, and collagen disease head the list and are statistically far more common than the numerous but infrequent stragglers.

Fortunately, we did not have to consider the ponderous questions of exploratory laparotomy and therapeutic trials. These are "last resort" decisions, and often difficult to make. Therapeutic trials are especially risky, because you often do more harm than good when treating almost blindly with antibiotics, NSAIDs, or steroids. But sometimes your hand may be forced.

Intern This case bothers me. Do not you feel we should have had the answer sooner?

MD Yes, I do. It bothers me, too. I think we may

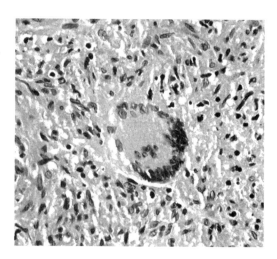

▶ **Figure 22.5.** Caseating granulomas in liver showing necrosis and typical Langhans' giant cell.

have proceeded too slowly, and I must accept responsibility for that. The cluster of fever, a positive PPD finding, and an elevated alkaline phosphatase level should have directed our inquiry more rapidly into a liver biopsy. Most of the studies could have been bypassed. There are indeed some diseases associated with fever where speedy diagnosis is essential to prevent rapid deterioration. This is especially true for miliary tuberculosis, infective endocarditis, and intra-abdominal infection.

In the future, when confronted with diagnostic problems of this sort, try to form an early hypothesis by clustering a few clues. Then do a directed or selective study. For example, if your patient with fever just returned from an African safari, do a blood smear for malaria. If your patient with fever just had an appendectomy or complicated bowel surgery, look for intra-abdominal suppuration with a computed tomographic scan, a gallium scan, or an ultrasound study. It would be senseless to request a PPD skin test or an antinuclear antibody titer. So rather than use a general checklist for all causes of FUO, evaluate the problem as it exists in a specific clinical setting. If your initial hypothesis is not supported by selected studies, you may have to formulate a new one.

In this regard, the key clue may often be found in the history—previous illnesses or surgery, drugs, or alcohol, social and occupational history, hobbies, travel, and animal exposure.

If no hypothesis is feasible, then you must resort to an orderly battery of tests and studies for an FUO.

Hospitalized cases can be quite complicated. Often the clinical setting offers many possible causes for fever. Suppose you have a 60-year-old man who had a mitral valve replacement performed 5 days ago. He begins to have fever. Because of the surgery it is still difficult for him to cough and clear his chest. There is a catheter in his bladder because he is having trouble voiding; an intravenous catheter is in place for fluids and electrolytes; and he is being given two antibiotics, either of which sometimes causes fever. On examination there are signs of a left pleural effusion.

Based on this information, you may postulate suppurative thrombophlebitis at the intracatheterization site, infective endocarditis, infected incision, acute urinary tract infection, pneumonia, empyema, pulmonary embolus, and drug fever. With these presumptions, you would then order the appropriate confirmatory tests and actions. It would be farfetched to hunt for collagen disease or cancer under these circumstances.

By the way, recheck our patient's fundi for choroid tubercles.

Intern The next patient we would like you to see has a problem that was very easy to solve. Just by looking at her, I could tell. . . .

Questions

1. In general, therapeutic trials are frowned upon, but if the patient is deteriorating, and no diagnosis has been made, you might try:
   (a) antibiotics if endocarditis is suspected.
   (b) steroids if collagen-vascular disease is suspected.
   (c) isoniazid and adjunctive therapy if miliary tuberculosis is suspected.
   (d) antimetabolites if lymphoma is suspected.

2. In miliary tuberculosis, which of the following circumstances is excluded?
   (a) Enlarged liver and spleen
   (b) Signs of meningeal irritation
   (c) Leukopenia and anemia
   (d) Leukemia-like blood picture
   (e) Normal chest radiograph
   (f) Abnormal chest radiograph
   (g) Positive PPD skin test finding
   (h) Negative PPD skin test finding

3. Which of the following questions is important in trying to determine the cause of an FUO?
   (a) Have you been bitten by a rat in the past 2 months?
   (b) Do any other members of your family suffer from recurrent fevers?
   (c) Do you have shaking chills?
   (d) Are you of Indian extraction?

Answers

1. **(a) and (c) are correct.** For example, a young patient with a heart murmur and fever who appears ill may be given intelligent antibiotic treatment even if an etiologic agent is not identified, and you are suspicious but not certain. There are definite risks. So too if miliary tuberculosis is suspected but not identified as such. But steroids are nonspecific in their action, may mask most diseases, and

may make the patient susceptible to others. Their use is therefore inadvisable in almost all instances. Suspected lymphomas should not be treated without a tissue diagnosis, even if it necessitates laparotomy.

2. **None is correct** because all are possible. Widespread miliary involvement can enlarge the liver and spleen, cause meningitis, and involve the bone marrow. It may replace the bone marrow, causing leukopenia and anemia, or irritate the bone marrow, causing a leukemoid reaction. If miliary spread results from a caseous hilar node eroding a pulmonary vein, the chest radiographic finding may remain normal until miliary lesions in the lung coalesce and become radiologically visible. On the other hand, the chest radiographic finding may be abnormal from the start because it may show re-infection tuberculosis. The PPD skin test result is usually positive, although it is sometimes negative if the patient is debilitated, anergic, immunosuppressed, or overwhelmed.

3. **(a), (b), and (c) are correct.** Rat-bite fever can be caused by either *Spirillum minus* or *Streptobacillus moniliformis*. Fever in another member of the family suggests FMF, especially if the extraction is Italian, Sephardic Jewish, or Arab. Shaking chills suggest malaria, sepsis, or abscess formation somewhere. Whether the patient is Asian Indian or American Indian seems to have no bearing if he or she lives here.

COMMENT The principal technique used here was the traditional exhaustive one. A complete data base was needed, and even then the problem remained unsolved. Fever was the key clue because other symptoms were too vague, and the conclusive clue resided in the liver biopsy. Bayes' mathematics again proved that common diseases deserve prime consideration, and that even uncommon manifestations of common diseases must be kept in mind before thinking of the rare.

Note the unreliability of statistics as demonstrated by the fact that causes for FUO will vary with both its definition and the vigor of diagnostic study during the first week. Further variability hinges on whether the patient is female, young, or old—and whether your population subset does or does not contain Mediterraneans who get FMF, underprivileged persons who are more susceptible to tuberculosis, addicts who are prone to endocarditis, or soldiers returning from the tropics who may harbor the malaria *Plasmodium*.

The order, speed, urgency, cost, and danger of studies received careful consideration in a patient who was not desperately ill, and in whom tincture of time was an important ingredient in mandating that a definite diagnosis be made before giving treatment—which is usually a good idea. But in this case, a more rapid, hypothesis-driven approach would have been more advisable. The physician's zeal for teaching and the intern's thirst for learning and passion for thoroughness may not have been in the best interests of the patient and health care costs. *(P.C.)*

Suggested Readings

Barbado FJ, Vazquez JJ, Pena JM, et al. Pyrexia of unknown origin: Changing spectrum of diseases in two consecutive series. Postgrad Med J 1992;68:884–887.

Kazanjian PH. Fever of unknown origin: Review of 86 patients treated in community hospitals. Clin Infect Dis 1992;15:968–973.

Knockaert DC, Vanneste LJ, Vanneste SB, et al. Fever of unknown origin in the 1982: An update of the diagnostic spectrum. Arch Intern Med 1992;152:51–55.

Appendix: Final Diagnoses

Listed below are the final diagnoses for the 86 cases in Section 2. In each instance, the initial presentation resulted in diagnostic closure only after the formulation of a differential diagnosis, the application of a full range of clinical reasoning processes, and the appropriate consideration of each diagnostic contender.

Chapter 12: Hematologic Problems

Case 1: Weakness and Joint Pains
Diagnosis: Iron deficiency anemia; carcinoma of the cecum
Case 2: Mild Asymptomatic Anemia
Diagnosis: Excessive blood donation
Case 3: Bleeding Gums and Bruising
Diagnosis: Autoimmune thrombocytopenic purpura
Case 4: Lethargy and Confusion
Diagnosis: Pernicious anemia
Case 5: A Family Affair
Diagnosis: von Willebrand's disease
Case 6: Cough, Fever, then Fatigue
Diagnosis: Glucose-6-phosphate dehydrogenase deficiency
Case 7: Neck Lumps
Diagnosis: Hodgkin's disease
Case 8: Elevated Hematocrit
Diagnosis: Polycythemia vera
Case 9: Backache, Weakness, Nosebleeds
Diagnosis: Multiple myeloma
Case 10: Jaundice, Weakness, Pallor
Diagnosis: Acute lymphocytic leukemia
Case 11: Leg Pain
Diagnosis: Hypercoagulability

Chapter 13: Endocrine Problems

Case 12: A Thyroid Nodule
Diagnosis: Thyroid adenoma
Case 13: Glycosuria
Diagnosis: Diabetes mellitus
Case 14: Weakness, Anxiety, Sweating
Diagnosis: Functional hypoglycemia
Case 15: Obesity and Hirsutism
Diagnosis: Obesity, hypertension, diabetes
Case 16: Nervousness and Weight Loss
Diagnosis: Hyperthyroidism
Case 17: Polyuria and Polydipsia
Diagnosis: Compulsive water drinking
Case 18: Hypercalcemia
Diagnosis: Parathyroid adenoma
Case 19: Compounded Confusion
Diagnosis: Pharmaceutical error
Case 20: Amenorrhea and Galactorrhea
Diagnosis: Prolactinoma
Case 21: Weak and Shaky Spells
Diagnosis: Pheochromocytoma
Case 22: A Fat Problem
Diagnosis: Hypertriglyceridemia

Chapter 14: Cardiovascular Problems

Case 23: Abnormal ECG
Diagnosis: Aortic regurgitation
Case 24: Severe Substernal Tightness
Diagnosis: Acute myocardial infarction
Case 25: Systolic Murmur
Diagnosis: Aortic stenosis
Case 26: High Blood Pressure
Diagnosis: Essential hypertension
Case 27: Dyspnea on Exertion
Diagnosis: Congestive heart failure
Case 28: Coma and T-wave Inversion
Diagnosis: Subarachnoid hemorrhage
Case 29: Sharp Chest Pains
Diagnosis: Chest pain, cause undetermined

Chapter 20: Neurologic Problems

Case 71: Headache
Diagnosis: Tension headaches
Case 72: Dizziness
Diagnosis: Vertebral artery thrombosis
Case 73: Convulsions
Diagnosis: Parasagittal meningioma
Case 74: Paralysis
Diagnosis: Cerebral thrombosis

Chapter 21: Geriatric Problems

Case 75: Incontinence
Diagnosis: Incontinence, idiopathic
Case 76: Nocturia and Frequency
Diagnosis: Benign prostatic hypertrophy
Case 77: Demented or Depressed
Diagnosis: Alzheimer's disease

Case 78: Erectile Dysfunction
Diagnosis: Impotence, mixed cause
Case 79: Falls
Diagnosis: Falls—multifactorial

Chapter 22: Multisystem Problems

Case 80: Weakness, Weight Loss, Anorexia
Diagnosis: Carcinoma of the prostate
Case 81: The Great Imitator
Diagnosis: AIDS, multiple infections
Case 82: Fainting Spells
Diagnosis: Sick sinus syndrome
Case 83: Strange Behavior
Diagnosis: Barbiturate withdrawal
Case 84: Fatigue
Diagnosis: Chronic fatigue syndrome
Case 85: Sudden Coma
Diagnosis: Barbiturate overdose
Case 86: Prolonged Fever
Diagnosis: Miliary tuberculosis

Figure Credits

Figure 1.4 Modified from Brant WE, Helms CA. Fundamentals of diagnostic radiology. 1st ed. Baltimore: Williams & Wilkins, 1994:1174.

Figure 6.2 Reprinted with permission from Burnside JW. Adams' physical diagnosis. 15th ed. Baltimore: Williams & Wilkins, 1974:87.

Figure 6.3 Reprinted with permission from Barclay L. Clinical geriatric neurology. 1st ed. Baltimore: Williams & Wilkins, 1993:156.

Figure 7.5 Reprinted with permission from Burnside JW. Adams' physical diagnosis. 15th ed. Baltimore: Williams & Wilkins, 1974:69.

Figure 9.1 Reprinted with permission from Brant WE, Helms CA. Fundamentals of diagnostic radiology. 1st ed. Baltimore: Williams & Wilkins, 1994:575.

Figure 9.2 Reprinted with permission from Brant WE, Helms CA. Fundamentals of diagnostic radiology. 1st ed. Baltimore: Williams & Wilkins, 1994:575.

Figure 9.3 Reprinted with permission from Brant WE, Helms CA. Fundamentals of diagnostic radiology. 1st ed. Baltimore: Williams & Wilkins, 1994:347.

Figure 9.4 Reprinted with permission from Brant WE, Helms CA. Fundamentals of diagnostic radiology. 1st ed. Baltimore: Williams & Wilkins, 1994:118.

Figure 9.6 Reprinted with permission from Brant WE, Helms CA. Fundamentals of diagnostic radiology. 1st ed. Baltimore: Williams & Wilkins, 1994:98.

Figure 10.2 Reprinted with permission from Takasugi JE, Rapaport S, Shaw C. Superior sulcus tumors: the role of imaging. J Thorac Imaging 1989;4:41–48.

Figure 10.4 Reprinted with permission from Brant WE, Helms CA. Fundamentals of diagnostic radiology. 1st ed. Baltimore: Williams & Wilkins, 1994:691.

Figure 10.5 Reprinted with permission from Brant WE, Helms CA. Fundamentals of diagnostic radiology. 1st ed. Baltimore: Williams & Wilkins, 1994:706.

Figure 13.2 Courtesy of Diabetic Retinopathy Study (DRS) Research Group.

Figure 13.6 Reprinted with permission from Becker KL. Principles and practice of endocrinology and metabolism. 2nd ed. Philadelphia: Lippincott-Raven, 1995:1807.

Figure 13.7 Reprinted with permission from Brant WE, Helms CA. Fundamentals of diagnostic radiology. 1st ed. Baltimore: Williams & Wilkins, 1994:1196.

Figure 13.10 Reprinted with permission from Burnside JW. Adams' physical diagnosis. 15th ed. Baltimore: Williams & Wilkins, 1974:64.

Figure 13.11 Reprinted with permission from Becker KL. Principles and practice of endocrinology and metabolism. 2nd ed. Philadelphia: Lippincott-Raven, 1995:1388.

Figure 15.5 Reprinted with permission from Brant WE, Helms CA. Fundamentals of diagnostic radiology. 1st ed. Baltimore: Williams & Wilkins, 1994:571.

Figure 15.8 Reprinted with permission from Light RW. Pleural diseases. 3rd ed. Baltimore: Williams & Wilkins, 1995:19.

Figure 15.10 Reprinted with permission from Brant WE, Helms CA. Fundamentals of diagnostic radiology. 1st ed. Baltimore: Williams & Wilkins, 1994:433.

Figure 15.11 Reprinted with permission from George RB, Light RW, Matthay MA, et al. Chest medicine. 3rd ed. Baltimore: Williams & Wilkins, 1995:118.

Figure 15.13 Reprinted with permission from Brant WE, Helms CA. Fundamentals of diagnostic radiology. 1st ed. Baltimore: Williams & Wilkins, 1994:979.

Figure 15.15 Reprinted with permission from George RB, Light RW, Matthay MA, et al. Chest medicine. 3rd ed. Baltimore: Williams & Wilkins, 1995:307.

Figure 15.16 Reprinted with permission from George RB, Light RW, Matthay MA, et al. Chest medicine. 3rd ed. Baltimore: Williams & Wilkins, 1995:333.

Figure 16.1 Reprinted with permission from Brant WE, Helms CA. Fundamentals of diagnostic radiology. 1st ed. Baltimore: Williams & Wilkins, 1994:716.

Figure 16.2 Reprinted with permission from Kaplowitz N. Liver and biliary diseases. 2nd ed. Baltimore: Williams & Wilkins, 1996:255.

Figure 16.5 Reprinted with permission from Brant WE, Helms CA. Fundamentals of diagnostic radiology. 1st ed. Baltimore: Williams & Wilkins, 1994:703.

Figure 16.12 Reprinted with permission from George RB, Light RW, Matthay MA, et al. Chest medicine. 3rd ed. Baltimore: Williams & Wilkins, 1995:453.

Figure 17.1 Reprinted with permission from Brant WE, Helms CA. Fundamentals of diagnostic radiology. 1st ed. Baltimore: Williams & Wilkins, 1994:774.

Figure 17.10 Modified from Berk T, Anderson RJ, McDonald KM, et al. Clinical disorders of water metabolism. Kidney Int 1976;10:117–132.

Figure 18.1 Reprinted with permission from Brant WE, Helms CA. Fundamentals of diagnostic radiology. 1st ed. Baltimore: Williams & Wilkins, 1994:535.

Figure 19.2 Reprinted with permission from Burnside JW. Adams' physical diagnosis. 15th ed. Baltimore: Williams & Wilkins, 1974:97.

Figure 21.1 Reprinted with permission from Brant WE, Helms CA. Fundamentals of diagnostic radiology. 1st ed. Baltimore: Williams & Wilkins, 1994:809.

Figure 21.3 Reprinted with permission from Rowland LP. Merritt's textbook of neurology. 9th ed. Baltimore: Williams & Wilkins, 1996:379.

Figure 22.1 Courtesy of Albert Saltzman, MD

Figure 22.2 Reprinted with permission from Brant WE, Helms CA. Fundamentals of diagnostic radiology. 1st ed. Baltimore: Williams & Wilkins, 1994:446.

Table Credits

Table 16.14 Reprinted with permission from Sleisinger MH, Fordtran JS. Gastrointestinal disease: pathophysiology, diagnosis, management. 5th ed. Philadelphia: WB Saunders, 1994:241.

Table 17.8 Modified from Hays RM, Levine SD. Pathophysiology of water metabolism. In: Brenner BM, Rector FC, eds. The kidney. 2nd ed. Philadelphia: WB Saunders, 1981.

Table 17.9 Modified from Hays RM, Levine SD. Pathophysiology of water metabolism. In: Brenner BM, Rector FC, eds. The kidney. 2nd ed. Philadelphia: WB Saunders, 1981.

Index

Page numbers in *italics* indicate figures. Page numbers followed by 't' indicate tables.

About The Author

Paul Cutler, the author of *Problem Solving in Clinical Medicine,* is certified by the American Board of Internal Medicine and is a Fellow of the American College of Physicians. After 20 years in the private practice of general internal medicine, he lived and worked for years in North Africa and Central Asia where he treated patients and developed clinical training programs for medical students and house staffs. Thereafter, he became Associate Dean, Professor of Medicine and Physiology, and head of the division of General Internal Medicine at the University of Texas Health Sciences Center at San Antonio, where at various times he directed the intensive care unit, the emergency department, the outpatient department, and developed courses in Physical Diagnosis and Introduction to Clinical Medicine. Many times he was selected as the outstanding instructor and his courses were chosen as "the best of the year."

In 1985, he returned to his alma mater as Clinical Professor of Medicine at the Jefferson Medical College of the Thomas Jefferson University in Philadelphia, and additionally served for 11 years as the Dean and Chief Academic Officer of the St. George's University School of Medicine in Grenada, where he played a role in the establishment and development of a widely accredited international medical school.

During his entire professional life, Dr. Cutler has been actively involved in the teaching of medical students and house officers. He bears membership in the University of Pennsylvania chapter of Phi Beta Kappa and the Jefferson Medical College chapter of Alpha Omega Alpha. Currently, he is Honorary Clinical Professor of Medicine at Jefferson, and Dean Emeritus at St. George's.